HANDBOOK OF GERIATRIC NURSING CARE

SECOND EDITION

HANDBOOK OF GERIATRIC NURSING CARE

SECOND EDITION

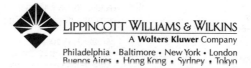

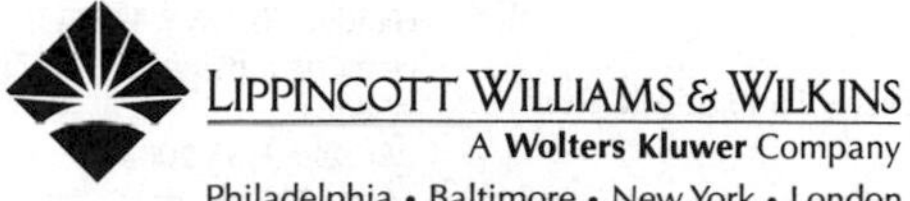

Philadelphia • Baltimore • New York • London
Buenos Aires • Hong Kong • Sydney • Tokyo

STAFF

Publisher
Judith A. Schillling McCann, RN, MSN

Editorial Director
David Moreau

Clinical Director
Joan M. Robinson, RN, MSN

Senior Art Director
Arlene Putterman

Clinical Editor
Joanne Bartelmo, RN, MSN

Editors
Jaime L. Stockslager (senior associate editor), Liz Schaeffer

Copy Editors
Kimberly Bilotta, Scotti Cohn, Tom DeZego, Heather Ditch, Dolores Matthews, Elizabeth Mooney, Judith Orioli, Dona Perkins, Carolyn Peterson, Marcia Ryan, Dorothy Terry, Pamela Wingrod

Designers
Lesley Weissman-Cook (design project manager), Donna S. Morris

Ilustrators
John Carlance, Kevin Curry, Jean Gardner, Linda Gist, Frank Grobelny, Jacalyn Bove Facciolo, Bob Jackson, Dimitri Karetnikov, Michael Morrison, Judy Newhouse, Srdjan Nickolich, Nancy Lou Makris, Bob Neumann, Eileen Rudnick, Lauren Simeone, Mary Stangl, Larry Ward

Electronic Production Services
Diane Paluba (manager), Joyce Rossi Biletz (senior desktop assistant), Richard Eng

Manufacturing
Patricia K. Dorshaw (manager), Beth Janae Orr

Editorial Assistants
Danielle J. Barsky, Beverly Lane, Linda Ruhf

Indexer
Karen C. Comerford

HGNC2 - D N O S

04 03 02 10 9 8 7 6 5 4 3 2 1

Library of Congress Cataloging-in-Publication Data

Handbook of geriatric nursing care.—2nd ed.
p. ; cm.
Includes bibliographical references and index.
1. Geriatric nursing—Handbooks, manuals, etc.
[DNLM: 1. Nursing Care—methods—Aged—Handbooks. 2. Geriatric Nursing—methods—Handbooks. WY 49 H2354 2003] I. Title: Geriatric nursing care. II. Lippincott Williams & Wilkins.
RC954 .H33 2003
618.97'0236—dc21
ISBN 1-58255-143-X (pbk. : alk. paper)
2002010338

Contents

Contributors

Bertha L. Almendarez, RN, MSN
Chairperson,
Vocational Nurse Education
Del Mar College
Corpus Christi, Tex.

Jane Ashley, RN, PhD
Associate Professor
Boston College
Chestnut Hill, Mass.

Kathleen M. Baldwin, RN, PhD, ANP, CCRN, CEN, GNP
Associate Professor
Director of Graduate Studies
Texas Christian University,
Harris School of Nursing
Fort Worth

Barbara Broome, PhD, RN, CNS
Chair, Community and Mental Health
University of South Alabama,
College of Nursing
Mobile

Mona M. Counts, CRNP, PhD, FAANP, FNAP
Elouise Ross Eberly Professor
Pennsylvania State University,
School of Nursing
University Park

Janet M. Farahmand, EdD, CGN
Adjunct Professor
Neumann College,
Division of Nursing and Health Sciences
Aston, Pa.
Immaculata (Pa.) College

Mary Jo Gerlach, RN, MSN
Assistant Professor, Adult Nursing, Retired
Medical College of Georgia,
School of Nursing
Athens

Richard M. Keller, RN, NHA, RN,C, CRRN, MSN
Independent Consultant
Hospice Registered Nurse
Grandview Hospital Hospice
Sellersville, Pa.

Elaine Bishop Kennedy, RN, EdD
Professor, Nursing
Wor-Wic Community College
Salisbury, Md.

Lynda A. Mackin, RN, MS, ANP, CNS, CS
Assistant Clinical Professor
University of California,
School of Nursing
San Francisco

Ellen J. Mangin, CRNP, WOCN, CS
Nurse Practitioner
Rydal Park
Rydal, Pa.

Lisa A. Salamon, RNC, MSN
Clinical Nurse Specialist
Cleveland Clinic Foundation

Marilyn J. Vontz, RN, PhD
Nurse Educator
Bryan School of Nursing
Lincoln, Nebr.

We extend special thanks to the following people, who contributed to the previous edition:

Beverly Sigl Felten, RN, MS, APNP, CS

Peg Gray-Vickrey, RN,C, DNSc

Gladys Purvis, RN, MSN, CCRN

Janet C. Ross-Kerr, RN, PhD

Foreword

There's no argument that primary care, acute care, extended care, adult day health care, home health care, and hospice care are distinct practice areas. However, as nurses in these settings, we understand that we primarily care for elderly patients and that this care requires specialized knowledge and skills. We also know that, in many cases, care of older patients extends to some, if not all, of these practice areas. For example, a newly admitted participant to an adult day health care program may have experienced a surgical hospital admission, a stay on an extended care unit, and home health care before admission to the day care program. With each successive admission, older patients' care and discharge plans become more and more complex. To help the nurse provide the best care for geriatric patients, a quick and practical reference on the crucial aspects of clinical care of older adults — one that cuts across care settings — is essential.

Handbook of Geriatric Nursing Care, Second Edition, quickly and concisely covers a multitude of topics affecting older adults, including information on the most common geriatric diseases and disorders, such as heart failure, Alzheimer's disease, and diabetes; medical treatments, such as cataract removal, implantable cardioverter-defibrillators, and hip replacement; and nursing procedures, such as ostomy care, pain management, and bowel retraining.

Nurses who care for older patients need to understand the differences between normal physiologic changes associated with aging and changes associated with disease. The practical guide to physiologic changes of aging, the quick reference to age-adjusted laboratory values, and the notes on pharmacodynamic changes with advanced age that can be found in *Handbook of Geriatric Care* highlight these important differences, helping to make differentiating easier and helping you provide the most exemplary care.

In addition to your own hands-on care, you increasingly share the care of your older patients with their family members. Enabling caregivers to do their jobs well usually includes teaching an array of complex skills to individuals who have minimal knowledge of health care concepts. All of the topics covered in this handy reference are explained in concise and understandable language that can easily be used as a springboard for discussions with caregivers.

For busy clinicians — and aren't we all — the inclusion in this book of key nursing diagnoses, expected outcomes, and relevant nursing interventions helps facilitate care planning that's specialized for the older patient. *Drug alert* logos warn about common drug reactions in elderly patients, and *Cultural diversity* logos explain how cultural differences may factor into your care.

In addition, because nurses often lead initiatives — such as exercise programs, community-wide immunization efforts, and nutrition screening programs — aimed at keeping older citizens healthy and independent, this latest edition includes *Staying well* sidebars that specifically address care issues involving illness prevention and health promotion. Also included in this edition are new or expanded entries on such relevant topics as end-of-life care, sexuality, and suicide.

I've always thought that one of the best indicators of a text's usefulness is the amount of wear shown on its pages. There's no doubt in my mind that this newest edition of the *Handbook of Geriatric Care* will be worn and tattered from frequent use long before the next edition appears.

Shirley S. Travis, RN, PhD, CS
President
National Gerontological Nursing Association
Dean W. Colvard Distinguished Professor of Nursing
College of Nursing and Health Professions
Faculty Associate
Center for Professional and Applied Ethics
University of North Carolina at Charlotte

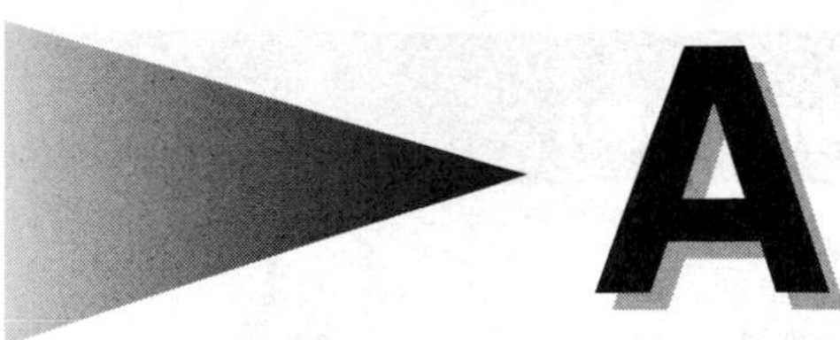

Abdominal aortic aneurysm

An abnormal dilation in the arterial wall, an abdominal aortic aneurysm typically occurs in the aorta between the renal arteries and the iliac branches. The aneurysm, which develops slowly, can be fusiform (spindle shaped) or saccular (pouchlike). First, a focal weakness in the muscular layer of the aorta (tunica media), caused by degenerative changes, allows the inner layer (tunica intima) and outer layer (tunica adventitia) to stretch outward. Then, blood pressure within the aorta progressively weakens the vessel walls and enlarges the aneurysm.

Abdominal aneurysms most commonly affect hypertensive white men ages 50 to 80. About 95% of them are caused by arteriosclerosis or atherosclerosis. The rest are linked to cystic medial necrosis, trauma, syphilis, or other infections. Most patients with an abdominal aneurysm are asymptomatic until the aneurysm enlarges and compresses surrounding tissue. As a result, these aneurysms are typically detected inadvertently through routine X-rays.

More than half of all patients with an untreated abdominal aneurysm die of hemorrhage and shock from aneurysmal rupture within 2 years of diagnosis. More than 85% die within 5 years.

Signs and symptoms

Enlarged aneurysm

- Gnawing, generalized, steady abdominal pain or lower back pain that's unaffected by movement
- Gastric or abdominal fullness caused by pressure on GI structures
- Sudden onset of severe abdominal pain or lumbar pain that radiates to the flank and groin resulting from pressure on lumbar nerves (may signify enlargement and imminent rupture)
- Severe and persistent abdominal and back pain, mimicking renal or ureteral colic (if the aneurysm ruptures into the peritoneal cavity)
- GI bleeding with massive hematemesis and melena (if the aneurysm ruptures into the duodenum)
- Hypotension (if the aneurysm ruptures)
- Pulsating mass in the periumbilical area (if the patient isn't obese)
- On auscultation, systolic bruit over the aorta caused by turbulent blood flow in the widened arterial segment
- On palpation, tenderness over the affected area (If you feel a pulsatile mass, avoid deep palpation to locate it. The pressure could cause a rupture.)

Diagnostic tests

- *Abdominal ultrasonography* or *echocardiography* can determine the size, shape, and location of the aneurysm.
- *Anteroposterior and lateral X-rays* of the abdomen can detect aortic calcification.
- *Computed tomography scan* can note the aneurysm's effect on nearby organs.

Endovascular grafting for repair of AAA

Endovascular grafting is a minimally invasive procedure for the patient who requires repair of an abdominal aortic aneurysm (AAA). Endovascular grafting reinforces the walls of the aorta to prevent rupture and prevents expansion of the size of the aneurysm.

The procedure is performed with fluoroscopic guidance, whereby a delivery catheter with an attached compressed graft is inserted through a small incision into the femoral or iliac artery over a guidewire. The delivery catheter is advanced into the aorta, where it is positioned across the aneurysm. A balloon on the catheter expands the graft and affixes it to the vessel wall. The procedure generally takes 2 to 3 hours to perform. Patients are instructed to walk the first day after surgery and discharged from the hospital in 1 to 3 days.

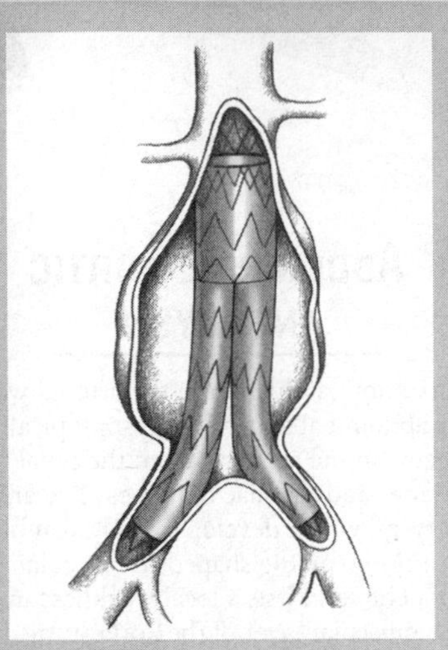

- *Aortography* can show the condition of the vessels proximal and distal to the aneurysm as well as the extent of the aneurysm's progression. Be aware that this test may underestimate the aneurysm's diameter because it shows only the flow channel and not the surrounding clot.

Treatment

An abdominal aneurysm usually requires resection of the aneurysm and Dacron graft replacement of the aortic section. If the aneurysm is small and produces no signs or symptoms, surgery may be delayed while the physician monitors its progression through regular physical examinations and ultrasonography. Large or symptomatic aneurysms risk rupture and need immediate repair. (See *Endovascular grafting for repair of AAA.*)

In acute dissection, emergency treatment before surgery includes resuscitation with fluid and blood replacement, I.V. propranolol to reduce myocardial contractility, I.V. nitroprusside to reduce and maintain blood pressure at 100 to 120 mm Hg systolic, and analgesics (usually morphine for older adults) to relieve pain. An arterial line and an indwelling urinary catheter help monitor the patient's condition.

Drug alert **Because of propranolol's CNS penetration and nonselective action, it may not be the beta-adrenergic blocker of choice for the elderly. Monitor older patients receiving propranolol carefully for signs and symptoms of bradycardia, heart failure, hypotension, bronchospasm, and GI effects.**

Key nursing diagnoses and outcomes

Anxiety related to possible aneurysm rupture

Treatment outcome: The patient will show fewer physical signs of anxiety.

Risk for injury related to possible aneurysm rupture

Treatment outcome: The patient will understand the prescribed medical regimen and the importance of follow-up care.

Ineffective (cardiopulmonary) tissue perfusion related to hemorrhage caused by aneurysm rupture

Treatment outcome: The patient will demonstrate adequate tissue perfusion, as evidenced by stable vital signs, adequate urine output (≥30 ml/hour) and capillary refill of ≤ 2 seconds.

Nursing interventions

- Allow the patient to express his fears and concerns about the diagnosis. Offer him and his family psychological support.
- If the patient's condition is or becomes acute, expect him to be admitted to the intensive care unit (ICU). If he's being admitted to the ICU, help ease his fears about the threat of impending rupture and any planned surgery.
- Administer ordered medications to control aneurysm progression as well as analgesics to relieve pain.
- Prepare the patient for elective surgery, as indicated, or emergency surgery, if rupture occurs. In an emergency, the patient may need a pneumatic antishock garment to protect him as he's moved to surgery.
- Assess the patient's vital signs, especially blood pressure, every 4 hours or more frequently, depending on the severity of his condition.
- Evaluate kidney function by obtaining blood samples for blood urea nitrogen, creatinine, and electrolyte levels. Measure his intake and output.
- Monitor complete blood count for evidence of blood loss, reflected in decreased hemoglobin level, hematocrit, and red blood cell count.
- If the patient's condition is acute, obtain an arterial sample for arterial blood gas analysis, as ordered, and monitor cardiac rhythm. Insert an arterial line for continuous blood pressure monitoring. Assist with insertion of a pulmonary artery line to assess hemodynamic balance.
- Observe the patient for signs of rupture, which could be fatal immediately. Watch closely for any signs of acute blood loss: decreasing blood pressure; increasing pulse and respiratory rates; cool, clammy skin; restlessness; and decreased alertness.

PATIENT TEACHING

- Take time to answer any questions the patient or family members may have about his condition or treatment.
- For patients undergoing complex abdominal surgery (I.V. lines, endotracheal and nasogastric intubation, and mechanical ventilation), explain the surgical procedure and the expected postoperative care in the ICU.
- Tell the patient to take all drugs as prescribed and to carry a list of them at all times, in case of an emergency.
- Tell the patient not to push, pull, or lift heavy objects until the physician approves.

ABUSE AND NEGLECT

Abuse and neglect are serious and prevalent problems for older people in home, community, and institutional settings. The National Elder Abuse Incidence Study (NEAIS) reports that approximately 450,000 elderly persons in domestic settings were abused or neglected in 1996. The NEAIS also found that an additional 101,000 elderly were subject to self-neglect. In almost 90% of incidents, the abuser is a family member. Two-thirds of the perpetrators are adult children or spouses of the abused.

These problems affect people of both sexes, good or frail health, and all racial, ethnic, and socioeconomic groups. Frail older people who live alone are particularly vulnerable to self-neglect, and those who become dependent on others for care are at higher risk for abuse by either a family member or a caregiver who may be under intense strain.

Older people are given inadequate care for other reasons, such as the caregiver's ignorance, disability, poverty, lack of access to care, or poor training. It's up to professionals who care for aging adults to determine when inadequate care is actually due to abuse or neglect.

Although abuse and neglect of older people is not a new phenomenon, it has received more attention recently. Yet, despite growing awareness among health care professionals, abuse remains extremely difficult to detect for many reasons: denial of the extent of the problem in society, ignorance of signs and symptoms, difficulty in identifying abuse without obvious signs of battering, ignorance of reporting laws and procedures, and ageism (ignoring an older person's reports of abuse because he's labeled "demented").

In other cases, the abused older adult may be unwilling or unable to report the problem for fear of retaliation, not having his basic needs met, and being institutionalized or abandoned. When the abusive person is an offspring, the parent may be reluctant to report the abuse because of shame and embarrassment and the feeling that he has failed as a parent. Finally, in some cases the older person is physically unable to report the abuse because of illness or such impairments as dementia or aphasia.

Classifications

Official definitions and categories of elder *abuse* vary from state to state and among agencies. The U.S. Department of Health and Human Services defines abuse as "the willful infliction of injury, unreasonable confinement, intimidation, or punishment with resulting physical harm or pain or mental anguish, or deprivation by an individual, including a caretaker, of goods or services that are necessary to attain or maintain physical, mental, and psychosocial well-being." It defines *neglect,* on the other hand, as any "failure to provide goods and services necessary to avoid physical harm, mental anguish, or mental illness." It's neglect, for example, when an older person doesn't receive adequate care and is left in soiled clothing for extended periods of time.

Common elements of these definitions of abuse are:

- an action against another individual
- committed knowingly
- causing harm to that individual.

Neglect, specifically, contains the following common elements:

- failure to provide treatment, care, goods, or a service
- which omission leads to harm for that individual.

The absence of standard definitions makes it even more urgent that you be vigilant for signs of abuse and neglect as you assess and treat older adults. Look for:

- physical abuse
- psychological abuse
- exploitation
- physical neglect
- psychological neglect
- self-neglect
- violation of rights.

Risk factors

What specific characteristics put an older person at risk for mistreatment? Studies have shown that cognitive impairment (for example, dementia) and shared living arrangements are the risk factors most likely to predispose older people to mistreatment. The extreme psychological and physical demands placed on a caregiver by a cognitively impaired person, who may exhibit aggressive, disruptive, and hostile behaviors, expose the older adult to mistreatment by a fatigued and demoralized caregiver. And shared living arrangements increase the opportunities to develop stress and tension, which can escalate to episodes of abuse, particularly if an older person is heavily dependent on a caregiver.

What specific characteristics put a caregiver at risk for mistreating an older person? Many abusers have a history of family violence, alcoholism or drug addiction, or mental illness. Additionally, abusers may be unduly dependent on the older person for either housing or financial support. Isolation also may contribute to abuse. In many cases, the caregiver has no support system of family or friends with whom she can share her concerns, and the elder also has no family, friends, or neighbors who visit.

Identifying abuse and neglect

Researchers have suggested that a geriatric interdisciplinary team, consisting of a physician, a nurse, and a social worker, can detect signs of elder abuse more effectively than a single health care professional. Using a systematic approach, as provided by a written protocol, for example, can also help the assessment process.

The identification process begins when a health care professional first comes in contact with an older person. The most common settings are the emergency department, the physician's office, and the home. Each setting requires different skills for detecting and assessing abuse and neglect. For example, an older person who arrives in the emergency department because of an urgent problem may have overt signs of physical abuse, such as bruises, making detection easier. But a visit to the physician's office may take place when overt signs of physical abuse are less noticeable or have healed, making abuse harder to detect. The home health care nurse, on the other hand, has the advantage of observing the older person in his own surroundings but must complete the initial evaluation without another team member's assessment and opinion.

In any setting, psychological abuse and exploitation are more difficult to identify than physical abuse. Self-neglect is similarly challenging to identify and usually involves a number of ethical considerations, including preserving the patient's autonomy and privacy.

Interview topics

The initial interview is conducted in a private setting by either a physician, a nurse, or a person from the home care environment, such as a social worker or another team member. Both the older person and the caregiver are interviewed.

Certain clues should alert you to suspect elder abuse or neglect. For example, an older person who seeks medical care long after an injury has occurred may be an abuse victim. Lacerations and fractures that have healed without appropriate medical treatment may indicate abuse. Additionally, you may suspect abuse and neglect when a caregiver insists on providing the older person's medical history rather than allowing the person to speak for himself or when a caregiver provides implausible explanations for illnesses or injuries or insists that the older person is "accident prone."

Also, suspect elder neglect if frail or cognitively impaired older people are not accompanied to appointments by their caregivers. Repeated hospital admissions, numerous emergency department visits, and readmissions for medical noncompliance may also be indicators of elder abuse or neglect.

Comprehensive assessment

After the interviews of the older person and the caregiver, a comprehensive assessment is conducted. This includes preassessment strategies (obtaining consent, gathering any necessary equipment) and an evaluation of functional, cognitive, and psychosocial domains. An evaluation for dementia is also part of the cognitive assessment.

In cases of suspected abuse and neglect, the older person may be unable to provide a thorough history. To identify mistreatment, you'll need astute observation skills, use of pertinent assessment tools, and accurate documentation. Some states have specific documentation guidelines, but the medical record should be clear and explicit and should include the following:

- chief complaint and description of the abusive event or neglectful situation, using the patient's own words, whenever possible, rather than the interviewer's assessment
- complete medical history
- relevant social history
- detailed description of any injuries, including type, number, size, location, stages of healing, color, resolution, possible causes, and any explanations given (including, where applicable, a body chart or drawing showing the location and nature of the injuries and evidence of any old injuries that may have resulted from abuse)
- your opinion on whether the injuries were adequately explained
- results of all pertinent laboratory and other diagnostic procedures
- color photographs and imaging studies, if applicable
- if the police were called, the name of the investigating officer and any actions taken
- quotes or verbatim comments made by the patient.

Functional assessment

Begin the functional assessment by evaluating activities of daily living (ADLs). A recommended tool is the Katz Index of Activities of Daily Living, developed in 1963. ADLs include bathing, dressing, grooming, eating, toileting, walking, transferring, and maintaining bowel and bladder continence. Instrumental ADLs, more sophisticated levels of function, should also be assessed. These include the capacity to shop, prepare meals, perform housework, handle finances, use the telephone, take medications, and arrange transportation. An older adult who is dependent on a caregiver for any ADLs or instrumental ADLs may be at increased risk for abuse because of the added strain placed on the caregiver.

Evaluating your patient's living arrangements may uncover possible financial abuse, particularly if a caregiver is financially dependent on the older adult. Directly ask the older person if the current living arrangements are satisfactory. Ask who else lives in the home. If the older adult owns the home, determine if the caregiver is living there out of choice or necessity. Find out if the older person or caregiver requires cohabitation or if it's a mutually agreed upon arrangement.

Cultural diversity **Be aware of possible cultural influences on living arrangements. Sharing a home with an adult child is more common among certain ethnic groups. For example, many elderly black people live with family members, and approximately three-fourths of Hispanic older adults live with a family member.**

Finally, assess the older person's support services. An informal network of family and friends can provide valuable services for an older person, as can neighbors, church members, and community service workers. Ask the person how often friends and neighbors visit. Inquire about any religious-affiliated sources of support. Suspect psychological abuse or neglect when a caregiver leaves an older person alone for long periods of time, ignores his needs for companionship, prevents his friends from visiting, or fails to inform the older person of changes in routines or plans.

Determine if formal services, such as visiting nurse services, are needed and in place. If there's a discrepancy between need and services provided, suspect financial or material abuse or neglect. For example, note situations in which an older person needs, wants, and can afford services, but the caregiver is not providing them. Also, suspect financial abuse or neglect if unnecessary services are being provided or exorbitant prices are being charged.

Physical examination

When you perform the physical examination, use a standard examination form and begin by describing the person's general appearance. A physically abused or neglected older person may exhibit:

- unshaven or uncombed hair
- poor skin hygiene
- unkempt or unclean body
- patches of hair missing
- foul odor
- unexplained bruises or bruises in various stages of healing
- burns from cigarettes, ropes, or chains
- injuries reflecting the outline of an object, such as a belt or handprint
- explanations that don't match the injury.

Use a head-to-toe approach, moving downward on the body so that you don't miss any important indicators:

- Start with the face, noting any bruises, and then move to the neck, checking for handprints. These markings may indicate physical abuse. Document how old the bruises seem to be and whether the patient has injuries in different stages of resolution.
- Proceed down the body, paying attention to injuries in unusual locations.
- Check the upper inner arms and thighs for bruises.
- Check bony prominences for skin breakdown, the coccyx for pressure ulcers, and the heels of both feet for signs of ulcers; positive findings may reflect the effects of physical immobility or they may signal neglect.
- Assess for dehydration and malnutrition. Signs of physical neglect may include weight loss, poor skin turgor, poor personal hygiene, and failure to comply with medical treatment.

After the physical examination and before meeting with the older person and caregiver, hold a brief interdisciplinary meeting. The meeting is to ensure that all team members who participated in the evaluation agree with the findings and to formulate recommendations for halting the abuse or neglect. The team members should individualize the recommendations, based on the needs and strengths of the older person and his caregiver, rather than trying to fit the older adult into an established care plan.

Diagnostic tests

Inform the older adult and caregiver about any ordered laboratory tests or X-ray procedures. Diagnostic tests that may rule out suspected abuse or neglect include:

- *X-rays* for fractures
- *computed tomography scan* of the head to detect neurologic changes or head trauma
- *blood tests,* including complete blood count, serum electrolyte levels, coagulation studies, iron studies, vitamin B_{12} levels, thyroid hormone levels, drug toxicology screening, and screening for tertiary syphilis, hepatitis, and anemia
- *urinalysis* if a urinary tract infection is suspected (For males, obtain a voided specimen; for females, consider a straight catheterization specimen.)

Formulating interventions

True geriatric patient care means respecting the older person, helping him define realistic goals, and then providing the support he needs to achieve those goals. In choosing interventions for abuse, you should be guided primarily by the following criteria: the safety needs of the patient; his rights to self-determination, autonomy, and freedom of choice; and the legal requirements for reporting abuse and neglect.

Various social and legal interventions can be used to either stop current mistreatment or reduce the risk of potential abuse or neglect. Each intervention has advantages and limitations. Aside from weighing the practical pros and cons, the health care team will also need to consider the ethical implications of various interventions and ensure that the older person maintains his autonomy in the decision-making process.

Ethical dilemmas are situations requiring a choice between what seem to be two equally desirable or undesirable alternatives. An example of a desirable choice would be having to decide which grown child an older adult will live with, when both children want him but live in different states. An example of an undesirable choice would be deciding whether to move to a nursing home or remain in an abusive situation. In such situations, your role is to help the older person understand all his options and to support him in his decision.

Four important considerations

You need to answer four critical questions in order to create the most appropriate treatment plan for an abused or neglected older adult.

- Is abuse or neglect suspected?
- Is your geriatric patient in immediate danger?
- Is he willing to accept services voluntarily?
- Does he have the capacity to make decisions?

IS ABUSE OR NEGLECT SUSPECTED?

If the answer is no (after interviews and comprehensive assessment), but the health care team has found inadequate care or the potential for abuse and neglect, the team develops a treatment and follow-up plan based on the identified needs and strengths of the older person and any caregiver involved. The plan typically includes referrals to a home health care agency, legal services, hotlines, and other community resources. However, if the inadequate care is related to a caregiver, the caregiver should be referred to appropriate training and self-help programs. You should then review the proposed service plan with the older person (and caregiver if one is involved) and formulate a contract for care and follow-up.

If abuse is suspected, you are legally obligated to report it. Reporting mechanisms vary from state to state, so consult specific state laws. Reporting mechanisms may also vary if the abused older person lives in a long-term facility. The Older Americans Act of 1978 established a Long-Term Care Ombudsman program that investigates all complaints made by residents against a nursing facility.

IS THE PATIENT IN IMMEDIATE DANGER?

Ensuring a mistreated patient's safety should be your first concern. If you believe imminent danger *does not* exist, devise a service plan and negotiate its acceptance with the patient and the caregiver.

If imminent danger *does* exist, you must arrange to have the older person removed from the dangerous setting immediately. If he has significant injuries due to physical abuse, hospitalization achieves this goal. If hospitalization is not an option, devise a plan of immediate separation. Adult Protective Services (APS) staff members will work with you to place an abused older person in a safe environment, such as a foster home, an adult group home, or a nursing facility, if he can't remain in his home or is living in the home of the abuser. In certain cases, however, the older person can remain at home, if support services are provided. For example, an older person who is malnourished due to self-neglect secondary to a new diagnosis of early dementia may be able to remain at home with support from a helpful neighbor, Meals On Wheels, a daily telephone-call program, and adult day-care services.

WILL THE PATIENT ACCEPT THE SERVICE PLAN? The ultimate goal of the service plan is to achieve a level of care that is satisfactory to the older person. Exercising his right of self-determination, he may choose to remain in an abusive situation. However, if you have good negotiating skills, present enough easily understood information, and demonstrate respect and compassion, you can usually persuade him to take at least one step toward improving his situation. An older adult may be more willing to accept services when he's informed enough to help in decision making.

DOES THE PATIENT HAVE THE CAPACITY TO MAKE DECISIONS?

Whenever an abused older person refuses services, his competence to make decisions must be evaluated to ensure his safety. This is especially important when dealing with cognitively impaired people who can't speak for themselves.

When an older patient *does* have decision-making capacity, isn't in imminent danger, and refuses services, you must honor this choice. In such cases, document in the medical record the service plan, the patient's refusal, the evaluation of his capacity to make decisions, any educational instructions given, the follow-up plan, and the referral to APS. Give him emergency numbers to call and a list of suitable community agencies, in case he decides to take advantage of them. Finally, send a report of the situation and the team's follow-up recommendations to the physician.

When the older person *does not* have decision-making capacity, isn't in imminent danger, and refuses services, you must intervene on his behalf by reporting the situation to APS. In some states, APS will begin an investigation within 24 hours for emergency situations and, otherwise, within 3 working days. You may use various legal interventions, such as arranging for a guardian, depending on the individual case.

Social interventions

When the suspected cause of abuse or neglect is primarily social in nature, the social worker becomes the lead person on the interdisciplinary team and works most directly with the older person and caregiver. The other team members stay involved to monitor health issues and provide support for the social interventions as needed.

Each service plan is developed to match the identified needs and strengths of both the abused and the abuser and should include the following:

- identified needs (such as meal preparation, help with household chores, socialization, transportation, and periodic safety checks)
- goals that meet the needs (such as Meals On Wheels, homemaker services, participation in social groups, transportation services, and visits by a social worker or visiting nurse to check on safety)
- actions of all involved
- time line for achievement of goals
- follow-up review date.

The patient's social needs and use of appropriate services are evaluated regularly, either by telephone or periodic follow-up visits with the patient or the involved community professionals.

The older person's financial resources and the availability of community-based resources, particularly for homebound patients, are pertinent when you select social interventions. If the patient is eligible for Medicaid, the social worker can help him obtain and complete Medicaid forms. If he's not eligible for Medicaid, the social worker can tell him about other available financial resources. If community-based support services aren't available, the patient may have to begin planning for long-term care in a nursing facility.

Legal interventions

Although various legal interventions can be used to help abused older people, taking legal action requires serious and careful thought to avoid infringing on the older adult's rights and freedoms. Experts recommend that you consider four questions when suggesting a specific legal option:

- Is the older adult unable to make or carry out decisions about major issues (such as health care, housing, living arrangements, and sale or management of property and money) on his own behalf?
- Is there a risk to his health and safety?
- Is there a risk of theft or loss of property or money because he is unable to act effectively on his own behalf?
- Do the actions that someone else would have to take on the older adult's behalf require legal authority?

You always should try to implement the least restrictive legal interventions—those that least limit an older person's right to make decisions and that least restrict his personal freedoms. For example, if guardianship is necessary, consider using a limited guardianship, for only specific areas of asset management and personal decision making, rather than a full guardianship.

Special considerations

Educational sessions for elderly people, family members, and the community on various issues of elder care may be helpful in preventing and detecting abuse.

ACUTE RENAL FAILURE

Acute renal failure, the sudden interruption of renal function, may be caused by obstruction, reduced circulation, or renal parenchymatous disease. Your patient may be at increased risk for renal failure because of his already decreased renal function combined with chronic illnesses, such as diabetes mellitus and hypotension.

Acute renal failure is classified as prerenal, intrarenal, or postrenal, and normally passes through three distinct phases: oliguric, diuretic, and recovery. It's usually reversible with medical treatment. If not treated, it may progress to end-stage renal disease, uremia, and death.

Each of the three types of acute renal failure has a separate cause. Prerenal failure results from conditions that diminish blood flow to the kidneys. Between 40% and 80% of all cases of acute renal failure are caused by prerenal azotemia. Intrarenal failure (also called intrinsic or parenchymal renal failure) results from damage to the kidneys themselves, usually from acute tubular necrosis. Postrenal failure results from bilateral obstruction of urine outflow. (See *Causes of acute renal failure.*)

Ischemic acute tubular necrosis can lead to renal shutdown. Electrolyte imbalance, metabolic acidosis, and other severe effects follow as the patient becomes increasingly uremic and renal dysfunction disrupts other body systems. If left untreated, the patient will die. Even with treatment, the older patient is particularly susceptible to volume overload, precipitating acute pulmonary edema, hypertensive crisis, hyperkalemia, and infection. (See *Preventing acute renal failure,* page 12.)

Signs and symptoms

- History of a disorder known to cause renal failure
- Fever and chills
- GI problems, such as anorexia, nausea, vomiting, diarrhea, constipation, and vague, diffuse abdominal pain
- Central nervous system (CNS) problems, such as headache, irritability, altered level of consciousness (drowsiness, confusion), seizures, and coma

Causes of acute renal failure

Acute renal failure can be classified as prerenal, intrarenal, or postrenal. All conditions that lead to prerenal failure impair renal perfusion, resulting in decreased glomerular filtration rate and increased proximal tubular reabsorption of sodium and water. Intrarenal failure follows damage to the kidneys themselves; postrenal failure follows obstruction of urine flow. The causes of each type of renal failure are listed below.

Prerenal failure

Cardiovascular disorders
- Arrhythmias
- Cardiac tamponade
- Cardiogenic shock
- Heart failure
- Myocardial infarction

Volume depletion
- Burns
- Dehydration
- Diuretic abuse
- Hemorrhage
- Hypovolemic shock
- Trauma

Peripheral vasodilation
- Antihypertensive drugs
- Sepsis

Renovascular obstruction
- Arterial embolism
- Arterial or venous thrombosis
- Tumor

Severe vasoconstriction
- Disseminated intravascular coagulation
- Malignant hypertension
- Vasculitis

Intrarenal failure

Acute tubular necrosis
- Ischemic damage to renal parenchyma from unrecognized or poorly treated prerenal failure
- Nephrotoxins, including analgesics, anesthetics, antibiotics, heavy metals, radiographic contrast media, and organic solvents
- Pigment release, such as crush injury, myopathy, sepsis, transfusion reaction

Other parenchymal disorders
- Acute glomerulonephritis
- Acute interstitial nephritis
- Acute pyelonephritis
- Bilateral renal vein thrombosis
- Malignant nephrosclerosis
- Papillary necrosis
- Periarteritis nodosa
- Renal myeloma
- Sickle cell disease
- Systemic lupus erythematosus
- Vasculitis

Postrenal failure

Bladder obstruction
- Anticholinergic drugs such as benztropine mesylate
- Infection
- Bladder tumor

Ureteral obstruction
- Blood clots
- Calculi
- Edema
- Inflammation
- Necrotic renal papillae
- Retroperitoneal fibrosis or hemorrhage
- Surgery
- Tumor
- Uric acid crystals

Urethral obstruction
- Prostatic hyperplasia or tumor
- Strictures

Preventing acute renal failure

Preventive measures for acute renal failure include:
- aggressively restoring fluid volume to patients recovering from major surgery, trauma, burns, or an infection such as cholera
- carefully monitoring drug administration to help prevent nephrotoxicity
- monitoring blood levels and adjusting medication dosages accordingly in order to limit damage to the kidney
- allopurinol and forced diuresis for patients at high-risk such as those undergoing cancer chemotherapy.

▶ Urine output of less than 400 ml/24 hours (if oliguric) or less than 100 ml/24 hours (if anuric)
▶ Petechiae and ecchymoses
▶ Hematemesis
▶ Uremic frost and breath odor
▶ Dry mucous membranes
▶ Muscle weakness
▶ Tachycardia or arrhythmias
▶ Bibasilar crackles upon pulmonary auscultation
▶ Peripheral edema

Diagnostic tests

▶ *Blood tests* show elevated blood urea nitrogen, serum creatinine, and potassium levels and low blood pH, bicarbonate, hematocrit, and hemoglobin levels.
▶ *Urinalysis* shows casts, cellular debris, decreased specific gravity and, in glomerular diseases, proteinuria and urine osmolality close to serum osmolality. The urine sodium level is under 20 mEq/L if oliguria is caused by decreased perfusion and above 40 mEq/L if it's caused by an intrarenal problem.
▶ *Creatinine clearance test* measures the glomerular filtration rate and allows for an estimate of the number of remaining functioning nephrons.
▶ *Electrocardiogram* (ECG) shows tall, peaked T waves, a widening QRS complex, and disappearing P waves if hyperkalemia is present.
▶ *Imaging studies* that help determine the cause of renal failure include kidney ultrasonography, plain films of the abdomen, kidney-ureter-bladder radiography, excretory urography, renal scan, retrograde pyelography, computed tomography scans, and nephrotomography (radiologic contrast agents are contraindicated in the older adult who has only one functioning kidney).

Treatment

The patient should eat foods high in calories and low in protein, sodium, and potassium, with supplemental vitamins and restricted fluids. Early initiation of diuretic therapy during the oliguric phase may be helpful.

Meticulous electrolyte monitoring is essential to detect hyperkalemia. If hyperkalemia occurs, acute therapy may include hypertonic glucose-and-insulin infusions and sodium bicarbonate, administered I.V., and sodium polystyrene sulfonate by mouth or enema to remove potassium from the body.

If these measures fail to control uremic signs and symptoms, hemodialysis or peritoneal dialysis may be required.

Key nursing diagnoses and outcomes

Excess fluid volume related to decreased ability of the kidneys to excrete water and sodium

Treatment outcome: The patient will regain and maintain normal fluid volume with alleviation of acute renal failure.

Risk for infection related to renal dysfunction

Treatment outcome: The patient will show no signs or symptoms of infection.

Risk for injury related to potential for hyperkalemia
Treatment outcome: The patient will show no signs or symptoms of hyperkalemia.

Nursing interventions

- Use infection-control measures during care because the patient with acute renal failure is highly susceptible to infection. Don't allow staff members or visitors with upper respiratory tract infections to come into contact with the patient. Also, use standard precautions when handling all blood and body fluids.
- Replace blood components as ordered.

Key point **Don't use whole blood for an older patient with acute renal failure because he may be prone to heart failure and unable to tolerate the extra fluid volume. Packed red blood cells deliver the necessary blood components without added volume.**

- Maintain proper electrolyte balance. Avoid administering medications that contain potassium.
- Maintain nutritional status. Provide a diet high in calories and low in protein, sodium, and potassium, with vitamin supplements (water-soluble vitamins are dialyzed out of the patient during treatment). Give anorexic patients small, frequent meals.
- Prepare the patient for hemodialysis or peritoneal dialysis, as indicated.
- Provide emotional support to the patient and his family members or friends.
- Measure and record intake and output of all fluids, including wound drainage, nasogastric tube output, and diarrhea.
- Weigh the patient daily. You may also need to measure abdominal girth every day. Mark the skin with indelible ink so that measurements can be taken in the same place.
- Monitor vital signs, keeping in mind that the older patient with an infection may be afebrile. Watch for and report signs and symptoms of pericarditis (pleuritic chest pain, tachycardia, and pericardial friction rub), inadequate renal perfusion (hypotension), and acidosis.
- Prevent complications of immobility by encouraging frequent coughing and deep breathing and by performing passive range-of-motion exercises.
- Provide frequent mouth care.
- Provide perineal care to reduce the risk of ascending urinary tract infection in women and to protect skin integrity caused by frequent loose, irritating stools.
- Administer any prescribed medications after hemodialysis is completed.
- Use appropriate safety measures, such as side rails and restraints, because the patient with CNS involvement may become dizzy or confused.
- Watch for signs and symptoms of hyperkalemia (malaise, anorexia, paresthesia, muscle weakness, and ECG changes), and report them immediately.
- Assess the patient frequently, especially during emergency treatment to lower potassium levels. If he receives hypertonic glucose-and-insulin infusions, monitor potassium and glucose levels.

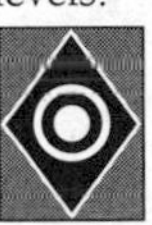

Drug alert **Large doses of sodium polysterene sulfonate may cause fecal impaction and intestinal obstruction. It's best to administer sodium polysterene using sorbital 70% as a vehicle. Make sure the patient doesn't retain it and become constipated. This can lead to bowel perforation.**

PATIENT TEACHING

- Reassure the patient and his family by clearly explaining all diagnostic tests, treatments, and procedures.

- Tell the patient about his prescribed medications, and stress the importance of complying with the regimen.
- Stress the importance of following the prescribed diet and fluid allowance.
- Instruct the patient to weigh himself daily and report changes of 3 lb (1.4 kg) or more immediately.
- Advise the patient against overexertion. If he becomes dyspneic or short of breath during normal activity, tell him to report it to his physician.
- Teach the patient how to recognize edema, and tell him to report this finding to his physician.

ADULT RESPIRATORY DISTRESS SYNDROME

Adult respiratory distress syndrome (ARDS) is a process of acute inflammatory lung injury that can affect both medical and surgical patients. ARDS causes acute life-threatening respiratory failure and is associated with various acute pulmonary injuries. It begins with increased permeability of the alveolocapillary membrane. Fluid accumulates in the lung interstitium, alveolar spaces, and small airways, causing the lung to stiffen. Ventilation becomes impaired, preventing adequate oxygenation of pulmonary capillary blood. Severe ARDS can cause intractable and fatal hypoxemia; however, people who recover may have little or no permanent lung damage.

Older adults, who have decreased lung elasticity and fewer functioning capillaries because of aging, are more likely to develop ARDS after a pulmonary incident. In older people, ARDS usually arises from various respiratory and nonrespiratory insults, including aspiration of gastric contents, sepsis (usually gram-negative), trauma, oxygen toxicity, and shock. It can also occur with pneumonia, microemboli, and disseminated intravascular coagulation. Drug overdose, blood transfusion, inhalation of smoke or chemicals, ingestion of hydrocarbons, pancreatitis, and near drowning are less common causative factors.

Mortality rates for patients with ARDS appear high because many older patients have chronic underlying health problems that contribute to the patient's (or family's) decision to withdraw support measures.

Key point The older person may appear to be doing well following an initial ARDS episode. Signs and symptoms may not appear until 2 to 3 days later. In addition, many older people have chronic underlying health problems. The activity and extent of these conditions may influence patient-family decisions to withdraw support measures, thereby contributing to higher mortality.

After the syndrome is triggered, altered permeability of the alveolocapillary membrane causes fluid to accumulate in the interstitial space. If the pulmonary lymphatics can't remove this fluid, interstitial edema develops. The fluid collects in the peribronchial and peribronchiolar spaces, producing bronchiolar narrowing. Hypoxemia occurs as a result of fluid accumulation in alveoli and subsequent alveolar collapse, causing the shunting of blood through nonventilated lung regions. In addition, regional differences in compliance and airway narrowing cause regions of low ventilation and inadequate perfusion, which also contribute to hypoxemia.

Overwhelming hypoxemia, if uncorrected, results in hypotension, decreasing urine output, respiratory and metabolic acidosis and, eventually, ventricular fibrillation or standstill. (See *What happens in ARDS*.)

Signs and symptoms

Early stages

- Rapid respiratory rate
- Use of accessory muscles
- Apprehension

What happens in ARDS

This flowchart shows the process and progress of adult respiratory distress syndrome (ARDS).

Injury reduces normal blood flow to the lungs, allowing platelets to aggregate.

▼

These platelets release substances, such as serotonin, bradykinin and, especially, histamine, that inflame and damage the alveolar membrane and later increase capillary permeability. At this early stage, signs and symptoms of ARDS are undetectable.

▼

Histamines and other inflammatory substances increase capillary permeability, allowing fluid to shift into the interstitial space. As a result, the patient may experience tachypnea, dyspnea, and tachycardia.

▼

As capillary permeability increases, proteins and more fluid leak out, increasing interstitial osmotic pressure and causing pulmonary edema. At this stage, the patient may experience increased tachypnea, dyspnea, and cyanosis. Hypoxia (usually unresponsive to increased fraction of inspired oxygen), decreased pulmonary compliance, and crackles and rhonchi may also develop.

▼

Fluid in the alveoli and decreased blood flow damage surfactant in the alveoli, reducing the cells' ability to produce more. Without surfactant, alveoli collapse, impairing gas exchange. Look for thick frothy sputum and marked hypoxemia with increased respiratory distress.

▼

The patient breathes faster, but sufficient oxygen (O_2) can't cross the alveolocapillary membrane; carbon dioxide (CO_2), however, crosses more easily and is lost with every exhalation. Both O_2 and CO_2 levels in the blood decrease. Look for increased tachypnea, hypoxemia, and hypocapnia.

▼

Pulmonary edema worsens. Meanwhile, inflammation leads to fibrosis, which further impedes gas exchange. The resulting hypoxemia leads to metabolic acidosis. At this stage, look for increased partial pressure of arterial carbon dioxide, decreased pH and partial pressure of arterial oxygen, decreased bicarbonate levels, and mental confusion

- Restlessness
- Cyanosis
- Grunting with respiratory effort

Late stages

- Mental sluggishness
- Motor dysfunction
- Tachycardia
- Possible transient increase in arterial blood pressure
- Crackles and rhonchi from fluid accumulation

Diagnostic tests

- *Arterial blood gas* (ABG) *analysis* initially shows a decreased partial pressure of arterial oxygen ($Pa{O_2}$) (less than 60 mm Hg) and decreased partial pressure of arterial carbon dioxide ($Pa{CO_2}$) (less than 35 mm Hg) on room air. The resulting pH usually reflects respiratory alkalosis. As ARDS becomes more severe, ABG levels show respiratory acidosis ($Pa{CO_2}$ more than 45 mm Hg) and metabolic acidosis (bicarbonate less than 22 mEq/L) and a decreasing $Pa{O_2}$ despite oxygen therapy.
- *Pulmonary artery catheterization* helps identify the cause of pulmonary edema by evaluating pulmonary artery wedge pressure (PAWP); allows collection of pulmonary artery blood, which shows decreased oxygen saturation, reflecting tissue hypoxia; measures pulmonary artery pressure; and measures cardiac output (CO) by thermodilution techniques.
- *Serial chest X-rays* may initially be normal or may show bilateral infiltrates. In later stages, a ground-glass appearance is present and, eventually (as hypoxemia becomes irreversible), "white-outs" of both lung fields occur.

Treatment

When possible, treatment is designed to correct the underlying cause of ARDS and to prevent progression and potentially fatal complications of hypoxemia and respiratory acidosis.

Current strategies for treating ARDS include ventilatory support and pharmacologic options. Ventilatory support options, such as permissive hypercapnea, pressure targeted ventilation, use of positive end-expiratory pressure (PEEP), tracheal gas insufflation, patient positioning, high frequency ventilation, liquid ventilation, or extracorporeal life support minimize iatrogenic lung injury by maintaining transalveolar pressure levels below 30 mm Hg. Pharmacologic options, such as antiadhesion molecular therapy, PGE 1, ketoconazole, antioxidants, pentoxifylline, lisofylline, or use of nitric oxide help to modulate the inflammatory process.

Key nursing diagnoses and outcomes

Anxiety related to potential for ARDS to develop into acute respiratory failure and possible death

Treatment outcome: The patient will demonstrate diminished physical signs and symptoms of anxiety.

Impaired gas exchange related to direct or indirect lung injury

Treatment outcome: The patient will demonstrate adequate gas exchange with therapy, as evidenced by ABG values that return to normal and restoration of normal respiratory function.

Nursing interventions

- Frequently assess the patient's respiratory status. Note respiratory rate, rhythm, and depth, and be alert for inspiratory retractions. Watch for dyspnea and accessory muscle use. Listen for adventitious or diminished breath sounds. Check for clear, frothy sputum (indicating pulmonary edema).
- Closely monitor the patient's heart rate and blood pressure. Watch for arrhythmias that may result from hypoxemia, acid-base disturbances, or electrolyte imbalance.

▶ If the patient is on mechanical ventilation, drain any condensate from the tubing promptly to ensure maximum oxygen delivery.
▶ Maintain a patent airway by suctioning. Use sterile, nontraumatic technique. Ensure adequate humidification to help liquefy tenacious secretions.
▶ Suction only as needed to maintain PEEP. High-frequency jet ventilation may also be required.
▶ Check ventilator settings frequently and monitor peak airway pressures. Monitor ABG levels; document and report changes in arterial oxygen saturation as well as metabolic and respiratory acidosis and PaO_2 changes.
▶ Because PEEP may lower CO, check for hypotension, tachycardia, and inadequate urine output.
▶ Provide other means of communication for the patient on mechanical ventilation.
▶ With pulmonary artery catheterization, know the desired PAWP level, check readings as indicated, and watch for decreasing mixed venous oxygen saturation.
▶ Frequently evaluate the patient's serum electrolyte levels. Measure intake and output, and weigh the patient daily.
▶ Administer medications, such as diuretics, steroids, sedatives, analgesics, and neuromuscular blocking agents, as ordered. Monitor and record the patient's response to the medications. Be aware of dose changes or adjustments that must be made for the elderly.
▶ Provide emotional support. Answer the patient's and family members' questions as fully as possible to allay their fears and concerns.
▶ Reposition the patient often. Prone positioning may help improve oxygenation.
▶ Note and record any changes in respiratory status, temperature, or blood pressure that may indicate a deteriorating condition. Notify the physician if changes occur.
▶ Administer tube feedings and parenteral nutrition as ordered.
▶ To promote health and prevent fatigue, arrange for alternate periods of rest and activity.

PATIENT TEACHING

▶ Explain the disorder to the patient and his family. Tell them which signs and symptoms may occur. Also, explain all procedures and treatments.
▶ Orient the patient and family members to the unit and hospital surroundings. Provide them with simple explanations and demonstrations of treatments.
▶ Tell the recuperating patient that recovery will take some time and that he'll feel weak for a while. Urge him to share his concerns with staff members.
▶ Explain to the patient the need for adequate oxygenation; urge him to tell you if he's unable to breathe adequately.
▶ Tell the patient and family members that regular evaluation of the patient's oxygenation may require blood tests.
▶ Stress that the patient needs rest to maintain adequate gas exchange.
▶ Emphasize the importance of suctioning and positioning to encourage the patient's participation in his care.
▶ Explain the need for mechanical ventilation to maintain oxygenation. Be sure to explain how the patient will be weaned off the ventilator at the appropriate time.

ADVANCE DIRECTIVES

To prevent patients from needlessly worrying about relying on others to make decisions if they become unable to speak for themselves, most states and the District of Columbia have adopted some type of advance directive, a document that expresses the patient's wishes in writing while he is competent. Many states recognize more than one form of advance directive, giving patients choices to suit their individual needs and circumstances.

Living wills

A living will is a directive from a competent individual to medical personnel and family members regarding the treatment he is to receive if he becomes seriously ill and incompetent. It isn't applicable while the patient is competent and capable of making his wishes known. Typically, the language of a living will is broad and vague. It gives little direction to the health care provider concerning the circumstances and actual time that the declarant wishes the living will to be honored.

Living wills are typically not legally enforceable; medical practitioners may choose to abide by the patient's wishes or to ignore them as they see fit. Because these documents don't protect practitioners from criminal or civil liability, many physicians have refused to follow a living will's direction for fear that family members or the state would file charges of wrongful death.

Natural death acts

To protect medical practitioners from potential civil and criminal lawsuits and to ensure that the patient's wishes are followed when he's no longer able to express them, most states have enacted some form of natural death act. These documents are living wills that *are* legally enforceable. Recognizing that some physicians may be unwilling to follow the directive, several of these laws require the physician to make a reasonable effort to transfer the patient to a physician who will abide by the patient's wishes.

The provisions of natural death acts vary greatly from state to state. Generally, people over age 18 may sign a natural death act if they are of sound mind and capable of understanding the purpose of the document. The document usually calls for withholding or withdrawing life-sustaining treatment should the patient ever be in a terminal state. In most states, the natural death act must be in written form, signed by the patient, and witnessed by two people age 18 or older. However, some states permit oral invocation of a natural death act by a patient or allow another person to invoke a natural death act for the patient.

Some states also specify that the witnesses to the natural death act not be related to the patient by blood or marriage; not be entitled to any portion of the patient's estate by will or intestacy; not be directly financially responsible for the patient's medical care; not be the attending physician, his employee, or an employee of the facility in which the declarant is a patient; and not be the same person who signed the declaration because the patient was unable to do so. Other states incorporate some of these restrictions.

The forms of natural death acts also vary from state to state. For states that have no set form, private organizations have suggested formats for these special living wills.

Once signed and witnessed, most natural death acts are effective until revoked, although some states require that they be reexecuted every 5 years or another stated time frame. It may be advisable for the declarant to review, redate, and re-sign the natural death act every year or so. This assures family members and health care providers that the directions contained in the document reflect the declarant's current wishes.

The natural death act may be revoked by physical destruction or defacement, by a written revocation, or by an oral statement indicating the declarant's wish to revoke it. Some states place fewer restrictions on revocation, for example, allowing the document to be revoked without regard to the patient's mental condition.

If a valid natural death act exists, it's effective only when the person becomes qualified — that is, when he is diagnosed with a terminal condition and the use of life-support systems would only prolong the death process. Most states require that two physicians certify in writing that any procedures and treatments will not prevent the ultimate death of the patient but will only serve to postpone death in a patient with no chance of recovery. Medications and procedures used to prevent the patient's suffering and to provide comfort are excluded from this definition.

Special considerations

When caring for an older adult, ask if the patient has an advance directive; if he does, obtain a copy for his chart. If the patient doesn't have an advance directive, provide him with information necessary to complete one. If the patient isn't able to complete a written advanced directive but can verbalize his wishes, a health care provider should document the patient's wishes in the medical record.

AGE DISCRIMINATION

Older adults make up the most stereotyped age-group. Normal aging and the changes associated with it are rarely viewed as positive — or even natural. We describe most changes as losses, such as a loss of tissue elasticity or a decrease in blood flow. We regard aging as a series of inevitable, negative events that a person must tolerate. In addition, we often mention aging changes and disease conditions in the same breath.

Some of the myths, misconceptions, and negative stereotypes about older people stem from our culture's values and beliefs. Our youth-oriented society values intelligence, strength, self-reliance, and productivity — characteristics rarely attributed to older adults. Many people perceive older adults as being senile and sick and making few worthwhile contributions to society. Portrayals of elderly people in movies, television, advertisements, and other media compound this image.

Cultural diversity **Although some societies devalue older adults, viewing them as obsolete and worthless, others — as in Japan — revere their aged, esteeming their advanced knowledge, wisdom, and skills.**

While seemingly harmless, such images perpetuate negative ideas about aging that can affect the quality of care that health care workers provide to older adults. Stereotyping can affect all aspects of care planning and implementation — for example, a nurse regularly delaying response to an older patient's call bell. It can influence salaries — nurses working in nursing homes typically make less money than those working in other facilities. It can also affect policy and program development. (See *Dispelling common myths about aging,* page 20.)

Demographic realities

In 1999, 31 million older adults — those age 65 and older — accounted for approximately 12.7% of the U.S. population. By the year 2030, older adults are projected to make up about 20% of the U.S. population. In fact, the fastest growing segment of the older population is over age 75.

In 1999, there were 20.2 million older women and 14.3 million older men in the United States, a ratio of 141 women to 100 men. The 65 to 74 age group was 8 times larger in 1999 than in 1900, the 75 to 84 age group was 16 times larger and the 85 and older age group was 34 times larger.

The most rapid increase will occur from 2005 to 2030, as the baby boom generation reaches age 65. By 2030, there will be about 70 million older persons — more than twice their number in 1999.

Dispelling common myths about aging

Here are some common misconceptions about aging and the facts to help dispel them.

Myth	Fact
Most older people are senile or demented.	*Senility* is an inaccurate term used to refer to dementing conditions that are always caused by pathologic changes. Most people age 65 and older aren't mentally disturbed. Significant, progressive, cognitive impairments are a consequence of disease that affects less than 5% of people ages 65 to 74 and about 25% of people older than age 85.
Most old people feel miserable and depressed most of the time.	Studies of happiness, morale, and life satisfaction reveal that most older people are just as happy as when they were younger. Only about one-third of older people show signs and symptoms of depression.
Older people can't work as effectively as younger people.	On the contrary, studies show that older workers produce more consistent output and have less job turnover, fewer accidents, and less absenteeism than younger workers.
Older people can't learn complex new skills, and they experience a decline in intellectual ability.	Older adults are capable of learning new things, but the speed at which they process information is slower. Healthy older adults show no decline and sometimes show improvement in some cognitive skills, such as wisdom, judgment, creativity, and common sense. Most show a slight and gradual decline in other cognitive skills, such as abstraction, calculation, and verbal comprehension.
Most older people are sick and need help with daily activities.	In fact, 80% of older people are healthy enough to carry on their normal lifestyle. About 15% have chronic health conditions that interfere with their daily lives, and another 5% are institutionalized.
Older people are set in their ways and can't change.	People tend to become more stable in their attitudes as they age, but they adapt to many social changes and changes in lifestyle. In fact, older people may be required to change more frequently than when they were younger because of major events in their lives.

Fear of aging

Most people don't know enough about the realities of aging; they fear death and, therefore, fear growing older. *Gerontophobia* refers to this fear and the refusal to accept older people into the mainstream of society.

Anyone — regardless of age — can experience gerontophobia, which sometimes causes strange behavior, such as teenagers buying antiwrinkle cream, 30-year-olds considering face lifts, and long-term marriages dissolving so that one spouse can pursue someone younger.

The extreme forms of gerontophobia are ageism and age discrimination. Like other forms of prejudice, they result from ignorance about a group of people who are different from ourselves.

Ageism, the dislike of aging and older persons, rests on a belief that aging makes people unattractive, unintelligent, and unproductive; it's an emotional prejudice.

Age discrimination goes beyond emotion; it's the practice of treating people differently simply because of their age. Refusing to hire older people, barring them from bank loans, and limiting the types or amounts of health care provided, despite laws prohibiting such actions, are examples of age discrimination.

Definitions of aging

Aging is defined as the time from birth to the present for a living individual, as measured in specific units. *Old* is defined as having lived for a long time and is generally synonymous with negative terms, such as *ancient, antiquated,* and *timeworn.*

However, the way these terms are used depends largely on the speaker's age and experiences. Children don't describe themselves as aging, but they happily proclaim how old they are. For adults, aging is negatively associated with being old, and old age is commonly described as any age several years beyond the speaker's.

The process of aging is a complex one that can be described chronologically, physiologically, and functionally.

Chronological age refers to the number of years a person has lived. Easy to identify and measure, it's the most commonly used objective method. In the United States, old age is sometimes classified in three chronological categories:

- young-old (ages 65 to 74)
- middle-old (ages 75 to 84)
- old-old (age 85 and older).

In addition, chronological age serves as a criterion in society for entitlement to certain activities, such as driving, employment, and the collection of retirement benefits. With the passage of the Social Security Act and the establishment of Medicare, age 65 became the minimum age of eligibility for retirement benefits. Therefore, 65 is the accepted age for becoming a senior citizen in the United States. Many people, however, are challenging this determination.

Physiologic age refers to the determination of age by body function. Although age-related changes affect everyone, it's impossible to pinpoint exactly when these changes occur. That's why physiologic age isn't useful in determining a person's age.

Functional age refers to a person's ability to contribute to society and benefit others and himself. It's based on the fact that not all individuals of the same chronological age function at the same level. Many people may be chronologically older but remain physically fit, mentally active, and productive members of society. Others may be chronologically young, but physically or functionally old.

Changing attitudes

Society is slowly adjusting its attitudes about aging as the number of older adults increases and new roles for them emerge. Increasingly, we see the individual as continually evolving, with the potential for ongoing self-development and contributions to others, regardless of age. More positive attitudes about old age now exist among older people themselves and among many younger people, better educated people, and those who have had contact with healthy older adults.

Among health care professionals, attitudes about aging are changing as well. A good example is the emphasis of the American Nurses Association (ANA) on holistic care and treatment of older patients. The new attitude recognizes the need for nurses to address not only age-related diseases but also associated aspects and problems — physiologic, pathologic, psychological, economic, and sociologic — to maximize their nursing capabilities. The ANA's standards of gerontological nursing provide general guidelines for the nursing care of

ANA standards of professional gerontological nursing performance

The American Nurses Association (ANA) has developed eight standards to help focus your care of older adults.

Standard I: Quality of care
The gerontological nurse systematically evaluates the quality of care and effectiveness of nursing practice.

Standard II: Performance appraisal
The gerontological nurse evaluates her own nursing practice in relation to professional practice standards and relevant statutes and regulations.

Standard III: Education
The gerontological nurse acquires and maintains current knowledge applicable to nursing practice.

Standard IV: Collegiality
The gerontological nurse contributes to the professional development of peers, colleagues, and others.

Standard V: Ethics
The gerontological nurse's decisions and actions on behalf of older adults are determined in an ethical manner.

Standard VI: Collaboration
The gerontological nurse collaborates with the older adult, the older adult's caregivers, and all members of the interdisciplinary team to provide comprehensive care.

Standard VII: Research
The gerontological nurse interprets, applies, and evaluates research findings to inform and improve gerontological nursing practice.

Standard VIII: Resource utilization
The gerontological nurse considers factors related to safety, effectiveness, and cost in planning and delivering patient care.

Adapted from *Scope and Standards of Gerontological Clinical Nursing Practice,* 2nd edition. American Nurses Association, 2001, with permission of the publisher.

older adults. The standards address the nursing process and emphasize the patient's involvement in decision making and goal setting. (See *ANA standards of professional gerontological nursing performance.*)

Special considerations

People are beginning to view aging as a normal part of the developmental process, a lifelong continuum that begins at conception and culminates with death. As a health care professional, you're in a prime position to help make this final phase rewarding and meaningful for the older adults in your care.

ALCOHOL ABUSE

Alcohol abuse is a prevalent but frequently unrecognized condition in the elderly. Research suggests that of the estimated 10 million alcoholics in the United States, approximately 3 million are over age 60.

50-75% of older alcoholics experience an early onset of alcohol abuse. Early-onset alcoholics typically start to abuse alcohol in their thirties and forties. They're generally less well-adjusted and have more physical and psychological problems than late-onset alcoholics.

In late-onset alcoholism, individuals typically don't begin drinking until they're age 60 or older. They tend to be reactive drinkers who begin drinking as a result of stresses and losses associated with aging. (See *Stressors that lead to alcoholism in older adults*.)

Alcoholics who are elderly are more likely to have additional psychiatric problems, including anxiety disorders, major depression, and organic mental syndrome.

The older alcoholic may suffer permanent damage in a relatively short period because of the normal physiologic changes connected with aging and because less alcohol is needed to cause toxicity. Hepatotoxicity, nephrotoxicity, GI toxicity, and cerebral toxicity put the patient at risk for permanent cognitive impairment, decreased liver and kidney function, and GI damage leading to ulcers and hemorrhage.

Alcohol can increase the metabolism of other drugs, such as anticonvulsants (Dilantin), anticoagulants (Coumadin), and antidiabetic drugs (such as DiaBeta, Glucotrol, or Avandia). The combination of alcohol and diuretics can lower blood pressure, which is already compromised and may be labile in an older person. Motor, sensory, verbal, and global deficits are marked in alcoholics and very marked in older alcoholics.

Other physical complications may include the following:

- *Organic mental syndrome* is related to active alcohol abuse. Signs and symptoms include confusion, memory loss, decreased verbal fluency, and loss of visual-spatial and problem-solving skills. Signs and symptoms subside after 3 to 4 weeks of abstinence.
- *Wernicke's encephalopathy*, which occurs secondary to thiamine deficiency, is marked by true delirium with clouding of alertness, focal neurologic deficits, ataxia, and ophthalmoplegia.
- *Korsakoff's syndrome* is characterized by profound anterograde and retrograde amnesia, although sensorium and verbal fluency are intact.
- *Alcoholic polyneuropathy* causes decreased sensation in the extremities, fine motor dysfunction, and weakness, especially in the lower extremities and hands. When slight to moderate, it usually resolves almost completely within 6 months of alcohol abstinence and rehabilitation.
- *Alcoholic dementia* may be diagnosed if organic mental syndrome does not clear up after alcohol abstinence lasting 3 weeks. In this case, the patient will demonstrate symptoms of memory loss, aphasia, and apraxia.
- *Marchiafava-Bignami disease* is a rare disorder that causes demyelination of the corpus callosum in chronic alcoholics (predominantly males). Nutritional factors may be involved. Signs and symptoms include progressive intellectual deterioration, confusion, hallucinations, emotional disturbances, tremors, and rigidity. The patient may recover after several months, but the disease may also progress to seizures,

Stressors that lead to alcoholism in older adults

Researchers believe that many older people start drinking heavily as a response to the stresses of aging. These include:

- physical changes that can cause immobility, isolation, loss of health and, sometimes, chronic pain
- emotional losses, such as the loss of spouse, friends, family, and coworkers
- loss of purpose, identity, fulfillment, and self-esteem associated with working
- feeling of helplessness
- loss of routine
- boredom
- financial worries.

coma, and death. Although it first appeared among red wine drinkers in Italy, Marchiafava-Bignami disease has been reported in many other countries and with many other alcoholic beverages.

Signs and symptoms

Alcoholism

- Problems in self-care
- Signs of trauma, such as frequent falls, accidents, bruising, or fractures
- Infections
- Sensory alterations
- Insomnia or chronic fatigue associated with poor sleep
- Urinary incontinence
- Noticeable deterioration in cognitive function, including confusion and short-term memory loss
- Complaints of anxiety and requests for or use of antianxiety agents, hypnotics, or sedatives
- In the postoperative patient, unexplained agitation, anxiety, and confusion or a new onset of seizure activity, especially without a history of cerebrovascular disease
- Multiple spider nevi
- GI problems, such as gastritis, peptic ulcers, hemorrhage, loss of appetite, weight loss, and malnutrition
- Gait disturbances (caused by thiamine deficiency)
- Cardiovascular signs and symptoms, such as peripheral edema, arrhythmias, and cardiomegaly
- Signs and symptoms of liver damage, such as jaundice and ascites
- Peripheral neuropathy and tremors
- Palmar erythema and hepatomegaly in late-stage alcohol dependence

The patient history may include loss of a spouse, financial duress, isolation due to immobility, recent retirement, and lack of close relatives.

Alcohol withdrawal

- Tachycardia
- Hypertension
- Shortness of breath
- Headache
- Nausea
- Irritability
- Psychomotor agitation
- Sleep disturbances
- Alcohol withdrawal syndrome (delirium tremens) in severe withdrawal

Diagnostic tests

- *Gamma glutamyltransferase* (GGT) is particularly sensitive to the effects of alcohol; elevated GGT levels may persist for more than 60 hours following moderate alcohol intake. Levels above 24 U/L in females and above 37 U/L in males may indicate alcohol abuse.
- *Aspartate aminotransferase* levels above 20 U/L may indicate acute hepatic disease.
- *Mean corpuscular volume* (MCV), the hematocrit–red blood cell (RBC) count ratio, indicates the size of RBCs and helps to diagnose anemia, a consequence of alcoholism. Normal MCV is 80 to 96 μm^3.
- *Blood tests* may indicate malabsorption of folate, vitamin B (thiamine), vitamin B_{12}, and fat (in approximately one-half of all alcohol abusers).

Malabsorption may result from mucosal damage in the intestine, increased GI motility, and reduced biliary and pancreatic secretions. Accelerated osteoporotic changes may also occur.

Assessment tools

The following assessment tools help to evaluate alcohol abuse:

- The *Michigan Alcohol Screening Test* (MAST) consists of a 25-item questionnaire. It's easy to use because it takes less than 10 minutes to complete, requires no special training to administer, is suitable for administration in various settings, and has a high level of validity. The most recent variation of this test is the MAST-G, developed to evaluate late-onset alcoholism in older adults. (See *MAST-G: Alcoholism screening test for older adults.*)

MAST-G: Alcoholism screening test for older adults

Use this tool, known as MAST-G, to help assess your older patient for possible alcohol abuse. Score each "yes" answer with one point; give each "no" answer a zero. Five or more "yes" responses indicate that the patient has an alcohol problem.

	YES (1)	NO (0)
1. After drinking, have you ever noticed an increase in your heart rate or beating in your chest?	1	
2. When talking with others, do you ever underestimate how much you actually drink?		0
3. Does alcohol make you sleepy so that you often fall asleep in your chair?	1	
4. After a few drinks, have you sometimes not eaten or been able to skip a meal because you didn't feel hungry?		0
5. Does having a few drinks help decrease your shakiness or tremors?	1	
6. Does alcohol sometimes make it hard for you to remember parts of the day or night?		0
7. Do you have rules for yourself that you won't drink before a certain time of the day?		0
8. Have you lost interest in hobbies or activities you used to enjoy?		0
9. When you wake up in the morning, do you ever have trouble remembering part of the night before?		0
10. Does having a drink help you sleep?	1	
11. Do you hide your alcohol bottles from family members?		0
12. After a social gathering, have you ever felt embarrassed because you drank too much?		0
13. Have you ever been concerned that drinking might be harmful to your health?	1	
14. Do you like to end your evening with a nightcap?		0
15. Did you find that your drinking increased after someone close to you died?	1	
16. In general, would you prefer to have a few drinks at home rather than go out to social events?		0
17. Are you drinking more now than in the past?		0
18. Do you usually take a drink to relax or calm your nerves?	1	
19. Do you drink to take your mind off your problems?		0
20. Have you ever increased your drinking after experiencing a loss in your life?	1	
21. Do you sometimes drive when you've had too much to drink?		0
22. Has a doctor or a nurse ever said they were worried or concerned about your drinking?		0
23. Have you ever made rules to manage your drinking?		0
24. Does having a drink help when you feel lonely?	1	

Adapted with permission from Beresford, T.P. "Alcoholism in the Elderly," *International Review of Psychiatry* 5:477-83, 1993.

The CHARM questionnaire

These five questions, using the acronym CHARM, outline an interview to assess older adults for substance abuse:

C = Cut down or quit drinking, ever?
H = How do you use your alcohol? Any rules?
A = Anyone concerned about your drinking?
R = Relief of problems when you use?
M = More drinking than you intended?

- The *CHARM and CAGE questionnaires* are brief, unscored surveys that provide some standardization for health histories. The CHARM questionnaire uses the acronym CHARM to elicit information about alcohol and prescription drug use in older patients. (See *The CHARM questionnaire.*) The CAGE questionnaire, which asks only four questions, is very effective in identifying alcoholics in clinical settings.
- The *Diagnostic and Statistical Manual of Mental Disorders,* 4th edition, Text Revision *(DSM-IV-TR),* cites seven criteria for establishing a diagnosis of substance dependence. Three or more of the seven criteria must be manifested at any one time in the same year to establish a diagnosis of dependence. Researchers of geriatric alcoholism, however, think that applying the *DSM-IV-TR* criteria to older people is difficult because the emphasis is on consequences that they don't experience.

Although these assessment tools are excellent and proven, they merely provide a standard framework for health histories. Remember that denial may distort the patient's responses to the questions, thus invalidating the findings.

Treatment

Late-onset alcoholics have a better prognosis than other alcoholics if they receive treatment. Unfortunately, by the time the older person is treated for dependence, permanent damage has already occurred in many cases.

Once the person has decided to stop drinking, the health care team must carefully manage the withdrawal process to achieve detoxification. (Detoxification in a treatment center is necessary only if the patient has a medical illness that requires monitoring.) Another important step is identifying sources of stress and helping patients find ways to regain control over their lives.

The Johnson method detailed in *I'll Quit Tomorrow: A Practical Guide to Alcohol Treatment* has been a favored approach in home care. In this approach, family members and others with influence over the patient confront him with the facts about his addiction and the behavior it causes. The goal is to encourage the patient to confront the consequences of his behavior and thus motivate him to seek help. The Johnson method differs from the Alcoholics Anonymous (AA) approach in that the support team doesn't wait for the patient to hit "rock bottom" before beginning interventions.

For physical signs and symptoms

The standard therapy for alcoholism is detoxification, administration of vitamin C and B-complex vitamins (especially thiamine), and fluid replacement. Treatment of coexisting psychiatric disorders (such as anxiety and affective disorder) and cognitive impairment may be necessary during acute withdrawal.

Benzodiazepines lorazepam and oxazepam are the drugs of choice for short-term administration to patients undergoing drug withdrawal.

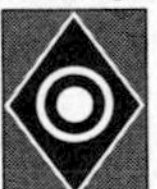

Drug alert The dosage of benzodiazepines for older adults is one-half to one-third the normal adult dosage. Because these drugs may raise problems of their own regarding dependence and

compliance, their use must be closely monitored. Alprazolam is the benzodiazepine of choice because of its short duration of action. Diazepam is a drug that should be avoided because of its long duration of action.

Some researchers advocate using chlordiazepoxide to treat signs and symptoms of alcohol withdrawal in older adults because it produces a smoother withdrawal without cumulative sedation and promotes less dependence than long-acting benzodiazepines such as diazepam. Others oppose treatment with benzodiazepines unless the patient has significant withdrawal signs, such as marked diaphoresis, tremors, agitation, or cardiac irregularities such as tachycardia.

Clonidine patches may be substituted for benzodiazepines in moderate withdrawal cases. Clonidine controls autonomic nervous system excitation, insomnia, and anxiety but doesn't inhibit the tremors of alcohol withdrawal syndrome.

Detoxification should be achieved, if possible, without the use of disulfiram because of the risk of liver damage. If the patient is debilitated, thiamine treatment should begin. The thiamine should be administered before any I.V. dextrose to avoid Wernicke's encephalopathy caused by depletion of marginal stores of thiamine. Thiamine should then be given orally along with multivitamins.

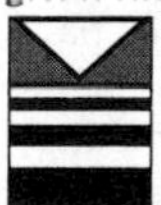

Key point Because the older patient may be more sensitive to these drugs, withdrawal may take longer (weeks or months) and be more severe than in younger adults.

Withdrawal may also be more severe if the patient is experiencing concomitant malnutrition, physical illness, emotional stress, depression, social isolation, or fatigue.

For psychological signs and symptoms

By working cooperatively with the physician, family members, home health care agencies, social agencies, and senior citizen centers, you may be able to help the patient develop a positive attitude toward life and reduce his need to drink. In the institutional setting, you'll need to surrender some of your control over the patient and make him responsible for his addiction. For long-term success, the recovering patient must learn to fill the place alcohol once occupied in his life with something constructive.

AA programs encourage the patient to learn about his disease, confront his denial, change his attitudes and lifestyle, and make a commitment to recovery. Some older adults find this program unappealing because of the stigma surrounding stereotypical alcoholics. One way to deal with this reluctance is to help older people form their own AA chapter.

Other treatments include adverse conditioning, which associates alcohol with negative sights, smells, tastes, and thoughts to evoke negative reinforcement, and behavioral psychotherapy, which establishes behavioral goals and a time frame in which to complete them. The goals may range from total abstinence to holistic networking (group treatment through the support of others).

The psychosocial approach is the most widely used in treatment programs for older adults because it addresses, through talk therapy, the social and psychological stressors associated with aging. This approach can center on the individual, group, or family and can take place within the patient's facility. Geriatric group programs restore their members' capacity to enter into relationships, improve self-image and communication, and provide catharsis.

Day-treatment programs developed specifically for older alcoholics have been particularly successful because of the program structure. These programs focus on three areas: primary health needs and risk reduction; education about the physical, emotional, and psychosocial needs of the older patient; and skill-building in individual coping and socialization.

Inpatient programs, some of which embrace the AA philosophy, also are available. These programs, designed for older alcoholics, typically last 90 to 120 days and deal with the older person's special problems, including physical disabilities, cognitive impairment, aphasia, and sensory deficits. They also provide physical therapy, occupational therapy, special diets, and adaptive equipment. These programs provide sufficient time to integrate new information and make the behavioral changes necessary to achieve sobriety.

Key nursing diagnoses and outcomes

Imbalanced nutrition: Less than body requirements related to alcohol consumption and poor dietary habits

Treatment outcomes: The patient will improve nutritional status and decrease alcohol consumption.

Anxiety related to loss of control and personal crisis

Treatment outcome: The patient will report feelings of relief and control over actions.

Powerlessness related to alcohol addiction

Treatment outcome: The patient will verbalize control over his addiction.

Risk for injury related to alteration in perception

Treatment outcomes: The patient will remain free from injury and injure no others.

Nursing interventions

- Orient the patient to reality because he may have hallucinations and may try to harm himself or others. Minimize noise and shadows to decrease the incidence of delusions and hallucinations. Avoid using restraints unless necessary to protect the patient or others.
- Monitor the patient for signs and symptoms of depression or impending suicide.
- Use a multidisciplinary approach, which is essential to provide the support that even healthy older people lack. Support groups, such as AA, can offer large-print materials and peer support and can fill the gaps that exist in treatment after acute detoxification.
- Once the motivation process has begun, focus your long-term goals on increasing the patient's socialization and support network, improving his diet, and implementing an exercise program.
- Approach the patient in a nonthreatening way. Limit sustained eye contact, which he may perceive as threatening. Listen attentively, respond with empathy, and explain all procedures even if the patient is verbally abusive.
- Before you confront the patient, evaluate his level of denial, significant relationships, history of alcohol abuse, and social and recreational activities engaged in before abuse. Also assess the support team's knowledge and beliefs about alcoholism because their attitudes toward alcoholics can significantly affect the patient's outcome.
- Help the patient accept his drinking problem and the need for abstinence.
- Encourage positive health behaviors, and offer emotional support in a calm, nonjudgmental manner.
- Present various treatment options. Avoid being vague. Be prepared for rationalization as a defense, and be ready to offer rebuttals to the excuses the patient may offer to avoid seeking help. You'll need to break down the patient's

defenses to motivate him to seek help before he suffers permanent damage.

- Refer the patient to AA, and offer to arrange a visit from an AA member. Explain how this organization can provide the support he'll need to abstain from alcohol.
- Refer spouses of alcoholics to Al-Anon and adult children of alcoholics to the National Association for Children of Alcoholics. These organizations provide support to family members.

PATIENT TEACHING

- Make sure family members are aware of the patient's addiction.
- Educate the patient and his family members about his illness, and emphasize that the patient must abstain from alcohol for the rest of his life.
- Make family members and the patient aware that the effects of alcohol involve all senses and that all the patient's perceptions may be incorrect. Remind family members that, because his reported perceptions may be incorrect, his actions may be inappropriate.
- Teach the family and patient the need for improved dietary habits as related to the deficits caused by alcohol consumption. Provide information on wholesome diets and encourage nutritional counseling.
- Encourage family members to monitor the patient's alcohol use and be aware of when his motor functions are not stable.
- Recommend removal of available car keys when the patient is under the influence of alcohol or in the midst of withdrawal.
- Remind family members and the patient that relapse may occur, but that help will always be available.

ALZHEIMER'S DISEASE

A chronic condition characterized by declining intellectual capacity, Alzheimer's disease (AD) is the most common form of dementia. This progressive degenerative disorder of the cerebral cortex (especially the frontal lobe) causes gradual loss of memory with loss of at least one other cognitive function, such as language, abstraction, or spatial orientation.

Because this is a primary progressive dementia, the prognosis for a person with AD is poor. Typically, patients die of debilitating brain disease 2 to 15 years after the onset of signs and symptoms. The average duration of the illness before death is 8 years. In 1997, 2.32 million people in the U.S. were suffering from AD. It's projected that this number will quadruple in the next 50 years, by which time 1 in 45 Americans will be afflicted with the disease.

The cause of AD is unknown. However, several factors are thought to be closely connected to this disease. They include neurochemical factors, such as deficiencies of the neurotransmitters acetylcholine, somatostatin, substance P, and norepinephrine; viral factors such as slow-growing central nervous system viruses; trauma; and genetic factors.

Some researchers believe that up to two-thirds of AD cases may stem from genetic abnormalities that in some way interact with other factors to cause the disorder. Age also has been identified as a possible factor. Approximately 43% of persons with AD are between ages 75 and 85. 4.3% are 75 years old, 8.5% are 80 years old, 16% are 85 years old, and 28.5% are 90 years old.

In this disorder, complications include injury from the patient's own violent behavior or from wandering or unsupervised activity; pneumonia and other infections, especially if the person doesn't exercise enough; malnutrition and dehydration, especially if the patient refuses or forgets to eat; and aspiration.

Signs and symptoms

Early stages

- Forgetfulness and subtle memory loss without loss of social skills and behavior patterns
- Difficulty learning and remembering new information
- General deterioration in personal hygiene and appearance
- Inability to concentrate
- Impaired sense of smell

Late stages

- Difficulty with abstract thinking and activities that require judgment
- Severe deterioration of memory, language, and motor function (may eventually result in loss of coordination and an inability to speak or write)
- Use of meaningless words and nonsensical phrases
- Repetitive actions and restlessness
- Negative personality changes, such as irritability, depression, paranoia, hostility, and combativeness
- Labile emotions: inappropriate laughter or crying, mood swings, and sudden angry outbursts
- Sleep disturbances
- Disorientation
- Misperception of environment, misidentification of objects and people
- Impaired stereognosis (inability to recognize and understand the form and nature of objects by touching them)
- Complaints of stolen or misplaced objects
- Overdependence on caregivers
- Gait disorders leading to falls
- Urinary or fecal incontinence
- Tremors, twitching, and seizures
- Positive snout reflex (determined by tapping or stroking the patient's lips or the area just under the nose; grimacing or puckering the lips is a positive sign for AD in an adult.)

Diagnostic tests

AD is diagnosed by exclusion. Various tests, such as those described below, rule out other disorders. However, the diagnosis can't be confirmed until death, when pathologic findings come to light at autopsy.

- *Positron emission tomography* measures the metabolic activity of the cerebral cortex and may help confirm early diagnosis.
- *Computed tomography scanning* in some patients shows progressive brain atrophy in excess of that which occurs in normal aging.
- *Magnetic resonance imaging* may permit evaluation of the condition of the brain and rule out intracranial lesions as the source of dementia.
- *Electroencephalography* allows evaluation of the brain's electrical activity and may show slowing of brain waves in the late stages of the disease. This diagnostic test also helps identify tumors, abscesses, and other intracranial lesions that might cause the patient's signs and symptoms.
- *Cerebrospinal fluid analysis* may help determine if the patient's signs and symptoms are caused by a chronic neurologic infection.
- *Cerebral blood flow studies* may reveal abnormalities in blood flow to the brain.
- *Neuropsychology testing* is a battery of tests designed to assess cognitive ability and reasoning. They can help differentiate AD from other types of dementia.

Treatment

No cure or definitive treatment exists for AD. Drugs that attempt to reduce the rate of cognitive decline in people with AD include donepezil, rivastigmine and tacrine.

Other treatments include cerebral vasodilators, such as ergoloid mesylates, isoxsuprine, and cyclandelate, to enhance the brain's circulation; hyperbaric oxygen to increase oxygenation to the brain; psychostimulators, such as methylphenidate, to enhance the patient's mood; and antidepressants if depression seems to exacerbate the dementia.

Key nursing diagnoses and outcomes

Imbalanced nutrition: Less than body requirements related to patient's forgetfulness

Treatment outcome: The patient will consume a well-balanced diet provided by the caregiver.

Disturbed thought processes related to progressive deterioration of the cerebral cortex

Treatment outcome: The patient will demonstrate appropriate interventions, reorientation techniques, and coping skills.

Risk for trauma related to negative personality changes and confusion

Treatment outcome: The patient will remain safe and protected from injury.

Nursing interventions

- Administer ordered medications, and note their effects. If the patient has trouble swallowing, crush tablets and open capsules and mix them with a semisoft food. Always check with the pharmacist before crushing tablets or opening capsules because some drugs shouldn't be altered. Ask the prescriber to order a liquid form of the drug if available.
- Monitor the patient's eating habits, and note his ability to feed himself and swallow safely.
- Monitor the patient's fluid and food intake to detect imbalances.
- Establish an effective communication system with the patient and his family members to help them adjust to the patient's altered cognitive abilities.
- Provide emotional support to the patient and family members or friends. Encourage them to talk about their concerns. Listen to them, and answer their questions honestly.
- Use a soft tone and a slow, calm manner when speaking to the patient. Allow him sufficient time to answer because his thought processes are slow, impairing his ability to communicate verbally.
- Protect the patient from injury by providing a safe, structured environment. Provide rest periods between activities because these patients tire easily.
- Encourage the patient to exercise as ordered to help maintain mobility.
- Because the patient may be disoriented or have impaired neuromuscular function, take him to the bathroom at least every 2 hours and make sure he knows the location of the bathroom.
- Assist the patient with hygiene and dressing as necessary. Many patients with AD are incapable of performing these tasks.
- Monitor the patient's neurologic function, including his emotional and mental states and motor capabilities, for changes indicating further deterioration.
- Inspect the patient's skin for evidence of trauma, such as bruises or skin breakdown.
- Evaluate the family member's or caregiver's ability to manage the patient if he's living at home.
- Encourage sufficient fluid intake and adequate nutrition. Provide assistance with menu selection, and allow the patient to feed himself as much as he can. Provide a well-balanced diet with adequate fiber. Avoid stimulants, such as coffee, tea, cola, and chocolate. Give the patient semisolid foods if he has dysphagia. Insert and care for a nasogastric tube or a gastrostomy tube for feeding, as ordered.

PATIENT TEACHING

- Teach the patient's family members about the disease. Explain that the cause of AD is unknown. Review the signs and symptoms of the disease with them. Be sure to explain that AD progresses, but at an unpredictable rate, and that the patient will eventually suffer complete memory loss and total physical deterioration.

▶ Refer the family to support groups, such as the Alzheimer's Association. Set up an appointment with the social service department, which will help the family assess its needs.

▶ Encourage patient independence, and allow ample time for the patient to perform tasks.

▶ Advise the family to provide the patient with exercise. Suggest physical activities, such as walking or light housework, that occupy and satisfy the patient.

▶ Encourage the family to allow the patient as much independence as possible while ensuring his and others' safety. Tell them to create a routine for all the patient's activities, which will avoid confusion. If the patient becomes belligerent, advise family members to remain calm and to try distracting him.

▶ Stress the importance of an adequate diet. Instruct the family members to limit the number of foods on the patient's plate so that he won't have to make decisions. If the patient has coordination problems, tell the family to cut up his food and to provide finger foods, such as fruit and sandwiches. Suggest using plates with rim guards, built-up utensils, and cups with lids and spouts.

AMPUTATION

Performed to preserve function in a remaining part or, at times, to prevent death, amputation is a radical treatment for severe trauma, gangrene, cancer, vascular disease, congenital deformity, or thermal injury. It can take one of two basic forms. In a closed, or flap, amputation (the most commonly performed type), the surgeon uses skin flaps to cover the bone stump. In an open, or guillotine, amputation (a rarely performed emergency operation), the surgeon cuts the tissue and bone flush, leaving the wound open. A second operation completes repair and stump formation. Amputation may be performed at a number of sites, depending on the nature and extent of injury. (See *Common levels of amputation*.)

Implementation

The patient receives a general anesthetic (or perhaps a local anesthetic for a finger or toe amputation). In the closed technique, the surgeon incises the tissue to the bone, leaving sufficient skin to cover the stump end. He usually controls bleeding above the level of amputation by tying off the bleeding vessels with suture ties. He then saws the bone (or resects a joint), files the bone ends smooth and rounded, and removes the periosteum up about ½″ (1.3 cm) from the bone end. After ligating all vessels and dividing the nerves, he sutures opposing muscles over the bone end and to the periosteum to provide better muscle control and circulation. Next, he sutures the skin flaps closed. Placement of an incisional drain and a soft dressing completes the procedure.

In a below-the-knee amputation, the surgeon may order a rigid dressing applied over the stump in the operating room. This enables immediate postoperative fitting of a prosthesis and helps prevent contractures.

In an emergency, or guillotine, amputation, the surgeon makes a perpendicular incision through the bone and all tissue. He leaves the wound open, applying a large bulky dressing.

Complications

Amputation can lead to complications, including infection at the stump site, contractures in the remaining limb part (if exercise of the limb part is delayed), skin breakdown from improper care of the stump, or an ill-fitting prosthetic device. Phantom pain (a sensation of pain, itching, or numbness in the area of amputation, even though the limb or digit has been removed) commonly develops after a major amputation and can occur as late as 2 to 3 months afterward. The patient may also suffer depression over limb loss, which may be severe enough to interfere with self-care and require psychiatric therapy.

Common levels of amputation

Review the following list for common types and levels of amputation:

- partial foot: removal of one or more toes and part of the foot
- total foot: removal of the foot below the ankle joint
- ankle (Syme's amputation): removal of the foot at the ankle joint
- below-the-knee: removal of the leg 5″ to 7″ (12.5 to 18 cm) below the knee
- knee disarticulation: removal of the patella, with the quadriceps brought over the end of the femur, or fixation of the patella to a cut surface between the condyles (known as the Gritti-Stokes amputation)
- above-the-knee: removal of the leg from 3″ (7.5 cm) above the knee
- hip disarticulation: removal of both the leg and hip or the leg and pelvis
- hemipelvectomy: removal of a leg and half of the pelvis
- fingers: removal of one or more fingers at the hinge or condyloid joints
- wrist disarticulation: removal of the hand at the wrist
- below-the-elbow: removal of the lower arm about 7″ below the elbow
- elbow disarticulation: removal of the lower arm at the elbow
- above-the-elbow: removal of the arm from 3″ above the elbow.

Key nursing diagnoses and outcomes

Disturbed body image related to loss of limb or digit

Treatment outcome: The patient will accept his altered body image.

Risk for infection related to improper stump care

Treatment outcome: The patient will exhibit no signs and symptoms of infection (blistering, redness, or pain), abrasions, or delayed tissue and skin healing at stump site.

Acute pain related to surgery and phantom pain

Treatment outcome: The patient will experience complete disappearance of phantom pain.

Nursing interventions

When caring for an amputation patient, your major roles include preparing the patient for surgery and providing care and instruction after the amputation.

Before surgery

- If time permits, review the physician's explanation of the scheduled amputation, answering any questions the patient may have.
- Remember that the patient faces not only the loss of a body part, with an attendant change in body image, but also the threat of loss of mobility and independence. Keep in mind, too, that loss of a limb or digit can be emotionally devastating to the patient; be sure to provide emotional support.
- If possible, arrange for the patient to meet with a well-adjusted amputee, who can provide additional reassurance and encouragement.
- Discuss postoperative care and rehabilitation measures. Demonstrate appropriate exercises to strengthen the remaining portion of the limb and maintain mobility. Such exercises may include active hip extension and abduction, and adduction for an above-the-knee amputation. Follow the physician's

or physical therapist's directions in explaining such exercises.

▶ The patient may be fitted with a prosthesis while hospitalized, but he will probably require more time to heal and so will be discharged before being fitted. Explain to him that the duration between amputation and fitting of the prosthesis varies, depending on wound healing, muscle tone, and overall stump condition. Stress that good stump care can speed this process and help ensure a better fit for the prosthesis. If possible, show him the types of prostheses available for his type of amputation and explain how they work.

▶ Point out the possibility of phantom limb sensation. Explain that the patient may "feel" sensations of pain, itching, or numbness in the area of amputation, even though the limb or digit has been removed. Reassure him that these sensations, although inexplicable, are common and should eventually disappear.

▶ As ordered, administer broad-spectrum antibiotics to minimize the risk of infection.

After surgery

▶ After the patient returns from surgery, monitor his vital signs frequently until they're stable. Be particularly alert for bleeding through the dressing. Notify the physician if any bleeding occurs.

▶ If ordered, elevate the stump on a pillow or other support for 24 to 48 hours; be aware, however, that this could lead to contractures. Check dressings frequently and change them as necessary. Assess drain patency, and note the amount and character of drainage.

▶ Assess for pain, and provide analgesics and other pain-control measures as needed. Because movement may be painful and interfere with therapy, give analgesics about 30 minutes before scheduled exercises or ambulation. Keep in mind that morphine is the drug of choice for older adults. Distinguish stump pain from phantom limb sensation; severe, unremitting stump pain may indicate infection or other complications.

▶ Keep the stump properly wrapped with elastic compression bandages. A properly applied bandage is essential to stump care; it supports soft tissue, controls edema and pain, and shrinks and molds the stump into a cone-shaped form to allow a good fit for the prosthesis. Rewrap the stump at least twice a day to maintain tightness. As an alternative to bandages, the physician may order that the patient wear a stump shrinker, a custom-fitted elastic stocking, that fits snugly over the stump.

▶ If a rigid plaster dressing has been applied, care for it as you would a plaster cast for a fracture or severe sprain. Keep it from getting wet, and observe its margin for skin irritation and excessive or malodorous drainage, which may indicate infection. As the stump shrinks, the plaster dressing may loosen or fall off. If this occurs, notify the physician and wrap the stump in an elastic compression bandage until he can replace the dressing.

▶ Emphasize the need for proper body alignment and regular physical therapy to condition the stump and prevent contractures and deformity. Encourage frequent ambulation, if possible, and a program of active or passive range-of-motion exercises, as ordered.

▶ If the patient is bedridden, encourage him to turn from side to side and to assume an alternate position — usually on his stomach from time to time throughout the day. Frequent position changes will stretch the hip flexor muscles and prevent contractures.

PATIENT TEACHING

▶ If the patient has had a leg amputation, instruct him not to prop his stump on a pillow to avoid hip flexion contracture.

▶ If the patient has had a below-the-knee amputation, tell him to keep the knee extended to prevent hamstring contracture.

▶ Instruct the patient with a partial arm amputation to keep his elbow extended and shoulder abducted.

▶ If possible, give the patient information about available prostheses. Keep in mind his advanced age and physical condition as well as the complexity and cost of the device. The older adult patient may require a prosthesis that provides extra stability even if it means sacrificing some flexibility.

▶ Throughout recovery and rehabilitation, encourage the patient to adopt a positive outlook toward resuming an independent lifestyle. Emphasize that the prosthesis should allow him to lead a full and active life with few restrictions on activity. If he seems overly despondent or depressed, consider referring him to psychological counseling or social services.

Home care instructions include the following:

▶ Instruct the patient to examine his stump daily, using a handheld mirror to visualize the entire area. Tell him to watch for and report swelling, redness, or excessive drainage as well as increased pain. Also, instruct him to note and report any skin changes on the stump, including rashes, blisters, or abrasions.

▶ Explain that good stump hygiene will prevent irritation, skin breakdown, and infection. Tell the patient to wash the stump daily with mild soap and water and then rinse and gently dry it. Suggest that he wash the stump at night and bandage it when dry because bandaging a wet stump may lead to skin maceration or infection. Advise against applying body oil or lotion to the stump because this can interfere with proper fit of the prosthesis.

▶ Teach the patient how to apply a stump dressing. Teach him to change dressings frequently, as necessary, and to maintain sterile technique. Explain that as the wound heals, he'll need to change the dressing less often.

▶ As appropriate, show the patient how to properly wrap his stump with elastic bandages or how to slip on a stump shrinker. If he's using bandages, show him how to apply them with even, moderate pressure, avoiding overtightness that could impair circulation. Suggest that he apply the bandages when he awakens in the morning and rewrap the stump at least twice a day to maintain proper compression. If he's using a shrinker, suggest that he have two available; one can be worn while the other is being washed. Explain that he'll need to use elastic bandages or a stump shrinker at all times (except when bathing or exercising) until postoperative edema completely subsides and the prosthesis is properly fitted. Even after he adjusts to the prosthesis, he may need to continue nighttime bandaging for many years.

▶ Instruct the patient to apply a clean stump sock before attaching his prosthesis. Advise him never to wear a stump sock that has any tears, holes, mends, or seams; these could cause skin irritation. Explain that as the stump shrinks over time, he may need to apply two stump socks to ensure a snug fit of the prosthesis. Tell him to notify the physician if he needs more than two socks for proper fit or if his prosthesis feels loose for any other reason.

▶ Review proper care of the prosthesis. Instruct the patient never to immerse it in water, which could weaken its leather joints or hinges. Tell him to clean the device with soap and water each night before bedtime and to let it dry overnight.

▶ If appropriate, refer the patient to a local support group.

ANEMIA, IRON DEFICIENCY

Anemia is fairly common in the older adult population, probably due to underlying predisposing conditions, such as malnutrition and chronic infections. The prognosis after replacement therapy is favorable.

Iron deficiency anemia is caused by an inadequate supply of iron for optimal formation of red blood cells (RBCs), which produces smaller (microcytic) cells with less color on staining. Body stores of iron, including plasma iron, decrease, as does transferrin, which binds with and transports iron. Insufficient body stores of iron lead to a depleted RBC mass and, in turn, to a decreased hemoglobin concentration (hypochromia) and decreased oxygen-carrying capacity of the blood. (See *Understanding iron absorption and storage*.)

Iron deficiency can result from any of the following:

- inadequate dietary intake of iron or a poorly balanced diet
- iron malabsorption, as in chronic diarrhea, partial or total gastrectomy, and malabsorption syndromes such as celiac disease
- blood loss secondary to drug-induced GI bleeding (from anticoagulants, aspirin, steroids) or due to hemorrhage from trauma, GI ulcers, malignant tumors, and varices
- intravascular hemolysis-induced hemoglobinuria or paroxysmal nocturnal hemoglobinuria
- mechanical erythrocyte trauma caused by a prosthetic heart valve or vena cava filter.

Possible complications of this disorder include infection and pneumonia. Another complication is bleeding, which may be identified by ecchymotic areas on the skin, hematuria, and gingival bleeding. Plummer-Vinson syndrome can occur in severe cases.

The most significant complication of iron deficiency anemia is caused by overreplacement of iron with oral or I.M. supplements. Hemochromatosis (excessive iron deposits in tissue) can result, affecting the liver, heart, pituitary gland, and joints.

Signs and symptoms

- May be asymptomatic for years
- Fatigue
- Headaches
- Inability to concentrate
- Shortness of breath (especially on exertion)
- Pica (uncontrollable urge to eat strange things, such as clay, starch, and ice)
- Increased frequency of infections
- In chronic anemia, dysphagia, neuromuscular effects (vasomotor disturbances, paresthesia, and neuralgic pain), glossitis (red, swollen, smooth, shiny, and tender tongue), angular stomatitis, and spoonshaped, brittle nails
- In late stages, tachycardia (caused by decreased oxygen perfusion and increased cardiac output)

Diagnostic tests

- *Blood studies* may reveal the following:
  - low hemoglobin levels (less than 12 g/dl in males, less than 10 g/dl in females)
  - low hematocrit (less than 47 ml/dl in males, less than 42 ml/dl in females)
  - low serum iron levels, with high binding capacity
  - low serum ferritin levels
  - low RBC count, with microcytic and hypochromic cells (in early stages, RBC count may be normal)
  - decreased mean corpuscular hemoglobin (in severe anemia).
- *Bone marrow studies* reveal depleted or absent iron stores and normoblastic hyperplasia.
- *GI studies,* such as guaiac stool tests, barium swallow and enema, endoscopy, and sigmoidoscopy, rule out or confirm

whether bleeding is causing the iron deficiency.

Diagnosis must rule out other forms of anemia, such as those caused by thalassemia minor, cancer, and chronic inflammatory, hepatic, and renal disease.

Treatment

Before treatment can begin, the underlying cause of anemia must be determined. Then iron replacement therapy—consisting of an oral iron preparation or a combination of iron and ascorbic acid (which enhances iron absorption)—can begin. In rare cases, iron may have to be administered I.M.—for instance, if the patient is noncompliant with the oral preparation, if he needs more iron than he can take orally, if malabsorption prevents adequate iron absorption, or if a maximum rate of hemoglobin regeneration is desired.

Total-dose I.V. infusions of supplemental iron can be administered to older patients with severe iron deficiency anemia. The patient should receive this painless infusion of iron dextran in normal saline solution over 8 hours. To minimize the risk of an allergic reaction to iron, an I.V. test dose should be given first.

Key nursing diagnoses and outcomes

Imbalanced nutrition: Less than body requirements related to dietary deficiency of iron

Treatment outcomes: The patient will increase his daily dietary intake of iron to meet the recommended daily allowance and will express relief from the signs or symptoms of iron deficiency anemia.

Fatigue related to decreased tissue oxygenation caused by decreased hemoglobin

Treatment outcome: The patient will regain his normal energy level.

Understanding iron absorption and storage

Essential to erythropoiesis, iron is abundant throughout the body. Two-thirds of total body iron is found in hemoglobin; the other third, mostly in the reticuloendothelial system (liver, spleen, and bone marrow), with small amounts in muscle, serum, and body cells.

Adequate dietary ingestion of iron and recirculation of iron released from disintegrating red blood cells maintain iron supplies. The duodenum and upper part of the small intestine absorb dietary iron. Such absorption depends on gastric acid content, the amount of reducing substances (ascorbic acid, for example) present in the alimentary canal, and dietary iron intake. If iron intake is deficient, the body gradually depletes its iron stores, causing decreased hemoglobin and, eventually, signs and symptoms of iron deficiency anemia.

Nursing interventions

- Administer iron supplements as ordered. Use the Z-track injection method when administering iron I.M. to prevent skin discoloration, scarring, and irritating iron deposits in the skin. (See *How to inject iron solutions*, page 38.)
- If the patient is receiving iron I.V., monitor the infusion rate carefully. Stop the infusion and begin supportive treatment immediately if the patient shows signs and symptoms of an allergic reaction. Also, watch for dizziness and headache and for thrombophlebitis around the I.V. site.
- Monitor the patient's compliance with the prescribed iron replacement therapy.
- Monitor the patient for iron replacement overdose.

How to inject iron solutions

For deep I.M. injections of iron solutions, use the Z-track technique to avoid subcutaneous (S.C.) irritation and discoloration from leaking medication.

Choose a 19G to 20G, 2″ to 3″ needle. After drawing up the solution, change to a fresh needle to avoid tracking the solution through the S.C. tissue. Draw 0.5 cc of air into the syringe as an air lock.

Displace the skin and fat at the injection site (in the upper outer quadrant of the buttocks only) firmly to one side. Clean the area, and insert the needle. Aspirate to check for entry into a blood vessel. Inject the solution slowly, followed by the 0.5 cc of air in the syringe. Wait 10 seconds, then pull the needle straight out, and release the skin tissues.

Apply direct pressure to the site, but don't massage it. Caution the patient against vigorous exercise for 15 to 30 minutes.

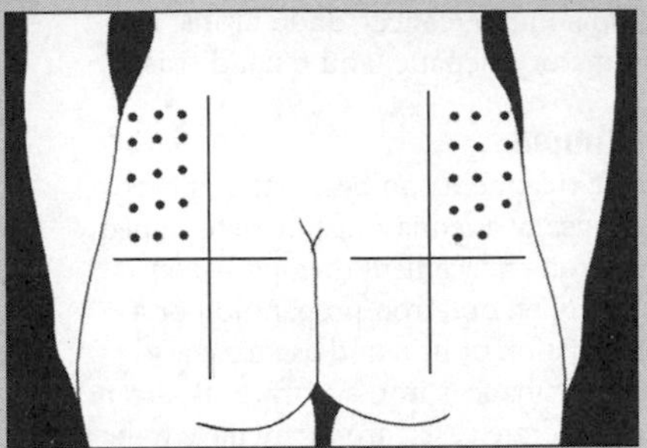

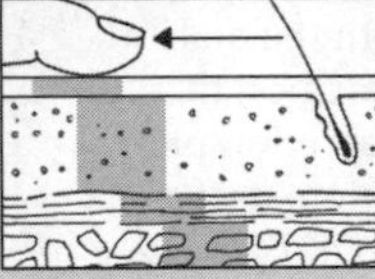

1. Displace tissues.

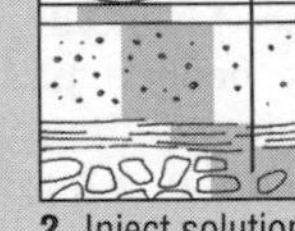

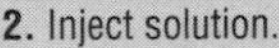

2. Inject solution.

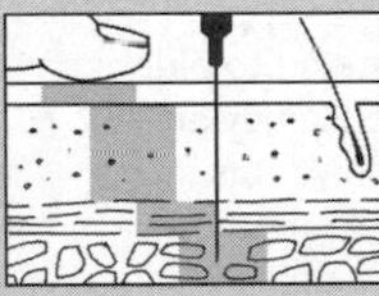

3. Wait 10 seconds.

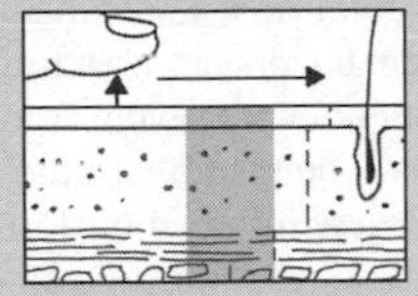

4. Release tissues.

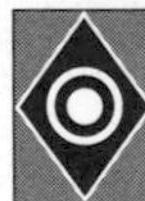

Drug alert Excessive iron replacement may cause such signs and symptoms as diarrhea, fever, severe stomach pain, nausea, and vomiting. Notify the physician promptly if the patient experiences any of these, and administer the prescribed treatments. For this acute condition, treatment may include iron-binding agents (deferoxamine), induced vomiting to produce alkalinization, and anticonvulsants.

▶ Monitor the patient's complete blood count and serum iron and ferritin levels regularly.

▶ Assess the family's dietary habits for iron intake, noting the influence of childhood eating patterns, cultural food preferences, and family income on adequate nutrition.

▶ Evaluate the patient's drug history. Certain drugs, such as pancreatic enzymes and vitamin E, may interfere with iron metabolism and absorption; aspirin, steroids, and other drugs may cause GI bleeding.

▶ Provide oxygen therapy as necessary to help prevent and reduce hypoxia.

▶ Provide frequent rest periods to decrease physical exhaustion. Plan activities so that the patient has sufficient rest between them.

▶ As ordered, administer analgesics for headache and other discomfort.

▶ Because a sore mouth and tongue make eating painful, ask the dietitian to give the patient nonirritating foods. If these symptoms make talking difficult, supply a pad and pencil or some other communication aid. Provide diluted mouthwash or, in especially severe conditions, swab the patient's mouth with tap water or warm saline solution. An oral anesthetic diluted in saline solution may also be used.

- Monitor the patient for signs and symptoms of decreased perfusion to vital organs: dyspnea, chest pain, dizziness, and signs of neuropathy such as tingling in the extremities.
- Monitor the patient's pulse rate often; tachycardia indicates that his activities are too strenuous.

PATIENT TEACHING

- Reinforce the physician's explanation of the disorder, and answer any questions. Make sure the patient understands the prescribed treatments and possible complications.
- Advise the patient not to stop therapy, even if he feels better, because replacement of iron stores takes time.
- Inform the patient that milk or an antacid interferes with absorption, but that vitamin C can increase absorption. Tell him to drink liquid supplemental iron through a straw to prevent staining his teeth.
- Tell the patient to report any adverse effects of iron therapy, such as nausea, vomiting, diarrhea, and constipation, which may indicate the need for a dosage adjustment or supplemental stool softeners.
- Teach the patient to schedule activities with rest periods that may be adjusted as his anemia is adjusted.
- Because an iron deficiency may recur, explain the need for regular checkups and compliance with prescribed treatments. (See *Preventing iron deficiency anemia*.)

Staying well

Preventing iron deficiency anemia

In order to help your patient prevent iron deficiency anemia, make sure to address the following teaching points:

- Teach the basics of a nutritionally balanced diet: red meats, green vegetables, eggs, milk, and whole wheat, iron-fortified bread. Explain that no food in itself contains enough iron to treat iron deficiency anemia; an average-sized person with anemia would have to eat at least 10 lb (4.5 kg) of steak daily to receive therapeutic amounts of iron.
- Warn the patient to guard against infections because his weakened condition may increase his susceptibility. Stress the importance of meticulous wound care, periodic dental checkups, good hand-washing technique, and other measures to prevent infection. Also, tell him to report any signs or symptoms of infection, including temperature elevation and chills.

ANGIOPLASTY, PERCUTANEOUS TRANSLUMINAL CORONARY

A nonsurgical alternative to coronary artery bypass grafting, percutaneous transluminal coronary angioplasty (PTCA) uses a balloon-tipped catheter to open coronary vessels narrowed by arteriosclerosis. This procedure, performed in the cardiac catheterization laboratory under local anesthesia, relieves pain due to angina and myocardial ischemia.

Cardiac catheterization usually accompanies PTCA to assess the stenosis

Performing PTCA

Percutaneous transluminal coronary angioplasty (PTCA) is a procedure that opens an occluded coronary artery without opening the chest. It's performed in the cardiac catheterization laboratory after coronary angiography confirms the presence and location of the occlusion. As soon as the occlusion is located, the physician threads a guide catheter through the patient's femoral artery and into the coronary artery under fluoroscopic guidance, as shown in the first illustration.

When the guide catheter's position at the occlusion site is confirmed by angiography, the physician carefully introduces into the catheter a double-lumen balloon that's smaller than the catheter lumen. He then directs the balloon through the lesion, where a marked pressure gradient will be obvious. The physician alternately inflates (as shown in the second illustration) and deflates the balloon until an angiogram verifies successful arterial dilation and the pressure gradient has decreased.

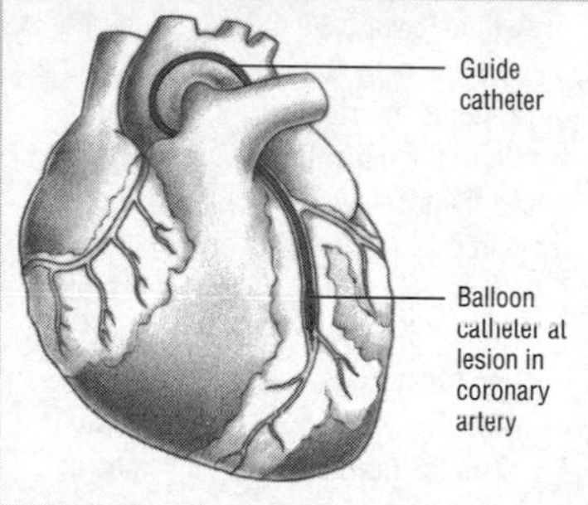

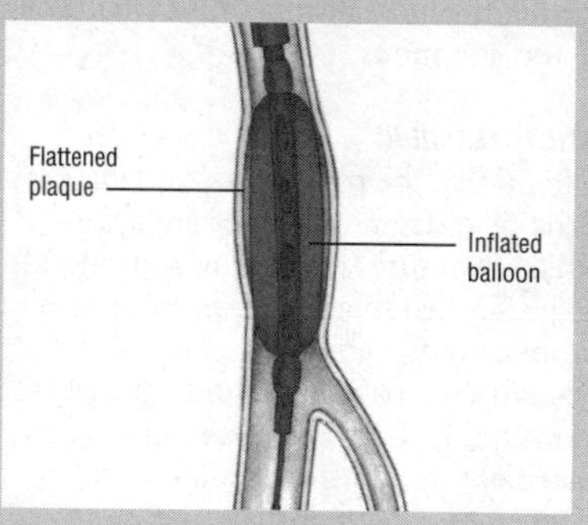

and the efficacy of the angioplasty. Catheterization is used as a visual tool to direct the balloon-tipped catheter through the vessel's area of stenosis. As the balloon is slowly inflated, the plaque is compressed against the vessel wall, allowing coronary blood to flow more freely. (See *Performing PTCA*.)

PTCA provides an alternative for older patients who are poor surgical risks because of chronic medical problems. It's also useful for patients who have total coronary occlusion, unstable angina, and plaque buildup in several areas and for those with poor left ventricular function.

The ideal candidate for PTCA has a single- or double-vessel blockage excluding the left main coronary artery with at least 50% proximal stenosis. The lesion should be discrete, uncalcified, concentric, and not located near a bifurcation.

Be aware that PTCA is contraindicated in left main coronary artery disease, especially when the patient is a poor surgical risk; in patients with variant angina or critical valvular disease; and in patients with vessels occluded at the aortic wall orifice.

Supplies

- Povidone-iodine solution
- Local anesthetic
- I.V. solution and tubing
- Electrocardiogram (ECG) monitor and electrodes
- Oxygen
- Nasal cannula
- Shaving supplies or depilatory cream

- Sedative
- Pulmonary artery (PA) catheter
- Contrast medium
- Emergency medications
- Heparin for injection
- 5-lb (2.3-kg) sandbag
- Introducer kit for PTCA catheter
- Sterile gown, gloves, and drapes
- Optional: nitroglycerin, soft restraints

Implementation

Before angioplasty

- Check the patient's history for allergies; if he has had allergic reactions to shellfish, iodine, or contrast media, notify the physician.
- Administer aspirin the evening before the procedure to prevent platelet aggregation, as ordered.

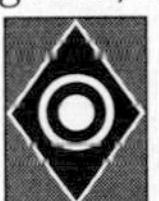

Drug alert Patients over age 60 may be more susceptible to the toxic effects of aspirin. The effects of aspirin on renal prostaglandins may cause fluid retention and edema, a significant drawback for older patients and those with heart failure.

- Make sure that the patient signs a consent form.
- Restrict food and fluids for at least 6 hours before the procedure or as ordered.
- Ensure that the results of coagulation studies, a complete blood count, serum electrolyte studies, and blood typing and crossmatching are available.
- Insert an I.V. line in case emergency medications are needed.
- Shave hair from the insertion site (groin or brachial area), or use a depilatory cream. Then clean the area with povidone-iodine solution.
- Give the patient a sedative, as ordered.
- Take baseline peripheral pulses in all extremities.

During angioplasty

- When the patient arrives at the cardiac catheterization laboratory, apply ECG electrodes and ensure I.V. line patency.
- Administer oxygen through a nasal cannula.
- The physician will put on a sterile gown and gloves. Open the sterile supplies.
- The physician prepares the site and injects a local anesthetic. If the patient doesn't already have a PA catheter in place, the physician may insert one now.
- The physician inserts a large guide catheter into the artery and sutures it in place. Then he threads an angioplasty catheter through the guide catheter. An angioplasty catheter is thinner and longer and has a balloon at its tip. Using a thin, flexible guide wire, he then threads the catheter up through the aorta and into the coronary artery to the area of stenosis.
- He injects a contrast medium through the angioplasty catheter and into the obstructed coronary artery to outline the lesion's location and help assess the blockage. He also injects heparin to prevent the catheter from clotting, and intracoronary nitroglycerin to dilate coronary vessels and prevent spasm, if needed.
- He inflates and deflates the catheter's balloon for gradually increasing periods of time and pressure. The expanding balloon compresses the atherosclerotic plaque against the arterial wall, expanding the arterial lumen. Because balloon inflation deprives the myocardium distal to the inflation area of blood, the patient may experience angina during the process. If balloon inflation fails to decrease the stenosis, a larger balloon may be used.
- The physician removes the angioplasty catheter but leaves the guide catheter in place in case he must repeat the procedure to open an occluded vessel. The guide catheter is usually removed 8 to 24 hours after the procedure.

After angioplasty

▶ Because coronary spasm may occur during or after PTCA, monitor the ECG for ST-segment and T-wave changes, and take vital signs frequently.

Key point **Be alert for signs and symptoms of ischemia, which requires emergency coronary revascularization.**

▶ When the patient returns to the unit, he may be receiving I.V. heparin or nitroglycerin. If there is bleeding at the catheter insertion site, he may also have a sandbag on the insertion site to prevent a hematoma.

▶ Assess the patient's vital signs every 15 minutes for the first hour, then every 30 minutes for 4 hours, unless his condition warrants more frequent checking.

▶ Assess peripheral pulses distal to the catheter insertion site as well as the color, sensation, temperature, and capillary refill of the affected extremity.

▶ Monitor ECG rhythm and arterial pressures.

▶ Instruct the patient to remain in bed for 8 hours and to keep the affected extremity straight; if the patient is restless and moving his extremities, apply soft restraints if necessary. Elevate the head of the bed 15 to 30 degrees.

▶ Assess the catheter site for hematoma, ecchymosis, and hemorrhage. If an area of expanding hematoma appears, mark the site and alert the physician. If bleeding occurs, locate the artery and apply manual pressure; then notify the physician.

▶ Administer I.V. fluids as ordered—usually 100 ml/hour—to promote excretion of the contrast medium. Be sure to assess for signs of fluid overload (distended neck veins, atrial and ventricular gallops, dyspnea, pulmonary congestion, tachycardia, hypertension, and hypoxemia).

▶ After the physician removes the catheter, apply direct pressure for at least 10 minutes and monitor the site frequently.

▶ After angioplasty, serial angiograms help determine the effectiveness of treatment.

Complications

The most common complication of PTCA is prolonged angina. PTCA can also cause coronary artery perforation, balloon rupture, reocclusion (necessitating a coronary artery bypass graft), myocardial infarction, pericardial tamponade, hematoma, hemorrhage, reperfusion arrhythmias, and closure of the vessel.

Coronary spasm may occur during or after PTCA. For this reason, monitor the ECG for ST-segment and T-wave changes, and take vital signs frequently. Coronary artery dissection may occur with no early signs or symptoms, and it can cause restenosis of the vessel.

Patient teaching

Before angioplasty

▶ Explain the procedure to the patient and family members to reduce the patient's fear and promote cooperation.

▶ Inform the patient that the procedure lasts from 1 to 4 hours and that he may feel some discomfort from lying on a hard table for that long.

▶ Tell him that a catheter will be inserted into an artery or a vein in his groin and that he may feel pressure as the catheter moves along the vessel.

▶ Reassure him that although he'll be awake during the procedure, he'll be given a sedative. Explain that the physician or nurse may ask him how he's feeling and that he should tell them if he experiences any angina.

▶ Explain that the physician will inject a contrast medium to outline the lesion's location. Warn the patient that he may feel a hot, flushing sensation or transient nausea during the injection.

After angioplasty

▶ Instruct the patient or a family member to call the physician if there's any bleeding or bruising at the arterial puncture site.

- Explain the necessity of taking all prescribed medications, and ensure that the patient or family member understands their intended effects.
- Tell the patient that he can resume normal activity. Most patients experience an increased cardiac tolerance.
- Instruct the patient to return for a stress thallium imaging test and follow-up angiography, as recommended by his physician.

Documentation

Note the patient's tolerance of the procedure and his condition after it, including vital signs and the condition of the insertion site and the extremity. Also document any complications and interventions as well as your patient teaching.

ANXIETY

Many psychosocial stressors, such as an impending serious diagnostic test, a sudden financial reversal, or the severe illness of a family member, can trigger an anxiety reaction. Drugs can also cause anxiety signs and symptoms, especially in older adults, who may be taking several medications.

In many cases, the signs and symptoms of anxiety resemble those of depression; a person who's depressed is likely to be anxious as well. Many physical disorders are marked by signs and symptoms of anxiety, such as heart failure, pulmonary embolism, irritable bowel syndrome, and peptic ulcers.

Signs and symptoms

- Anxious mood, irritability, and anticipation of the worst
- Tachycardia, palpitations, chest pain, faintness
- Tension, restlessness, inability to relax, trembling, or increased startle response
- Chest pressure or constriction, choking feeling, dyspnea
- Constipation, nausea, vomiting, difficulty swallowing, abdominal fullness or pain, diarrhea, weight loss
- Urinary frequency or urgency, impotence or frigidity
- Dry mouth, flushing, pallor, tendency to sweat
- Aches and pains, twitching, stiffness, myoclonic jerking movements, unsteady voice, increased muscle tone
- Tinnitus, blurred vision, feeling of weakness
- Insomnia
- Difficulty concentrating, poor memory

Diagnostic tests

Laboratory tests must exclude organic causes of the patient's signs and symptoms, such as hyperthyroidism, pheochromocytoma, coronary disease, paroxysmal atrial tachycardia, and Ménière's disease.

Treatment

Treatment depends on the cause of anxiety. Antianxiety drugs, such as benzodiazepines, are effective in controlling anxiety; however, they aren't recommended for older patients. Buspirone, a nonbenzodiazepine, is the drug of choice in treating anxiety in older patients.

Complimentary therapies, such as pet therapy and music therapy, have also been effective in reducing anxiety in older adults. Mental health facilities, chaplains, social workers, family physicians, and other mental health practitioners may be able to assist with treatment.

Key nursing diagnoses and outcomes

Disturbed thought processes related to anxiety

Treatment outcome: The patient's thought processes will improve with the treatment of anxiety.

Ineffective coping related to anxiety

Treatment outcome: The patient will develop effective coping mechanisms to manage his anxiety.

Nursing interventions

- Carefully assess the patient to ensure that his anxiety is not a symptom of an underlying disease process, such as pain or hypoxia.
- Encourage the patient to verbalize his feelings and fears.
- Ask him what coping skills he has used to deal successfully with stress in the past.
- Administer antianxiety drugs as ordered, and note their effectiveness.
- Ask the patient which drugs he's taking. Anxiety symptoms can result from the use of various drugs, including caffeine, thyroid hormone, aminophylline, oral antidiabetic drugs, nonsteroidal anti-inflammatory drugs, steroids, cardiac glycosides, and selective serotonin reuptake inhibitors. It's better to ask the physician to substitute another drug with fewer anxiety-producing adverse effects than to add drugs just to treat anxiety signs and symptoms.
- Alcohol is a common method of self-treatment for anxiety, but not a benign one. Be sure to ask your patient about his alcohol use — what type he drinks (beer, wine, whiskey), approximately how much per day, and for how long. One martini a day for 30 years may easily have serious consequences.

PATIENT TEACHING

- Teach the patient coping mechanisms to deal with specific situations that create anxiety.
- Urge family members to help the patient deal with or decrease his anxiety.
- Refer the patient and family members to a mental health facility, counselor, or specific person who may help the patient cope with anxiety.

AORTIC STENOSIS

In aortic stenosis, the opening of the aortic valve becomes narrowed and the left ventricle exerts increased pressure to drive blood through the opening. The added workload increases the demand for oxygen, while diminished cardiac output reduces coronary artery perfusion, causes ischemia of the left ventricle, and leads to heart failure.

Evidence of aortic stenosis may not appear until the patient reaches ages 50 to 70, even though the lesion has been present since childhood. Incidence increases with age, and the disorder is the most significant valvular lesion seen among older adults. About 80% of patients with aortic stenosis are male.

Aortic stenosis may be caused by congenital aortic bicuspid valve (associated with coarctation of the aorta), congenital stenosis of pulmonary valve cusps, rheumatic fever or, in older patients, atherosclerosis.

The disorder leads to left-sided heart failure, usually after age 70. It typically occurs within 4 years after the onset of signs and symptoms and is fatal in up to two-thirds of patients. Sudden death, possibly caused by an arrhythmia, occurs in up to 20% of patients, usually around age 60.

Signs and symptoms

- May be asymptomatic for years
- Dyspnea on exertion
- Fatigue
- Exertional syncope
- Angina
- Palpitations
- On palpation, diminished carotid pulses and alternating pulse on palpation
- On auscultation, systolic ejection murmur (at least grade 3 or 4) that disappears when the valve calcifies, a split S_2 as stenosis becomes more severe, and an S_4 (a normal finding in older people)

- In left-sided heart failure, orthopnea, paroxysmal nocturnal dyspnea, peripheral edema, and apex of heart displaced inferiorly and laterally
- In pulmonary hypertension, a systolic thrill that's palpable at the base of the heart, at the jugular notch, and along the carotid arteries (occasionally palpable only during expiration and when the patient leans forward)

Diagnostic tests

- *Cardiac catheterization* reveals the pressure gradient across the valve (indicating the obstruction's severity), increased left ventricular end-diastolic pressures (indicating left ventricular function), and the location of the left ventricular outflow obstruction.
- *Chest X-rays* show valvular calcification; left ventricular enlargement; pulmonary vein congestion; and, in later stages, left atrial, pulmonary artery, right atrial, and right ventricular enlargement.
- *Echocardiography* demonstrates a thickened aortic valve and left ventricular wall and, possibly, coexistent mitral valve stenosis.
- *Electrocardiography* (ECG) reveals left ventricular hypertrophy. In advanced stages, the patient exhibits ST-segment depression and T-wave inversion in standard leads I and aV_L and in the left precordial leads. Up to 10% of patients have atrioventricular and intraventricular conduction defects.

Treatment

Treatment of aortic stenosis includes cardiac glycosides, a low-sodium diet, diuretics and oxygen to treat heart failure, nitroglycerin to help relieve angina, valve replacement (when valves become calcified and patients become symptomatic or are at risk for developing left-sided heart failure), and percutaneous balloon aortic valvuloplasty, which is useful in older patients with severe calcifications. This procedure may improve left ventricular function so that the patient can tolerate valve replacement surgery.

Key nursing diagnoses and outcomes

Ineffective (cardiopulmonary) tissue perfusion related to decreased coronary artery perfusion and increased demand for oxygen

Treatment outcome: The patient will show no ischemic changes on the ECG.

Decreased cardiac output related to narrowed opening of aortic valve

Treatment outcome: The patient will express the importance of following the prescribed diet, taking medications as ordered, and adhering to activity guidelines.

Excess fluid volume related to left-sided heart failure

Treatment outcome: The patient will display no signs or symptoms of fluid overload, such as shortness of breath, distended neck veins, edema, sudden unexplained weight gain, and crackles on lung auscultation.

Nursing interventions

- Allow the patient to express his fears and concerns about the disorder, its impact on his life, and any impending surgery. Reassure him as needed.
- If the patient needs bed rest, stress its importance. Assist him with bathing if necessary. Provide a bedside commode because using a commode puts less stress on the heart than using a bedpan. Offer diversionary activities that aren't physically demanding.
- Alternate periods of activity and rest to prevent extreme fatigue and dyspnea.
- Keep the patient's legs elevated while he sits in a chair to improve venous return to the heart.
- If necessary, place the patient in an upright position to relieve dyspnea.
- Administer oxygen as needed to prevent tissue hypoxia.

- Keep the patient on a low-sodium diet. Consult with a dietitian to ensure that he receives foods that he likes while adhering to the diet restrictions.
- After cardiac catheterization, apply firm pressure to the catheter insertion site, usually in the groin. If the site bleeds, remove the pressure dressing, apply firm pressure, and contact the physician. Monitor the insertion site every 15 minutes for at least 6 hours for signs of bleeding. Also, monitor the patient for chest pain, and assess his vital signs, heart rhythm, and peripheral pulses distal to the insertion site. Notify the physician of any changes in the patient's condition.
- Monitor the patient's weight and intake and output for signs of fluid overload.
- Evaluate the patient's activity tolerance and degree of fatigue.
- Monitor the patient's ECG for ischemic changes.
- Regularly assess the patient's cardiopulmonary function. Notify the physician if sudden or significant changes occur.
- Observe the patient for complications and adverse reactions to drug therapy.

PATIENT TEACHING

- Advise the patient to plan for periodic rest in his daily routine to prevent undue fatigue.
- Teach the patient about diet restrictions, medications, signs and symptoms that should be reported, and the importance of consistent follow-up care.
- Tell the patient to elevate his legs whenever he sits.

APPENDECTOMY

With rare exception, the only effective treatment of acute appendicitis is appendectomy, the surgical removal of an inflamed vermiform appendix. Commonly performed as an emergency procedure, this surgery aims to prevent imminent rupture or perforation of the appendix. When completed before these complications can occur, appendectomy is generally effective and uneventful.

Implementation

With the patient under general anesthesia, the surgeon makes an incision in the right lower abdominal quadrant, using McBurney's (muscle-splitting) incision to expose the appendix (called "open appendectomy"). He ligates the base of the appendix and places a purse-string suture in the cecum. Then he removes any excess fluid or tissue debris from the abdominal cavity and closes the incision. The use of laparoscopy for diagnosis and removal of the appendix is a safe and common approach, even in acute cases.

If the appendix perforates, the surgeon may drain the abdominal cavity by inserting one or more Penrose drains or abdominal sump tubes (or both) before closing the incision, or he may leave the incision open. The open incisional wound then heals by secondary intention through granulation and epithelialization.

Complications

If the appendix ruptures or perforates before surgery, its infected contents spill into the peritoneal cavity, possibly causing peritonitis — the most common and deadly complication of appendicitis, with a mortality of 10%.

An appendectomy usually causes few complications postoperatively if the appendix is removed before inflammation has progressed to the point of perforation. Potential complications include infection at the surgical site and paralytic ileus. If the appendix has ruptured before surgery, requiring drainage postoperatively, complications are more likely. These include local or general peritonitis, paralytic ileus, intestinal obstruction, and secondary abcesses in the pelvis or liver or under the diaphragm.

Key nursing diagnoses and outcomes

Risk for infection related to potential for peritonitis or formation of secondary abscesses following an appendectomy performed for a ruptured appendix

Treatment outcome: The patient will show no other signs or symptoms of infection.

Acute pain related to surgical incision or infectious process postoperatively (or both)

Treatment outcome: The patient will report a decrease in incisional pain in 24 hours and eventually become pain-free.

Risk for deficient fluid volume related to temporary cessation of oral intake caused by appendectomy

Treatment outcome: The patient will exhibit no signs or symptoms of dehydration, such as dry mucous membranes, poor skin turgor, thirst, and decreased urine output.

Nursing interventions

When preparing for or managing a patient with an open appendectomy, expect to implement the following interventions.

Before surgery

- Typically, you'll have little time to prepare the patient for an appendectomy. Begin by reassuring him that the surgery will relieve his pain and won't interfere with normal GI functioning.
- Briefly explain the surgery, and answer any questions the patient and his family might have. Explain that before surgery he'll receive prophylactic antibiotics to prevent infection and I.V. fluids to maintain blood pressure during surgery. He may have a nasogastric (NG) tube inserted to decompress the stomach and reduce postoperative nausea and vomiting, and he'll be given a sedative and general anesthetic. Tell him that he'll awaken from general anesthesia with a dressing over the surgical site and possibly several drains in the incision; the drains will remain in place for 3 to 5 days.
- Assure the patient that recovery is usually rapid; if no complications occur, he should be walking and gradually resuming oral foods the day after surgery. He can expect to be discharged after 3 days and return to his normal activity level in 2 to 4 weeks.
- While awaiting surgery, place the patient in Fowler's position to reduce pain. Avoid giving analgesics, which can mask the pain that indicates impending rupture. Also, never apply heat to the abdomen or give cathartics or enemas; these measures could trigger rupture.
- Ensure that the patient or a responsible family member has signed a consent form.

After surgery

- After the patient awakens from anesthesia, place him in Fowler's position to decrease the risk of any contaminated peritoneal fluid infecting the upper abdomen. Monitor his vital signs and record intake and output for 2 days after surgery. Auscultate the abdomen for bowel sounds, indicating the return of peristalsis.
- Regularly check the dressing for drainage, and change it as necessary. If abdominal drains are in place, check and record the amount and nature of drainage and maintain drain patency. Also, check drainage from the NG tube and suction as necessary.
- Encourage ambulation within 12 hours after surgery, if possible. Assist the patient as necessary. Also, encourage coughing, deep breathing, and frequent position changes to prevent pulmonary complications. On the day after surgery, remove the NG tube and gradually resume oral foods and fluids, as ordered.
- Throughout the recovery period, assess the patient closely for signs and symptoms of peritonitis. Watch for and

report continuing pain and fever, excessive wound drainage, hypotension, tachycardia, pallor, weakness, and other signs and symptoms of infection and fluid and electrolyte loss. If peritonitis develops, expect to assist with emergency treatment, including GI intubation, parenteral fluid and electrolyte replacement, and antibiotic therapy.

▶ After a laparoscopic appendectomy, assess the three or four small abdominal incisions and dressings. Prepare to ambulate the patient within 6 hours. Anticipate discharge in 1 to 2 days.

PATIENT TEACHING

▶ Tell the patient to watch for and immediately report fever, chills, diaphoresis, nausea, vomiting, and abdominal pain.

▶ Teach the patient about wound care as necessary.

▶ After a laparoscopic appendectomy, instruct the patient to resume normal activities in about 8 to 10 days.

▶ Encourage the patient to keep his scheduled follow-up appointments to monitor healing and detect any complications.

APPENDICITIS

Appendicitis is an inflammation of the vermiform appendix, a small, fingerlike projection attached to the cecum just below the ileocecal valve. Although the appendix has no known function, it does regularly fill and empty itself of food. Appendicitis occurs when the appendix becomes inflamed from ulceration of the mucosa or obstruction of the lumen.

Appendicitis may occur at any age and affects both sexes equally; about 10% of elderly people hospitalized with acute abdominal pain and tenderness are diagnosed with appendicitis. Since the advent of antibiotics, the incidence and mortality of appendicitis have declined. If untreated, this condition is invariably fatal.

Appendicitis probably results from an obstruction of the appendiceal lumen, caused by a fecal mass, stricture, barium ingestion, or viral infection. This obstruction sets off an inflammatory process that can lead to infection, thrombosis, necrosis, and perforation.

The most common and perilous complication of appendicitis occurs when the appendix ruptures or perforates. When this happens, the infected contents spill into the abdominal cavity, causing peritonitis. Other complications include appendiceal abscess and pyelophlebitis.

Signs and symptoms

Early stage

▶ Abdominal pain (may be generalized initially but within a few hours becomes localized in right lower abdomen [McBurney's point])

▶ Anorexia

▶ Nausea and vomiting

Signs and symptoms may be vague in the older adult, leading to a delayed diagnosis.

Late stage

▶ Malaise

▶ Constipation or diarrhea (rare)

▶ Low-grade fever (because core temperature of older people is lower, a temperature of 99° F [37.2° C] may be significant)

▶ Bent-over posture to reduce right lower quadrant pain, bent-up right knee to decrease pain when in a supine position

▶ On palpation, tenderness in the right lower abdominal quadrant that worsens upon gentle percussion or when the patient is asked to cough; rebound tenderness; and spasm of the abdominal muscles

▶ Tenderness in the flank if the appendix is positioned retrocecally or in the pelvis

Key point Keep in mind that abdominal rigidity and tenderness worsen as the condition progresses. Sudden cessation of abdominal pain signals perforation or infarction.

Diagnostic tests

- *Blood studies* show a moderately elevated white blood cell (WBC) count, with increased numbers of immature cells.
- *Contrast studies* indicate failure of the contrast agent to fill the appendix, signaling appendicitis.

Diagnosis must rule out illnesses with similar signs and symptoms: bladder infection, diverticulitis, gastritis, ovarian cyst, pancreatitis, renal colic, and uterine disease.

Treatment

Appendectomy is the only effective treatment. If peritonitis develops, treatment involves GI intubation, parenteral replacement of fluids and electrolytes, and administration of antibiotics.

Key nursing diagnoses and outcomes

Risk for deficient fluid volume related to nausea and vomiting caused by appendicitis

Treatment outcome: The patient will maintain normal fluid volume, as evidenced by normal blood pressure and urine output and adequate hydration.

Risk for infection related to potential for ruptured or perforated appendix

Treatment outcome: The patient will exhibit a WBC count and temperature that return to normal and remain normal.

Acute pain related to inflammation of the vermiform appendix

Treatment outcome: The patient will become pain-free after surgery.

Nursing interventions

- Monitor the patient's vital signs. Measure intake and output to assess for fluid imbalance.
- Evaluate the severity and location of abdominal pain. Notify the physician immediately if pain suddenly ceases (signifying that the appendix has ruptured).
- Observe the patient for complications, such as peritonitis, appendiceal abscess, and pylephlebitis.
- Make sure the patient with suspected or known appendicitis receives nothing by mouth until surgery is performed.
- Administer I.V. fluids to prevent dehydration. Never administer cathartics or enemas because they may rupture the appendix.
- Don't administer analgesics until the diagnosis is confirmed because they mask signs and symptoms. Once the diagnosis is confirmed, analgesics may be given (I.V. morphine sulfate is the drug of choice for severe acute pain in older adults).
- Place the patient in Fowler's position to reduce pain. Never apply heat to the right lower abdomen; this may cause the appendix to rupture.
- Once the diagnosis is confirmed, prepare the patient for surgery.
- If peritonitis occurs, nasogastric drainage may be necessary to decompress the stomach and reduce nausea and vomiting. If so, record drainage and provide proper mouth and nose care. Expect to administer antibiotic therapy.

PATIENT TEACHING

- Teach the patient what happens in appendicitis.
- Explain why analgesic administration may be delayed, and reassure the patient that an analgesic will be administered as soon as possible.
- Tell the patient that assuming Fowler's position may help relieve his pain.
- Emphasize the importance of notifying a health care professional if pain is

suddenly relieved without medical or surgical treatment.

▶ Help the patient understand the required surgery and its possible complications.

AROMATHERAPY

Aromatherapy refers to the inhalation or application of essential oils distilled from various plants. Those who use aromatherapy say it's effective in reducing stress, preventing disease, and even treating certain illnesses—both physical and psychological.

Aromatherapy is popular in Europe, where essential oils are inhaled, massaged into the skin, or placed in bath water to create pleasant sensations, promote relaxation, or treat specific ailments. Aromatherapy can be used—either alone or with other therapies, such as massage or herbal therapy—to treat bacterial and viral infections, anxiety, pain, muscle disorders, arthritis, herpes simplex, herpes zoster, skin disorders, premenstrual syndrome, headaches, and indigestion. When absorbed by body tissues, these oils are thought to interact with hormones and enzymes to produce changes in blood pressure, pulse rate, and other physiologic functions. (See *Therapeutic effects of essential oils.*)

Aromatherapy may be self-administered or administered by a trained aromatherapist. In the United States, where interest in aromatherapy has skyrocketed, several organizations train and certify people as aromatherapists. These organizations can also provide information to interested laymen and health care providers, referrals to aromatherapists, and sources for obtaining essential oils.

Although there's no scientific evidence indicating that aromatherapy prevents or cures disease, nurses trained in aromatherapy may recommend specific oils as adjuncts to conventional therapies, teach patients how to use these oils, and administer treatment themselves.

Implementation

▶ Besides the appropriate essential oil, aromatherapy may require other supplies, depending on how the oil is administered (for example, massage, inhalation, a bath, or diffusion).

▶ Massage requires a carrier oil and, for a full body massage, a massage table. Massage involves diluting the essential oil in the appropriate carrier oil and applying it to the exposed body part or the entire body using massage techniques.

▶ Inhalation requires a bowl of hot water and a large towel. With the towel draped over his head, the patient leans over a bowl of steaming water that contains a few drops of the essential oil. The patient inhales the vapors for few minutes.

▶ A bath requires a tub filled with warm water. The patient adds a few drops of essential oil to the surface of the bath water and then soaks in the tub for 10 to 20 minutes, inhaling the vapors as he soaks.

▶ Diffusion requires a micromist or candle diffuser or a ceramic ring that can be placed on a light bulb. This method involves placing a few drops of the essential oil in the diffuser and turning on the heat source to diffuse microparticles of the oil into the air. The average treatment is 30 minutes.

Special considerations

▶ Citrus oils shouldn't be applied before exposure to the sun. Advise patients to avoid applying cinnamon or clove oil on the skin. Be aware that certain oils—such as basil, fennel, lemongrass, rosemary, and verbena—may cause irritation if the patient has sensitive skin. If such irritation develops, advise him to stop using these oils. Also, high doses of certain oils—such as wintergreen, sage, aniseed, thyme, lemon, fennel, clove,

Therapeutic effects of essential oils

The chart below lists some popular essential oils and the traditional indications for which practitioners use them.

Essential oil	Traditional therapeutic uses
Chamomile *(Anthemis nobilis)*	■ Anti-inflammatory, antifungal, and antibacterial effects ■ Relieving mental or physical stress ■ Balancing body and mind
Eucalyptus *(Eucalyptus radiata)*	■ Antiviral and expectorant effects ■ Relieving nausea and motion sickness ■ Clearing the sinuses ■ Soothing irritable bowel ■ Stimulant effect
Geranium *(Pelargonium x asperum)*	■ Antiviral and antifungal effects ■ Stimulating metabolism in the skin ■ Improving cell regeneration ■ Improving circulation ■ Relieving pain ■ Improving vital organ function
Lavender *(Lavandula angustifolia)*	■ Anti-inflammatory and antibacterial effects ■ Treating burns, insect bites, and minor injuries ■ Soothing stomachache and colic ■ Relieving toothache and teething pain ■ Relieving mental or physical stress
Peppermint *(Mentha piperita)*	■ Antibacterial and antiviral effects ■ Decongestant and expectorant effects ■ Relieving nausea and motion sickness ■ Soothing irritable bowel ■ Stimulant effect
Rosemary *(Rosmarinus officinalis)*	■ Antibacterial, antifungal, and antiviral effects ■ Restoring energy and alleviating stress ■ Improving cell regeneration
Tea tree *(Melanleuca alternifolia)*	■ Anti-inflammatory, antibacterial, and antiviral effects ■ Treating burns, insect bites, and minor injuries ■ Providing calmness and sedation

cinnamon, camphor, and cedar wood—can result in nonlethal poisoning.

▶ Different administration methods require specific safety precautions. When using inhalation therapy, the patient should keep his face far enough from the water's surface to avoid a burn injury. When using the diffusion method, he should be at least 3′ (1 m) away from the diffuser.

▶ Aromatherapy is contraindicated during pregnancy because it poses a toxic risk to the mother and fetus. It should be used with caution in infants and children younger than age 5 because many essential oils are toxic to patients in this age-group.

▶ Caution patients to keep essential oils away from the eyes and mucous membranes to avoid irritation. If contact occurs, the patient should flush with plenty of water; if flushing doesn't relieve the pain, he should seek medical attention.

ARTERIAL OCCLUSIVE DISEASE

An obstruction or narrowing of the lumen of the aorta and its major branches, arterial occlusive disease interrupts blood flow, usually to the legs and feet. This disorder may affect the carotid, vertebral, innominate, subclavian, mesenteric, and celiac arteries.

Arterial occlusive disease is more common in males than in females. The prognosis depends on the location of the occlusion, the development of collateral circulation to counteract reduced blood flow and, in acute disease, the time elapsed between the development of the occlusion and its removal.

The most common cause of acute arterial occlusion is obstruction of a major artery by a clot. The occlusive mechanism may be endogenous, resulting from emboli formation, thrombosis, or plaques, or exogenous, resulting from trauma or fracture. Chronic arterial occlusive disease is a common complication of atherosclerosis.

Predisposing factors include smoking; aging; conditions such as hypertension, hyperlipidemia, and diabetes mellitus; and family history of vascular disorders, myocardial infarction, or cerebrovascular accident. (See *Maintaining vascular health.*)

Occlusions may be acute or chronic and, in many cases, cause severe ischemia, skin ulceration, and gangrene.

Signs and symptoms

▶ Sudden and localized pain in the affected arm or leg (most common symptom)

▶ Pallor (from vasoconstriction distal to the occlusion)

▶ Pulselessness distal to the occlusion

▶ Paralysis and paresthesia in the affected arm or leg (from disturbed nerve endings or skeletal muscles)

▶ Poikilothermy (temperature changes that occur distal to the occlusion, making the skin feel cool)

Specific signs and symptoms vary, depending on the vessel involved. (See *Detecting arterial occlusive disease,* page 54.)

Diagnostic tests

▶ *Arteriography* demonstrates the type, location, and degree of obstruction and the establishment of collateral circulation. It's particularly useful in chronic disease and in the evaluation of candidates for reconstructive surgery.

▶ *Ultrasonography* and *plethysmography* are noninvasive tests that, in acute disease, show decreased blood flow distal to the occlusion.

▶ *Doppler ultrasonography* typically reveals a relatively low-pitched sound and a monophasic waveform.

▶ *Segmental limb pressures and pulse volume measurements* help evaluate the location and extent of the occlusion.

▶ *Ophthalmodynamometry* helps determine the degree of obstruction in the internal carotid artery by comparing ophthalmic artery pressure with brachial artery pressure on the affected side. More than a 20% difference between pressures suggests arterial insufficiency.

▶ *Electroencephalography* and a *computed tomography scan* may be necessary to rule out brain lesions.

Treatment

In mild chronic disease, treatment includes smoking cessation, control of hypertension, walking, and foot and leg care.

In carotid artery occlusion, treatment includes antiplatelet therapy, possibly beginning with dipyridamole and aspirin. In intermittent claudication caused by chronic arterial occlusive disease, pentoxifylline may be given to improve blood flow through the capillaries. This drug is particularly useful for poor surgical candidates.

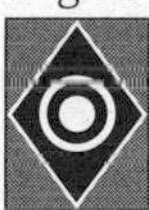

Drug alert **Because of increased bioavailability and decreased excretion, older adults are at higher risk for drug toxicity from pentoxifylline. Clinical signs of toxicity include flushing, hypotension, seizures, somnolence, loss of consciousness, fever, and agitation. Adverse reactions (headache, dizziness, angina, dyspepsia, nausea, vomiting, flatus, and bloating) may also be more common.**

In obstruction caused by a thrombus, treatments include thrombolytics, such as urokinase, streptokinase, and alteplase, to dissolve clots and relieve the obstruction.

Acute arterial occlusive disease usually requires surgery, such as embolectomy, in which a balloon-tipped Fogarty catheter is used to remove thrombotic material from the artery. Embolectomy is used mainly for mesenteric, femoral, or popliteal artery occlusion.

Thromboendarterectomy involves the opening of the artery and removal of the obstructing thrombus and the medial layer of the arterial wall. Plaque deposits will remain intact. Thromboendarterectomy is usually performed after angiography and is commonly used in conjunction with autogenous vein or Dacron bypass surgery (femoropopliteal or aortofemoral).

Percutaneous transluminal coronary angioplasty uses fluoroscopy and a special balloon catheter to dilate the stenosis or occluded artery to a predetermined diameter without overdistending it. Laser surgery uses an excimer or a hot-tip laser to obliterate the clot and plaque by vaporizing it.

Patch grafting involves removal of the thrombosed arterial segment and replacement with an autogenous vein or Dacron graft. Bypass grafting diverts blood flow through an anastomosed autogenous or woven Dacron graft to bypass the thrombosed arterial segment.

Depending on the condition of the sympathetic nervous system, lumbar sympathectomy may be used as an adjunct to reconstructive surgery. Amputation may be necessary if arterial reconstructive surgery fails or if gangrene, uncontrollable infection, or intractable pain develops. Other treatments include heparin to prevent emboli (for embolic occlusion) and bowel resection after restoration of blood flow (for mesenteric artery occlusion).

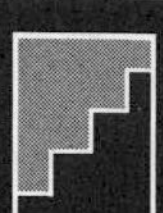

Staying well

Maintaining vascular health

To help your patient maintain vascular health, teach the following points:

- Tell the patient to engage in low-impact exercise at least three times a week.
- If the individual uses tobacco products, recommend smoking cessation therapies or programs.
- Discuss how to lower the amount of fat in the patient's diet.
- For post-menopausal women, recommend discussing hormonal replacement therapy with the family physician.
- Provide information about weight reduction and maintaining a healthy diet.

Detecting arterial occlusive disease

A patient with arterial occlusive disease may have various signs and symptoms, depending on which portion of the vasculature is affected by the disorder.

Site of occlusion	Signs and symptoms
Internal and external carotid arteries	Transient ischemic attacks (TIAs) due to reduced cerebral circulation produce unilateral sensory or motor dysfunction (transient monocular blindness, hemiparesis), possible aphasia or dysarthria, confusion, decreased mentation, and headache. These recurrent clinical features usually last for 5 to 10 minutes but may persist for up to 24 hours and may herald a cerebrovascular accident. Absent or decreased pulsation with an auscultatory bruit over the affected vessels.
Vertebral and basilar arteries	TIAs of brain stem and cerebellum produce binocular visual disturbances, vertigo, dysarthria, and falling down without loss of consciousness. Less common than carotid TIA.
Innominate (brachiocephalic) artery	Signs and symptoms of vertebrobasilar occlusion. Indications of ischemia (claudication) of right arm; possible bruit over right side of neck.
Subclavian artery	Subclavian steal syndrome characterized by the backflow of blood from the brain, through the vertebral artery on the same side as the occlusion, and into the subclavian artery distal to the occlusion; clinical effects of vertebrobasilar occlusion and exercise-induced arm claudication. Possible gangrene, usually limited to the digits.
Mesenteric artery	Bowel ischemia, infarct necrosis, and gangrene; sudden, acute abdominal pain; nausea and vomiting; diarrhea; leukocytosis; shock due to intraluminal fluid and plasma loss.
Aortic bifurcation (saddle-block occlusion, a medical emergency associated with cardiac embolization)	Sensory and motor deficits (muscle weakness, numbness, paresthesia, paralysis) and ischemia (sudden pain; cold, pale legs with decreased or absent peripheral pulses) in legs.
Iliac artery (Leriche's syndrome)	Intermittent claudication of lower back, buttocks, and thighs, relieved by rest; absent or reduced femoral or distal pulses; shiny, scaly skin, subcutaneous tissue loss, and no body hair on affected limb; nail deformities; increased capillary refill time; blanching of feet on elevation; possible bruit over femoral arteries; impotence in males.
Femoral and popliteal arteries (associated with aneurysm formation)	Intermittent claudication of the calves on exertion; ischemic pain in feet; pretrophic pain (heralds necrosis and ulceration); leg pallor and coolness; shiny, scaly skin, subcutaneous tissue loss, and no body hair on affected limb; nail deformities; increased capillary refill time; blanching of feet on elevation; gangrene; no palpable pulses distal to occlusion. Auscultation over affected area may reveal a bruit.

Key nursing diagnoses and outcomes

Activity intolerance related to exercise-induced pain and ischemia in the lower extremities

Treatment outcome: The patient will perform self-care activities to tolerance level.

Ineffective (peripheral or cerebral) tissue perfusion related to reduced blood flow

Treatment outcome: The patient will demonstrate adequate tissue perfusion, as evidenced by the presence of peripheral pulses, normal skin temperature and color in the extremities, absence of pain, and orientation to time, person, and place.

Acute pain related to peripheral ischemia in the lower extremities

Treatment outcome: The patient will become pain-free after treatment.

Nursing interventions

- Perform range-of-motion exercises to the affected extremity, as tolerated.
- Regularly assess the patient's circulatory status by checking for the most distal pulses and inspecting his skin color and temperature for evidence of aortic, iliac, femoral, or popliteal artery involvement. Compare findings to earlier assessments and observations.
- Evaluate the patient's neurologic status regularly for evidence of carotid, innominate, vertebral, or subclavian artery involvement. Watch for changes in level of consciousness, pupil size, and muscle strength.
- Monitor the patient for severe abdominal pain and change in bowel function by performing abdominal assessment for evidence of mesenteric artery involvement. Increasing abdominal distention and tenderness may indicate extension of bowel ischemia with resulting gangrene, or it may indicate peritonitis.
- Check the patient for signs and symptoms of fluid and electrolyte imbalance. Monitor his intake and output for signs of renal failure (urine output of less than 30 ml/hour) in an acute arterial occlusive episode involving the mesenteric artery or aorta.
- If the patient has experienced an embolus occlusion, expect to administer heparin or thrombolytics by continuous infusion drip, as ordered.
- During an acute episode, reposition the affected leg often to prevent pressure on any one area until surgery is performed. Strictly avoid elevating or applying heat to the affected leg.
- Pace the patient's self-care activities to avoid pain and fatigue.
- Prepare the patient experiencing an acute episode for surgery. Explain the surgical procedure to the patient and family members. Answer any questions to reduce anxiety.
- Prevent trauma to the affected extremity. Use minimal-pressure mattresses, heel protectors, a foot cradle, or a footboard to reduce pressure that could lead to skin breakdown. Keep the arm or leg warm, but never use heating pads. Check the temperature of the patient's bath water before allowing him to wash the affected extremity. If the patient is wearing socks, remove them frequently to check his skin.
- Avoid using restrictive clothing such as antiembolism stockings.
- Administer analgesics, as ordered, to relieve pain.

PATIENT TEACHING

- Advise the patient to pace his activities to avoid pain and fatigue.
- Tell the patient constipation is a common adverse effect of analgesics. Encourage a high-fiber diet.
- Tell the patient to avoid temperature extremes. If he must go outside in the cold, remind him to dress warmly and take special care to keep his feet warm.
- When preparing the patient for discharge, tell him to watch for signs and symptoms of recurrence (pain, pallor, numbness, paralysis, absence of pulse)

that can result from graft occlusion or occlusion at another site. Caution against wearing constrictive clothing, crossing his legs, or wearing garters. Tell him to avoid bumping injuries to affected limbs.

- Advise the patient to wear sturdy, properly fitting shoes. Refer him to a podiatrist for any foot problems.
- Warn the patient to avoid all tobacco products.
- Instruct him to wash his feet daily, and inspect them for signs and symptoms of injury or infection. Remind him to report any abnormalities to the physician.

ART THERAPY

Art therapy is the creative use of various expressive media to help a person deal with thoughts, emotions, life changes, personal issues, and conflicts often buried deep within his subconscious. If the patient can externalize his feelings for examination and reflection, he may discover meaning and insight, release, and transformation. Such discovery enhances integration of the whole person and supports growth, change, and the healing process.

Creative activities may include drawing, painting, sculpting, and making collages (from cuttings from recycled newspapers, magazines, catalogs, greeting cards, or calendars). Mask making is a powerful and popular form of expression used commonly in groups or as individual healing rituals. Puppetry is another form of artistic therapy. It requires fashioning of a hand puppet, several puppets or marionettes, and perhaps even a stage, scenery, or puppet theater. Photography, videography, and computer-generated art are newer forms of art therapy.

Some conditions in which art therapy is useful are posttraumatic stress disorder, substance abuse and addictions, catastrophic illness (cancer, acquired immunodeficiency syndrome), chronic pain or disease, prolonged hospitalization or treatment, extensive surgery, loss of voice (through surgery, tracheostomy, intubation), aging and loss of roles, and chronic fatigue and immune dysfunction syndrome.

Implementation

- Make sure the patient is physically capable of carrying out the artistic activity. Medications, a weakened condition, inflamed or painful joints in hands or fingers, or neurologic damage can impair the patient's ability. Someone who is physically unable to manipulate media may still participate in the making of a collage — for example, by choosing pictures, words, or materials for someone else to cut and paste or by indicating the position of cutouts and colors. Also, computer programs may be available to create art with adapted controls.
- Explain the creative procedure to the patient and get his agreement. Assess the patient for special equipment or needs.
- Collect and prepare all necessary materials.
- Provide a quiet and comfortable environment and arrange a clean, flat surface on which the patient can work.
- Reassure the patient that he doesn't need to know how to draw or have any previous knowledge or training in art. Stick figures can get his message across effectively.
- Assess the patient's prior art knowledge and his experience with various media. A patient may be intimidated by a creative activity that appears too complex, or he might consider a more simplistic project demeaning.
- Praise any and all efforts, and be careful not to make suggestions about colors or forms. Remain nonjudgmental and supportive.
- If the patient has certain signs and symptoms of a disease, encourage him to draw a picture representing himself in relation to this. You may suggest that the

patient draw himself in the past, present, and future, or in terms of before disease, with disease, and after treatment.

- Allow the patient time to complete the drawing to his satisfaction. Sometimes it's important for the patient to draw every small detail and search for just the right color.
- When the drawing is complete, allow the patient to show the drawing and tell you about it. Listen attentively. There may be a healing story involved, or perhaps the patient will come upon new insights. You may want to point out certain details.
- Repeat back to the patient what he has said to validate the meaning. Be supportive of the patient's efforts, and summarize the experience for him.
- Notice how the patient represents his size in relation to other figures or objects. Is the entire body drawn? What are the dominant colors and shapes? Is there a smile or frown drawn on the face? What is the overall mood?
- Strong emotions may surface as a patient explores and connects with underlying emotions. If the patient shows signs of agitation or uncontrolled emotion, end the session and reassure him that it's normal to have strong feelings and it's appropriate to express them. Refer the patient to other health care professionals, as appropriate.
- If a patient is especially proud of an art work, arrange to have it displayed (with the patient's permission) so that others may admire it, thereby adding a source of acknowledgment for the patient.

Special considerations

Some older patients may not be open to participating in art therapy, either because they're shy and self-conscious or just not interested. Don't insist, but instead work on building a trusting therapeutic relationship. The patient may be open to participation in the future.

ASPIRATION PNEUMONIA

Aspiration pneumonia results from the inhalation of a foreign substance, such as vomitus or food particles, into the pulmonary system. In older people, this disorder commonly results from impaired swallowing and a diminished gag reflex, which may occur after a cerebrovascular accident or any prolonged illness. It may also occur in patients receiving enteral tube feedings.

Depending on the type and extent of the aspirated substance, the patient may suffer either mild lung damage, with minimal inflammation and compromise to respiration and oxygenation, or severe damage, resulting in destruction of alveolar function, pulmonary edema, and respiratory failure.

Aspirated substances commonly are grouped according to their physical properties (liquid or solid, large or particulate, acidic or alkalotic, and infectious or noninfectious). The qualities of the aspirated content have direct clinical implications for both morbidity and care requirements.

Signs and symptoms

- Vomitus or particulate matter in the oropharynx
- Bronchospasm
- Chest pain
- Coughing
- Cyanosis
- Dyspnea
- Fever
- Hypotension
- Minimal sputum production
- Crackles or rhonchi
- Tachycardia
- Wheezing over the tests affected area
- Changes in LOC or cognition

Diagnostic tests

- *Chest X-rays* show alveolar and interstitial infiltrates 12 to 24 hours after the aspiration.

▶ *Blood and sputum cultures and gram staining* can identify causative organisms.
▶ *Computed tomography scan* helps to differentiate the infiltrate from the surrounding area.
▶ *Bronchoscopy* may be necessary to collect specimens and identify obstruction
▶ *Arterial blood gas analysis* reveals decreased partial pressure of arterial oxygen; as the patient hyperventilates, partial pressure of arterial carbon dioxide decreases and pH increases. As ventilation becomes compromised, carbon dioxide is retained, causing a decrease in pH.
▶ *Pulse oximetry* may show a reduced level of arterial oxygen saturation.

Treatment

Antimicrobial therapy varies with the causative agent. Therapy should be reevaluated early in the course of treatment. Supportive measures include humidified oxygen therapy for hypoxemia, mechanical ventilation for respiratory failure, a high-calorie diet, adequate fluid intake, bed rest, and analgesics to relieve pleuritic chest pain. Patients who are on mechanical ventilation may require positive end-expiratory pressure to facilitate oxygenation.

Key nursing diagnoses and outcomes

Impaired gas exchange related to decreased availability of lung tissue for gas exchange

Treatment outcome: The patient will exhibit no signs and symptoms of hypoxia, such as a change in level of consciousness, restlessness, or dyspnea.

Risk for infection related to potential for sepsis, lung abscess, and other complications

Treatment outcome: The patient will remain free from signs and symptoms of a secondary infection.

Ineffective airway clearance related to thick sputum production

Treatment outcome: The patient will maintain a patent airway.

Nursing interventions

▶ Promote pulmonary hygiene — including frequent coughing and deep-breathing exercises, incentive spirometry, chest physiotherapy, and gravitational drainage — to mobilize secretions.
▶ Change the patient's position every 2 hours to enhance ventilation and perfusion.
▶ If the disease is unilateral, maintain the healthy lung in a dependent position (which can dramatically increase oxygenation).
▶ Schedule the patient's activities at appropriate intervals to decrease his demands for oxygen.
▶ Assess the patient for signs of pulmonary edema (decreased oxygen saturation, urine output that is less than intake, respiratory distress, increasing edema, crackles, rhonchi, and wheezing).

For patients receiving enteral tube feedings

▶ Keep the head of the patient's bed elevated 30 to 40 degrees.
▶ Check tube placement prior to feeding, and measure residual volume prior to feeding. Stop feeding and notify the physician if the residual volume exceeds 100 ml or is twice the hourly rate of a continuous feeding.
▶ Stop the feeding if the patient becomes nauseous or vomits and when transferring or repositioning the patient.

PATIENT TEACHING

▶ Educate the patient and his family about aspiration pneumonia and its consequences.
▶ If the patient has difficulty swallowing, teach him the "chin-tuck and swallow" technique. Inform the patient and family members that adding thickening agents to liquids helps in swallowing.

Also instruct the patient to avoid multi-textured foods (such as thin soups with pieces of meat or vegetable) because they are more difficult to swallow.

▶ If the patient is receiving enteral feedings, explain the importance of positioning him with his head up at least 30 to 40 degrees.

ASSESSMENT, FUNCTIONAL

A functional assessment is used to evaluate the older adult's overall well-being and self-care abilities. It will help you identify individual needs and care deficits, provide a basis for developing a care plan that enhances the abilities of a patient with coexisting disease and chronic illness, and provide feedback about treatment and rehabilitation. You can use the information to identify and match the patient's needs to such services as housekeeping, home health care, and day care to help the patient maintain independence.

Numerous tools are available to help you perform a methodical functional assessment. Some of the more widely used methods are discussed below.

Assessment tools

Katz Index

The Katz Index of Activities of Daily Living is a widely used tool for evaluating a patient's ability to perform daily personal care activities. This tool ranks the patient's ability to perform six functions: bathing, dressing, toileting, transfer, continence, and feeding. It describes his functional level at a specific point in time and objectively scores his performance on a three-point scale. (See *Katz Index of Activities of Daily Living,* pages 60 and 61.)

Lawton Scale

Another widely used tool is the Lawton Scale for Instrumental Activities of Daily Living. This tool evaluates the patient's ability to perform more complex personal care activities needed to support independent living, such as the ability to use the telephone, shop, do laundry, manage finances, take medications, and prepare meals. Each activity is rated on a three-point scale, ranging from independence, to needing some help, to complete disability. (See *Lawton Scale for Instrumental Activities of Daily Living,* page 62.)

Key point When using the Lawton scale, make sure you evaluate the patient in terms of safety. For example, a person may be able to cook a small meal for himself but may leave the stove burner on after cooking.

Barthel Index

The Barthel Index also helps to assess a patient's capacity for self-care. It evaluates 10 items: feeding, moving from wheelchair to bed and returning, performing personal toilet, getting on and off the toilet, bathing, walking on a level surface or propelling a wheelchair, going up and down stairs, dressing and undressing, maintaining bowel continence, and controlling bladder. Each item is scored according to the degree of assistance needed; over time, results reveal improvement or decline.

OARS Social Resource Scale

The Older Americans Research and Service Center (OARS) Social Resource Scale is a multidimensional assessment tool developed at Duke University in 1978. It evaluates level of function in five areas: social resources, economic resources, physical health, mental health, and activities of daily living. The tool takes about 1 hour to complete and requires training to use it correctly.

Katz Index of Activities of Daily Living

EVALUATION FORM Name James Collins Date March 13, 2002

For each area of functioning listed below, check the description that applies. (The word assistance means supervision, direction, or personal assistance.)

Bathing: Sponge bath, tub bath, or shower.

☑ Receives no assistance (gets into and out of tub by self, if tub is usual means of bathing).	☐ Receives assistance in bathing only one part of the body (such as the back or leg).	○ Receives assistance in bathing more than one part of the body (or not bathed).

Dressing: Gets outer garments and underwear from closets and drawers and uses fasteners, including suspenders, if worn.

☑ Gets clothes and gets completely dressed without assistance.	☐ Gets clothes and gets dressed without assistance except for tying shoes.	○ Receives assistance in getting clothes or in getting dressed, or stays partly or completely undressed.

Toileting: Goes to the room termed "toilet" for bowel movement and urination, cleans self afterward, and arranges clothes.

☑ Goes to toilet room, cleans self, and arranges clothes without assistance. (May use object for support, such as cane, walker, or wheelchair and may manage night bedpan or commode, emptying it in the morning.)	○ Receives assistance in going to toilet room or in cleaning self or arranging clothes after elimination or in use of night bedpan or commode.	○ Doesn't go to the toilet room for the elimination process.

Transfer

☑ Moves into and out of bed and chair without assistance (May use object, such as cane or walker for support.)	○ Moves into or out of bed or chair with assistance.	○ Doesn't get out of bed.

Continence

☐ Controls urination and bowel movement completely by self.	✓○ Has occasional accidents.	○ Supervision helps keep control of urination or bowel movement, or catheter is used, or is incontinent.

Feeding

☑ Feeds self without assistance.	☐ Feeds self except for assistance in cutting meat or buttering bread.	○ Receives assistance in feeding or is fed partly or completely through tubes or by I.V. fluids.

Evaluator: P. Rasteni, RN

☑ Indicates independence ✓○ Indicates dependence

Katz Index of Activities of Daily Living *(continued)*

A: Independent in all six functions.
B: Independent in all but one of these functions.
C: Independent in all but bathing and one additional function.
D: Independent in all but bathing, dressing, and one additional function.
E: Independent in all but bathing, dressing, toileting, and one additional function.
F: Independent in all but bathing, dressing, toileting, transferring, and one additional function.
G: Dependent in all six functions.

Other: Dependent in at least two functions but not classifiable as C, D, E, or F.

Adapted with permission from Katz, S., et al. "Studies of Illness in the Aged: The Index of ADL—A Standardized Measure of Biological and Psychosocial Function," *JAMA* 185:914-19, 1963.

Minimum Data Set

In an attempt to improve the quality of care in extended care facilities, the federal government instituted major reforms through the Omnibus Budget Reconciliation Act (OBRA) of 1981 and its 1987 amendments. A standardized assessment tool called the Minimum Data Set was developed to make assessment more consistent and reliable throughout the country. Its use is required in all extended care facilities that receive federal funding. (See *Minimum Data Set tracking form*, pages 63 to 82.)

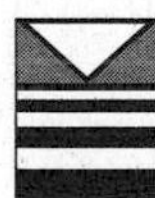

Key point To stress the importance of timely assessment, OBRA established time limits that institutions must follow: The physical portion of the assessment must be completed by a licensed nurse within 24 hours of a patient's admission, and the entire assessment must be completed within 4 days. OBRA also mandates that the total assessment be revised and updated whenever a significant change occurs in a patient's mental or physical condition.

Documentation

Document all assessment findings according to your facility's policy.

ASSESSMENT, PHYSICAL

A comprehensive health assessment of the older person focuses on current health status, including a review of body systems, medical history, diet regimen, and ability to function in the environment. This information establishes the person's baseline health status, allowing you to evaluate any improvement or decline in his condition over time and to determine the need for support services.

Obtaining the health history

The health history and interview, the first phase of the health assessment, provide a subjective account of the older adult's present and past health status. They also initiate your relationship and establish the patient's well-being as your primary concern. The information you obtain from the health history alerts you to key areas of focus for the physical examination. Talking with the older person about health concerns increases his health awareness and helps you identify any knowledge deficits and launch your patient teaching. Because the patient may overlook some important health information, you must interview him methodically and also gather information from family members or friends.

Lawton Scale for Instrumental Activities of Daily Living

Name *Julia Lawson* Rated by *Kathy Mitchell, RN* Date *March 28, 2002*

1. Can you use the telephone?
- without help ③
- with some help 2
- completely unable 1

2. Can you get to places beyond walking distance?
- without help ③
- with some help 2
- not without special arrangements 1

3. Can you go shopping for groceries?
- without help ③
- with some help 2
- completely unable 1

4. Can you prepare your own meals?
- without help ③
- with some help 2
- completely unable 1

5. Can you do your own housework?
- without help 3
- with some help ②
- completely unable 1

6. Can you do your own handyman work?
- without help 3
- with some help ②
- completely unable 1

7. Can you do your own laundry?
- without help ③
- with some help 2
- completely unable 1

8a. Do you take medicines or use any medications?
- Yes ①
(If yes, answer Question 8b.)
- No 2
(If no, answer Question 8c.)

8b. Do you take your own medicine?
- without help (in the right doses at the right times) ③
- with some help (if someone prepares it for you and/or reminds you to take it) 2
- completely unable 1

8c. If you had to take medicine, could you do it?
- without help (in the right doses at the right time) 3
- with some help (if someone prepared it for you and reminded you to take it) 2
- completely unable 1

9. Can you manage your own money?
- without help ③
- with some help 2
- completely unable 1

The Lawton Scale evaluates more sophisticated functions than the activities of daily living index. Patients or caregivers can complete the form in a few minutes. The first answer in each case—except for 8a—indicates independence; the second indicates capability with assistance; and the third, dependence. In this version the maximum score is 29, although scores have meaning only for a particular patient, as when declining scores over time reveal deterioration. Questions 4 to 7 tend to be gender specific; modify them as necessary.

Adapted with permission from Lawton, M.P., and Brody, E.M. "Assessment of Older People: Self-Maintaining and Instrumental Activities of Daily Living," *The Gerontologist* 9(3):179-186, Autumn 1969.

Cultural Diversity Be alert to your patient's cultural background during the interview. Don't confuse cultural differences with abnormal behavior. For example, an Asian patient may not look you in the eye when speaking and may answer "yes" inappropriately to a direct question—either out of deference or a fear of giving offense. Using first names, touching, and other methods useful with most patients may be considered inappropriate by an Asian patient, who may react negatively or not respond at all. Before drawing conclusions, try to evaluate the

(Text continues on page 83.)

Minimum Data Set tracking form

Numeric identifier ____________

MINIMUM DATA SET (MDS) — VERSION 2.0
FOR NURSING HOME RESIDENT ASSESSMENT AND CARE SCREENING
BASIC ASSESSMENT TRACKING FORM

SECTION AA. IDENTIFICATION INFORMATION

1.	RESIDENT NAME⊙	Amy / J. / Gaston a. (First) b. (Middle Initial) c. (Last) d. (Jr/Sr)	
2.	GENDER⊙	1. Male 2. Female	2
3.	BIRTHDATE⊙	1 2 — 3 0 — 1 9 3 2 Month Day Year	
4.	RACE/ ETHNICITY⊙	1. American Indian/Alaskan native 2. Asian/Pacific Islander 3. Black, not of Hispanic origin 4. Hispanic 5. White, not of Hispanic origin	5
5.	SOCIAL SECURITY⊙ AND MEDICARE NUMBERS⊙ (C in first box if non med. no.)	a. Social Security Number 0 4 1 — 2 4 — 0 0 0 0 b. Medicare number (or comparable railroad insurance number) ☐☐☐☐☐☐☐☐☐☐☐☐	
6.	FACILITY PROVIDER NUMBER⊙	a. State No. ☐☐☐☐☐☐☐☐☐☐☐☐☐☐☐ b. Federal No. ☐☐☐☐☐☐☐☐☐☐☐☐	
7.	MEDICAID NO. ["+" if pending, "N" if not a Medicaid recipient] ⊙	N ☐☐☐☐☐☐☐☐☐☐☐☐☐	
8.	REASONS FOR ASSESSMENT	(Note—Other codes do not apply to this form) **a. Primary reason for assessment** 1. Admission assessment (required by day 14) 2. Annual assessment 3. Significant change in status assessment 4. Significant correction in status assessment 5. Quarterly 10. Significant correction of prior quarterly assessment 0. NONE OF THE ABOVE ***b. Codes for assessments required by Medicare PPS or the State*** 1. Medicare 5 day assessment 2. Medicare 30 day assessment 3. Medicare 60 day assessment 4. Medicare 90 day assessment 5. Medicare readmission/return 6. Other state required assessment 7. Medicare 14 day assessment 8. Other Medicare required assessment	a. 1 b.

⊙= Key items for computerized resident tracking
☐ = When box blank, must enter number or letter
☐a. = When letter in box, check if condition applies

GENERAL INSTRUCTIONS
Complete this information for submission with all full and quarterly assessments (Admissions, Annual, Significant Change, State or Medicare required assessments, or Quarterly Reviews, etc.)

(continued)

Minimum Data Set tracking form *(continued)*

9.	Signature of Persons who Completed a Portion of the Accompanying Assessment or Tracking Form

I certify that the accompanying information accurately reflects resident assessment or tracking information for this resident and that I collected or coordinated collection of this information on the dates specified. To the best of my knowledge, this information was collected in accordance with applicable Medicare and Medicaid requirements. I understand that this information is used as a basis for ensuring that residents receive appropriate and quality care, and as a basis for payment from federal funds. I further understand that payment of such federal funds and continued participation in the government-funded health care programs is conditioned on the accuracy and truthfulness of this information, and that I may be personally subject to or may subject my organization to substantial criminal, civil, and/or administrative penalties for submitting fake information. I also certify that I am authorized to submit this information by this facility on its behalf.

Signature and Title	Sections	Date
a. Christine Gaslo, RN, MSN	AT	4/2/02
b.		
c. James Shaw, RN, BSN	AA	4/2/02
d.		
e.		
f.		
g.		
h.		
i.		
j.		
k.		
l.		

Minimum Data Set tracking form *(continued)*

MINIMUM DATA SET (MDS) — VERSION 2.0
FOR NURSING HOME RESIDENT ASSESSMENT AND CARE SCREENING
BACKGROUND (FACE SHEET) INFORMATION AT ADMISSION

SECTION AB. DEMOGRAPHIC INFORMATION

1.	DATE OF ENTRY	Date the stay began: Note — Does not include readmission if record was closed at time of temporary discharge in hospital, etc, in such cases, use prior admission date 0 4 — 0 1 — 2 0 0 2 Month Day Year	
2.	ADMITTED FROM (AT ENTRY)	1. Private home/apt. with no home health services 2. Private home/apt. with home health services 3. Board and care/assisted living/group home 4. Nursing home 5. Acute care hospital 6. Psychiatric hospital, MR/DD facility 7. Rehabilitation hospital 8. Other	1
3.	LIVED ALONE (PRIOR TO ENTRY)	0. No 1. Yes 2. In other facility	0
4.	ZIP CODE OF PRIOR PRIMARY RESIDENCE	1 4 0 0 0	
5.	RESIDENTIAL HISTORY 5 YEARS PRIOR TO ENTRY	(Check all settings resident lived in during 5 years prior to date of entry given in item AB1 above) Prior stay at the nursing home Stay in other nursing home Other residential facility — board and care home, assisted living, group home MH/psychiatric setting MR/DD setting NONE OF THE ABOVE.	a. b. c. d. e. f. ✓
6.	LIFETIME OCCUPATION(S) (Put "/" between two occupations)	T E A C H E R	
7.	EDUCATION (Highest Level Completed)	1. No schooling 2. 8th grade/less 3. 9-11 grades 4. High school 5. Technical or trade school 6. Some college 7. Bachelor's degree 8. Graduate degree	8
8.	LANGUAGE	(Code for correct response) a. Primary Language 0. English 1. Spanish 2. French 3. Other b. If other, specify	0
9.	MENTAL HEALTH HISTORY	Does resident's RECORD indicate any history of mental retardation, mental illness, or developmental disability problem? 0. No 1. Yes	0
10.	CONDITIONS RELATED TO MR/DD STATUS	(Check all conditions that are related to MR/DD status that were manifested before age 22, and are likely to continue indefinitely) Not applicable — no MR/DD (Skip to AB11) MR/DD with organic condition Down's syndrome Autism Epilepsy Other organic condition related to MR/DD MR/DD with no organic condition	a. ✓ b. c. d. e. f.
11.	DATE BACKGROUND INFORMATION COMPLETED	0 4 — 0 3 — 2 0 0 2 Month Day Year	

(continued)

Minimum Data Set tracking form *(continued)*

SECTION AC. CUSTOMARY ROUTINE

1.	CUSTOMARY ROUTINE (In year prior to DATE OF ENTRY to this nursing home, or year last in community if now being admitted from another nursing home)	(Check all that apply. If all information UNKNOWN, check last box only.)	
		CYCLE OF DAILY EVENTS	
		Stays up late at night (e.g. after 9 pm)	a.
		Naps regularly during day (at least 1 hour)	b. ✓
		Goes out 1+ days a week	c.
		Stays busy with hobbies, reading, or fixed daily routine	d. ✓
		Spends most of time alone or watching TV	e.
		Moves independently indoors (with appliances, if used)	f.
		Use of tobacco products at least daily	g.
		NONE OF THE ABOVE	h.
		EATING PATTERNS	
		Distinct food preferences	i.
		Eats between meals all or most days	j. ✓
		Use of alcoholic beverage(s) at least weekly	k.
		NONE OF ABOVE	l.
		ADL PATTERNS	
		In bedclothes most much of day	m.
		Wakens to toilet all or most nights	n. ✓
		Has irregular bowel movement pattern	o.
		Showers for bathing	p.
		Bathing in PM	q. ✓
		NONE OF THE ABOVE	r.
		INVOLVEMENT PATTERNS	
		Daily contact with relatives/close friends	s. ✓
		Usually attends church, temple, synagogue (etc.)	t.
		Finds strength in faith	u. ✓
		Daily animal companion/presence	v.
		Involved in group activities	w.
		NONE OF THE ABOVE	x.
		UNKNOWN — Resident/family unable to provide information	y.

SECTION AD. FACE SHEET SIGNATURES

SIGNATURES OF PERSONS COMPLETING FACE SHEET

James Shaw, RN, BSN

Christine Gaslo, RN, MSN 04/03/02

I certify that the accompanying information accurately reflects resident assessment or tracking information for this resident and that I collected or coordinated collection of this information on the dates specified. To the best of my knowledge, this information was collected in accordance with applicable Medicare and Medicaid requirements. I understand that this information is used as a basis for ensuring that residents receive appropriate and quality care, and as a basis for payment from federal funds. I further understand that payment of such federal funds and continued participation in the government-funded health care programs is conditioned on the accuracy and truthfulness of this information, and that I may be personally subject to or may subject my organization to substantial criminal, civil, and/or administrative penalties for submitting fake information. I also certify that I am authorized to submit this information by this facility on its behalf.

Signature and Title	Sections	Date
a. *Christine Gaslo, RN, MSN*	A-T	4/03/02
b.		
c.		
d.		
e.		
f.		
g.		

Minimum Data Set tracking form *(continued)*

MINIMUM DATA SET (MDS) — VERSION 2.0
FOR NURSING HOME RESIDENT ASSESSMENT AND CARE SCREENING

FULL ASSESSMENT FORM

(Status in last 7 days, unless other time frame indicated)

SECTION A. IDENTIFICATION INFORMATION

1.	RESIDENT NAME	Amy / J. / Gaston a. (First) b. (Middle Initial) c. (Last) d. (Jr/Sr)	
2.	ROOM NUMBER	4 0 2	
3.	ASSESSMENT REFERENCE DATE	a. Last day of MDS observation period 0 4 — 0 3 — 2 0 0 2 Month Day Year b. Original (0) or corrected copy of form (enter number of correction)	
4a.	DATE OF REENTRY	Date of reentry from most recent temporary discharge to a hospital in last 90 days (or since last assessment or admission if less than 90 days) __ __ — __ __ — __ __ __ __ Month Day Year	
5	MARITAL STATUS	1. Never married 3. Widowed 5. Divorced 2. Married 4. Separated	3
6.	MEDICAL RECORD NO.	M M 0 0 0 9 9 2 2 6 8 1	
7.	CURRENT PAYMENT SOURCES FOR N.H. STAY	(Billing Office to indicate; check all that apply in last 30 days) Medicaid per diem a. ☐ VA per diem f. ☐ Medicare per diem b. ☒ Self or family pays for full per diem g. ☒ Medicare ancillary part A c. ☐ Medicaid resident liability or Medicare co-payment h. ☐ Medicare ancillary part B d. ☐ Provide insurance per diem (including co-payment) i. ☐ CHAMPUS per diem e. ☐ Other per diem j. ☐	
8.	REASONS FOR ASSESSMENT (Note: If this is a discharge or reentry assessment, only a limited subset of MDS items must be completed)	a. Primary reason for assessment 1. Admission assessment (required by day 14) 2. Annual assessment 3. Significant change in status assessment 4. Significant correction of prior full assessment 5. Quarterly review assessment 6. Discharged—return not anticipated 7. Discharged—return anticipated 8. Discharged prior to completing initial assessment 0. NONE OF THE ABOVE b. Codes for assessments required for Medicare PPS or the State 1. Medicare 5 day assessment 2. Medicare 30 day assessment 3. Medicare 60 day assessment 4. Medicare 90 day assessment 5. Medicare readmission/return assessment 6. Other state required assistance 7. Medicare 14 day assessment 8. Other Medicare required assessment	1
9.	RESPONSIBILITY/ LEGAL GUARDIAN	(Check all that apply) Legal guardian a. ☐ Durable power attorney/financial d. ☐ Other legal oversight b. ☐ Family member responsible e. ☐ Durable power of attorney/health care c. ☒ Patient responsible for self f. ☐ NONE OF THE ABOVE g. ☐	
10.	ADVANCED DIRECTIVES	(For those items with supporting documentation in the medical record, check all that apply) Living will a. ☒ Feeding restrictions f. ☐ Do not resuscitate b. ☐ Medication restrictions g. ☐ Do not hospitalize c. ☐ Other treatment restrictions h. ☐ Organ donation d. ☐ NONE OF THE ABOVE i. ☐ Autopsy request e. ☐	

(continued)

Minimum Data Set tracking form *(continued)*

SECTION B: COGNITIVE PATTERNS

1.	COMATOSE	(Persistent vegetative state/no discernible consciousness) 0. No 1. Yes (If yes, skip to section G)	0
2.	MEMORY	(Recall of what was learned or known) a. Short-term memory OK—seems/appears to recall after 5 minutes 0. Memory OK 1. Memory problem	1
		b. Long-term memory OK—seems/appears to recall long past 0. Memory OK 1. Memory problem	1
3.	MEMORY/ RECALL ABILITY	(Check all that resident was normally able to recall during last 7 days) Current season a. Location of own room b. That he/she is in a nursing home d. Staff names/faces c. NONE OF THE ABOVE are recalled e.	e. X
4.	COGNITIVE SKILLS FOR DAILY DECISION-MAKING	(Made decisions regarding tasks of daily life) 0. INDEPENDENT—decisions consistent/reasonable 1. MODIFIED INDEPENDENCE—some difficulty in new situations only 2. MODERATELY IMPAIRED—decisions poor, cues/supervision required 3. SEVERELY IMPAIRED—never/rarely made decisions	2
5.	INDICATORS OF DELIRIUM—PERIODIC DISOR-DERED THINKING/ AWARENESS	(Code for behavior in the last 7 days.) [Note: Accurate assessment requires conversations with staff and family who have direct knowledge of the resident's behavior over this time]. 0. Behavior not present 1. Behavior present, not of recent onset 2. Behavior present, over last 7 days appears different from resident's usual functioning (e.g., new onset or worsening)	
		a. EASILY DISTRACTED—(e.g., difficulty paying attention; gets sidetracked)	1
		b. PERIODS OF ALTERED PERCEPTION OR AWARENESS OF SURROUNDINGS—(e.g., moves lips or talks to someone not present, believes he/she is somewhere else; confuses night and day)	0
		c. EPISODES OF DISORGANIZED SPEECH—(e.g., speech is incoherent, nonsensical, irrelevant, or rambling from subject to subject; loses train of thought)	0
		d. PERIODS OF RESTLESSNESS—(e.g., fidgeting or picking at skin, clothing, napkins, etc; frequent position changes; repetitive physical movements or calling out)	0
		e. PERIODS OF LETHARGY—(e.g., sluggishness; staring into space; difficult to arouse; little body movement)	0
		f. MENTAL FUNCTION VARIES OVER THE COURSE OF THE DAY—(e.g., sometimes better, sometimes worse; behaviors sometimes present, sometimes not)	0
6.	CHANGE IN COGNITIVE STATUS	Resident's cognitive status, skills, or abilities have changes as compared to status of 90 days ago (or since last assessment if less than 90 days) 0. No change 1. Improved 2. Deteriorated	0

Minimum Data Set tracking form *(continued)*

SECTION C: COMMUNICATION/HEARING PATTERNS

No.	Item	Description	Code
1.	HEARING	(With hearing appliance, if used) 0. HEARS ADEQUATELY—normal talk, TV, phone 1. MINIMAL DIFFICULTY when not in quiet setting 2. HEARS IN SPECIAL SITUATIONS ONLY—speaker has to adjust tonal quality and speak distinctly 3. HIGHLY IMPAIRED absence of useful hearing	1
2.	COMMUNICATION DEVICES/ TECHNIQUES	(Check all that apply during last 7 days) Hearing aid, present and used Hearing aid, present and not used regularly Other receptive comm. techniques used (e.g., lip reading) NONE OF THE ABOVE	a. b. c. d. X
3.	MODES OF EXPRESSION	(Check all used by resident to make needs known) Speech a. X Writing messages to express or clarify needs b. American sign language or Braille c. Signs/gestures/sounds d. Communication board e. Other f. NONE OF THE ABOVE g.	
4.	MAKING SELF UNDER-STOOD	(Expressing information content—however able) 0. UNDERSTOOD 1. USUALLY UNDERSTOOD—difficulty finding words or finishing thoughts 2. SOMETIMES UNDERSTOOD—ability is limited to making concrete requests 3. RARELY/NEVER UNDERSTOOD	1
5.	SPEECH CLARITY	(Code for speech in the last 7 days) 0. CLEAR SPEECH—distinct, intelligible words 1. UNCLEAR SPEECH—slurred, mumbled words 2. NO SPEECH—absence of spoken words	0
6.	ABILITY TO UNDER-STAND OTHERS	(Understanding verbal information content—however able) 0. UNDERSTANDS 1. USUALLY UNDERSTANDS—may miss some part/intent of message 2. SOMETIMES UNDERSTANDS—responds adequately to simple, direct communication 3. RARELY/NEVER UNDERSTANDS	2
7.	CHANGE IN COMMUNI-CATION/ HEARING	Resident's ability to express, understand, or hear information has changed as compared to status of 90 days ago (or since last assessment if less than 90 days) 0. No change 1. Improved 2. Deteriorated	0

SECTION D: VISION PATTERNS

No.	Item	Description	Code
8.	VISION	(Ability to see in adequate light and with glasses if used) 0. ADEQUATE—sees dine detail, including regular print in newspapers/books 1. IMPAIRED—sees large print, but not regular print in newspapers/books 2. MODERATELY IMPAIRED—limited vision; not able to nee newspaper headlines, but can identify objects 3. HIGHLY IMPAIRED—object identification in question, but eyes appear to follow objects 4. SEVERELY IMPAIRED—no visions or sees only light, colors, or shapes; eyes do not appear to follow objects	0
9.	VISUAL LIMITATIONS/ DIFFICULTIES	Side vision problems—decreased peripheral vision (e.g., leaves food on one side of tray, difficulty traveling, bumps into people and objects, misjudges placement of chair when seating self) Experiences any of following: sees halos or rings around lights; sees flashes of light; sees "curtains" over eyes NONE OF THE ABOVE	 X
10.	VISUAL APPLIANCES	Glasses; contact lenses; magnifying glass 0. No 1. Yes	1

(continued)

Minimum Data Set tracking form *(continued)*

SECTION E: MOOD AND BEHAVIOR PATTERNS

1.	INDICATORS OF DEPRES-SION, ANXIETY, SAD MOOD	(Code for indicators observed in last 30 days, irrespective of the assumed cause) 0. Indicator not exhibited in last 30 days 1. Indicator of this type exhibited up to five days a week 2. Indicator of this type exhibited daily or almost daily (6, 7 days a week)	
		Verbal expressions of distress	
		a. Resident made negative statements—e.g., "Nothing matters; Would rather be dead; What's the use; Regrets having lived so long; Let me die"	0
		b. Repetitive questions—e.g., "Where do I go; What do I do?"	0
		c. Repetitive verbalizations—e.g., calling out for help, (God help me")	0
		d. Persistent anger with self or others—e.g., easily annoyed, anger at placement in nursing home; anger at care received	0
		e. Self deprecation—e.g., "I am nothing; I am of no use to anyone"	0
		f. Expressions of what appear to be unrealistic fears—e.g., fear of being abandoned, left alone, being with others	0
		g. Recurrent statements that something terrible is about to happen—e.g., believes he or she is about to die, have a heart attack	0
		h. Repetitive health complaints—e.g., persistently seeks medical attention, obsessive concern with body functions	0
		i. Repetitive anxious complaints/concerns (non-health related) e.g., persistently seeks attention/reassurance regarding schedules, meals, laundry, clothing, relationship issues.	0
		SLEEP CYCLE ISSUES	
		j. Unpleasant mood in the morning	0
		k. Insomnia/change in usual sleep pattern	0
		SAD, APATHETIC, ANXIOUS APPEARANCE	
		l. Sad, pained, worried facial expressions—e.g., furrowed brows	0
		m. Crying, tearfulness	0
		n. Repetitive physical movements—e.g., pacing, hand wringing, restlessness, fidgeting, picking	0
		LOSS OF INTEREST	
		o. Withdrawal from activities of interest—e.g., no interest in long standing activities or being with family/friends	0
		p. Reduced social interaction	0
2.	MOOD PERSIS-TENCE	One or more indicators of depressed, sad or anxious mood were not easily altered by attempts to "cheer up," console, or reassure the resident over last 7 days 0. No mood indicators 1. Indicators present, easily altered 2. Indicators present, not easily altered	0
3.	CHANGE IN MOOD	Resident's mood status has changed as compared to status 90 days ago (or since last assessment if less than 90 days) 0. No change 1. Improved 2. Deteriorated	0

			(A)	(B)
4.	BEHAVIORAL SYMPTOMS	(A) Behavioral symptom frequency in last 7 days 0. Behavior not exhibited in last 7 days 1. Behavior of this type occurred 1 to 3 days in last 7 days 2. Behavior of this type occurred 4 to 6 days, but less than daily 3. Behavior of this type occurred daily (B) Behavioral symptom alterability in last 7 days 0. Behavior not present OR behavior was easily altered 1. Behavior was no easily altered		
		a. WANDERING (moved with no rational purpose, seemingly oblivious to needs or safety	0	0
		b. VERBALLY ABUSIVE BEHAVIORAL SYMPTOMS (others were threatened, screamed at, cursed at)	0	0
		c. PHYSICALLY ABUSIVE BEHAVIORAL SYMPTOMS (others were hit, shoved, scratched, sexually abused)	0	0
		d. SOCIALLY INAPPROPRIATE/DISRUPTIVE BEHAVIORAL SYMPTOMS (made disruptive sounds, noisiness, screaming, self-abusive acts, sexual behavior or disrobing in public, smeared/threw food/feces, hoarding, rummaged through others' belongings	0	0
		e. RESISTS CARE (resisted taking medications/injections, ADL assistance or eating)	0	0
5.	CHANGE IN BEHAVIORAL SYMPTOMS	Resident's behavior status has changed as compared to status of 90 days ago (or since last assessment if less than 90 days) 0. No change 1. Improved 2. Deteriorated		0

Minimum Data Set tracking form *(continued)*

SECTION F: PSYCHOSOCIAL WELL-BEING

1.	SENSE OF INITIATIVE/ INVOLVE-MENT	At ease interacting with others	a. X
		At ease doing planned or structured activities	b.
		At ease doing self-initiated activities	c.
		Establishes own goals	d.
		Pursues involvement in life of facility (e.g. makes/keeps friends; involved in group activities; responds positively to new activities; assists at religious services)	e.
		Accepts invitations into most group activities	f. X
		NONE OF ABOVE	g.
2.	UNSETTLED RELATION-SHIPS	Covert/open conflict with or repeated criticism of self	a.
		Unhappy with roommate	b.
		Unhappy with residents other than roommate	c.
		Openly expresses anger with family/friends	d. X
		Absence of personal contact with family/friends	e.
		Recent loss of close family member/friend	f.
		Does not adjust easily to change in routines	g.
		NONE OF ABOVE	h.
3.	PAST ROLES	Strong identification with past roles and life status	a.
		Expresses sadness/anger/empty feeling over lost role/status	b. X
		Resident perceives that daily routine (customary routine, activities) is very different from prior pattern in the community	c.
		NONE OF ABOVE	d.

SECTION G: PHYSICAL FUNCTIONING AND STRUCTURAL PROBLEMS

1. (A) ADL SELF-PERFORMANCE — (Code for resident's PERFORMANCE OVER ALL SHIFTS during last 7 days — Not including setup)

0. INDEPENDENT — No help or oversight — OR — Help/oversight provided only 1 or 2 times during last 7 days
1. SUPERVISION — Oversight, encouragement or cueing provided 3 or more times during last 7 days — OR — Supervision (3 or more times) plus physical assistance provided only 1 or 2 times during last 7 days
2. LIMITED ASSISTANCE — Resident highly involved in activity; received physical help in guided maneuvering of limbs or other nonweight bearing assistance 3 or more times — OR — More help provided only 1 or 2 times during last 7 days
3. EXTENSIVE ASSISTANCE — While resident performed part of activity, over last 7-day period, help of following type(s) provided 3 or more times:
   — Weight-bearing support
   — Full staff performance during part (but not all) of last 7 days
4. TOTAL DEPENDENCE — Full staff performance of activity during entire 7 days
5. ACTIVITY DID NOT OCCUR during entire 7 days

(B) ADL SUPPORT PROVIDED — (Code for MOST SUPPORT PROVIDED OVER ALL SHIFTS during last 7 days; code regardless of resident's self-performance classification)

0. No setup of physical help from staff
1. Setup help only
2. One person physical assist
3. Two+ persons physical assist
8. ADL activity itself did not occur during entire 7 days

			(A) SELF-PERF	(B) SUPPORT
a.	BED MOBILITY	How resident moves to and from lying position, turns side to side, and positions body while in bed	3	3
b.	TRANSFER	How resident moves between surfaces — to/from: bed, chair, wheelchair, standing position (EXCLUDE to/from bath/toilet)	4	3
c.	WALK IN ROOM	How resident walks between locations in his/her room	4	2
d.	WALK IN CORRIDOR	How resident walks in corridor on unit	4	3
e.	LOCOMO-TION ON UNIT	How resident moves between locations in his/her room and adjacent corridor on same floor. If in wheelchair, self-sufficiency once in chair	4	2
f.	LOCOMO-TION OFF UNIT	How resident moves to and returns from off unit location (e.g. areas set aside for dining, activities, or treatments). If facility has only one floor, how resident moves to and from distant areas on the floor. If in wheelchair, self-sufficiency once in chair.	4	2

(continued)

Minimum Data Set tracking form *(continued)*

SECTION G: PHYSICAL FUNCTIONING AND STRUCTURAL PROBLEMS *(continued)*

			(A)	(B)
g.	DRESSING	How resident puts on, fastens, and takes off all items of street clothing, including donning/removing prosthesis	4	3
h.	EATING	How resident eats and drinks (regardless of skill). Includes intake of nourishment by other means (e.g., tube feeding, total parenteral nutrition)	2	2
i.	TOILET USE	How resident uses the toilet room (or commode, bedpan, urinal); transfer on/off toilet, cleanses, changes pad, manages ostomy or catheter, adjusts clothes	4	3
j.	PERSONAL HYGIENE	How resident maintains personal hygiene, including combing hair, brushing teeth, shaving, applying makeup, washing/drying face, hands, and perineum (EXCLUDE baths and showers)	4	2
2.	BATHING	How resident takes full-body bath/shower, sponge bath, and transfers in/out of tub/shower (EXCLUDE washing of back and hair.) Code for most dependent in self-performance and support. (A) BATHING SELF-PERFORMANCE codes appear below 0.Independent—No help provided 1.Supervision—Oversight help only 2.Physical help limited to transfer only 3.Physical help in part of bathing activity 4.Total dependence 8.Activity itself did not occur during entire 7 days (Bathing support codes are as defined in Item 1, code B above)	4	3
3.	TEST FOR BALANCE (see training manual)	(Code for ability during the last 7 days) 0.Maintained position as required in test 1.Unsteady, but able to rebalance self without physical support 2.Partial physical support during test 3.Not able to attempt test without physical help		
		a. Balance while standing		3
		b. Balance while sitting—position, trunk control		2
4.	FUNCTIONAL LIMITATION IN RANGE OF MOTION (see training manual)	(Code for limitations during last 7 days that interfered with daily functions or placed resident at risk of injury) (A) RANGE OF MOTION: 0.No limitation; 1.Limitation on one side; 2Limitation on both sides (B) VOLUNTARY MOVEMENT: 0.No loss; 1.Partial loss; 2.Full loss	(A)	(B)
		a. Neck	1	1
		b. Arm—including shoulder or elbow	1	1
		c. Hand—including wrist or fingers	1	1
		d. Leg—including hip or knee	1	1
		e. Foot—including ankle or toes	1	1
		f. Other limitation or loss	0	0
5.	MODES OF LOCOMOTION	(Check all that apply during last 7 days) Cane/walker/crutch — a. Wheeled self — b. Other person wheeled — c. Wheelchair primary mode of locomotion — d. X NONE OF THE ABOVE — e.		
6.	MODES OF TRANSFER	(Check all that apply during last 7 days) Bedfast all or most of the time — a. X Bed rails used for bed mobility or transfer — b. Lifted manually — c. Limited mechanically — d. Transfer aid (e.g., side board, trapeze, cane, walker, brace) — e. NONE OF THE ABOVE — f.		

Minimum Data Set tracking form *(continued)*

SECTION G: PHYSICAL FUNCTIONING AND STRUCTURAL PROBLEMS *(continued)*

7.	TASK SEGMENTATION	Some or all of ADL activities were broken into subtasks during last 7 days so that resident could perform them. 0. No 1. Yes	0
8.	ADL FUNCTIONAL REHABILITATION POTENTIAL	Resident believes he/she is capable of increased independence in at least some ADLs	
		Direct care staff believe resident is capable of increased independence in at least some ADLs	
		Resident able to perform tasks/activity but is very slow	
		Difference in ADL Self-Performance or ADL Support, comparing mornings to evening	
		NONE OF THE ABOVE	0
9.	CHANGE IN ADL FUNCTION	Resident's ADL self-performance status has changed as compared to status of 90 days ago (or since last assessment if less than 90 days) 0. No change 1. Improved 2. Deteriorated	0

SECTION H: CONTINENCE IN LAST 14 DAYS

1.	CONTINENCE SELF-CONTROL CATEGORIES (Code for resident's PERFORMANCE OVER ALL SHIFTS) 0. CONTINENT— Complete control [Includes use of indwelling urinary catheter or ostomy device that does not leak urine or stool] 1. USUALLY CONTINENT— BLADDER, incontinent episodes once a week or less; BOWEL, less than weekly 2. OCCASIONALLY INCONTINENT—BLADDER, 2 or more times a week but nor daily; BOWEL, once a week 3. FREQUENTLY INCONTINENT—BLADDER, tended to be incontinent daily, but some control present (e.g., on day shift); BOWEL, 2-3 times a week. 4. INCONTINENT— Had inadequate control BLADDER, multiple daily episodes; BOWEL, all (or almost all) of the time				
a.	BOWEL CONTINENCE	Control of bowel movement, with appliance or bowel continence programs, if employed			2
b.	BLADDER CONTINENCE	Control of urinary bladder function (if dribbles, volume insufficient to soak through underpants), with appliances (e.g., foley) or continence programs, if employed			2
2.	BOWEL ELIMINATION PATTERN	Bowel elimination pattern regular—at least one movement every three days	a. X	Diarrhea	c.
		Constipation	b.	Fecal impaction	d.
				NONE OF THE ABOVE	e.
3.	APPLIANCES AND PROGRAMS	Any scheduled toileting plan	a.	Did not use toilet room/commode/urinal	f.
		Bladder retraining program	b.	Pads/briefs used	g. X
		External (condom) catheter	c.	Enemas/irrigation	h.
		Indwelling catheter	d.	Ostomy present	i.
		Intermittent catheter	e.	NONE OF THE ABOVE	j.
4.	CHANGE IN URINARY CONTINENCE	Resident's urinary continence has changed as compared to status of 90 days ago (or since last assessment if less than 90 days) 0. No change 1. Improved 2. Deteriorated			0

(continued)

Minimum Data Set tracking form *(continued)*

SECTION I: DISEASE AND DIAGNOSES

Check only those diseases that have a relationship to current ADL status, cognitive status, mood and behavior status, medical treatments, nursing monitoring, or risk of death. (Do not list inactive diagnoses)

1. DISEASES (If none apply, CHECK the NONE OF ABOVE box)

Disease	Box	Disease	Box
ENDOCRINE/METABOLIC/ NUTRITIONAL		Hemiplegia/Hemiparesis	v.
		Multiple sclerosis	w.
Diabetes mellitus	a.	Paraplegia	x.
Hyperthyroidism	b.	Parkinson's disease	y.
Hypothyroidism	c. X	Quadriplegia	z.
HEART/CIRCULATION		Seizure disorder	aa.
Arteriosclerotic heart disease (ASHD)	d.	Transient ischemic attack (TIA)	bb.
		Traumatic brain injury	cc.
Cardiac dysrhythmias	e.	PSYCHIATRIC/MOOD	
Congestive heart failure	f.	Anxiety disorder	dd.
Deep vein thrombosis	g.	Depression	ee.
Hypertension	h.	Manic depression (bipolar disease)	ff.
Hypotension	i.		
Peripheral vascular disease	j. X	Schizophrenia	gg.
Other cardiovascular disease	k.	PULMONARY	
MUSCULOSKELETAL		Asthma	hh.
Arthritis	l.	Emphysema/COPD	ii.
Hip fracture	m.	SENSORY	
Missing limb (e.g., amputation)	n.	Cataracts	jj.
Osteoporosis	o.	Diabetic retinopathy	kk.
Pathological bone fracture	p.	Glaucoma	ll.
NEUROLOGICAL		Macular degeneration	mm.
Alzheimer's disease	q.	OTHER	
Aphasia	r.	Allergies	nn.
Cerebral palsy	s.	Anemia	oo.
Cerebrovascular accident (stroke)	t.	Cancer	pp.
		Renal failure	qq.
Dementia other than Alzheimer's disease	u. X	NONE OF ABOVE	rr.

2. INFECTIONS (If none apply, CHECK the NONE OF ABOVE box)

Infection	Box	Infection	Box
Antibiotic resistant infection (e.g., Methicillin resistant staph)	a.	Septicemia	g.
		Sexually transmitted diseases	h.
Clostridium difficile (c. diff.)	b.	Tuberculosis	i.
Conjunctivitis	c. X	Urinary tract infection in last 30 days	j.
HIV infection	d.	Viral hepatitis	k.
Pneumonia	e.	Wound infection	l.
Respiratory infection	f.	NONE OF THE ABOVE	m.

3. OTHER CURRENT OR MORE DETAILED DIAGNOSES AND ICD-9 CODES

	Diagnosis	ICD-9 code
a.	*Hypertension*	402.11
b.		
c.		
d.		
e.		

Minimum Data Set tracking form *(continued)*

SECTION J: HEALTH CONDITIONS

1.	PROBLEM CONDITIONS	(Check all problems present in last 7 days unless other time frame is indicated) INDICATIONS OF FLUID STATUS Weight gain or loss of 3 or more pounds within a 7 day period Inability to lie flat due to shortness of breath Dehydrated; output exceeds input Insufficient fluid; did NOT consume all/almost all liquids provided during last 3 days OTHER Delusions	a. b. c. d. e.	Dizziness/Vertigo Edema Fever Hallucinations Internal bleeding Recurrent lung aspirations in last 90 days Shortness of breath Syncope (fainting) Unsteady gait Vomiting NONE OF ABOVE	f. g. h. i. j. k. l. m. n. o. p. X
2.	PAIN SYMPTOMS	(Code the highest level of pain present in the last 7 days) a. FREQUENCY with which resident complains or shows evidence of pain 0. No pain (skip to J4) 1. Pain less than daily 2. Pain daily	2	b. INTENSITY of pain 1. Mild pain 2. Moderate pain 3. Times when pain is horrible or excruciating	
3.	PAIN SITE	(If pain present, check all sites that apply in last 7 days) Back pain Bone pain Chest pain while doing usual activities Headache Hip pain	a. X b. c. d. e. X	Incisional pain Joint pain (other than hip) Soft tissue pain (e.g., lesion, muscle) Stomach pain Other	f. g. h. i. j.
4.	ACCIDENTS	(Check all that apply) Fell in past 30 days Fell in past 31-180 days	a. b.	Hip fracture in last 180 days Other fracture in last 180 days NONE OF ABOVE	c. d. e. X
5.	STABILITY OF CONDITIONS	Conditions/diseases make resident's cognitive, ADL, mood or behavior patterns unstable—(fluctuating, precarious, or deteriorating) Resident experiencing an acute episode or a flare-up of a recurrent or chronic problem End-stage disease, 6 or fewer months to live NONE OF ABOVE			a. b. c. d. X

(continued)

Minimum Data Set tracking form *(continued)*

SECTION K: ORAL/NUTRITIONAL STATUS

1.	ORAL PROBLEMS	Chewing problem	a.
		Swallowing problem	b.
		Mouth pain	c.
		NONE OF ABOVE	d. X
2.	HEIGHT AND WEIGHT	Record (a.) height in inches and (b.) weight in pounds. Base weight on most recent measure in last 30 days; measure weight consistently in accord with standard facility practice—e.g., in a.m. after voiding, before meal, with shoes off, and in nightclothes a. HT 9 (in.) 7 0 b. WT 9 (lb.) 1 8 0	
3.	WEIGHT CHANGE	a. Weight loss—5% or more in last 30 days; or 10% or more in last 180 days 0. No 1. Yes	0
		b. Weight gain—5% or more in last 30 days; or 10% or more in last 180 days 0. No 1. Yes	0
4.	NUTRITIONAL PROBLEMS	Complains about the taste of many foods	a.
		Regular or repetitive complaints of hunger	b.
		Leaves 25% or more of food uneaten at most meals	c.
		NONE OF THE ABOVE	d. X
5.	NUTRITIONAL APPROACHES	(Check all that apply in last 7 days)	
		Parenteral/IV	a.
		Feeding tube	b.
		Mechanically altered diet	c.
		Syringe (oral feeding)	d.
		Therapeutic diet	e. X
		Dietary supplement between meals	f.
		Plate guard, stabilized built-up utensil, etc.	g.
		On a planned weight change program	h.
		NONE OF ABOVE	i.
6.	PARENTERAL OR ENTERAL CARE	(Skip to Section L if neither 5a nor 5b is checked) a. Code the proportion of total calories the resident received through parenteral or tube feedings in the last 7 days 0. None 3. 51% to 75% 1. 1% to 25% 4. 76% to 100% 2. 26% to 50%	0
		b. Code the average fluid intake per day by IV or tube in last 7 days 0. None 3. 1001 to 1500 cc/day 1. 1 to 500 cc/day 4. 1501 to 2000 cc/day 2. 501 to 1000 cc/day 5. 2001 or more cc/day	0

SECTION L: ORAL/DENTAL STATUS

1.	ORAL STATUS AND DISEASE PREVENTION	Debris (soft, easily movable substances) present in mouth prior to going to bed at night	a.
		Has dentures or removable bridge	b. X
		Some/all natural teeth lost—does not have or does not use dentures (or partial plates)	c.
		Broken, loose, or carious teeth	d.
		Inflamed gums (gingiva); swollen or bleeding gums; oral abscesses; ulcers or rashes	e.
		Daily cleaning of teeth/dentures or daily mouth care—by resident or staff	f. X
		NONE OF THE ABOVE	g.

Minimum Data Set tracking form *(continued)*

SECTION M. SKIN CONDITION

1.	ULCERS (Due to any cause)	(Record the number of ulcers at each ulcer stage—regardless of cause. If none present at a stage, record "0" (zero). Code all that apply during last 7 days. Code 9=9 or more.) [Requires full body exam.]	Number at stage
		a. Stage 1. A persistent area of skin redness (without a break in the skin) that does not disappear when pressure is relieved.	1
		b. Stage 2. A partial thickness loss of skin layers that presents clinically as an abrasion, blister, or shallow crater.	0
		c. Stage 3. A full thickness of skin is lost, exposing the subcutaneous tissues - presents as a deep crater with or without undermining adjacent tissue.	0
		d. Stage 4. A full thickness of skin and subcutaneous tissue is lost, exposing muscle or bone.	0
2.	TYPE OF ULCER	(For each type of ulcer, code for the highest stage in the last 7 days using scale in item M1—i.e., 0=none; stages 1, 2, 3, 4)	
		a. Pressure ulcer—any lesion caused by pressure resulting in damage of underlying tissue	1
		b. Stasis ulcer—open lesion caused by poor circulation in the lower extremities	0
3.	HISTORY OF RESOLVED ULCERS	Resident had an ulcer that was resolved or cured in LAST 90 DAYS 0. No 1. Yes	0
4.	OTHER SKIN PROBLEMS OR LESIONS PRESENT	(Check all that apply during last 7 days)	
		Abrasions, bruises	a.
		Burns (second or third degree)	b.
		Open lesions other than ulcers, rashes, cuts (e.g., cancer lesions)	c.
		Rashes—e.g., intertrigo, eczema, drug rash, heat rash, herpes zoster	d.
		Skin desensitized to pain or pressure	e.
		Skin tears or cuts (other than surgery)	f.
		Surgical wounds	g.
		NONE OF THE ABOVE	h. X
5.	SKIN TREAT-MENTS	(Check all that apply during last 7 days)	
		Pressure relieving device(s) for chair	a. X
		Pressure relieving device(s) for bed	b. X
		Turning/repositioning program	c. X
		Nutrition or hydration intervention to manage skin problems	d. X
		Ulcer care	e.
		Surgical wound care	f.
		Application of dressings (with or without topical medications) other than to feet	g.
		Application of ointments/medications (other than to feet)	h.
		Other preventative or protective skin care (other than to feet)	i.
		NONE OF THE ABOVE	j.
5.	FOOT PROBLEMS AND CARE	(Check all that apply during last 7 days)	
		Resident has one or more foot problems—e.g., corns, calluses, bunions, hammer toes, overlapping toes, pain, structural problems	a.
		Infection of the foot—e.g., cellulitis, purulent drainage	b.
		Open lesions on the foot	c.
		Nails/calluses trimmed during last 90 days	d.
		Received preventative or protective foot care (e.g., used special shoes, inserts, pads, toe separators)	e.
		Application of dressings (with or without topical medications)	f.
		NONE OF ABOVE	g. X

(continued)

Minimum Data Set tracking form *(continued)*

SECTION N: ACTIVITY PURSUIT PATTERNS

1.	TIME AWAKE	(Check appropriate time periods over last 7 days) Resident awake all or most of time (i.e. naps no more than one hour per time period) in the: Morning a. X — Evening c. Afternoon b. — NONE OF ABOVE d.	
(If resident is comatose, skip to Section O)			
2.	AVERAGE TIME INVOLVED IN ACTIVITIES	(When awake and not receiving treatments or ADL care) 0. Most—more than 2/3 of time — 2. Little—less than 1/3 of time 1. Some—from 1/3 to 2/3 of time — 3. None0	
3.	PREFERRED ACTIVITY SETTINGS	(Check all settings in which activities are preferred) Own room a. X Day/activity room b. — Outside facility d. Inside NH/off unit c. — NONE OF ABOVE e.	
4.	GENERAL ACTIVITY PREFER-ENCES (adapted to resident's current abilities)	(Check all PREFERENCES whether or not activity is currently available to resident) Cards/other games a. — Trips/shopping g. Crafts/arts b. — Walking/wheeling outdoors h. Exercise/sports c. — Watching TV i. X Music d. X — Gardening or plants j. Reading/writing e. — Talking or conversing k. Spiritual/religious activities f. — Helping others l. NONE OF ABOVE m.	
5.	PREFERS CHANGE IN DAILY ROUTINE	Code for resident preferences in daily routines 0. No change — 1. slight change — 2. Major change	
		a. Type of activities in which resident is currently involved	
		b. Extent of resident involvement in activities	

SECTION O: MEDICATIONS

1.	NUMBER OF MEDICA-TIONS	(Record the number of different medications used in the last 7 days; enter "0" if none used)	4
2.	NEW MEDICA-TIONS	(Resident currently receiving medications that were initiated during the last 90 days) 0. No — 1. Yes	0
3.	INJECTIONS	(Record the number of DAYS injections of any type received during the last 7 days; enter "0" if none used.)	0
4.	DAYS RECEIVED THE FOLLOWING MEDICATION	(Record the number of DAYS during last 7 days; enter "0" if not used. Note—enter "1" for long-acting meds used less than weekly) a. Antipsychotic — d. Hypnotic b. Antianxiety — e. Diuretic c. Antidepressant	X

Minimum Data Set tracking form *(continued)*

SECTION P: SPECIAL TREATMENTS AND PROCEDURES

1. SPECIAL TREATMENTS, PROCEDURES, AND PROGRAMS

a. SPECIAL CARE—Check treatments or programs received during the last 14 days

TREATMENTS		PROGRAMS	
Chemotherapy	a.	Ventilator or respirator	l.
Dialysis	b.	Alcohol/drug treatment program	m.
IV medication	c.	Alzheimer's/dementia special care unit	n. X
Intake/output	d.	Hospice care	o.
Monitoring acute medical condition	e.	Pediatric unit	p.
Ostomy care	f.	Respite care	q.
Oxygen therapy	g.	Training skills required to return to the community (e.g., taking medications, house work, shopping, transportation, ADLs)	r.
Radiation	h.	NONE OF ABOVE	s.
Suctioning	i.		
Tracheostomy care	j.		
Transfusions	k.		

b. THERAPIES - Record the number of days and total minutes each of the following therapies was administered (for at least 15 minutes a day) in the last 7 calendar days (Enter 0 if none or less than 15 min. daily)
[Note—count only post admission therapies]
(A) = # of days administered for 15 minutes or more
(B) = total # of minutes provided in last 7 days

	DAYS (A)	MIN (B)
a. Speech - language pathology and audiology services	0	
b. Occupational therapy	0	
c. Physical therapy	1	
d. Respiratory therapy	0	
e. Psychological therapy (by any licensed mental health professional)	0	

2. INTERVENTION PROGRAMS FOR MOOD, BEHAVIOR, COGNITIVE LOSS

(Check all interventions or strategies used in the last 7 days—no matter where received)

Special behavior symptom evaluation program	a. X
Evaluation by a licensed mental health specialist in last 90 days	b.
Group therapy	c.
Resident-specific deliberate changes in the environment to address mood/behavior patterns—e.g., providing bureau in which to rummage	d. X
Reorientation—e.g., cueing	e.
NONE OF ABOVE	f.

3. NURSING REHABILITATION/ RESTORATIVE CARE

Record the NUMBER OF DAYS each of the following rehabilitation or restorative techniques or practices was provided to the resident for more than or equal to 15 minutes per day in the last 7 days
(Enter 0 if none or less than 15 min. daily.)

a. Range of motion (passive)	1	f. Walking	
b. Range of motion (active)		g. Dressing or grooming	
c. Splint or brace assistance		h. Eating or swallowing	
TRAINING AND SKILL PRACTICE IN:		i. Amputation/prosthesis care	
d. Bed mobility		j. Communication	
e. Transfer		k. Other	

(continued)

Minimum Data Set tracking form *(continued)*

SECTION P: SPECIAL TREATMENTS AND PROCEDURES *(continued)*

4.	DEVICES AND RESTRAINTS	(Use the following codes for last 7 days) 0. Not used 1. Used less than daily 2. Used daily	
		Bed rails a. —Full bed rails on all open sides of bed	0
		b. —Other types of side rails used (e.g., half rail, one side)	1
		c. Trunk restraint	0
		d. Limb restraint	0
		e. Chair prevents rising	0
5.	HOSPITAL STAY(S)	Record number of times resident was admitted to hospital with an overnight stay in last 90 days (or since last assessment if less than 90 days). (Enter 0 if no hospital admissions)	0
6.	EMERGENCY ROOM (ER) VISIT(S)	Record number of times resident visited ER without an overnight stay in last 90 days (or since last assessment if less than 90 days.) (Enter 0 if no ER visits)	0
7.	PHYSICIAN VISITS	In the LAST 14 DAYS (or since admission if less than 14 days in facility) how many days has the physician (or authorized assistant or practitioner) examined the resident? (Enter 0 if none)	1
8.	PHYSICIAN ORDERS	In the LAST 14 DAYS (or since admission if less than 14 days in facility) how many days has the physician (or authorized assistant or practitioner) changed the resident's orders? Do not include order renewals without change. (Enter 0 if none)	0
9.	ABNORMAL LAB VALUES	Has the resident had any abnormal lab values during the last 90 days (or since admission)? 0. No 1. Yes	0

SECTION Q: DISCHARGE POTENTIAL AND OVERALL STATUS

1.	DISCHARGE POTENTIAL	a. Resident expresses/indicates preference to return to the community 0. No 1. Yes	0
		b. Resident has a support person who is positive towards discharge 0. No 1. Yes	0
		c. Stay projected to be of a short duration—discharge projected within 90 days (do not include expected discharge due to death) 0. No 2. Within 31-90 days 1. Within 30 days 3. Discharge status uncertain	0
2.	OVERALL CHANGE IN CARE NEEDS	Resident's overall self-sufficiency has changed significantly as compared to status of 90 days ago (or since last assessment if less than 90 days) 0. No change 1. Improved—receives fewer supports, needs less restrictive level of care 2. Deteriorated—receives more support	2

SECTION R: ASSESSMENT INFORMATION

1.	PARTICIPATION IN ASSESSMENT	a. Resident:	0. No	1. Yes		1
		b. Family:	0. No	1. Yes	2. No family	1
		c. Significant other:	0. No	1. Yes	2. None	0

2. SIGNATURE OF PERSON COORDINATING THE ASSESSMENT:

Christine Gaslo, RN, MSN

a. Signature of RN Assessment Coordinator (sign on above line)

b. Date RN Assessment Coordinator signed as complete

Month	Day	Year
04	03	2002

Minimum Data Set tracking form *(continued)*

SECTION T: THERAPY SUPPLEMENT FOR MEDICARE PPS

1.	SPECIAL TREATMENTS AND PROCEDURES	a. RECREATION THERAPY—Enter number of days and total minutes of recreation therapy administered (for at least 15 minutes a day) in the last 7 days (Enter 0 if none) (A) = # of days administered for 15 minutes or more (B) = total # of minutes provided in last 7 days	DAYS (A): 0 MIN (B):
		Skip unless this is a Medicare 5 day or Medicare readmission/ return assessment. b. ORDERED THERAPIES—Has physician ordered any of following therapies to begin FIRST 14 days of stay—physical therapy, occupational therapy, or speech pathology service? 0. No 1. Yes	1
		If not ordered, skip to item 2 c. Through day 15, provide an estimate of the number of days when at least 1 therapy service can be expected to have been delivered.	10
		d. Through day 15, provide an estimate of the number of therapy minutes (across the therapies) that can be expected to be delivered?	300
2.	WALKING WHEN MOST SELF SUFFICIENT	Complete item 2 if ADL self-performance score for TRANSFER (G.1.b.A) is 0, 1, 2 or 3 AND at least one of the following are present: • Resident received physical therapy involving gait training (P. 1.b.c) • Physical therapy was ordered for the resident involving gait training (T.1.b) • Resident received nursing rehabilitation for walking (P.3.f) • Physical therapy involving walking has been discontinued within the past 180 days Skip to item 3 if resident did not walk in last 7 days (FOR FOLLOWING FIVE ITEMS, BASE CODING ON THE EPISODE WHEN THE RESIDENT WALKED THE FARTHEST WITHOUT SITTING DOWN, INCLUDE WALKING DURING REHABILITATION SESSIONS.)	
		a. Furthest distance walked without sitting down during this episode. 0. 150+ feet 3. 10-25 feet 1. 51-149 feet 4. Less than 10 feet 2. 26-50 feet	
		b. Time walked without sitting down during this episode. 0. 1-2 minutes 3. 11-15 minutes 1. 3-4 minutes 4. 16-30 minutes 2. 5-10 minutes 5. 31+ minutes	
		c. Self-Performance in walking during this episode. 0. INDEPENDENT—No help or oversight 1. SUPERVISION—Oversight, encouragement or cueing provided 2. LIMITED ASSISTANCE—Resident highly involved in walking; received physical help in guided maneuvering of limbs or other nonweight bearing assistance 3. EXTENSIVE ASSISTANCE—Resident received weight bearing assistance while walking	
		d. Walking support provided associated with this episode (code regardless of resident's self-performing classification). 0. No setup or physical help from staff 1. Setup help only 2. One person physical assist 3. Two+ persons physical assist	
		e. Parallel bars used by resident in association with this episode. 0. No 1. Yes	
3.	CASE MIX GROUP	Medicare ☐☐☐☐☐ State ☐☐☐☐☐	

(continued)

Minimum Data Set tracking form *(continued)*

SECTION V: RESIDENT ASSESSMENT PROTOCOL SUMMARY

Resident's Name: Amy J. Gaston	Medical Record No.: MM0009922681

1. Check if RAP is triggered.
2. For each triggered RAP, use the RAP guidelines to identify areas needing further assessment. Document relevant assessment information regarding the resident's status.
   - Describe:
     - — Nature of the condition (may include presence or lack of objective data and subjective complaints).
     - — Complications and risk factors that affect your decision to proceed to care planning.
     - — Factors that must be considered in developing individualized care plan interventions.
     - — Need for referrals/further evaluation by appropriate health professionals.
   - Documentation should support your decision-making regarding whether to proceed with a care plan for a triggered RAP and the type(s) of care plan interventions that are appropriate for a particular resident.
   - Documentation may appear anywhere in the clinical record (e.g., progress notes, consults, flow sheets, etc.).
3. Indicate under the Location of RAP Assessment Documentation column where information related to the RAP assessment can be found.
4. For each triggered RAP, indicate whether a new care plan, care plan revision, or continuation of current care plan is necessary to address the problem(s) identified in your assessment. The Care Planning Decision column must be completed within 7 days of completing the RAI (MDS and RAPs).

A. RAP PROBLEM AREA	(a) Check if triggered	Location and Date of RAP Assessment Documentation	(b) Care Planning Decision—check if addressed in care plan
1. DELIRIUM	☐		☐
2. COGNITIVE LOSS	X	progress notes	X
3. VISUAL FUNCTION	☐		☐
4. COMMUNICATION	X	progress notes	X
5. ADL FUNCTIONAL/ REHABILITATION POTENTIAL	☐		☐
6. URINARY INCONTINENCE AND INDWELLING CATHETER	☐		☐
7. PSYCHOSOCIAL WELL-BEING	☐		☐
8. MOOD STATE	☐		☐
9. BEHAVIORAL SYMPTOMS	☐		☐
10. ACTIVITIES	☐		☐
11. FALLS	☐		☐
12. NUTRITIONAL STATUS	☐		☐
13. FEEDING TUBES	☐		☐
14. DEHYDRATION/FLUID MAINTENANCE	☐		☐
15. DENTAL CARE	☐		☐
16. PRESSURE ULCERS	X	progress notes	X
17. PSYCHOTROPIC DRUG USE	☐		☐
18. PHYSICAL RESTRAINTS	☐		☐

B. James Shaw, RN, BSN
1. Signature of RN Coordinator for RAP Assessment Process

2. 04 (Month) – 03 (Day) – 2002 (Year)

Christine Saslo, RN, MSN
3. Signature of Person Completing Care Planning Decision

4. 04 (Month) – 03 (Day) – 2002 (Year)

effect of any cultural differences and react accordingly.

Current health status

The first part of the interview explores the person's chief complaint and his current health status. Ask the patient his full name, address, age, date of birth, birthplace, and contact persons in case of an emergency. Record your information on an appropriate patient history form. Next, record the reason for admission, ask the patient about any current medications and treatments, diet regimens, and list any devices the patient uses (cane, walker, hearing aid).

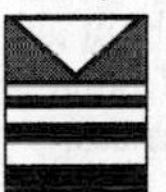

Key Point If the patient appears confused or is showing signs and symptoms of dementia, consider obtaining the patient's permission to include a spouse, child, or significant other in the interview.

Medical history

The medical history includes an overview of the person's general health status, a history of his adult illnesses, a record of past hospitalizations, the frequency of physician's visits, and previous use of medications and treatments and their purpose.

Review of body systems

When reviewing an older patient's body systems, keep in mind the physiologic changes normally associated with aging and the fact that older people commonly have an atypical disease presentation. For example, subtle changes in appetite and mental status may be their only signs and symptoms.

You can assess specific body areas and systems using either the head-to-toe approach or the major body system method. Both methods provide a systematic and organized framework, so choose the one that works best for you.

Performing the physical examination

The physical examination is the second component of the health assessment. Together with the health history, it helps you identify and evaluate your patient's strengths, weaknesses, capabilities, and limitations. Use inspection, palpation, percussion, and auscultation to gather objective patient data, which provide new information and help you validate the subjective data you obtained during the health history. Respect your patient's need for modesty; make sure the examination area is private, and explain how to put on the gown and drape.

General survey

Begin the physical examination with a general head-to-toe observation to gain an overall impression of your patient's status. This survey should include observations about:

- overall appearance, including skin, hygiene, grooming, and body build
- general mobility status
- level of consciousness (LOC), affect, and mood
- any overt signs of distress.
- vital signs (normal temperature in an older adult can range from 96° to 98.6° F [35.6° to 37° C]).

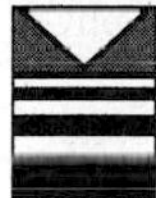

Key Point If an older person's normal body temperature is between 96° and 97° F., a reading of 98.6° F can be a significant elevation. In such cases, monitor the patient for other signs and symptoms of disease if his temperature is 98° F or above.

Skin

Inspect the skin of the scalp, head, neck, trunk, and limbs. Note the color, temperature, texture, tone, turgor, thickness, and moisture. Areas such as the knees or elbows may appear relatively darker because of sun exposure. Calloused areas may appear yellow.

Skin temperature can be described as cool, cold, warm, or hot. Use the ball of the hand to get an accurate assessment and to feel for symmetrical changes in temperature. Unilateral changes along with other clinical findings suggest a problem.

Skin turgor may be an unreliable sign of hydration in older people, who have less subcutaneous tissue. Check turgor by pinching the subcutaneous tissue at the forehead or over the xiphoid process and watching for a quick return to baseline.

Inspect the skin for the presence of tears, lacerations, scars, lesions, and ulcerations. Also, look for early signs of pressure ulcers such as local redness over pressure sites. Be alert to the common benign skin lesions found in older people, which must be differentiated from precancerous or malignant lesions. Note their size, pattern of distribution, shape, color, consistency, borders, and time of appearance. Any suspicious lesion warrants further evaluation.

Hair and nails

Inspect and palpate your patient's hair, noting color, quantity, distribution, and texture — fine, silky, or coarse. Hair thinning and sparseness are readily observed around the axillae and symphysis pubis.

Inspect fingernails and toenails, noting color, shape, thickness, presence of lesions, and capillary refill.

Some distortion of the normal flat or slightly curved nail surface is normal, but other changes in color, shape, or angle may indicate pathology.

Head and face

Inspect the head, noting size, contour, and symmetry. The size and shape of the skull shouldn't change with age. Soft-tissue swelling or bulging of the cranium may indicate recent head trauma.

Palpate the skull, noting tenderness, masses, or lesions. Localized enlargement of the cranium requires further evaluation.

Inspect the face and neck area for color and proportion. Color should be evenly distributed. Facial features should be in proportion to head size. Observe facial expression and movements.

Nose and mouth

Examine the external portion of the nose, noting any asymmetry or abnormality such as a structural deformity. Inspect the internal mucosa, noting color and any discharge, swelling, bleeding, or lesions. The area should be pink and moist with clear mucus and without any crusting or lesions. Palpate the frontal and maxillary sinuses for tenderness, which should not be present.

Inspect the mouth, beginning with the lips. Note color, symmetry, any lesions or ulceration, and hydration status. Dry, parched lips indicate dehydration. Note the presence of any dental appliances. Inspect the mouth with the appliance in place, noting the fit and observing for any sores or abscesses that may occur from friction. Inspect the mucosa, noting color, texture, hydration status, and any exudate. The mucosa and gums should be pink, smooth, and moist, but the mucosa of a dark-skinned person may be slightly bluish, a normal finding.

Palpate for lesions or nodules, noting any tenderness, pain, or bleeding. Inspect the gums for color, inflammation, lesions, and bleeding. They should be pink and moist. If your patient has his natural teeth, note the number and condition.

Observe the tongue, noting its color, size, texture, and coating. The tongue normally is pink to red, smooth, and free from involuntary movement. Assess the tongue's position; deviation to the right or left suggests a neurologic disorder. Observe the pharynx for signs of inflammation, discoloration, exudate, and lesions. The area should be pink to pale pink without discharge or lesions.

Eyes

When you examine an older person's eyes, keep in mind that ocular signs of aging can affect the appearance of the entire eye. You may see that the eyes sit deeper in the bony orbits, a normal finding that results from age-induced fatty tissue loss. Check eyebrow symmetry and distribution of hair.

Compare eyelid color to facial skin color; the lid should be free from color changes such as redness. Check for lesions or edema, and note the direction of the eyelashes. Determine whether the upper eyelid partially or completely covers the pupil, which indicates ptosis, an abnormal finding.

Inspect the lacrimal apparatus, noting any discharge, redness, edema, excessive tearing, or tenderness. Examine the sclera and conjunctiva. The sclera usually appears creamy white in color.

Inspect the pupils, noting size, shape, and reaction to light. Inspect the iris, noting any margin aberrations. You may see bilateral irregular iris pigmentation, with the normal pigment replaced by a pale brown color.

Test visual acuity with and without any corrective lenses, noting any differences. Perform an ophthalmoscopic examination to inspect the internal eye structures.

Ears

Inspect the auricle, noting color and any temperature changes, discharge, or lesions. Palpate the auricle for tenderness. Inspect the internal ear structures with an otoscope. Examine the external canal and tympanic membrane, and observe for the light reflex. Note any lesion, bulging of the tympanic membrane, cerumen accumulation, or (in an older male) hair growth.

To detect hearing loss early in an older person, always perform the Weber and Rinne tuning fork tests. Also, evaluate the patient's ability to hear and understand speech, in case you need to recommend rehabilitative therapy. If your patient wears a hearing aid, inspect it carefully for proper functioning.

Neck

Inspect the neck, noting scars, masses, and asymmetry. If masses are evident, gently palpate them, noting the consistency, size, shape, mobility, and tenderness. Repeat this for the lymph nodes.

Check the trachea for alignment. The trachea is normally located midline at the suprasternal notch. Note displacement and the presences of any masses. Inspect the thyroid gland while your patient takes a sip of water. Note any masses or bulging. Normally, the thyroid is invisible and not palpable.

Chest and respiratory system

Inspect the chest's shape and symmetry both anteriorly and posteriorly. Note the anteroposterior-to-lateral diameter.

During respirations, listen for inspiratory or expiratory wheezing, which may be audible from the oral airways.

Palpate the anterior and posterior chest for tenderness, masses, or lumps. Assess diaphragmatic excursion. Palpate the anterior and posterior chest symmetrically for tactile fremitus. Fremitus is usually most evident near the tracheal bifurcation.

Percuss the patient's lung fields anteriorly and posteriorly from bases to apices. Make certain to percuss in a symmetrical fashion for comparison. Normal lung fields will sound resonant on percussion. Bony prominences, organs, or consolidated tissue will sound dull.

Auscultate from the bases to the apices, anteriorly and posteriorly. Ask the patient to take some deep breaths, in and out, with his mouth open. You may hear diminished sounds at the lung bases because some of his airways are closed. Inspiration will be significantly more audible than expiration on auscultation of the lungs.

Cardiovascular system

Inspect and palpate the point of maximal impulse (PMI). In a young person, the PMI is located around the fifth or sixth, left intercostal space at the midclavicular line. In an older person, the PMI may be displaced downward to the left.

Using the ball of your hand, palpate over the aortic, pulmonic, and mitral areas for thrills, heaves, or vibrations. You may detect a palpable thrill in a person with valvular heart disease.

Auscultate the heart over the aortic, pulmonic, tricuspid, and mitral areas, and Erb's point. Listen for first and second heart sounds (S_1 and S_2) over each area, noting the intensity and splitting of S_1. Also, listen for extra diastolic heart sounds, or third and fourth heart sounds (S_3 and S_4), which you may be able to detect in an older adult. An S_3 heart sound is heard between S_1 and S_2, usually at the lower sternal border, and indicates ventricular decompensation. In an older adult, S_3 is not a reliable indicator of heart failure; it may be physiologic, or it may occur in response to an increased diastolic flow. An S_4 heart sound is heard after S_2 and before S_1. S_4 sounds are most audible over the heart's apex.

Assess the vessels of the head, neck, trunk, and extremities. Palpate the carotid arteries one at a time, pressing lightly to avoid obliterating the carotid pulse. Note the rate, rhythm, strength, and equality of both pulses. Auscultate each carotid artery for bruits — usually high-pitched sounds representing a narrowing of either the arterial or venous lumen.

Assess for jugular vein distention. Identify the level of venous pulsation and measure its height in relation to the sternal angle. A height exceeding 1⅛″ (3 cm) is considered abnormal and indicates right-sided heart failure.

Palpate the peripheral arteries, noting the rate, rhythm, strength, and equality of pulses. Also, note the presence of any bruits. In the older adult, expect arteries to be tortuous and appear kinked; they also may feel stiffer. However, the pulses should be symmetrical in strength.

Inspect the legs, noting color, temperature, edema, trophic changes of the toes, and any varicosities.

Using the ball of the hand, assess the temperature of the extremities; it should be equal bilaterally. Thrombosis is usually associated with a feeling of heat, but this response may be reduced in the older adult.

Check for edema, which is best assessed over bony prominences or the sacrum and typically pronounced in the most dependent areas of the body. Ascertain if the edema is pitting or nonpitting and grade the degree of edema.

GI system

Assessing an older adult's GI system is similar to examining a younger adult's, with two differences: Abdominal rigidity is less common in an older person, and abdominal distention is more common.

Inspect the abdomen, noting shape and symmetry and any scars, masses, pulsations, distention, or striae. The abdomen may be described as obese, scaphoid, or distended.

Auscultate all four quadrants for bowel sounds. Listen over the abdominal aorta for bruits.

Percuss to determine the presence of air or fluid, the size of the liver, and any bladder distention. Air in the large bowel will sound tympanic, whereas fluid will sound dull. Percuss the liver. The normal liver size at the midclavicular line is 2¼″ to 4¾″ (6 to 12 cm) in diameter. Also, percuss over the symphysis pubis toward the umbilicus, noting any change in percussion. Dullness in this area may indicate bladder distention.

Palpate the belly, noting any masses or tenderness on light or deep palpation. Watch for any peritoneal signs, such as rigidity or rebound tenderness. Masses in the lower quadrants may be impacted stool. Try to palpate the liver; normally it isn't palpable.

GU system

When you assess an older adult's genitourinary (GU) system, you'll use the same basic technique that you would with a younger patient.

When assessing the male genitalia, inspect the pubic hair, glans of the uncircumcised penis, penile shaft, scrotum, and inguinal canals for bulging masses, lesions, inflammation, edema, or discoloration. The pubic hair becomes sparse and gray with age. Palpate any lesions noting size, shape, consistency, and tenderness.

Palpate the testes for size, shape, consistency, and tenderness. Normally, in an older adult, the testes may be slightly smaller than adult size, but they should be equal, smooth, freely movable, and soft without nodules. Inspect and palpate the inguinal canal; you shouldn't observe any bulging.

When assessing the female genitalia, inspect the perineum for rash, lesion, or nodule. Examine the area for color, size, and shape. Inspect the vaginal orifice, and observe for any bulging of tissues or organs.

Perform an internal pelvic examination, if qualified. Take care to maximize your patient's comfort because the atrophic changes of the vaginal mucosa in the older female increase her discomfort during the pelvic examination. To examine the rectum, place the female patient in a side-lying position and the male patient bent over. Inspect the anus and overall skin surface characteristics. The area should be smooth and uninterrupted with coarse skin and slightly increased pigmented areas around the anus. Note any masses, nodules, lesions, or hemorrhoids.

Palpate the rectum using a gloved, lubricated finger, noting muscle tone. After withdrawing the finger, test any stool for blood. For males, assess the prostate gland. Note the size, consistency, shape, surface, and symmetry, and record any tenderness. The gland should be round, soft, nontender, free of masses, and about ¾" to 1½" (2 to 4 cm) in diameter.

Musculoskeletal system

Assessing the musculoskeletal system is vital in determining an older adult's overall ability to function. Limitations in range of motion (ROM), difficult ambulation, and diffused or localized joint pain can be detected easily during the physical examination.

During your assessment, be alert for signs of motor and sensory dysfunction: weakness, spasticity, tremors, rigidity, and various types of sensory disturbances. Observe the patient's walk, noting gait and posture. Gait reflects the integration of reflexes as well as motor function. Assess static balance and station by gently pushing on the patient's shoulders while he's standing.

Observe the patient's tandem walking to watch for any exaggerated ataxia and to observe the position of the head and neck in relation to shoulders and legs. Elicit Romberg's sign to evaluate posture and balance; it's positive if the patient sways.

Inspect the joints of the hands, wrists, elbows, shoulders, neck, hips, knees, and ankles. Note any joint enlargement, swelling, tenderness, crepitus, temperature changes, or deformities. Assess the foot for common deformities: hallux valgus, prolapsed metatarsals, and hammer toes.

Inspect each muscle group for atrophy, fasciculations, involuntary movements, and tremor. Move the joints through passive ROM exercises, and palpate the muscles for tone and strength.

Assess for rigidity and spasticity. Rigidity can be detected best in the wrist or elbow joint. Throughout the physical examination, ask the patient to show you how he buttons or zippers his clothing, allowing you to directly observe his ability to perform selected activities of daily living. Observe him grasping items, such as the doorknob or water faucets.

Neurologic system

The neurologic examination includes assessment of LOC or awareness, affect and mood, cognition, orientation, speech, general knowledge, memory, reasoning, object recognition and higher cognitive functions, cranial nerves, motor and sensory systems, and reflexes.

A number of screening tools are available to assess an older adult's cognitive status, such as the Mini-Mental State Examination, the Short Portable Mental Status Questionnaire, and the Mental Status Questionnaire.

Begin by observing your patient's general appearance, including mood, affect, and grooming. An older patient who seems depressed may require further evaluation; a number of assessment tools are available including the Geriatric Depression Scale. Note whether he is appropriately dressed, responds appropriately to questions, and is oriented to person, time, and place.

Note the patient's speech. Assess vocabulary and general knowledge level by discussing current news items or family events.

Assess the patient's memory — his immediate, recent, and remote recall. Assess immediate recall by naming a certain number of objects or reciting a group of numbers and having the patient repeat them immediately. To elicit recent memory, ask the patient about events that occurred in the past 24 to 48 hours. To assess remote memory, ask the patient to recall significant events that occurred many years ago.

Assess the patient's ability to reason. Ask him questions requiring judgment, insight, and abstraction. Also, assess object recognition. Point to two objects and ask the patient to identify each. The response is graded as normal or agnosia (the inability to name objects).

CRANIAL NERVES

Assess each cranial nerve sequentially, beginning with cranial nerve I and progressing to cranial nerve XII.

MOTOR AND SENSORY SYSTEMS

Evaluate muscle and joint function. Also, assess for rapid, rhythmic, alternating movements, which determine coordination. Observe your patient for the ability to repeat maneuvers and for smoothness in executing them. Expect the speed of response in an older person to be reduced.

Check your patient's ability to perceive pain, using the sharp and dull end of a safety pin; temperature, using hot and cold substances; touch, using a light touch of the hand; and vibration, using a vibrating tuning fork. Also, evaluate two-point discrimination and position sense. Perception should be accurate and symmetrical.

REFLEXES

You should assess an older adult's reflexes in the same manner as those in other age-groups. The plantar and Babinski's reflexes are important in assessing for upper motor neuron disease.

Documentation

Document all your assessment findings according to your facility's policy.

ASSISTED SUICIDE

Although suicide is no longer a crime in all 50 states, most states still prohibit assisted suicide. Some states treat assisted suicide harshly; others only prohibit causing suicide, not assisting with it. Washington, Oregon, and California have tried, through legislation, to pass assisted suicide statutes. Although these measures have either failed or are being challenged in the courts, they seem likely to pass at some future date. The Supreme Court may be the judiciary body that finally attempts to come to terms with this issue.

The Oregon Death with Dignity Act, passed by the voters in November 1994 and now under judicial review, would allow a physician to write a lethal drug prescription for a competent, terminally ill adult who is a resident of the state. Other provisions that would have to be met before the prescription was written include the following:

- Both the attending physician and a consulting physician must certify that the patient has no more than 6 months to live.
- The patient must make an oral and written request for the prescription, followed by a second oral request 15 days or more after the first requests.
- The attending physician must refer the patient for counseling if a psychological illness or depression is suspected.
- The physician must wait at least 48 hours after a third request before prescribing the medication.

Michigan has dealt with the assisted suicide issue extensively because of the actions of Dr. Jack Kevorkian. Michigan originally filed murder charges against Kevorkian, who has assisted dozens of gravely or terminally ill patients in ending their lives. The state then passed a statute "prohibiting one who has knowledge that a person intends to commit suicide from intentionally providing the physical means or participating in the physical act by which the person attempts or commits suicide," but the prohibition does not apply to "withholding or withdrawing (treatment) by a licensed health care professional." This law is currently being challenged.

The health care professional's role in this area is still developing. The American Nurses Association opposes assisted suicide as well as nurses' participation in either assisted or active euthanasia because it violates the ethical traditions embodied in the Code for Nurses (1994). However, the Michigan Nurses Association has come out in favor of legalizing assisted suicide for "competent persons whose suffering cannot be relieved or satisfactorily reduced with alternative strategies."

Special considerations

- If a patient asks you directly to assist with suicide, you must clearly refuse. If this occurs, reassure the patient that you care about him and will provide assistance through appropriate nursing interventions.
- Explore the possibility that the patient is expressing a need for greater pain control or for someone to talk to about fears of a terrible death.
- Refer the patient to a mental health practitioner to rule out the possibility that the patient is suffering from clinical depression.
- Arrange for a clergyman of the patient's faith or a social worker to speak with the patient.

ASSISTIVE DEVICES

Designed to maintain balance and stability, assistive devices such as canes and walkers must be individualized to the patient and his disorder. Older people should be encouraged to seek professional assistance when choosing a device rather than purchasing one from a medical equipment company. Improperly used or fitted equipment can lead to falls—a problem that is already common in the elderly population.

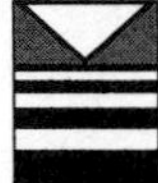

Key Point When assessing an individual with AD or Alzheimer's-like dementia, carefully evaluate the patient's ability to use the assistive device correctly. Also evaluate the patient's ability to remember to use the device. An assistive device can become a tripping hazard if it's used incorrectly, or if it's left out of place because the patient forgets to use it.

Canes

Indicated for the patient with one-sided weakness or injury, occasional loss of balance, or increased joint pressure, a cane provides balance and support for walking and reduces fatigue and strain on weight-bearing joints. Available in various sizes, the cane should extend from the greater trochanter to the floor and have a rubber tip to prevent slipping. Canes are contraindicated for the patient with bilateral weakness; such a patient should use a walker.

Although wooden canes are available, three types of aluminum canes are used most commonly. The standard aluminum cane—used by the patient who needs only slight assistance to walk—provides the least support. The T-handle cane—used by the patient with hand weakness—has a straight, shaped handle with grips and a bent shaft. It provides greater stability than the standard cane. Three- or four-pronged canes are used by the patient with poor balance or one-sided weakness and an inability to hold onto a walker with both hands. The base of these types of canes splits into three or four short, splayed legs and provides greater stability than a standard cane but considerably less than a walker.

Walkers

A walker consists of a metal frame with handgrips and four legs that buttresses the patient on three sides. One side remains open. Because this device provides greater stability and security than other ambulatory aids, it's recommended for the patient with insufficient strength and balance to use a cane or with weakness requiring frequent rest periods. Attachments for standard walkers and modified walkers help meet special needs.

Various types of walkers are available. The standard walker is used by the patient with unilateral or bilateral weakness or an inability to bear weight on one leg. It requires arm strength and balance. Platform attachments may be added to this walker for the patient with arthritic arms or a casted arm, who can't bear weight directly on his hand, wrist, or forearm. Wheels may be placed on the front legs of the standard walker to allow the extremely weak or poorly coordinated patient to roll the device forward, instead of lifting it.

Small skids or "skis" about 4″ in length can be applied to the rear legs of a standard walker that has wheels on the front legs. The skids prevent the rear legs from catching on carpets. Careful assessment of the patient is needed before applying wheels or skids to the legs of his walker. If improperly used, a walker can be a significant safety hazard.

The stair walker—used by the patient who must negotiate stairs without bilateral handrails—requires good arm strength and balance. Its extra set of handles extends toward the patient on the open side. The rolling walker—used by the patient with very weak legs—has four wheels and a seat. The reciprocal walker—used by the patient with very weak arms—allows one side to be advanced ahead of the other. Whenever possible, a patient should be trained to handle an assistive device by a therapist or nurse who is well-versed in their use.

Implementation

Canes

▶ Ask the patient to hold the cane on the uninvolved side 24″ to 26″ (61 to 66 cm) from the base of the little toe. If the cane is made of aluminum, adjust its height by pushing in the metal button on the shaft and raising or lowering the shaft; if it's wood, the rubber tip can be removed and excess length sawed off. At the correct height, the handle of the cane is level with the greater trochanter and allows approximately 15-degree flexion at the elbow. If the cane is too short, the patient will have to drop his shoulder to lean on it; if it's too long, he'll have to raise his shoulder and will have difficulty supporting his weight.

▶ To prevent falls during the learning period, guard the patient carefully by standing behind him slightly to his stronger side and putting one foot between his feet and your other foot to the outside of the uninvolved leg. If necessary, use a walking belt.

▶ Tell the patient to hold the cane on the uninvolved side to promote a reciprocal gait pattern and to distribute weight away from the involved side.

▶ Instruct the patient to hold the cane close to his body to prevent leaning, and to move the cane and the involved leg simultaneously, followed by the uninvolved leg.

▶ Encourage the patient to keep the stride length of each leg and the timing of each step (cadence) equal.

NEGOTIATING STAIRS

▶ Instruct the patient to always use a railing, if present, when going up or down stairs. Tell him to hold the cane with the other hand or to keep it in the hand grasping the railing. To ascend stairs, the patient should lead with the uninvolved leg and follow with the involved leg; to descend, he should lead with the involved leg and follow with the uninvolved one. Help the patient remember by telling him to use this mnemonic device: "The good goes up, and the bad goes down."

NEGOTIATING STAIRS WITHOUT A RAILING

▶ Instruct the patient to use the walking technique to ascend and descend the stairs but move the cane just before the involved leg. Thus, to ascend stairs, the patient should hold the cane on the uninvolved side, step with the uninvolved leg, advance the cane, then move the involved leg. To descend, he should hold the cane on the uninvolved side, lead with the cane, then advance the involved leg and, finally, the uninvolved leg.

USING A CHAIR

▶ To teach the patient to sit down, stand by his affected side and tell him to place the backs of his legs against the edge of the chair seat. Then tell him to move the cane out from his side and to reach back with both hands to grasp the chair's armrests. Supporting his weight on the armrests, he can then lower himself onto the seat. While he's seated, he should keep the cane hooked on the armrest or the chair back.

▶ To teach the patient to get up from a chair, stand by his affected side and tell him to unhook the cane from the chair and hold it in his stronger hand as he grasps the armrests. Then tell him to move his uninvolved foot slightly forward, to lean slightly forward, and to push against the armrests to raise himself upright.

▶ Warn the patient not to lean on the cane when sitting or rising from the chair to prevent falls.

▶ Supervise your patient each time he gets in or out of a chair until you're both certain he can do it alone.

Walkers

▶ Obtain the appropriate walker with the advice of a physical therapist, and adjust it to the patient's height. For correct positioning, the patient's elbows should be flexed at a 15-degree angle when standing comfortably within the walker with his hands on the grips. To adjust the walker, turn it upside down, and change the leg length by pushing in the button on each shaft and releasing it when the leg is in the correct position. Make sure the walker is level before the patient attempts to use it.

▶ Help the patient stand within the walker, and instruct him to hold the handgrips firmly and equally. Stand behind him, closer to the involved leg.

▶ If the patient has one-sided leg weakness, tell him to advance the walker 6″ to 8″ (15 to 20.5 cm) and to step forward with the involved leg and follow with the uninvolved leg, supporting himself on his arms. Encourage him to take equal strides. If he has equal strength in both legs, instruct him to advance the walker 6″ to 8″ and to step forward with either leg. If he can't use one leg, tell him to advance the walker 6″ to 8″ and to swing onto it, supporting his weight on his arms.

▶ If the patient is using a reciprocal walker, teach him the two- or four-point gait. If the patient is using a wheeled or stair walker, reinforce the physical therapist's instructions. Stress the need for caution when using a stair walker.

SITTING IN A CHAIR

▶ Instruct the patient to stand with the back of his stronger leg against the front of the chair, his weaker leg slightly off the floor, and the walker directly in front. Tell him to grasp the armrests on the chair one arm at a time while supporting most of his weight on the stronger leg. Tell him to lower himself into the chair and slide backward.

GETTING UP FROM A CHAIR

▶ With the walker in front of the chair, instruct the patient to slide forward in the chair. Place the back of his stronger leg against the seat; then advance the weaker leg. With both hands on the armrests, tell the patient to push himself to a standing position. Supporting himself with the stronger leg and the opposite hand, teach the patient to grasp the walker's handgrip with his freehand. Then have the patient grasp the free handgrip with his other hand.

▶ If the patient starts to fall, support his hips and shoulders to help maintain an upright position if possible.

Complications

A poorly fitted cane or walker or worn rubber tips can cause the patient to lose his balance and fall.

Patient teaching

▶ Explain the mechanics of cane and walker use to the patient.

▶ Demonstrate the technique, and then have the patient return the demonstration.

▶ Explain to the patient that rubber tips must be replaced when worn to reduce the risk of falling.

▶ Assist the patient or a family member in setting up a routine inspection schedule for the device's tips, movable parts, and locks.

Documentation

Record the type of cane or walker used, the amount of guarding required, the distance walked, and the patient's understanding and tolerance of ambulation.

ATRIAL FIBRILLATION

The most common arrhythmia in the older population — occurring in about 5% — atrial fibrillation is characterized by a lack of organized atrial activity and irregular timing of the ventricular response. If the ventricular response is too fast, the ventricle will not have a chance to fill, compromising the cardiac output.

In older adults, atrial fibrillation is more likely to be chronic than acute and usually signifies organic heart disease. As the body ages, the number of pacemaker cells decreases and myocardial fat, collagen, and elastin fibers increase. The sinus node, which is responsible for initiating atrial contraction, has 90% fewer cells at age 75 than at age 20.

Atrial fibrillation results from impulses in many circus reentry pathways in the atria. In atrial fibrillation, these impulses usually fire at a rate of 400 to 600 per minute, causing the atria to quiver rather than contract regularly. The most common predisposing factors in older people are hypertension, heart failure, alcohol use, cardiomyopathy, coronary artery disease, and mitral valve disease. Stimulants, such as nicotine and caffeine, as well as amyloidosis, sick sinus syndrome, and thyrotoxicosis may also trigger atrial fibrillation.

Signs and symptoms

- Commonly asymptomatic
- Complaints of heart racing or of feeling faint
- Irregular heart rate with no pattern to the irregularity of the pulse

Diagnostic tests

- *Electrocardiography* reveals an irregular tracing. The atrial rhythm is grossly irregular, with a rate of more than 400 per minute. The QRS complexes, which depict ventricular response, have a uniform configuration and duration but occur erratically. There are no discernible P waves, which depict atrial contraction in a normal heart rhythm, and there's no discernible PR interval. Instead, a wavy baseline, indicating quivering of the atria, is present between the QRS complexes.
- *Transesophageal echocardiography* should be done to rule out the presence of a clot in the atrium before cardioversion is considered

Treatment

Approximately one-third of older adults with atrial fibrillation have a controlled ventricular response and require no therapy.

If the patient is stable, drug therapy may include diltiazem, beta-adrenergic blockers, verapamil, digoxin, quinidine, procainamide, or amiodarone. However, drug therapy may become less effective over time.

Drug alert Older patients may need a lower dosage of quinidine because of their highly variable metabolism. Serum level monitoring is advised.

Radiofrequency catheter-induced ablation may be required for some patients with refractory atrial fibrillation that's uncontrolled by drugs. Cardioversion is another option if drug therapy isn't successful or if the arrhythmia is newly diagnosed. Because of the risks involved, the cause and duration of the rhythm, the size of the atria, and the risks of alternative therapy must be considered carefully.

Anticoagulation therapy is usually initiated with heparin, followed by maintenance warfarin therapy (atrial fibrillation is associated with 25% of cerebrovascular accidents [CVAs] in patients over age 65). Warfarin reduces the risk of CVA in these patients by 80%.

Key nursing diagnoses and outcomes

Decreased cardiac output related to decreased left ventricular filling time caused by atrial fibrillation

Treatment outcome: The patient will exhibit no signs or symptoms of decreased cardiac output, such as hypotension and altered tissue perfusion.

Anxiety related to potential for atrial fibrillation to become life-threatening

Treatment outcome: The patient will experience diminished physical symptoms of anxiety.

Cardiac monitoring

In your notes, document the date and time that monitoring begins and the monitoring leads used. Commit all rhythm strip readings to the record. Be sure to label the rhythm strip with the patient's name, his room number, and the date and time. Also, document any changes in the patient's condition.

1/8/02	07:20	Pt. on 5-lead electrode system. ECG strip
		shows Afib @ a ventricular rate of 96-120, QRS
		0.08, ventricular rate up to 130 @ 0710 hr. Dr.
		Cooper notified. Pt. asymptomatic. Peripheral
		pulses irregular; no edema noted. Heart
		irregular. No murmurs, gallops, or rubs. Pt.
		denied chest pain/discomfort. —— J. Steele, RN

ATRIAL FIBRILLATION

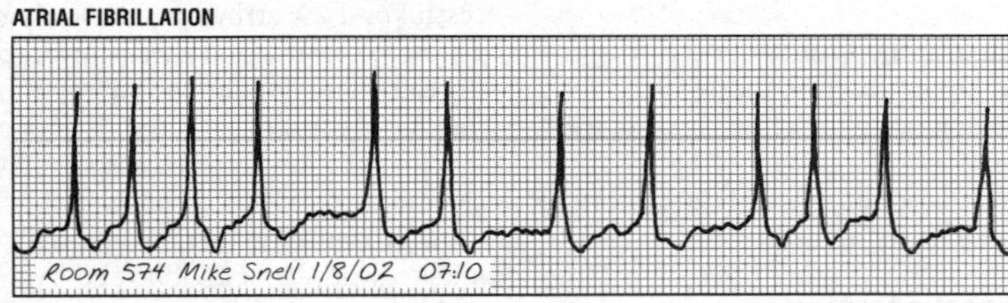

Nursing interventions

- Place the patient on a continuous heart monitor, and check his vital signs frequently. (See *Cardiac monitoring*.) Document any arrhythmia, and assess for hypotension or decreased urine output.
- Administer cardiac medications as ordered. Monitor digoxin and quinidine levels. If the person is receiving quinidine, document the QT interval before starting therapy and daily thereafter. A prolonged QT interval could lead to ventricular arrhythmias. Assist with cardioversion if ordered.

PATIENT TEACHING

- Teach the person about atrial fibrillation, its treatment, and any necessary lifestyle modifications.
- Explain that atrial fibrillation, if managed properly, usually won't interfere with normal activities. Encourage the patient to establish a regular exercise routine, under his physician's supervision, to improve his overall cardiovascular fitness. Remind him to avoid overexertion and to stop exercising immediately if he experiences dizziness, lightheadedness, dyspnea, or chest pain. Also, warn against driving or operating heavy machinery if the atrial fibrillation causes periodic dizziness or syncope.

▶ Emphasize the importance of taking medications as prescribed. Point out that medication can only control, not cure, the arrhythmia. Tell the person to continue taking antiarrhythmics and other prescribed drugs according to schedule, even if he's free from signs and symptoms. Advise him to call his physician if he experiences adverse reactions. Tell him not to stop any medication until he contacts his physician.

▶ If the person is taking digoxin, emphasize the importance of reporting any adverse effects and keeping follow-up appointments with his physician and appointments for blood testing.

▶ Teach him how to take his pulse, making sure that he is counting the beats for a full 60 seconds. Instruct him to call the physician if his heart rate is greater than 100 or less than 50. Instruct him to report any episodes of dizziness, syncope, or palpitations to the physician.

▶ Explain that caffeine and nicotine are stimulants that can increase the heart rate.

▶ If the person will be undergoing cardioversion, inform him that this procedure uses an electric current to restore the normal heart rate and relieve signs and symptoms. Instruct him to abstain from food and fluids for at least 8 hours before the procedure. Explain that he'll be given an I.V. sedative to induce sleep and that while he's asleep, an electric current will be delivered to his heart through paddles placed on his chest. Reassure him that he'll feel no pain or discomfort from the procedure and that he'll be able to eat and move about once the sedative has worn off. Inform him that he may notice a reddened area of skin where the paddles were placed. The area may feel tender and itchy for 1 to 2 days.

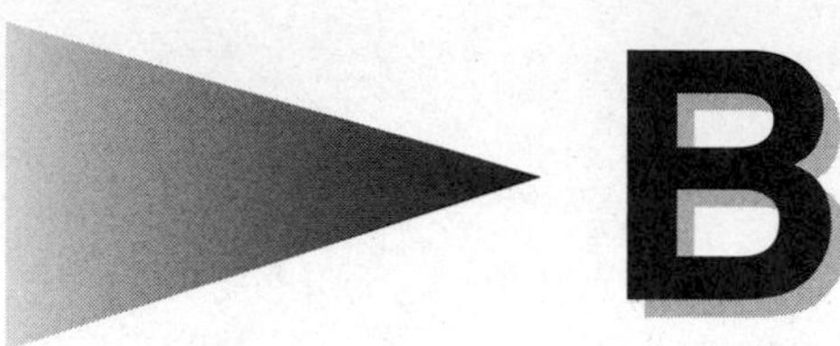

Basal cell epithelioma

A slow-growing, destructive skin tumor, basal cell epithelioma usually strikes people over age 40 and occurs two times more often in men than in women. It's the most common malignant tumor affecting whites and is most prevalent in blond, fair-skinned men.The two major types of basal cell epithelioma are noduloulcerative and superficial.

Prolonged sun exposure is the most common cause of basal cell epithelioma. Some 90% of tumors occur on sun-exposed areas of the body, but arsenic ingestion, radiation exposure, burns, immunosuppression and, rarely, vaccinations are other possible causes.

Although the pathogenesis is uncertain, some experts hypothesize that basal cell epithelioma originates when undifferentiated basal cells become cancerous instead of differentiating into sweat glands, sebum, and hair.

Signs and symptoms

- Small, smooth, pinkish, and translucent papules on forehead, eyelid margins, and nasolabial folds (early stage noduloulcerative); as lesions enlarge, centers become depressed and borders become firm, elevated (rodent ulcers)
- Multiple oval or irregularly shaped, lightly pigmented plaques on chest and back; may have sharply defined, slightly elevated, threadlike borders (superficial basal cell epithelioma)
- Waxy, sclerotic, yellow to white plaques without distinct borders on head and neck; may resemble small patches of scleroderma and may suggest sclerosing basal cell epitheliomas

The patient history may disclose prolonged exposure to the sun sometime in the patient's life or other risk factors for this disease.

Diagnostic tests

All types of basal cell epitheliomas are diagnosed by clinical appearance.

- *Incisional or excisional biopsy* and *histologic study* may help to determine the tumor type and histologic subtype.

Treatment

Depending on the size, location, and depth of the lesion, treatment may include curettage and electrodesiccation, chemotherapy, surgical excision, irradiation, or chemosurgery.

Curettage and electrodesiccation offer good cosmetic results for small lesions. Topical fluorouracil is commonly used for superficial lesions. This medication produces marked local irritation or inflammation in the involved tissue but no systemic effects.

Microscopically controlled surgical excision carefully removes recurrent lesions until a tumor-free plane is achieved. After removal of large lesions, skin grafting may be required. Irradiation is used if the tumor location requires it. It's also preferred for older or debilitated patients who might not tolerate surgery.

Chemosurgery may be necessary for persistent or recurrent lesions. It consists of periodic applications of a fixative paste (such as zinc chloride) and subsequent removal of fixed pathologic tissue. Treatment continues until tumor removal is complete. Cryotherapy, using liquid nitrogen, freezes the cells and kills them.

Key nursing diagnoses and outcomes

Disturbed body image related to facial disfigurement caused by lesions

Treatment outcomes: The patient will develop and express positive feelings about himself.

Fear related to the diagnosis of cancer

Treatment outcomes: The patient will express reduced fear and manifest no physical signs or symptoms of fear.

Impaired skin integrity related to ulceration caused by basal cell epithelioma or skin irritation from therapy

Treatment outcome: The patient will develop no skin breakdown from therapy.

Nursing interventions

- Watch for complications of treatment, including local skin irritation from topically applied chemotherapeutic agents and infection.
- If applicable, watch for radiation's adverse effects, such as nausea, vomiting, hair loss, malaise, and diarrhea.
- Listen to the patient's fears and concerns. Offer reassurance when appropriate. Remain with the patient during periods of severe stress and anxiety. Provide positive reinforcement for the patient's efforts to adapt.
- Arrange for the patient to interact with others who have a similar problem.
- Assess the patient's readiness for decision making; then involve him and his family members in decisions related to his care whenever possible.
- Provide reassurance and comfort measures when appropriate.

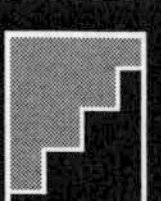

Staying well

Preventing skin cancer

To help your older patient prevent skin cancer, be sure to include these tips in your teaching:

- Instruct the patient to wear long sleeves, long pants, and a hat with a brim when he's out in the sun for an extended period of time — even if the day is overcast.
- Tell the patient to wear a sunscreen with SPF 35 or higher on all exposed skin areas when he's in the sun.
- Instruct the patient to avoid staying in swimming pools for long periods on sunny days, and tell him to wear water-resistant sunscreen while in the pool.
- Encourage the patient to inspect his skin for new and unusually shaped or colored lesions while he's bathing or dressing. The patient should report to his physician new lesions or old lesions that have changed shape or color.

PATIENT TEACHING

- Instruct the patient to eat frequent, small, high-protein meals. Advise him to include eggnog, pureed foods, and liquid protein supplements if the lesion has invaded the oral cavity and is causing eating difficulty.
- To prevent disease recurrence, tell the patient to avoid excessive sun exposure and to use a strong sunscreen to protect his skin from damage by ultraviolet rays.
- Advise the patient to relieve local inflammation from topical fluorouracil with cool compresses or with corticosteroid ointment.
- Instruct the patient with noduloulcerative basal cell epithelioma to wash his face gently when ulcerations and crusting occur; scrubbing too vigorously may cause bleeding.

- As appropriate, direct the patient and his family to hospital and community support services, such as social workers, psychologists, and cancer support groups. (See *Preventing skin cancer,* page 97.)

BENIGN PROSTATIC HYPERPLASIA

Most men over age 50 have some prostatic enlargement, known as benign prostatic hyperplasia (BPH). BPH becomes symptomatic when the prostate gland enlarges sufficiently to compress the urethra and cause some overt urinary obstruction. As the prostate enlarges, it may extend toward the bladder and obstruct urine outflow by compressing or distorting the prostatic urethra. BPH also may cause a weakening of the detrusor musculature that retains urine when the rest of the bladder empties. Depending on the size of the enlarged prostate, the age and health of the patient, and the extent of the obstruction, BPH may be treated surgically or symptomatically.

The cause of BPH isn't well understood. Some researchers theorize that the higher estrogen-androgen ratio that occurs with aging (declining serum testosterone levels and rising serum estrogen levels) stimulates prostatic enlargement.

Because BPH causes urinary obstruction, a patient may have one or more of the following complications:

- urine retention or incomplete bladder emptying, leading to urinary tract infection (UTI) or calculi
- bladder wall trabeculation
- detrusor muscle hypertrophy
- bladder diverticuli and saccules
- urethral stenosis
- hydronephrosis
- overflow incontinence
- acute or chronic renal failure
- acute postobstructive diuresis.

Signs and symptoms

Early stages

- Decreased urine stream caliber and force
- Interrupted urine stream
- Urinary hesitancy
- Difficulty starting urination
- Straining
- Feeling of incomplete voiding

Late stages

- Frequent urination with nocturia
- Dribbling
- Urine retention
- Incontinence
- Hematuria
- Visible midline mass above symphysis pubis
- Distended bladder upon palpation
- Enlarged prostate upon digital rectal examination

Diagnostic tests

- *Digital examinations,* routinely performed during a complete physical examination, can detect irregularities in size, shape, or tenderness of prostate tissue.
- *Excretory urography* may indicate urinary tract obstruction, hydronephrosis, calculi or tumors, and filling and emptying defects in the bladder.
- *Blood tests* reveal elevated blood urea nitrogen and serum creatinine levels, suggesting impaired renal function.
- *Urinalysis* and *urine culture* show hematuria, pyuria and, when the bacterial count exceeds 100,000/µl, UTI.
- *Prostate-specific antigen* levels are routinely drawn on men with prostatic symptoms to rule out prostate cancer.
- *Cystourethroscopy* is the definitive diagnostic measure when signs and symptoms are severe. It can show prostate enlargement, bladder wall changes, calculi, and a raised bladder and can help determine the best surgical treatment.

Treatment

BPH requires treatment only if the patient is significantly symptomatic or when complications, such as recurrent

UTI, persistent gross hematuria, or renal insufficiency, occur.

Alpha-adrenergic blockers, such as terazosin and doxazosin, relax the bladder neck and prostatic urethra. These drugs are also used for hypertension; adverse effects include hypotension, dizziness, headaches, and nasal congestion.

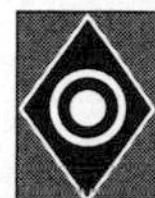

Drug alert The hypotensive effects of alpha-adrenergic blockers may be more pronounced in the older patient. Monitor blood pressure closely. In addition, monitor orthostatic blood pressures during the first week of drug therapy.

Finasteride blocks the conversion of testosterone to dihydrotestosterone within the prostate, preventing continued prostate growth. It must be taken for 6 to 12 months before the patient notices an improvement in signs and symptoms.

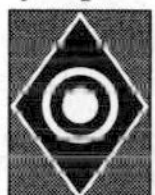

Drug alert Finasteride may decrease libido and cause impotence and ejaculatory dysfunction in older men, prompting decreased compliance.

Continuous drainage with an indwelling urinary catheter alleviates urine retention in high-risk patients. A transurethral resection may be performed if the prostate weighs under 2 oz (56.7 g). Weight is approximated by digital examination.

Transurethral needle ablation and transurethral microwave therapy are minimally invasive procedures that may be options for the older adult. Both procedures use heat through microwave energy to reduce the size of the prostate. Although the risk of morbidity is reduced with these procedures, the results are not as favorable as with transurethral resection. Electrovaporization of the prostate involves the use of a roller electrode to vaporize the prostate.

Other procedures involve open surgical removal of the prostate (prostatectomy). One of the following operations may be appropriate:

- suprapubic (transvesical) prostatectomy — most common operation; especially useful when prostatic enlargement remains within the bladder area
- perineal prostatectomy — usually performed for a large gland in an older patient; commonly results in impotence and incontinence
- retropubic (extravesical) prostatectomy — allows direct visualization; potency and continence usually maintained in about 50% of patients.

Key nursing diagnoses and outcomes

Impaired urinary elimination related to obstruction of the urethra

Treatment outcome: The patient will demonstrate skill in managing urine elimination problem.

Urge urinary incontinence related to obstruction of the urethra

Treatment outcomes: The patient will seek medical or surgical treatment, regain continence, and experience no complications of urinary incontinence (such as skin breakdown).

Nursing interventions

- Insert an indwelling urinary catheter for urine retention.
- Monitor intake and output.
- Avoid administering decongestants, tranquilizers, alcohol, antidepressants, or anticholinergics because these drugs can worsen obstruction.
- Monitor vital signs and daily weight.
- Monitor for signs of postobstructive diuresis (such as increased urine output and hypotension), which may lead to serious dehydration, lowered blood volume, shock, electrolyte losses, and anuria.
- Observe the patient for signs and symptoms of UTI, such as dysuria or changes in urine appearance, and obtain a urine specimen for culture and sensitivity.
- Administer antibiotics as ordered.

▶ Prepare the patient for diagnostic tests and surgery, as appropriate.

PATIENT TEACHING

▶ If an indwelling urinary catheter has been used to maintain urine flow until surgery can be done, the patient may experience urinary frequency, dribbling and, occasionally, hematuria after the catheter has been removed. Reassure him and his family that he'll gradually regain urinary control.

▶ Teach the patient to recognize the signs and symptoms of UTI. Urge him to immediately report these signs and symptoms to the physician because infection can worsen obstruction.

▶ Instruct the patient to follow the prescribed oral antibiotic regimen, and tell him the indications for using gentle laxatives.

▶ Urge the patient to seek medical care immediately if he can't void, passes bloody urine, or develops a fever.

▶ Advise the patient that it may take several months of medical therapy before symptoms improve; emphasize the importance of regular follow-up.

BIOFEEDBACK

A relatively new therapy, biofeedback refers to any modality that measures and immediately reports information about the patient's own physiologic processes. With biofeedback information, the patient can learn to consciously influence the measured body function, such as heart rate or blood pressure. The goal of biofeedback is to help him improve his overall health by consciously regulating bodily functions that are usually controlled unconsciously.

In this procedure, electrodes are attached to pertinent areas of the body to monitor such things as skeletal muscle activity, heart or brain wave activity, body temperature, or blood pressure. The electrodes feed information into a small monitoring box that reports the results by a sound or light that varies in pitch or brightness as the body function increases or decreases (the "feedback"). A biofeedback therapist leads the patient in mental exercises to help him regulate functions, such as body temperature, blood pressure, bladder control, or muscle tension, to reach the desired result. The patient eventually learns to control the body's inner mechanisms through mental processes.

The most common forms of biofeedback involve the measurement of muscle tension, skin temperature, electrical conductance or resistance of the skin, brain waves, and respiration. As advances in technology have made measurement devices more sophisticated, the applications of biofeedback have expanded. Sensors can now measure the activity of the internal and external rectal sphincters, the activity of the bladder's detrusor muscle, esophageal motility, and stomach acidity.

Some biofeedback treatments are accepted in traditional medicine. The American Medical Association, for instance, has endorsed electromyelogram biofeedback training for the treatment of muscle contraction headaches.

Biofeedback has a vast range of applications for prevention and health restoration. It is most successful in cases in which psychological factors play a role in the patient's health disturbance, such as sleep disorders and stress-related disorders. Patients with disorders arising from poor muscle control, such as incontinence, postural problems, back pain, and temporomandibular joint syndrome, also benefit. Biofeedback training has also been shown to benefit patients who have lost control of function as a result of brain or nerve damage or chronic pain disorders.

Improvement has also been seen in patients with heart dysfunctions, GI disorders, swallowing difficulties, esophageal dysfunction, tinnitus, eyelid twitching, fatigue, and cerebral palsy. Biofeedback isn't recommended for severe structural problems, such as broken bones or slipped disks.

Implementation

- You'll probably work with a trained biofeedback practitioner when conducting the session.
- Provide the patient with a private environment that is free from noise or other distractions.
- Gather the necessary equipment and wash your hands.
- Explain the procedure to the patient, and answer any questions he may have. If relaxation techniques or imagery will be used during the procedure, review this with the patient.
- Reassure the patient that biofeedback is not a test he has to pass, but a learning experience.
- Depending on the body function that will be monitored, clean and prepare the skin and attach the electrodes according to the manufacturer's instructions. The patient may experience a local skin irritation from the electrodes used in the biofeedback monitoring. Wash the skin well with soap and water to remove any leftover irritants, and pat it dry.
- Set the monitor where both you and the patient can easily see the results.
- Set a goal for the session with the patient, and review the information the patient will be seeing on the monitor.
- Turn on the monitor, and establish a baseline for the targeted body function.
- If goggles will be used, help the patient place them comfortably over his eyes.
- When the patient is ready, begin the session by starting the relaxation tapes or imagery sequence.
- At the close of the session, disconnect the monitor and remove the electrodes.
- Clean the patient's skin as needed.

BIPOLAR DISORDER

Also known as manic depressive illness and cyclical depression, bipolar disorder is characterized by cyclical mood changes from elation and euphoria to deep depression. The onset of bipolar disorder is usually between ages 20 and 30, but symptoms have been reported in late childhood and early adolescence. The cause of bipolar disorder is unclear, but hereditary, biological, and psychological factors may contribute.

Signs and symptoms

- Mood swings from hyperexcited euphoria to a moderate state, then to depression and psychomotor retardation
- Markedly changing mental status
- Confusion
- Agitation

Diagnostic tests

Diagnostic tests include those required to rule out an underlying disorder. Diagnosis can be confirmed if the patient meets the diagnostic criteria for bipolar disorder outlined in the *DSM-IV-TR*.

Treatment

Antipsychotic medication, such as haloperidol or thioridazine, is given for acute agitated behavior. Lithium carbonate is given to prevent recurrent manic episodes. Alternatively, valproic acid can be given to patients who don't tolerate lithium. Electroconvulsive therapy may be used if the patient can't tolerate lithium because of preexisting renal or cardiac disease.

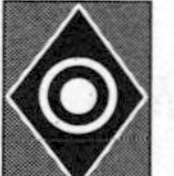

Drug alert **Concomitant use of lithium and thiazide diuretics may decrease renal excretion and enhance lithium toxicity. The dose of the diuretic may need to be reduced by 30%.**

Key nursing diagnoses and outcomes

Disturbed thought processes related to depression and mania

Treatment outcome: The patient will maintain controlled thought processes with treatment.

Disturbed sleep pattern related to episodes of mania

Treatment outcome: The patient will express feeling of being well rested.

Nursing interventions

- Monitor the patient for mood swings.
- Keep the patient in a safe, nonrestrictive environment.
- Administer medications as ordered, note their effectiveness, and monitor for adverse effects.
- Encourage the patient to seek counseling.
- Encourage follow-up care by a professional mental health practitioner.

PATIENT TEACHING

- Teach the patient and family members about the disease process, the treatment regimen, and possible adverse effects.
- Remind the patient to seek help if he feels out of control.
- Have family members or friends monitor the patient's behavior and report inappropriate actions to his mental health practitioner.
- Stress to the patient that this is a chronic condition and he shouldn't stop taking medications or therapies without first discussing it with his mental health practitioner.

BLADDER AND BOWEL RETRAINING

Habitual and automatic patterns of elimination are established as a person grows and develops. These patterns are influenced by various factors, such as diet, fluid intake, activity level, lifestyle, and advancing age.

In older people, two of the most common elimination problems are bladder and fecal incontinence. These problems may result from age- or disease-related changes in genitourinary or GI system function or, less commonly, from changes in other body systems, such as the musculoskeletal and nervous systems. If elimination problems are severe enough, they can have serious psychosocial effects and threaten the person's ability to live independently and to function and survive.

Incontinence commonly follows any loss or impairment of urinary or anal sphincter control. It may be transient or established. Urinary incontinence can have many causes, including confusion, depression, dehydration, fecal impaction, restricted mobility, urethral sphincter damage, certain drugs, and various disorders.

Although not usually a sign of serious illness, fecal incontinence can seriously impair an older patient's physical and psychological well-being. It may occur gradually (as in dementia) or suddenly (as in spinal cord injury). Most commonly, it results from fecal stasis and impaction accompanying reduced activity, inappropriate diet, untreated painful anal conditions, or chronic constipation. Fecal incontinence can also result from chronic laxative use; reduced fluid intake; neurologic deficits; pelvic, prostatic, or rectal surgery; and medications, such as antihistamines, psychotropics, and iron preparations.

A person with fecal incontinence might not be aware of the need to defecate. If he can't get to the bathroom or use a commode or bedpan on his own, he may lose rectal sensitivity from having to suppress the urge while waiting for help. Musculoskeletal changes also can affect a person's ability to assume a comfortable position, interfering with the frequency and effectiveness of bowel elimination. Social isolation, loss of independence, decreased self-esteem, and depression commonly follow incontinence problems.

Supplies

- Bedpan, urinal, toilet, or commode
- Toilet tissue
- Two washcloths
- Soap
- Gloves
- Towel
- Optional: linen-saver pad

Implementation

- Whether the patient reports urinary or fecal incontinence or both, you need to perform careful and continuing assessment to plan effective interventions. During your assessment, be sure to check for signs and symptoms of urinary tract infection.
- Be sure to schedule extra time to encourage and provide support for the patient and mitigate any feelings of shame, embarrassment, or powerlessness from loss of control.
- Praise the patient's successful efforts. Be sensitive to his feelings of embarrassment and self-consciousness.
- Always maximize the patient's level of independence while minimizing the risks to his self-esteem.

Bladder retraining

- To ensure healthful hydration and prevent urinary tract infection, be sure the patient maintains adequate daily fluid intake (eight to ten 8-oz [240-ml] glasses of fluid, if the patient's condition allows).
- To manage stress and urge incontinence, implement an exercise program to help strengthen the pelvic floor muscles. Biofeedback may be used to reinforce pelvic muscle contraction.
- To manage functional incontinence, frequently assess the patient's mental and functional status. Respond to his calls promptly, and help him get to the bathroom as quickly as possible.
- Encourage the patient to void every 2 hours. Once he can stay dry for 2 hours, increase the time between voidings by 30 minutes each day until he achieves a 3- to 4-hour voiding schedule.
- Have the patient empty his bladder completely before bedtime.

Bowel retraining

- Assess the patient to determine the usual time of day when a bowel movement occurs. To promote continence, you can then remind or help the patient to use the toilet or commode 15 to 20 minutes before that time. You might have to stay with him to make sure that he has a complete bowel movement.
- Have him contract his abdominal muscles or sway back and forth while on the toilet to help promote peristalsis.
- You may have to stay with a patient who has Alzheimer's disease and reinforce the need to stay on the toilet.
- Advise the patient to consume a fiber-rich diet, with raw, leafy vegetables (such as carrots and lettuce), unpeeled fruits (such as apples), and whole grains (such as wheat or rye breads and cereals). Bran cereals provide the best source of fiber.
- Encourage the patient to drink 2 to 3 qt (2 to 3 L) of fluid per day if his medical condition allows.
- Promote regular exercise by explaining how it helps to regulate bowel motility. Even a nonambulatory patient can perform some exercises while sitting or lying in bed.

Complications

Be alert for physiologic complications, such as skin breakdown and infection, especially in dual (urinary and fecal) incontinence.

Patient teaching

- Reassure the patient that periodic incontinent episodes do not mean the program has failed. Encourage persistence, tolerance, and a positive attitude.

- Teach the patient to gradually eliminate laxative use, if necessary. Point out that using over-the-counter laxatives to promote regular bowel movements can have the opposite effect and cause either constipation or incontinence over time. Suggest using natural laxatives, such as prunes or prune juice, instead.

Documentation

Record all bladder and bowel retraining efforts, noting scheduled bathroom times, food and fluid intake, and elimination amounts, as appropriate. Record the duration of continent periods. Note complications, including emotional problems and signs of skin breakdown and infection, and the treatment given. Also, document your patient teaching.

BLADDER CANCER

Benign or malignant tumors may develop on the bladder wall surface or grow within the wall itself and quickly invade underlying muscles. About 90% of bladder cancers are transitional cell carcinomas, arising from the transitional epithelium of mucous membranes. They may result from malignant transformation of benign papillomas. Less common bladder tumors include adenocarcinomas and squamous cell carcinomas.

Bladder tumors are most prevalent in people over age 50, are more common in men than in women, and occur more often in densely populated industrial areas. Bladder cancer is the fourth most common cause of cancer deaths in men over age 75.

Despite treatment, the patient with superficial disease has up to an 80% chance for recurrence. Only about 10% of superficial bladder cancers develop into invasive disease; in invasive disease, however, the patient's chances for metastasis are close to 90%. With treatment, about 50% of patients with invasive cancer experience a complete remission; 20% have a partial remission.

Certain substances, such as naphthylamine, tobacco, and nitrates, may predispose a person to transitional cell tumors. This places certain industrial workers (including rubber workers, weavers, aniline dye workers, hairdressers, petroleum workers, spray painters, and leather finishers) at high risk for developing bladder cancer. The latency period between exposure to the carcinogen and development of signs and symptoms is about 18 years.

Squamous cell carcinoma of the bladder is common in geographic areas in which schistosomiasis is endemic such as in Egypt. It's also associated with chronic bladder irritation and infection in people with renal calculi, indwelling urinary catheters, chemical cystitis that's caused by cyclophosphamide, and pelvic irradiation.

If bladder cancer progresses, complications include bone metastasis and problems resulting from tumor invasion of contiguous viscera.

Signs and symptoms

- Gross, painless, intermittent hematuria
- Suprapubic pain after voiding
- Bladder irritability
- Urinary frequency
- Nocturia
- Dribbling
- Flank pain, which can indicate an obstructed ureter

Key point **An older adult may not seek treatment for bladder irritability, urinary frequency, nocturia, and dribbling because he considers them normal changes of aging.**

Diagnostic tests

- *Cystoscopy* and *biopsy* confirm a bladder cancer diagnosis.

Cultural diversity **Performing a urologic examination or an invasive test such as cystoscopy can be problematic in Asian patients, who believe that the area between the waist and the knees is extremely personal and private.**

- *Excretory urography* can identify a large, early-stage tumor or an infiltrating tumor, delineate functional problems in the upper urinary tract, assess hydronephrosis, and detect rigid deformity of the bladder wall.
- *Urinalysis* detects blood and malignant cells in the urine.
- *Retrograde cystography* helps confirm a bladder cancer diagnosis.
- *Bone scan* detects metastasis.
- *Computed tomography scan* or *magnetic resonance imaging* defines the thickness of the involved bladder wall and any enlarged retroperitoneal lymph nodes.
- *Ultrasonography* can detect metastasis in tissues beyond the bladder and can also distinguish a bladder cyst from a bladder tumor.
- *Complete blood count* helps evaluate anemia, which is associated with bladder cancer.
- *Serum carcinoembryonic antigen level* is a tumor marker that is present with adenocarcinomas of the bladder.

Treatment

The type of treatment used depends on the stage of the cancer, the patient's lifestyle and other health problems, and his mental outlook. Surgery, chemotherapy, or radiation therapy may be used.

Superficial bladder tumors are typically removed cystoscopically by transurethral resection and electrically by fulguration. This approach usually is effective if the tumor hasn't invaded the muscle. If additional tumors develop, fulguration may have to be repeated every 3 months for years. Once the tumors penetrate the muscle layer or recur frequently, cystoscopy with fulguration is no longer an appropriate treatment choice.

Intravesical chemotherapy is used to treat superficial tumors (especially tumors in several sites) and to prevent tumor recurrence. This approach directly washes the bladder with drugs that fight the cancer, such as thiotepa, doxorubicin, and mitomycin. Intravesical administration of live, attenuated bacille Calmette-Guérin vaccine has also been effective in treating superficial bladder cancers, particularly primary and relapsed carcinoma in situ.

Tumors too large to be treated by cystoscopy require segmental bladder resection. This surgical approach removes a full-thickness section of the bladder and is practical only if the tumor isn't located near the bladder neck or ureteral orifices. Bladder instillation of thiotepa after transurethral resection may also be useful.

For patients with infiltrating bladder tumors, the treatment of choice is radical cystectomy. Treatment for patients with advanced bladder cancer includes cystectomy to remove the tumor, radiation therapy, and combination systemic chemotherapy with cisplatin, the most active agent. Other agents include methotrexate, vinblastine, and doxorubicin. In some instances, this combined treatment successfully arrests the disease.

Key nursing diagnoses and outcomes

Impaired urinary elimination related to changes in bladder function

Treatment outcome: The patient will maintain adequate urine elimination through natural or artificial means.

Fear related to potential radical changes in body image and possibly death from bladder cancer

Treatment outcomes: The patient will express reduced fear and demonstrate no physical signs of fear.

Acute pain related to urinary tract infection or cancer cell invasion to surrounding tissues
Treatment outcome: The patient will become pain-free after treatment.

Nursing interventions

- Monitor intake and output.
- Observe for signs of hematuria (reddish tint to gross bleeding) or infection (cloudy, foul smelling, with sediment present). The older adult with a urinary tract infection (UTI) may present with new onset of incontinence or worsening of incontinence as well as lethargy or confusion.
- Monitor laboratory tests, such as changes in white blood cell differential, indicating possible bone marrow suppression from chemotherapy.
- If treatment includes intravesical chemotherapy, watch closely for myelosuppression, chemical cystitis, and rash.
- If treatment includes chemotherapy, watch for complications from the particular drug regimen.
- Listen to the patient's fears and concerns; stay with him during episodes of severe stress and anxiety, and provide psychological support as needed.
- Encourage the patient to express his feelings and concerns about the extent of the cancer, the surgical procedure, an altered body image (especially if he undergoes urinary diversion surgery), and sexual dysfunction.
- Provide comfort measures for the patient.
- Administer analgesics as ordered, and monitor their effectiveness.

PATIENT TEACHING

- Tell the patient what to expect from the diagnostic tests. For example, make sure he understands that he may be anesthetized before he undergoes cystoscopy. After the test results are known, explain their implications to the patient and his family.
- Instruct the patient and family about the planned treatment. Teach them how to recognize and manage adverse effects of chemotherapy, if applicable.
- Teach the patient and family how to care for urinary diversions, if performed; arrange for home care follow-up if necessary.
- Stress the importance of notifying the physician if the patient develops signs and symptoms of UTI or other sudden changes in his condition.
- Refer the patient to the American Cancer Society as appropriate.

BLOOD SAMPLE COLLECTION

Performed to obtain a venous blood sample, venipuncture involves piercing a vein with a needle and collecting blood in a syringe or evacuated tube. Typically, venipuncture is performed using the antecubital fossa. If necessary, however, it can be performed on a vein in the wrist, the dorsum of the hand or foot, or another accessible location. Usually, laboratory personnel carry out the procedure in the hospital setting; however, a nurse may perform it occasionally.

Supplies

- Tourniquet
- Gloves
- Syringe or evacuated tubes and needle holder
- 70% isopropyl alcohol pad
- 20G or 21G needle for the forearm or 25G for the wrist, hand, ankle, and for the older patient with poor venous access
- Color-coded tubes containing appropriate additives
- Labels
- Laboratory request form
- 2″ × 2″ gauze pads
- Adhesive bandage

Implementation

▶ If you're using evacuated tubes, open the needle packet, attach the needle to its holder, and select the appropriate tubes.

▶ If you're using a syringe, attach the appropriate needle to it. Be sure to choose a syringe large enough to hold all the blood required for the test.

▶ Label all collection tubes clearly with the patient's name and room number, the physician's name, and the date and time of collection.

▶ Wash your hands thoroughly and put on gloves to prevent cross-contamination.

▶ Tell the patient that you're about to take a blood sample, and explain the procedure to ease his anxiety and encourage his cooperation. Ask him if he has ever felt faint, sweaty, or nauseated when having blood drawn.

▶ If the patient is on bed rest, ask him to lie supine, with his head slightly elevated and his arms at his sides. Ask the ambulatory patient to sit in a chair and support his arm securely on an armrest or table.

▶ Don't choose an extremity with a dialysis access or the affected arm of a mastectomy patient. Also, never draw a venous sample from an arm or leg already being used for I.V. therapy or blood administration because this may affect test results.

▶ Don't draw a venous sample from an infection site because this risks introducing pathogens into the vascular system. Likewise, avoid drawing blood from edematous areas, arteriovenous shunts, or sites of previous hematoma or vascular injury.

▶ If the patient has large, distended, highly visible veins, perform venipuncture without a tourniquet to minimize the risk of hematoma.

▶ If the patient has a clotting disorder or is receiving anticoagulant therapy, maintain firm pressure on the venipuncture site for at least 5 minutes after withdrawing the needle to prevent possible formation of a hematoma.

▶ Avoid using veins in the patient's legs for venipuncture, if possible, because this increases the risk of thrombophlebitis.

▶ Assess the patient's veins to determine the best puncture site. (See *Common venipuncture sites.*) Observe the skin for the vein's blue color, or palpate the vein for a firm rebound sensation.

▶ Tie a tourniquet 2″ (5 cm) proximal to the area chosen. By impeding venous return to the heart while still allowing arterial flow, a tourniquet produces venous dilation. If arterial perfusion remains adequate, you'll be able to feel the

Common venipuncture sites

The illustrations below show common anatomic locations of veins used for venipuncture. The most used sites are on the forearm, followed by those on the hand.

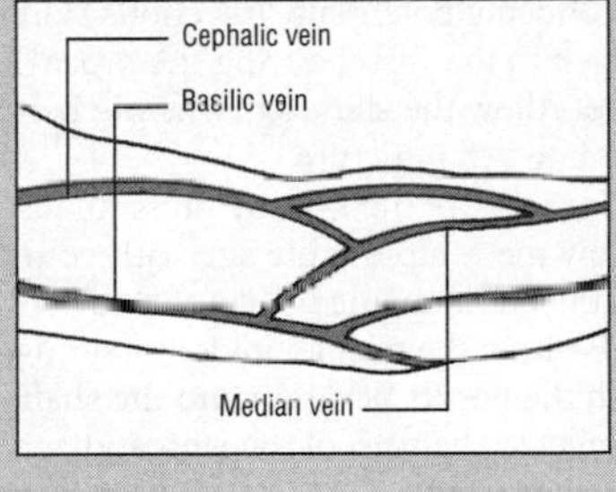

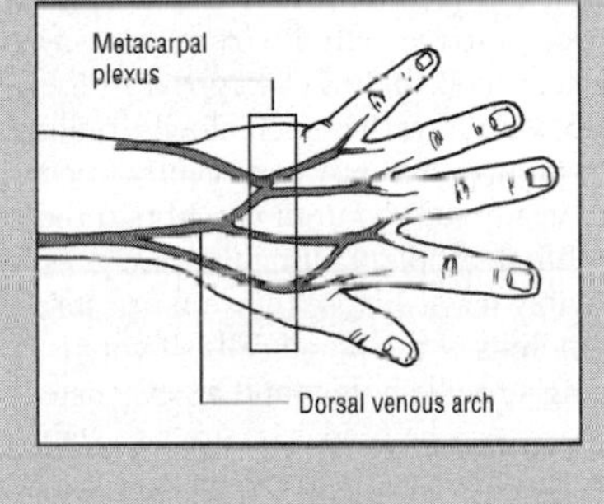

radial pulse. (If the tourniquet fails to dilate the vein, have the patient open and close his fist repeatedly. Then ask him to close his fist as you insert the needle and to open it again when the needle is in place.)

▶ Clean the venipuncture site with an alcohol pad. Wipe in a circular motion, spiraling outward from the site to avoid introducing potentially infectious skin flora into the vessel during the procedure. Allow the skin to dry before performing venipuncture.

▶ Immobilize the vein by pressing just below the venipuncture site with your thumb and drawing the skin taut.

▶ Position the needle holder or syringe with the needle bevel up and the shaft parallel to the path of the vein and at a 15-degree angle to the arm. Insert the needle into the vein. If you're using a syringe, venous blood will appear in the hub; withdraw the blood slowly, pulling the plunger of the syringe gently to create steady suction until you obtain the required sample. Pulling the plunger too forcibly may collapse the vein or cause hemolysis of the blood cells. If you're using a needle holder and an evacuated tube, grasp the holder securely to stabilize it in the vein, and push down on the collection tube until the needle punctures the rubber stopper. Blood will flow into the tube automatically.

▶ Remove the tourniquet as soon as blood flows adequately to prevent stasis and hemoconcentration, which can impair test results. If the flow is sluggish, leave the tourniquet in place longer, but always remove it before withdrawing the needle.

▶ Continue to fill the required tubes, removing one and inserting another. Gently rotate each tube as you remove it to help mix the additive.

▶ After you've drawn the sample, place a gauze pad over the puncture site, and slowly and gently remove the needle from the vein. When using an evacuated tube, remove it from the needle holder to release the vacuum before withdrawing the needle from the vein.

▶ Apply gentle pressure to the puncture site for 2 to 3 minutes or until bleeding stops. This prevents extravasation into the surrounding tissue, which causes hematoma.

▶ After bleeding stops, apply an adhesive bandage.

▶ If you've used a syringe, transfer the sample to a collection tube. Detach the needle from the syringe, open the collection tube, and gently empty the sample into the tube, being careful to avoid foaming, which may cause hemolysis.

▶ Finally, check the venipuncture site to make sure a hematoma hasn't developed. If it has, then apply warm soaks.

▶ Discard syringes, needles, and used gloves in the appropriate containers.

Complications

Hematoma at the needle insertion site is the most common complication of venipuncture. Infection may result from poor technique.

Patient teaching

▶ Explain the procedure to the patient. If appropriate, tell him why the sample is being collected.

▶ Inform the patient that there may be some bruising or tenderness at the venipuncture site after this procedure.

Documentation

Record the date, time, and site of venipuncture; the name of the test; the time the sample was sent to the laboratory; and any adverse effects the patient experiences, such as a hematoma or anxiety.

BLOOD TRANSFUSION

Whole blood transfusion replenishes acute massive blood loss and the oxygen-carrying capacity of the circulatory system. Transfusion of packed red blood cells (RBCs), from which 80% of the plasma has been removed, restores only the oxygen-carrying capacity. Both types of transfusion treat decreased hemoglobin levels and hematocrit.

Whole blood is usually transfused only when decreased levels result from hemorrhage; packed RBCs are transfused when such depressed levels do not require a large blood volume replacement to avoid possible fluid and circulatory overload. However, in the older patient, packed RBC transfusion can also lead to fluid and circulatory overload. (See *Transfusing blood and selected components*, pages 110 to 113.)

Both whole blood and packed RBCs contain cellular debris, necessitating in-line filtration during administration. (Washed packed RBCs—commonly used for patients previously sensitized by transfusions—are rinsed with a special solution that removes white blood cells and platelets, thus decreasing the chance of a transfusion reaction.)

Transfusion of plasma and its fractions serves various therapeutic purposes. For example, transfusion of platelets can correct an extremely low platelet count (below 10,000 to 20,000/µl), which can occur in patients with hematologic diseases, such as aplastic anemia and leukemia, and in those receiving antineoplastic chemotherapy. Usually, a large quantity of platelets—typically 4 U or more for an adult—is required to prevent or control bleeding.

Transfusion of fresh frozen plasma (FFP), which contains most clotting factors but no platelets, is ordered to treat an undetermined clotting factor deficiency, a specific factor deficiency when that factor alone isn't available, and factor deficiencies resulting from hepatic disease or blood dilution. Transfusion of FFP is the only treatment for factor V deficiency.

Although plasma functions as a blood-volume expander, plasma protein fraction (a 5% solution of selected proteins [albumin and some globulins] from pooled plasma in a buffered, stabilized saline diluent) and albumin (extracted from heat-treated, chemically processed plasma and available in 5% [isotonic] and 25% [hypertonic] preparations) are used more commonly. Both preparations also treat hypoproteinemia and hypoalbuminemia. Hypertonic albumin also reduces cerebral edema by drawing large amounts of extravascular fluid into the vascular system. Albumin transfusion is contraindicated in severe anemia because of the risk of cellular dehydration and should be administered cautiously in cardiac and pulmonary disease because of the risk of heart failure from circulatory overload.

Transfusion of cryoprecipitate, which forms when FFP thaws slowly, replaces missing clotting factors in hemophilia A, von Willebrand's disease, and fibrinogen and factor XIII deficiencies. However, transfusion of recombinant factor VIII (antihemophilia) is the long-term treatment of choice for hemophilia A because the amount of factor VIII per vial varies less than with cryoprecipitate. Recombinant factor VIII can also reduce the risk of transmitting viruses because it's genetically engineered, not a product of human blood.

Depending on facility policy, two nurses may have to identify the patient and blood product before administering a transfusion to prevent errors and a potentially fatal reaction. The procedure also usually requires a signed patient consent form.

Cultural diversity Jehovah's Witnesses oppose blood transfusions based on their interpretation of certain biblical passages. The courts have generally upheld their right to refuse treatment based on the constitutional guarantee of freedom of religion.

Standards established by the American Association of Blood Banks, in accordance with federal, state, and local regulations, allow a physician to order

(Text continues on page 112.)

Transfusing blood and selected components

Blood components	Indications
Whole blood Red blood cells (RBCs) and plasma components; processing removes most of the platelets and white blood cells (WBCs or leukocytes) *Volume: 500 ml*	■ To restore blood volume lost from hemorrhaging, trauma, or burns
Packed RBCs Same RBC mass as whole blood, but with 80% of the plasma removed *Volume: 250 ml*	■ To restore or maintain oxygen-carrying capacity ■ To correct anemia and blood loss that occurs during surgery ■ To increase RBC mass
Leukocyte-poor RBCs Same as packed RBCs with about 70% of the leukocytes removed *Volume: 200 ml*	■ Same as packed RBCs ■ To prevent febrile reactions from leukocyte antibodies ■ To treat immunocompromised patients
WBCs Whole blood with all the RBCs and about 80% of the supernatant plasma removed *Volume: usually 150 ml*	■ To treat sepsis that's unresponsive to antibiotics (especially if patient has positive blood cultures or a persistent fever exceeding 101° F [38.3° C]) and granulocytopenia (granulocyte count usually less than 500/µl)
Platelets Platelet sediment from RBCs or plasma *Volume: 35 to 50 ml/U; 1 U of platelets = 7×10^7 platelets*	■ To treat thrombocytopenia caused by decreased platelet production, increased platelet destruction, or massive transfusion of stored blood ■ To treat acute leukemia and marrow aplasia ■ To control active bleeding in a patient whose count is 50,000/µl or less ■ To prevent bleeding in a patient whose count is 20,000/µl or less ■ To improve platelet count preoperatively in a patient whose count is 100,000/µl or less

Crossmatching	Nursing considerations
■ ABO identical: Type A receives A; type B receives B; type AB receives AB; type O receives O ■ Rhesus factor (Rh) match necessary	■ Use a straight-line or Y-type I.V. set to infuse blood over 1 to 4 hours. ■ Avoid giving whole blood when the patient can't tolerate the circulatory volume. ■ Reduce the risk of a transfusion reaction by adding a microfilter to the administration set to remove platelets. ■ Warm blood if giving a large quantity.
■ Type A receives A or O ■ Type B receives B or O ■ Type AB receives AB, A, B, or O ■ Type O receives O ■ Rh match necessary	■ Use a straight-line or Y-type I.V. set to infuse blood over 1 to 4 hours. ■ Bear in mind that packed RBCs provide the same oxygen-carrying capacity as whole blood without the hazards of volume overload. ■ Give packed RBCs, as ordered, to prevent potassium and ammonia buildup, which may occur in stored plasma. ■ Avoid administering packed RBCs for anemic conditions correctable by nutritional or drug therapy. ■ Expect a 3% increase in hematocrit and a 1-g increase in hemoglobin per unit of packed RBCs.
■ Same as packed RBCs ■ Rh match necessary	■ Use a straight-line or Y-type I.V. set to infuse blood over 1 to 4 hours. ■ Use a 40-micron filter suitable for hard-spun, leukocyte-poor RBCs. ■ Other considerations are the same as those for packed RBCs.
■ Same as packed RBCs ■ Compatibility with human leukocyte antigen (HLA) preferable but not necessary unless patient is sensitized to HLA from previous transfusions ■ Rh match necessary	■ Use a straight-line I.V. set with a standard in-line blood filter to infuse over 1 to 2 hours. ■ Provide 1 U daily for 5 days, until infection resolves, or until the neutrophil count is greater than 500/ml. ■ As prescribed, premedicate with diphenhydramine. ■ Because a WBC infusion induces fever and chills, administer an antipyretic if fever occurs. However, don't discontinue the transfusion; instead, reduce the flow rate, as ordered, for patient comfort. ■ Agitate container to prevent WBCs from settling, thus preventing the delivery of a bolus infusion of WBCs. ■ Give transfusion with antibiotics (but not amphotericin B) to treat infection.
■ ABO compatibility unnecessary but preferable with repeated platelet transfusions ■ Rh match preferred	■ Use a component drip administration set to infuse over 15 to 30 minutes. ■ As prescribed, premedicate with antipyretics, antihistamines, or hydrocortisone, if the patient's history includes a platelet transfusion reaction. ■ Avoid administering platelets when the patient has a fever. ■ Prepare to draw blood for a platelet count, as ordered, 1 hour after the platelet transfusion to determine platelet transfusion increments. A unit of platelets should increase the platelet count by 5,000 to 10,000/µl. ■ Keep in mind that the physician seldom orders a platelet transfusion for conditions in which platelet destruction is accelerated, such as idiopathic thrombocytopenic purpura or drug-induced thrombocytopenia.

(continued)

Transfusing blood and selected components *(continued)*

Blood components	Indications
Fresh frozen plasma (FFP) Uncoagulated plasma separated from RBCs and rich in coagulation factors V, VIII, and IX *Volume: 200 to 250 ml*	■ To expand plasma volume ■ To treat postsurgical hemorrhage or shock ■ To correct an undetermined coagulation factor deficiency ■ To replace a specific factor when that factor alone isn't available ■ To correct factor deficiencies resulting from hepatic disease
Albumin 5% (buffered saline); albumin 25% (salt-poor) A small plasma protein prepared by fractionating pooled plasma *Volume: 5% = 12.5 g/250 ml; 25% = 12.5 g/ 50 ml*	■ To replace volume lost because of shock from burns, trauma, surgery, or infections ■ To replace volume and prevent marked hemoconcentration ■ To treat hypoproteinemia (with or without edema)
Factor VIII (cryoprecipitate) Insoluble portion of plasma recovered from FFP *Volume: About 30 ml (freeze-dried)*	■ To treat a patient with hemophilia A ■ To control bleeding associated with factor VIII deficiency ■ To replace fibrinogen or deficient factor VIII
Factors II, VII, IX, X complex (prothrombin complex) Lyophilized, commercially prepared solution drawn from pooled plasma	■ To treat a congenital factor V deficiency and other bleeding disorders resulting from an acquired deficiency of factors II, VII, IX, and X

transfusions of blood products (not whole blood) for home care patients. To qualify, a patient must be unable to leave his home without assistance and must have received previous transfusions without difficulties.

Supplies

- Blood administration set (filter and tubing with drip chamber for blood, or combined set). Straight-line and Y-type blood administration sets are commonly used.
- I.V. pole
- Gloves
- Face shield
- Alcohol pad
- Adhesive tape
- Whole blood, packed RBCs, plasma or plasma fraction
- 250 ml of normal saline solution

Crossmatching	Nursing considerations
■ ABO compatibility unnecessary but preferable with repeated transfusions ■ Rh match preferred	■ Use a straight-line I.V. set and administer the infusion rapidly. ■ Keep in mind that large-volume transfusions of FFP may require correction for hypocalcemia because citric acid in FFP binds calcium.
■ Unnecessary	■ Use a straight-line I.V. set with rate and volume dictated by the patient's condition and response. ■ Remember that reactions to albumin (fever, chills, nausea) are rare. ■ Avoid mixing albumin with protein hydrolysates and alcohol solutions. ■ Consider delivering albumin as a volume expander until the laboratory completes crossmatching for a whole blood transfusion. ■ Keep in mind that albumin is contraindicated in severe anemia and administered cautiously in cardiac and pulmonary disease because heart failure may result from circulatory overload.
■ ABO compatibility unnecessary but preferable	■ Use the administration set supplied by the manufacturer. Administer factor VIII with a filter. Standard dose recommended for treatment of acute bleeding episodes in hemophilia is 15 to 20 U/kg. ■ Half-life of factor VIII (8 to 10 hours) necessitates repeated transfusions at these intervals to maintain normal levels.
■ ABO and Rh match unnecessary	■ Administer with a straight-line I.V. set, basing dose on desired factor level and patient's body weight. ■ Recognize that a high risk of hepatitis accompanies this type of transfusion. ■ Arrange to draw blood for a coagulation assay to be performed before administration and at suitable intervals during treatment. ■ Keep in mind that this type of transfusion is contraindicated when the patient has hepatic disease resulting in fibrinolysis and when the patient has disseminated intravascular coagulation and isn't undergoing heparin therapy.

▶ Venipuncture equipment, if necessary (should include 18G catheter or 19G needle)

▶ Optional: gown, ice bag, warm compresses, leukocyte removal filter, or blood warmer

Implementation

▶ Make sure that the patient has signed an informed consent form before beginning transfusion therapy.

▶ Check the physician's order.

▶ If an I.V. line is already in place, check the insertion site for inflammation and the line for patency.

▶ If an I.V. line is not in place, perform a venipuncture, preferably using an 18G catheter or a 19G needle. Avoid using an existing line if the catheter or needle lumen is smaller than 20G. Central venous access devices also may be used.

Administering whole blood and packed cells

▶ Prepare the equipment when you're ready to start the infusion.

▶ Record the patient's baseline temperature and vital signs. Assess his skin for flushing, moisture, or rash.

▶ Obtain whole blood or packed RBCs from the blood bank within 30 minutes of the transfusion start time. Check the expiration date on the blood bag, and observe for abnormal color, RBC clumping, gas bubbles, and extraneous material. Return outdated or abnormal blood to the blood bank.

▶ Compare the name and number on the patient's wristband with those on the blood bag label. Check the blood bag identification number, ABO blood group, and rhesus factor compatibility. Also, compare the patient's blood bank identification number, if present, with the number on the blood bag. Identification of blood and blood products is performed at the patient's bedside by two licensed professionals according to facility policy.

▶ Put on gloves, and a face shield. Using a Y-type set, close all the clamps on the set. Then insert the spike of the line you're using for the normal saline solution into the bag of saline solution. Next, open the port on the blood bag, and insert the spike of the line you're using to administer the blood or cellular component into the port. Hang the bag of normal saline solution and the bag of blood or cellular component on the I.V. pole, open the clamp on the line of saline solution, and squeeze the drip chamber until it's half full. Then remove the adapter cover at the tip of the blood administration set, open the main flow clamp, and prime the tubing with saline solution.

▶ If you're administering packed RBCs with a Y-type set, you can add saline solution to the bag to dilute the cells by closing the clamp between the patient and the drip chamber and opening the clamp from the blood. Lower the blood bag below the saline container and let 30 to 50 ml of saline solution flow into the packed cells. Finally, close the clamp to the blood bag, rehang the bag, rotate it gently to mix the cells and saline solution, and close the clamp to the saline container.

▶ If administering whole blood, gently invert the bag several times to mix the cells.

▶ Using an alcohol pad, wipe the Y-injection port of the I.V. catheter.

▶ Attach the prepared blood administration set to the I.V. catheter, and flush it with normal saline solution.

▶ Then close the clamp to the saline solution, and open the clamp between the blood bag and the patient. Adjust the flow clamp closest to the patient to deliver the blood at the calculated drip rate.

▶ Remain with the patient, and watch for signs of a transfusion reaction. If such signs develop, stop the transfusion, record vital signs, infuse the saline solution at a keep-vein-open rate, and notify the physician at once. In the case of a transfusion reaction, both the blood bag and I.V. tubing must be returned to the blood bank for testing. If no signs of a reaction appear within 15 minutes, you'll need to adjust the flow clamp to the ordered infusion rate. Raising and lowering the blood bag to adjust the rate reduces the risk of hemolysis from pressure on the tubing. A unit of RBCs may be given over 1 to 4 hours, as ordered.

▶ If a hematoma develops at the I.V. site, immediately stop the infusion. Remove the needle or catheter. Notify the physician and expect to place ice on the site intermittently for 8 hours; then apply warm compresses. Promote reabsorption of the hematoma by elevating the affected limb and by having the patient gently exercise it.

If the transfusion stops, take the following steps as needed:

▶ Check that the I.V. container is at least 3′ (1 m) above the level of the I.V. site.

- Make sure that the flow clamp is open and that the blood completely covers the filter. If it doesn't, squeeze the drip chamber until it does.
- Gently rock the bag back and forth, agitating any blood cells that may have settled on the bottom.
- Untape the dressing over the I.V. site to check catheter placement. Reposition the catheter if necessary.
- Flush the line with saline solution and restart the transfusion. Using a Y-type set, close the flow clamp to the patient and lower the blood bag. Next, open the saline clamp and allow some saline solution to flow into the blood bag. Rehang the blood bag, open the flow clamp to the patient, and reset the flow rate.
- After completing the transfusion, you'll need to put on gloves and flush the filter and tubing with normal saline solution, if this is recommended by the manufacturer. Then remember to reconnect the original I.V. fluid or discontinue the I.V. infusion.
- Return the empty blood bag to the blood bank, and discard the tubing and filter.
- Record the patient's vital signs.
- Some microaggregate filters can be used for more than one unit of blood. Check the manufacturer's label. Always replace the filter and tubing if more than 1 hour elapses between transfusions. When administering multiple units of blood under pressure, use a blood warmer to avoid hypothermia.
- If the blood bag empties before the next one arrives, administer normal saline solution slowly. If you're using a Y-type set, close the blood-line clamp, open the saline-line clamp, and let the saline solution run slowly until the new blood arrives. Decrease the flow rate or clamp the line before attaching the new unit of blood.

Administering plasma, FFP, albumin, factor VIII concentrate, or prothrombin complex

- When transfusing a prothrombin preparation, carefully reconstitute it according to the manufacturer's directions if you did not receive it already prepared by the pharmacy.
- Positively identify the patient by carefully comparing the name and number on his wristband with the information on the laboratory slip. Follow your facility's policy for proper blood or blood product identification.
- Obtain baseline temperature and vital signs. Assess the patient's skin for flushing, moisture, or a rash.
- Attach the appropriate administration set to the plasma or plasma product and the needleless adapter to the tubing. Then prime the system.
- Using an alcohol pad, wipe the Y-injection port of the primary administration set. Then insert the needleless adapter from the plasma product administration set into the injection port, stop the saline infusion, and adjust the flow rate of the plasma or plasma product, as ordered.

Administering platelets or cryoprecipitate with a component drip set

- Positively identify the patient by carefully comparing the name and number on his wristband with the information on the laboratory slip. Follow your facility's policy for proper blood or blood product identification.
- Obtain baseline temperature and vital signs. Assess the patient's skin for flushing, moisture, and a rash.
- Open the port of the platelet or cryoprecipitate bag by pulling back the tabs. Then remove the protective cover of the administration set spike.
- Close the flow clamp and, using a twisting motion, insert the administration set spike into the port. Hang the bag, compress the drip chamber until fluid fully covers the filter, and open the clamp. Then prime the tubing and close

the clamp. Attach a needleless adapter to the end of the tubing.

▶ Using an alcohol pad, wipe the Y-injection port of the primary administration set. Then insert the needleless adapter from the component drip set into the injection port and stop the saline infusion.

▶ Completely open the flow clamp on the component drip set to administer the platelets or cryoprecipitate rapidly, preventing clumping or loss of activity.

Administering platelets or cryoprecipitate with a component syringe set

▶ After proper identification and assessment of the patient, close both clamps on the syringe set. Then open the port of the platelet or cryoprecipitate bag by pulling back the tabs. Next, remove the protective cover of the administration set spike.

▶ Using a twisting motion, insert the administration set spike into the port. Then attach the syringe to the luer-tip port.

▶ Open the clamp above the Y-connection, aspirate the contents of the bag into the syringe, and close the clamp. Then open the clamp below the Y-connection, hold the syringe upright, prime the tubing, and close the clamp.

▶ Using an alcohol pad, wipe the Y-injection port of the primary administration set.

▶ Insert the needle from the syringe set into the injection port, and stop the saline infusion. Depress the syringe plunger and rapidly administer the platelets or cryoprecipitate to prevent clumping or loss of activity.

▶ With either set, administer subsequent bags of platelets by removing the administration set spike and inserting it into a new bag. Remember, if you are using a drip set, close the clamp and attach a new bag before the drip chamber empties and air enters the line. If you are using a syringe set, close the clamp closest to the patient before aspiration.

▶ After completing the infusion, flush the line with 20 to 30 ml of saline solution, and discontinue the I.V. unless therapy is scheduled to continue; then, if appropriate, hang the original I.V. solution and adjust the flow rate, as ordered.

Complications

Despite increasingly accurate crossmatching precautions, transfusion reactions can occur. Mediated by immune or nonimmune factors, a transfusion reaction can accompany or follow I.V. administration of blood components. Its severity varies from mild (fever and chills) to severe (acute renal failure or complete vascular collapse and death), depending on the amount of blood transfused, the type of reaction, and the patient's general health.

Unlike a transfusion reaction, an infectious disease transmitted during a transfusion may go undetected until days, weeks, or even months later, when it produces signs and symptoms. Measures to prevent disease transmission include laboratory testing of blood products and careful screening of potential donors, neither of which is guaranteed.

Hepatitis C accounts for most post-transfusion hepatitis cases. The tests that detect hepatitis B and hepatitis C can produce false-negative results and may allow some hepatitis cases to go undetected.

When testing for antibodies to human immunodeficiency virus (HIV), keep in mind that antibodies don't appear until about 6 to 12 weeks after exposure. Donated blood is tested for HIV_1 antibodies, HIV_2 antibodies, and HIV_1 p24 antigen, but blood from a donor exposed to HIV who has not yet developed detectable antibodies could infect the recipient. The estimated risk of acquiring HIV from blood products varies from 1 in 450,000 to 1 in 660,000, depending on the source.

Many blood banks screen blood for cytomegalovirus (CMV). Blood with CMV is especially dangerous for an immunosuppressed, seronegative patient. Blood banks also test blood for syphilis, but the routine practice of refrigerating blood kills the syphilis organism and virtually eliminates the risk of transfusion-related syphilis.

Circulatory overload and hemolytic, allergic, febrile, and pyogenic reactions can result from any transfusion. Coagulation disturbances, citrate intoxication, hyperkalemia, acid-base imbalance, loss of 2,3-diphosphoglycerate, ammonia intoxication, and hypothermia can result from massive transfusion.

Patient teaching

- Explain the procedure to the patient to reduce fear and promote cooperation.
- Ask the patient to report any unusual sensations experienced during the transfusion such as chills, feelings of apprehension, chest or low back pain, and headache.

Documentation

Record the date and time of the transfusion, the type and amount of transfusion product, the patient's vital signs, your check of all identification data, and the patient's response. Document any transfusion reaction and treatment, according to your facility's policy.

BOWEL RESECTION WITH ANASTOMOSIS

Surgical resection of diseased intestinal tissue and anastomosis of the remaining segments helps treat localized obstructive disorders, including diverticulosis (with an area of acute diverticulitis or abscess formation), intestinal polyps, adhesions that cause bowel dysfunction, and malignant or benign intestinal lesions. It's the preferred surgical technique for localized bowel cancer but not for widespread carcinoma, which usually requires massive resection with creation of a temporary or permanent colostomy or an ileostomy.

Implementation

After the patient has received a general anesthetic, the surgeon makes the abdominal incision. The incision site varies, depending on the pathology's location. The surgeon limits the resection to the diseased area and a wide margin of surrounding normal tissue. After excising the diseased colonic tissue, the surgeon then anastomoses the remaining bowel segments to restore patency. End-to-end anastomosis provides the most physiologically sound junction and is the quickest to perform, but it requires that the approximated bowel segments be large enough to prevent postoperative obstruction at the anastomosis site. Side-to-side anastomosis minimizes the danger of obstruction, but this lengthy procedure may be contraindicated in an emergency. After the anastomosis is complete, the surgeon closes the incision and applies a sterile dressing.

Complications

Several complications can occur in a patient who has had a bowel resection with anastomosis. These include bleeding or leakage from the anastomosis site, peritonitis and resultant sepsis, postresection obstruction, and problems common to all patients undergoing abdominal surgery, such as wound infection and atelectasis.

Key nursing diagnoses and outcomes

Risk for infection related to anastomotic leak or spillage (or both) of intestinal contents into the abdominal cavity during surgery

Treatment outcome: The patient will experience no signs or symptoms of peritonitis, such as abdominal distention or increased abdominal pain.

Ineffective breathing pattern related to guarded respirations secondary to the abdominal incision

Treatment outcome: The patient will maintain adequate ventilation (as exhibited by normal respiratory rate and rhythm), clear breath sounds on auscultation, and normal arterial blood gas values postoperatively.

Nursing interventions

In caring for a patient undergoing bowel resection with anastomosis, your major roles include surgical preparation and postoperative care tailored to his condition.

Before surgery

- Explain that the surgery will remove a diseased portion of the patient's bowel and will connect the remaining healthy segments. Keep in mind that the patient and his family members will probably have many questions about the surgery and its effect on the patient's lifestyle. Take the time to listen to their concerns and to answer their questions.
- Discuss anticipated postoperative care measures. Tell the patient that he'll awaken from surgery with a nasogastric (NG) tube in place to drain air and fluid from the intestinal tract and prevent distention. Explain that when peristalsis returns, usually within 2 to 3 days, the tube will be removed. Tell him to anticipate ambulation on the first day after surgery to promote return of peristalsis. Also, prepare him for the presence of an I.V. line, which will provide fluid replacement, a urinary catheter, pneumatic compression boots or stockings to prevent venous stasis, and abdominal drains.
- To reduce the risk of postoperative atelectasis and pneumonia, teach the patient how to cough and deep-breathe properly and emphasize the need to do so regularly throughout the recovery period. Demonstrate incisional splinting to protect the sutures and reduce discomfort.
- Reassure the patient that pain medication will be available. Instruct him in the use of controlled analgesia if appropriate.
- Before surgery, as ordered, administer antibiotics to reduce intestinal flora and laxatives or enemas to remove fecal contents.
- Ensure that the patient or a responsible family member has signed a consent form.

After surgery

- For the first few days after surgery, carefully monitor intake and output and weigh the patient daily. Maintain fluid and electrolyte balance through I.V. replacement therapy, and check the patient regularly for signs and symptoms of dehydration, such as decreased urine output and poor skin turgor. Administer pain medication as needed.
- Keep the NG tube patent. Record the amount of drainage accumulated during each shift. Monitor for the return of peristalsis. Palpate the abdomen and ask the patient if he's been passing flatus.
- To detect possible complications, carefully monitor the patient's vital signs and closely assess his overall condition. Remember that anastomotic leakage may produce only vague signs and symptoms at first; watch for low-grade fever, malaise, slight leukocytosis, and abdominal distention and tenderness. Also, be alert for more extensive hemorrhage from acute leakage, and watch for signs and symptoms of hypovolemic shock (precipitous drop in blood pressure, tachycardia, respiratory difficulty, decreased level of consciousness) and bloody stool or wound drainage.
- Observe the patient for signs and symptoms of peritonitis or sepsis, caused by leakage of bowel contents into the abdominal cavity. Remember that older patients may be at increased risk for sepsis due to diminished immune response and poor nutrition. Sepsis also may result from wicking of colonic bacteria up the NG tube to the oral cavity;

to prevent infection, provide frequent mouth and tube care.

▶ Provide meticulous wound care, changing dressings often. Check dressings and drainage sites frequently for signs of infection (purulent drainage, foul odor) or fecal drainage. Also, watch for sudden fever, especially when accompanied by abdominal pain and tenderness.

▶ Regularly assess the patient for signs and symptoms of postresection obstruction. Examine the abdomen for distention and rigidity, auscultate for bowel sounds, and note passage of any flatus or feces.

▶ Encourage regular coughing and deep breathing to prevent atelectasis; remind him to splint the incision site as necessary.

▶ Once the patient regains peristalsis and bowel function, take steps to prevent constipation and straining during defecation — both of which can damage the anastomosis. Encourage him to drink plenty of fluids, and administer a stool softener or other laxatives, as ordered. Note and record the frequency and amount of all bowel movements as well as characteristics of the stool.

PATIENT TEACHING

▶ Tell the patient to record the frequency and character of bowel movements and to notify the physician of any changes in his normal pattern. Warn him against using laxatives without consulting his physician.

▶ Caution the patient to avoid abdominal straining and heavy lifting (anything over 10 lb [5 kg]) until the sutures are completely healed and the physician grants permission to do so.

▶ Instruct the patient to maintain the prescribed semibland diet until his bowel has healed completely (usually 4 to 8 weeks after surgery). In particular, urge him to avoid carbonated beverages and gas-producing foods.

▶ Because extensive bowel resection may interfere with the patient's ability to absorb nutrients from food, emphasize the importance of taking prescribed vitamin supplements.

BOWEL RESECTION WITH OSTOMY

A bowel resection with ostomy involves the excision of diseased bowel and the creation of a stoma on the outer abdominal wall to allow elimination of feces. This surgery is performed for such intestinal maladies as inflammatory bowel disease, familial adenomatous polyposis, diverticulitis, and especially advanced colorectal cancer, if conservative surgery and other treatments aren't successful or if the patient develops acute complications, such as obstruction, abscess, or fistula.

Depending on the nature and location of the problem, the surgeon will perform one of several types of procedures. For instance, some obstructions of the ascending, transverse, descending, or sigmoid colon require a colostomy with removal of the affected bowel segments. In many cases, cancer of the rectum mandates abdominal perineal resection, which involves wide resection of the rectum, surrounding tissues, and lymph nodes, with formation of a permanent colostomy. Perforated sigmoid diverticulitis, Hirschsprung's disease, rectovaginal fistula, and penetrating trauma commonly call for a temporary colostomy to interrupt the intestinal flow and allow healing of inflamed or injured bowel segments.

A small-bowel obstruction, on the other hand, may require resection and formation of an ileostomy from the proximal ileum. Severe, widespread colonic obstruction may require total or near-total removal of the colon and rectum and creation of an ileostomy. A permanent ileostomy requires that the patient wear a drainage appliance or pouch over the stoma to contain the constant fecal drainage.

Instead of a conventional stoma, patients with ulcerative colitis or familial adenomatous polyposis may be candidates for either of two surgical advances: the creation of an ileoanal reservoir or a Kock pouch. Both are continent diversions in which the patient retains stool until draining it. Both techniques eliminate the need to wear an external pouch or drainage bag.

Implementation

After the patient receives an anesthetic, the surgeon makes an incision in the abdominal wall. The location depends on the area of the bowel to be resected and the type of ostomy required. After excising the diseased bowel segment and, in the case of colon cancer, several more inches of bowel beyond the margins of the tumor, the surgeon creates the stoma used to drain fecal content. (See *Types of intestinal stomas*.)

For an abdominoperineal resection, the surgeon makes a low abdominal incision and divides the sigmoid colon. He brings the proximal end of the colon out through another, smaller abdominal incision to create an end stoma, which results in a permanent colostomy. He then makes a wide perineal incision and resects the anus, rectum, and distal portion of the sigmoid colon. He closes the abdominal wound and places one or more abdominal drains; he usually leaves the perineal wound open but may pack it with gauze or close it and place several wound drains.

For an ileostomy, the surgeon resects all or part of the colon and rectum (proctocolectomy). He creates a permanent ileostomy by bringing the end of the ileum out through a small abdominal incision, typically located in the right lower quadrant between the anterosuperior iliac spine and the umbilicus, and fashions a stoma.

For an ileoanal reservoir, the surgeon performs a colectomy and creates a loop or end stoma for a temporary ileostomy. He then strips the rectal mucosa to prevent recurrence of the disease, forms an internal pouch with a portion of the ileum, and performs a pouch-anus anastomosis. The temporary ileostomy is required to allow adequate healing of the internal pouch and all anastomosis sites and to allow for an increase in the capacity of the internal reservoir through postoperative fluid instillation. The ileostomy is closed after 3 to 4 months.

For a Kock pouch, the surgeon first performs a proctocolectomy, in which he removes the colon, the rectum, and the anus and closes the anus. He then constructs a reservoir from a loop of the terminal ileum that is folded and sutured together and then cut. A portion of the ileum is intussuscepted to form a nipple valve, and the upper part of the sutured and cut ileum is pulled down and sutured to form a pouch. The nipple valve, which shuts tight against pressure from a filled pouch, is used to create a stoma by pulling it through the abdominal wall and suturing it flush with the skin.

Both a standard colostomy and an end ileostomy have been created through a laparoscopic approach.

Complications

Patients undergoing ostomies are at risk for the same postoperative complications associated with abdominal surgery. Common complications of ostomies include hemorrhage, sepsis, ileus, and fluid and electrolyte imbalance from excessive drainage through the stoma. Skin excoriation may occur around the stoma from contact with acidic digestive enzymes in the drainage, and irritation may occur from pressure of the ostomy pouch. Ischemia, bleeding, and retraction can also occur with a new stoma.

Complications associated with the ileoanal reservoir include poor wound healing, sepsis, and pelvic abscess. The Kock pouch may result in an incompetent nipple valve, leading to leakage or difficulties with intubating the valve.

Types of intestinal stomas

The surgeon may construct a stoma from the large intestine in one of three ways: end, loop, or double-barrel.

End stoma

To form an end stoma, the surgeon pulls a section of the intestine through the outer abdominal wall, everts the section, and sutures it to the skin. An ostomy with an end stoma can be either temporary or permanent.

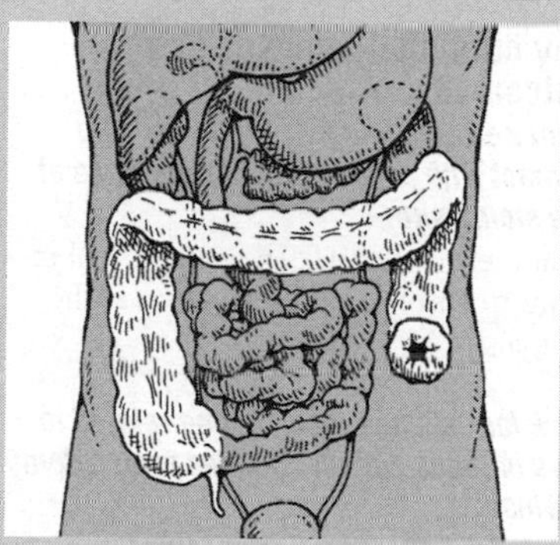

Loop stoma

To create a loop stoma, the surgeon brings a loop of intestine out through an abdominal incision to the abdominal surface and supports it with a rod or bridge (usually removed 5 to 7 days after surgery). He then opens the anterior wall of the bowel loop with a small incision to provide fecal diversion. The result is one stoma with a proximal, functioning limb and a distal, nonfunctioning limb. The surgeon then closes the wound around the exposed intestinal loop.

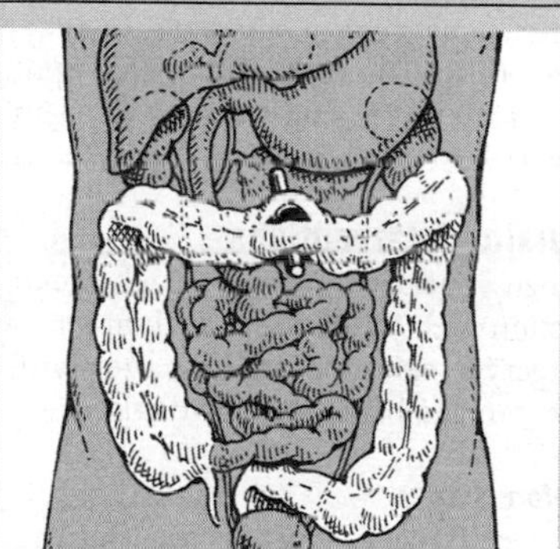

Double-barrel stoma

To create a double-barrel stoma, the surgeon divides the intestine and brings both the proximal and distal ends through the abdominal incision to the abdominal surface. He makes a small incision in the proximal stoma for fecal drainage. The distal stoma, also referred to as a mucous fistula, leads to the inactive intestine and is left intact.

Later, when the intestinal injury has healed or the inflammation has subsided, the colostomy is reversed and the divided ends of the intestine are anastomosed to restore intestinal integrity.

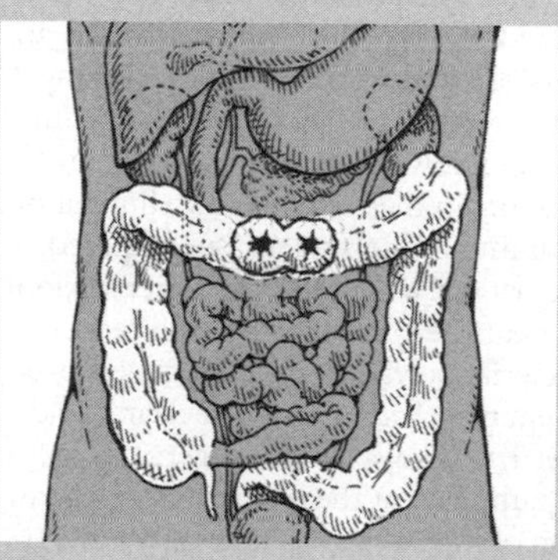

Ostomates commonly exhibit some degree of emotional and psychological problems, such as depression and anxiety, related to altered body image and worries about lifestyle changes associated with the stoma and ostomy pouch.

Key nursing diagnoses and outcomes

Impaired skin integrity related to skin contact with acidic digestive enzymes at the stoma site

Treatment outcome: The patient will remain free from skin breakdown at the stoma site.

Risk for deficient fluid volume related to loss of fluids and electrolytes from ostomy drainage

Treatment outcome: The patient will experience no signs or symptoms of dehydration, such as decreased urine output, poor skin turgor, and dry mucous membranes.

Nursing interventions

When your patient is to have a bowel resection with ostomy, prepare him for surgery, monitor his progress afterward, and provide home care instructions.

Before surgery

- If emergency surgery is necessary, briefly explain that the diseased or injured bowel portion will be repaired, if possible, and isolated to allow healing. Mention that a small portion of the unaffected bowel will be brought to an opening in the skin to allow elimination.
- If immediate surgery isn't required, the patient will need bowel preparation to clear the bowel of stool and reduce bacteria. Bowel preparation may consist of enemas, laxatives, and a clear liquid diet 1 to 2 days before surgery.
- Supplement the physician's explanation of the surgery as necessary and answer all questions in clear, simple terms. Explain all preoperative and postoperative procedures and equipment that the patient may encounter. Include family members or caregivers in your discussion, if appropriate.
- Prepare the patient for postoperative pain, and reassure the patient that analgesics will be provided.
- Describe the type of ostomy the patient will have and explain how fecal matter drains through it. Try using simple illustrations with your explanation. Discuss selection and use of ostomy appliances; if possible, show him the actual appliances. Prepare him for the foul smell and consistency of fecal drainage. This consistency varies, depending on the location of the stoma, from a constant watery stool with an ileostomy to a soft, semisolid stool with a colostomy in the descending colon.
- Inform the colostomy patient that he'll initially wear a pouch to collect fecal drainage. Point out that if the colostomy is placed in the descending or sigmoid colon, he may learn to control bowel movements by irrigating the colostomy. If he does learn bowel control, he may no longer need to use a pouch.
- Reassure the patient that once he becomes comfortable with the ostomy management routine, he should be able to resume his normal level of activity with few restrictions.
- Before surgery, arrange for a visit with an enterostomal therapist, who can provide more detailed information. The therapist can also help the patient select the best location for the stoma. If possible, arrange for the patient to meet with well-adjusted ostomy patients (from groups such as the United Ostomy Association) before undergoing surgery. These people can share their personal insights into the realities of living with and caring for a stoma.
- If chronic bowel disease has seriously compromised the patient's condition, evaluate his nutritional and fluid status for 3 to 4 days before surgery (if time permits). Typically, the patient will be receiving total parenteral nutrition (TPN) to prepare him for the physiolog-

ic stress of surgery. Record the patient's fluid intake and output and weight daily, and watch for early signs and symptoms of dehydration. Expect to draw periodic blood samples to determine hematocrit and hemoglobin levels. Be prepared to transfuse blood, if ordered.

▶ If the patient is on long-term, low-dose corticosteroid therapy, continue to administer the drug to prevent rebound adrenocortical insufficiency. Explain that the drug will be withdrawn gradually after surgery. Also, administer antibiotics, as ordered, to reduce intestinal flora.

▶ Ensure that the patient or a responsible family member has signed a consent form.

After surgery

▶ Encourage the patient to turn, cough, and deep breathe to prevent atelectasis.

▶ In the immediate postoperative period, carefully monitor the patient's intake and output. Maintain fluid and electrolyte balance, and watch for signs of dehydration: decreased urine output and electrolyte imbalance. (Poor skin turgor is not a good indicator in elderly people.) Provide analgesics, as ordered. Be especially alert for pain in the patient with an abdominoperineal resection because of the extent and location of the incisions.

▶ Note and record the color, consistency, and odor of fecal drainage from the stoma. If the patient has a double-barrel colostomy, check for mucus drainage from the inactive (distal) stoma. The nature of fecal drainage is determined by the type of ostomy surgery. Generally, the more colon tissue that is preserved, the more closely drainage will resemble normal stool. For the first few days after surgery, fecal drainage probably will be mucoid or liquid (and possibly slightly blood tinged) and mostly odorless. Report excessive blood or mucus content, which could indicate hemorrhage or infection.

▶ Observe the patient for signs and symptoms of peritonitis or sepsis, caused by leakage of bowel contents into the abdominal cavity. Remember that patients receiving antibiotics or TPN are at an increased risk for sepsis.

▶ Provide meticulous wound care, changing dressings often. Check dressings and drainage sites frequently for signs of infection (purulent drainage, foul odor) or fecal drainage. If the patient has had an abdominoperineal resection, monitor and record drainage from the perineal drains.

▶ Regularly check the stoma and the surrounding skin for irritation and excoriation, which may develop from contact with fecal drainage or from pressure caused by an overfilled or improperly fitted drainage pouch. Take measures to correct any such problems. Also, observe the stoma's appearance. The stoma should look smooth, cherry red, and slightly edematous; protrude approximately 2 cm from the abdominal wall; and be firmly adhered to the abdomen. Immediately report any purplish or black discoloration, retraction, or excessive swelling, which may indicate circulatory problems that could lead to ischemia.

▶ The patient with a Kock pouch will return from surgery with a catheter inserted in the stoma to drain fecal matter from the reservoir and prevent it from filling and placing pressure on the sutures. Be sure the catheter is connected to low intermittent suction or to straight drainage, as ordered. Check the patency of the catheter regularly, and irrigate it as ordered with 20 to 30 ml of normal saline solution every 2 to 4 hours to prevent obstruction. If no complications develop, the color of the pouch drainage will change 2 to 4 days after surgery from blood tinged to greenish brown, indicating the return of peristalsis. When this occurs, give the patient clear liquids and gradually introduce low-residue solids. Clamp and unclamp the pouch catheter to increase its capacity as ordered by the surgeon.

▶ During the recovery period, don't neglect the patient's emotional needs. Encourage him to express his feelings and concerns. If he's anxious and depressed, reassure him that these common postoperative reactions should fade as he adjusts to the ostomy. Continue to arrange for visits by an enterostomal therapist, if possible.

PATIENT TEACHING

▶ Instruct the patient with an ileostomy to change the drainage pouch every 3 to 7 days, or whenever it leaks. Emphasize the importance of maintaining meticulous skin care around the stoma site. Discuss dietary restrictions and suggestions for preventing stoma blockage, diarrhea, flatus, and odor. Explain the need for maintaining a high fluid intake to help ensure fluid and electrolyte balance.

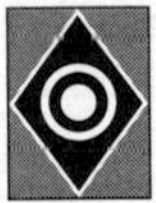

Drug alert Warn the patient to avoid alcohol, laxatives, and diuretics, which will increase fluid loss and may contribute to an imbalance. Tell him to report persistent diarrhea through the stoma, which can quickly lead to fluid and electrolyte imbalance. Patients with an ileostomy should avoid taking enteric-coated or capsule medications because these forms may not be absorbed.

▶ Teach the patient with an ileoanal reservoir how to temporarily manage an ileostomy and, after the pouch has healed and if needed, how to irrigate the pouch. Explain that after the ileostomy is reversed, perianal skin care with the use of skin sealants or moisture barriers is essential. Tell the patient that initially he will have 10 to 12 small-volume bowel movements daily but that they will decrease to approximately 6 a day as his diet is advanced and the reservoir expands. Inform him that some incontinence during the adaptation phase is common and that Kegel exercises will help strengthen the pelvic floor. Explain the signs and symptoms of inflammation of the reservoir, which include increased stool frequency, pelvic discomfort, fever, and malaise. Treatment usually involves antibiotics such as metronidazole.

▶ Explain to the patient with a Kock pouch that the catheter remains in place for 4 to 6 weeks after surgery. After it's removed, teach the patient how to empty the pouch by inserting a lubricated #28 French Silastic catheter through the stoma. He can empty the pouch while sitting or standing, though the latter position usually gives better results. Tell him he can also quicken drainage by contracting his abdominal muscles. Provide guidelines for draining the pouch. For example, immediately after surgery, the pouch usually holds 70 to 100 ml. One month later, it will hold about 200 ml. After 6 months, it will hold about 600 ml and need to be emptied three or four times a day. Be sure the patient knows to carry a catheter with him at all times. Between intubations, tell him to cover the stoma with gauze to prevent mucus from soiling his clothes. Before applying the gauze, he should wash the stomal area with warm water and dry it. Demonstrate how to irrigate the pouch. Suggest irrigation weekly or whenever undigested food obstructs drainage.

▶ Teach the colostomy patient how to apply, remove, and empty the pouch. If appropriate, teach the patient with a descending or sigmoid colostomy how to irrigate the ostomy with warm tap water to gain some control over elimination. Emphasize that continence can usually be achieved with dietary control and bowel retraining. Instruct him to change the appliance every 3 to 4 days and to wash the stoma site with warm water and soap without emollients to prevent skin irritation and excoriation.

▶ Tell the patient recovering from an abdominoperineal resection to take sitz baths to help relieve perineal discomfort. Instruct him to refrain from intercourse until the perineum heals.

- Encourage the ostomy patient to discuss his feelings about resuming sexual intercourse. Mention that the drainage pouch will not dislodge if the device is empty and fitted properly. Suggest avoiding foods and fluids for several hours before intercourse.
- Remind the patient and his family members that depression commonly occurs after ostomy surgery. Advise the patient to seek counseling, however, if depression persists or becomes severe.
- Ensure visiting nurse follow-up to reinforce teaching and provide initial assistance.

BREAST CANCER

Breast cancer is the most common cancer affecting women (although lung cancer accounts for more deaths). Although it may develop any time after puberty, more than 70% of breast cancer cases are diagnosed after age 50. Breast cancer strikes approximately 10% of all women. The 5-year survival rates show increasing improvement because of earlier diagnosis and better treatment.

The most reliable breast cancer detection method is monthly breast self-examination, annual professional examination, and regular mammography. Technical advances in mammography and enhanced imaging are responsible for an increase in the number of reported cases. Unfortunately, many older women don't receive regular mammograms, even when recommended by health care professionals, either because they're afraid or because they're embarrassed about exposing their breasts.

The causes of breast cancer remain elusive. Significant risk factors include gender (breast cancer is more likely to occur in women than in men), age older than 50 years, having a family history of breast cancer in first-degree relatives (such as a daughter, mother, or sister), early menarche (11 years or younger), nulliparity or first full-term pregnancy at age 30 or older, certain benign proliferative changes on breast biopsy, and $BRCA_1$ or RCA_2 gene mutations. Other probable risk factors being investigated include family history of breast cancer in second-degree relatives, late menopause, a high-fat diet, endometrial or ovarian cancer, radiation exposure, estrogen therapy, and excessive alcohol or tobacco use.

About half of all breast cancers develop in the upper outer quadrant, the section containing the most glandular tissue. The second most common cancer site is the nipple, where all the breast ducts converge. The next most common site is the upper inner quadrant, followed by the lower outer quadrant and, finally, the lower inner quadrant.

Growth rates vary. Theoretically, slow-growing breast cancer may take up to 8 years to become palpable at ⅜″. Breast cancer spreads by way of the lymphatic system and the bloodstream through the right side of the heart to the lungs and to the other breast, chest wall, liver, bone, and brain.

The estimated breast cancer growth rate is called its doubling time, or the time it takes malignant cells to double in number. Survival time is based on tumor size, the number of involved lymph nodes, the presence or absence of distant metastases, and the levels of estrogen and progesterone receptor proteins in the primary tumor.

Classified by histologic appearance and the lesion's location, breast cancer may be described in various ways.

- Adenocarcinoma arises from the epithelium of glandular tissue. This term describes the two most common types of breast cancer, infiltrating ductal carcinoma and infiltrating lobular carcinoma.
- Infiltrating (invasive) ductal carcinoma originates in the ducts and spreads to surrounding tissue. Examples include

tubular, medullary, mucinous, and papillary carcinomas.

▶ Infiltrating lobular carcinoma is a cancer that originates in the lobules and spreads to surrounding tissue.

▶ Carcinoma in situ refers to noninvasive cancer of either the ducts (such as intraductal carcinoma, including Paget's disease) or lobules.

Coupled with a staging system, these classifications provide a clearer picture of the cancer's extent. The most common system for staging, both before and after surgery, is the tumor, node, metastasis system which looks at the size of the tumor, the number of lymph nodes involved, and the extent of any metastasis.

Signs and symptoms

▶ Painless lump or mass in the breast

▶ Thickening of breast tissue

▶ Clear, milky, or bloody nipple discharge

▶ Nipple retraction

▶ Scaly, itchy skin around the nipple (Paget's disease)

▶ Skin changes, such as dimpling, peau d'orange, or inflammation

▶ Arm edema

Diagnostic tests

▶ *Mammography* can detect a tumor too small to palpate.

▶ *Fine-needle aspiration* and *excisional biopsy* provide cells for histologic examination to confirm the diagnosis.

▶ *Ultrasonography* can distinguish between a fluid-filled breast cyst and a solid mass.

▶ *Chest X-rays* can pinpoint metastases in the chest.

▶ *Scans of the bone, brain, liver, and other organs* can detect metastases to distant sites.

▶ *Blood tests*, such as alkaline phosphatase levels and liver function studies, can uncover distant metastases.

▶ *Hormonal receptor assay* can determine whether the tumor is estrogen- or progesterone-dependent.

Treatment

The choice of treatment usually depends on the stage of the cancer, tumor size, histologic appearance, lesion's location, patient's age and menopausal status, and disfiguring effects of surgery. Therapy may include any combination of surgery, radiation, chemotherapy, and hormone therapy.

Surgical options include lumpectomy, skin-sparing mastectomy, partial mastectomy, total mastectomy, and modified radical mastectomy. Removal of axillary lymph nodes is performed for staging purposes. Modified radical mastectomy has replaced radical mastectomy as the most extensively used surgical procedure for treating breast cancer.

Before or after tumor removal, primary radiation therapy may be effective for a patient who has a small tumor in early stages without distant metastases. Radiation therapy can also prevent or treat local recurrence. Furthermore, preoperative breast irradiation helps to sterilize the field, making the tumor more manageable surgically, especially in inflammatory breast cancer.

Chemotherapy relies on a combination of drugs, such as cyclophosphamide, 5-fluorouracil (5-FU) and paclitaxel, methotrexate, doxorubicin, vincristine, and prednisone. A typical regimen is cyclophosphamide, methotrexate, and fluorouracil. Chemotherapy is used for premenopausal and postmenopausal women.

Hormonal therapy blocks the uptake of estrogen and other hormones that may nourish breast cancer cells. For example, antiestrogen therapy (specifically tamoxifen, which is effective against tumors identified as estrogen receptor–positive) is used in postmenopausal women. Alternatively, the patient may receive antiandrogen (aminoglutethimide), androgen (fluoxymesterone), estrogen (diethylstilbestrol), or progestin (megestrol) therapy.

Key nursing diagnoses and outcomes

Imbalanced nutrition: Less than body requirements related to adverse effects of radiation or chemotherapy used to treat breast cancer

Treatment outcomes: The patient will maintain her weight, consume a well-balanced diet, and recover her appetite and GI function.

Decisional conflict related to multiple treatment options for breast cancer

Treatment outcome: The patient will make a well-informed decision about her breast cancer treatment.

Fear related to diagnosis of cancer and potential for metastatic breast disease

Treatment outcomes: The patient will express less fear and show fewer physical signs and symptoms of fear.

Nursing interventions

- Evaluate the patient's feelings about her illness, and determine her level of knowledge and expectations.
- Perform comfort measures to promote relaxation and relieve anxiety. Music therapy, religious practices, and reading may promote relaxation and alleviate anxiety.
- Administer analgesics as ordered, and monitor their effectiveness.
- Watch for treatment complications, such as nausea, vomiting, anorexia, leukopenia, thrombocytopenia, GI ulceration, and bleeding.
- Provide measures to relieve adverse effects of treatment.
- Monitor the patient's weight and nutritional intake for evidence of malnutrition. Encourage a high-protein diet. Dietary supplements may be indicated.
- Assess the patient's and family members' ability to cope, especially if the cancer is terminal. Refer them to the American Cancer Society if appropriate, and let them know hospice care is available if needed.

PATIENT TEACHING

- Provide clear, concise explanations of all procedures and prescribed treatments.
- Teach the patient or caregiver how to manage the adverse effects of treatment.
- Teach the patient how to examine her breasts and to perform monthly self-examinations. Many older women attribute associated breast changes to the normal changes of aging and need to be educated on normal changes versus changes that should be reported to the physician.
- Women who have had breast cancer in one breast are at higher risk for cancer in the other breast or for recurrent cancer in the chest wall. Therefore, urge the patient to continue examining the other breast and to comply with follow-up treatment.
- Refer the patient and family members to hospital and community support services.

BREAST SELF-EXAMINATION

The most reliable breast cancer detection method is regular breast self-examination (BSE), followed by immediate professional evaluation of any abnormality. As a woman ages, her breasts decrease in size and breast tissue is replaced with fat, which makes identification of palpable tumors easier. Through regular BSE, a woman can become familiar with the condition that's normal for her breasts and can more readily recognize any abnormalities. BSE is an easily learned procedure and is best performed 2 to 3 days after the menstrual period ends. Postmenopausal women should choose a day each month (such as the first day of the month) to perform the exam. (See *Teaching about breast self-examination,* pages 128 and 129.)

Teaching about breast self-examination

Teach your patient to conduct her own monthly self-examinations. Have her pick a date every month as a reminder to perform her examination.

Standing before a mirror

1. Have the patient undress to the waist and stand in front of a mirror, with her arms at her sides, as shown below. She should observe her breasts for any change in their shape or size and any puckering or dimpling of the skin.

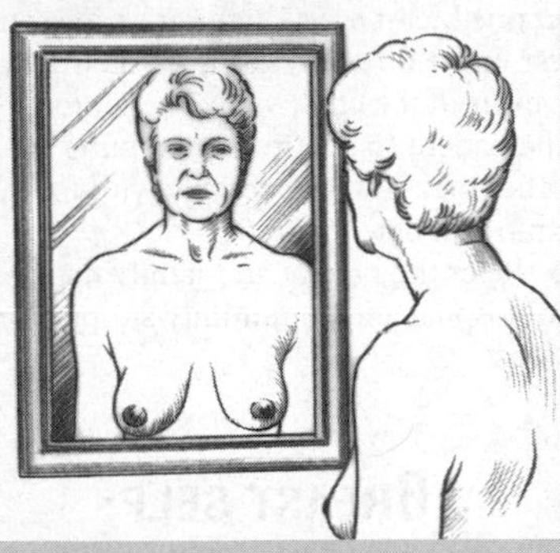

2. Have her raise her arms and press her hands together behind her head, as shown below. Then she should observe her breasts as she did before.

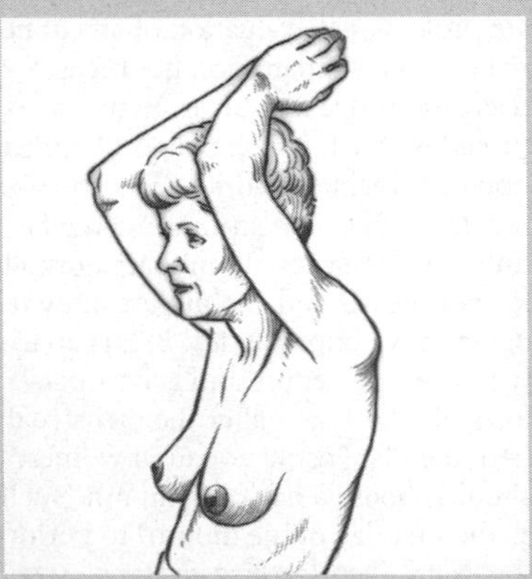

3. Next, have her press her palms firmly on her hips, as shown below, and observe her breasts again.

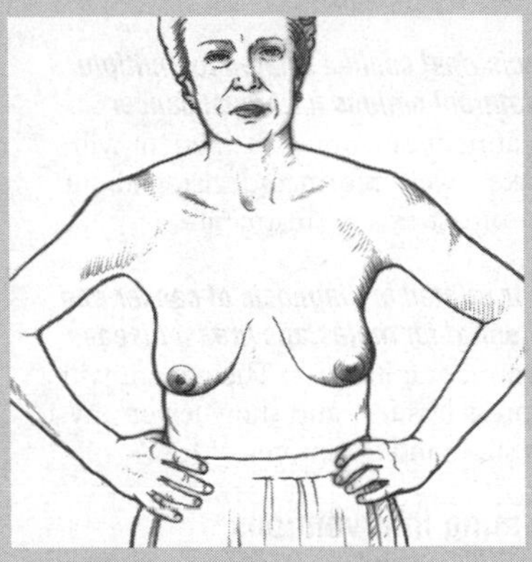

Lying down

1. Tell the patient that she should examine her breasts while lying flat on her back. Advise her to place a small pillow under her left shoulder, and to put her left hand behind her head, as shown below.

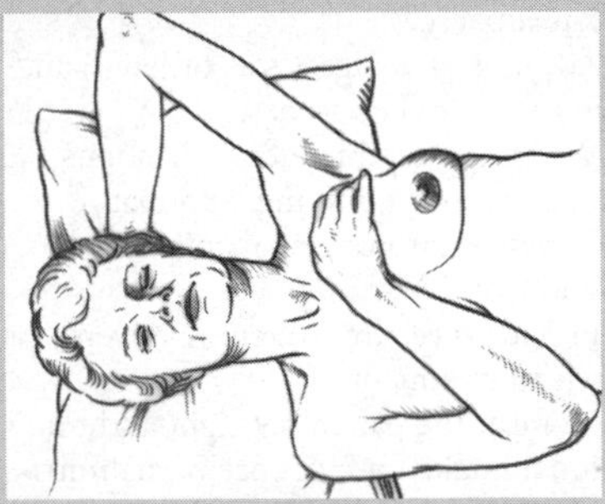

2. Instruct the patient to examine her left breast with her right hand, using a circular motion and progressing clockwise, until she has examined every portion. Explain that she'll notice a ridge of firm tissue in the lower

Teaching about breast self-examination *(continued)*

curve of her breast. Have her check the area under her arm, as shown below. Point out that she shouldn't be alarmed if she feels a small lump under her armpit that moves freely; this area contains lymph glands, which may become swollen when she's ill. Advise her to check the size of the lump daily and to call a physician or nurse if it doesn't go away in a few days or if it gets larger.

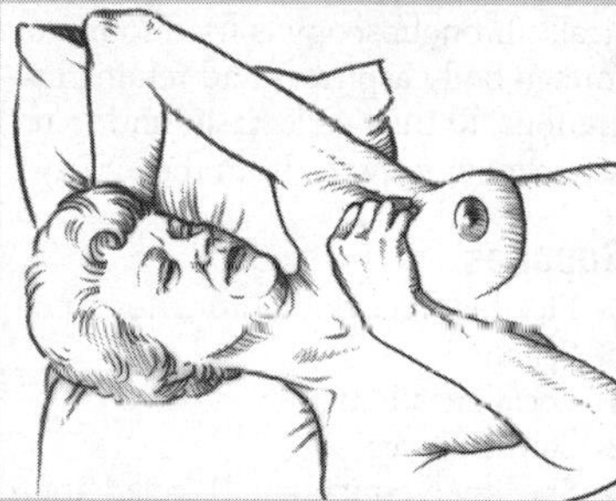

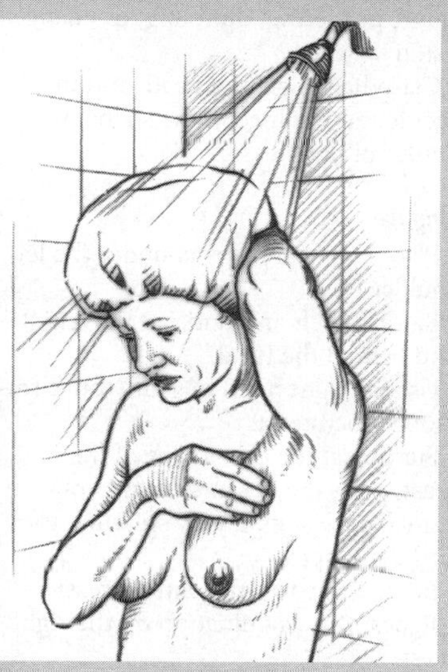

In the shower

Instruct the patient to lubricate her breasts with soap and water. Then, using the same circular motion, she should gently inspect both breasts with her fingertips, as shown top right.

What to do about lumps

Tell your patient not to panic if she feels a lump while examining her breasts. Reassure her that most lumps are not cancerous. Instruct her to note whether she can easily lift the skin covering it and whether the lump moves when she does so. Tell the patient to notify her physician or nurse after she has examined the lump. Advise her to describe how the lump feels (hard or soft) and whether it moves easily under the skin.

Finally, remind your patient that although self-examination is important, it's not a substitute for examination by her health care provider. The American Cancer Society recommends an annual clinical examination and an annual mammogram for women over age 50.

Supplies

- Shower
- Pillow or towel
- Mirror

Implementation

Standing in the shower

- Raise the right arm.
- Use the finger pads of the left hand to touch every part of the right breast.
- Feel gently for any lumps or changes under the skin. Begin at the outer edge of the breast. Move the fingers in small circles around the breast, gradually working toward the nipple. Squeeze the nipple gently and observe for any discharge.
- Raise the left arm and use the right hand to examine the left breast.

Standing before a mirror

- Place arms at sides.
- Inspect both breasts for unusual discharge, puckering, dimpling, or changes in skin texture.
- Clasp hands behind head, and inspect for any change in the shape or contour of the breasts.

Lying flat

- Place a pillow or towel under the left shoulder.
- Raise the left arm and put the left hand behind the head.
- Use the right hand to gently but firmly touch the breast.
- Starting at the outer edge of the breast, press the flat part of the fingers in small circles, gradually spiraling toward the nipple.
- Be sure to cover the entire breast.
- Repeat this examination on the right breast.

Standing and resting the arm

- Rest the left arm on a firm surface and with the right hand examine the left breast.
- Using the same circular motion, examine the area between the breast and underarm, and the underarm itself.
- Repeat this examination on the right breast.

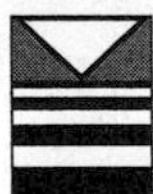

Key point If the patient has poor vision or tactile sensation, the BSE may need to be modified. Instruct the woman to use the palm of her hand in a sweeping motion from the chest wall to the nipple instead of the motion described above.

Patient teaching

- Teach the patient how to perform breast self-examination properly.
- Have the patient demonstrate the self-examination.

Documentation

Document patient teaching, and note the patient's understanding as shown in the return demonstration.

BRONCHOSCOPY

Bronchoscopy is used as both a diagnostic and therapeutic intervention.

Diagnostically, bronchoscopy is indicated for older adults experiencing hemoptysis and pneumonia. Therapeutically, bronchoscopy is used to remove foreign body aspirates and retained secretions, to treat atelectasis, and to resect benign growths from the airway.

Supplies

- Flexible fiber-optic bronchoscope
- Sedative
- Local anesthetic
- Sterile gloves
- Specimen containers (labeled appropriately)
- Sterile saline solution
- Handheld resuscitation bag with face mask
- Intubation equipment
- Pulse oximeter
- Suction setup
- Continuous cardiac monitor

Implementation

- Obtain a chest X-ray, prothrombin time or partial thromboplastin time, and an arterial blood gas analysis before performing the procedure.
- Attach the patient to a continuous cardiac monitor and apply a pulse oximeter.
- Place the patient in a supine position.
- Provide supplemental oxygen.
- Administer the sedation as ordered.
- After the physician sprays the local anesthetic agent into the patient's throat and it takes effect (usually in 1 to 2 minutes), the physician puts on sterile gloves and introduces the bronchoscope through the patient's nose or mouth.

Performing bronchoscopy

The bronchoscopic tube, inserted through the nostril into the bronchi, has four channels (see inset). Two light channels (A) provide a light source. One visualizing channel (B) permits the physician to see. One open channel (C) accommodates biopsy forceps, cytology brush, suctioning, lavage, anesthetic, or oxygen.

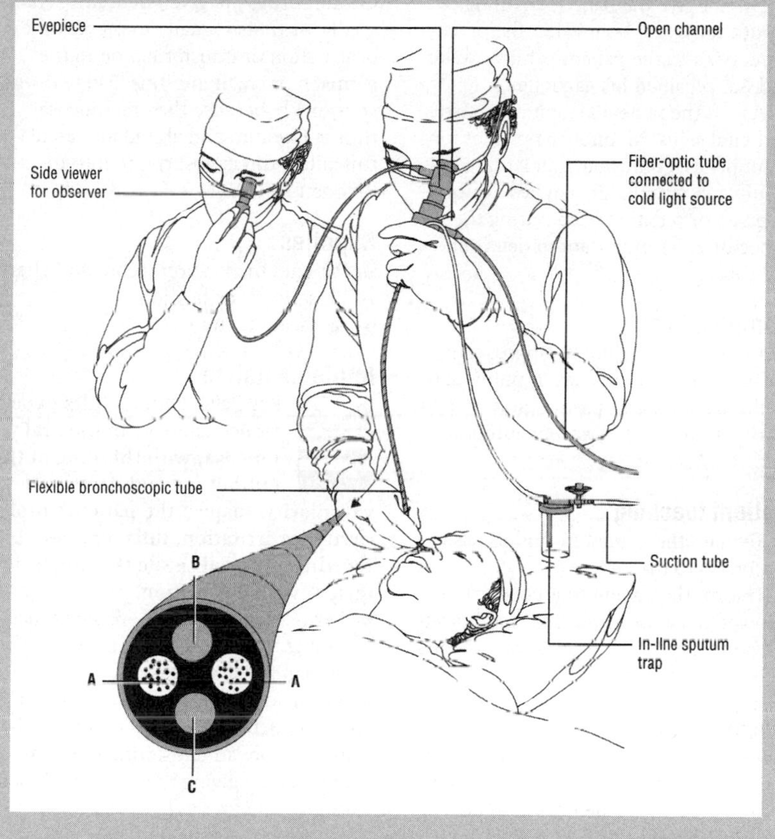

(See *Performing bronchoscopy*.) When the bronchoscope is just above the vocal cords, he flushes approximately 3 to 4 ml of 2% to 4% lidocaine through the inner channel of the scope to the vocal cords to anesthetize deeper areas. Then the physician inspects the anatomic structure of the trachea and bronchi, observes the color of the mucosal lining, and notes masses or inflamed areas. Next, he may use a biopsy forceps to remove a tissue specimen from a suspect area, a bronchial brush to obtain cells from the surface of a lesion, or a suction apparatus to remove either foreign bodies or mucous plugs. Bronchoalveolar lavage may also be performed to diagnose infectious causes of infiltrates in immunocompromised patients or to remove thickened secretions.

▶ After the tissue, mucus, or secretion is collected, place the specimens for microbiology, histology, and cytology in their respective labeled containers.

▶ Do not give the patient anything by mouth for 2 to 4 hours after the procedure, or until the patient is fully awake and has regained his gag reflex.

▶ Assess the patient's respiratory status and vital signs. Monitor the patient for hemoptysis, confusion, and lethargy. Confusion or lethargy may result from hypoxia or sedation used during the procedure. It's important to determine the cause.

Complications

Complications include laryngospasm, epistaxis, hemoptysis, fever, pulmonary infiltrates, bronchospasm, injury to dentition or vocal cords, and pneumothorax.

Patient teaching

▶ Explain the procedure and its associated risks to the patient.

▶ Inform the patient that he won't be allowed to eat or drink anything for 6 to 12 hours before the procedure and for 2 to 4 hours afterward.

Documentation

Document patient teaching, medications administered, and the patient's tolerance of the procedure. The physician performing the procedure should also include a note that describes exactly what was done during the procedure. Document the laboratory specimens that were obtained and how they were cared for.

BUCCAL, SUBLINGUAL, AND TRANSLINGUAL MEDICATION ADMINISTRATION

Certain drugs are given buccally, sublingually, or translingually to prevent their destruction or transformation in the stomach or small intestine. These drugs act quickly because the oral mucosa's thin epithelium and abundant vasculature allow direct absorption into the bloodstream.

Supplies

▶ Patient's medication record and chart

▶ Prescribed medication

▶ Medication cup

Implementation

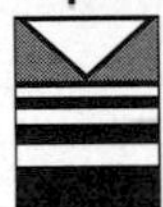

Key Point Older adults experience changes in the oral mucosa, with thinning of the epithelium and decreased vascularity. Inspect the patient's oral cavity for irritation, inflammation, or receding gingival tissue that might interfere with absorption.

▶ Verify the order on the patient's medication record by checking it against the physician's order on his chart.

▶ Wash your hands with warm water and soap. Check the label on the medication before administering it to make sure you'll be giving the prescribed medication.

▶ Confirm the patient's identity by asking his name and checking the name and room and bed number on his wristband.

Buccal and sublingual administration

▶ For buccal administration, place the tablet in the buccal pouch, between the cheek and gum. For sublingual administration, place the tablet under the patient's tongue. (See *Placing drugs in the oral mucosa.*)

- Caution him against chewing the tablet or touching it with his tongue to prevent accidental swallowing.
- Don't give liquids because some buccal tablets may take up to 1 hour to absorb. Eating, drinking, and smoking should be avoided until absorption is complete.
- Tell the angina patient to wet the nitroglycerin tablet with saliva and keep it under his tongue until it's fully absorbed.

Translingual administration

- To administer a translingual drug, tell the patient to hold the medication canister vertically, with the valve head at the top and the spray orifice as close to his mouth as possible.
- Instruct him to spray the dose onto his tongue by pressing the button firmly.

Complications

Some buccal medications may irritate the mucosa. The patient should alternate the sides of his mouth for repeat doses to prevent continuous irritation of the same site. Sublingual medications—erythrityl tetranitrate, for example—may cause a tingling sensation under the tongue. If the patient finds this annoying, try placing the drug in the buccal pouch instead.

Patient teaching

- Explain the procedure to the patient if he's never taken a drug buccally, sublingually, or translingually before.
- Instruct the patient to keep the medication in place until it dissolves completely to ensure absorption.
- Inform the older adult that he should not smoke before the drug has dissolved, because nicotine's vasoconstrictive effects slow absorption.

Documentation

Record the medication administered, the dose, the date and time, and the patient's reaction, if any.

Placing drugs in the oral mucosa

Buccal and sublingual administration routes allow some drugs, such as nitroglycerin or methyltestosterone, to enter the bloodstream rapidly without being degraded in the GI tract. To give a drug sublingually, place it under the patient's tongue, as shown below, and ask him to leave it there until it's dissolved.

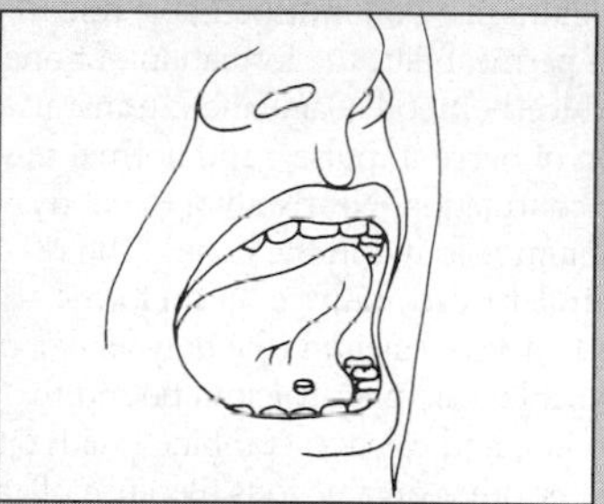

To give a drug buccally, insert it between the patient's cheek and teeth, as shown below. Ask him to close his mouth and hold the tablet against his cheek until the tablet is absorbed.

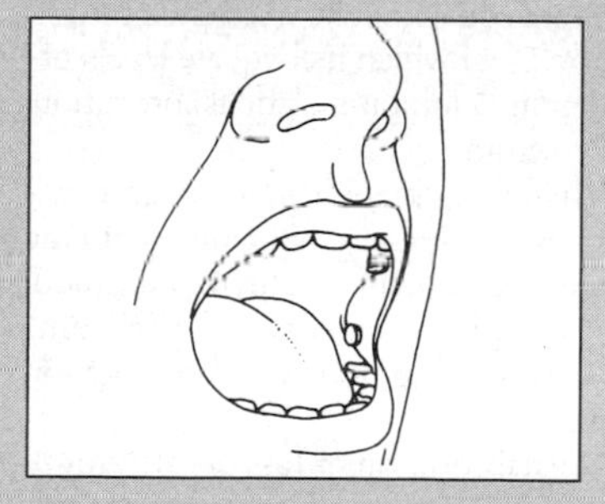

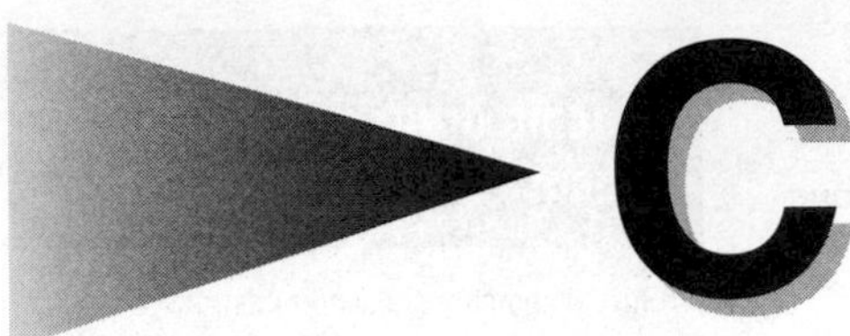

Calcium deficiency

Calcium plays an indispensable role in cell permeability, the formation of bones and teeth, blood coagulation, transmission of nerve impulses, and normal muscle contraction. Nearly all of the body's calcium is found in the bones. The remainder exists in three serum forms: ionized, or free, calcium (the only active, or available, calcium); calcium bound to protein; and calcium combined with citrate or other organic ions. Because of calcium's many important functions, a deficiency of this mineral, known as hypocalcemia, can cause serious—even lethal—effects.

Hypocalcemia may result from:

- inadequate intake of calcium and vitamin D, in which inadequate levels of vitamin D inhibit intestinal absorption of calcium
- hypoparathyroidism due to injury, disease, or surgery that reduces or eliminates secretion of parathyroid hormone (PTH), which is necessary for calcium absorption and normal serum calcium levels
- malabsorption or loss of calcium from the GI tract, caused by increased intestinal motility from severe diarrhea or laxative abuse, from inadequate levels of vitamin D or PTH, or from a reduction in gastric acidity
- severe infections or burns, in which diseased and burned tissue traps calcium from the extracellular fluid
- alkalosis, in which calcium forms a complex with bicarbonate, causing diminished levels of ionized calcium and inducing symptoms of hypocalcemia
- pancreatic insufficiency, which may cause malabsorption of calcium and subsequent calcium loss in feces; in acute pancreatitis, hypocalcemia varies in degree with the disorder's severity and is of unknown origin
- renal failure (polyuric phase) or use of loop diuretics, resulting in excessive excretion of calcium
- hypomagnesemia, which causes decreased PTH secretion and blocks the peripheral action of that hormone
- hyperphosphatemia, which causes calcium levels to decrease as phosphorus levels rise
- extensive administration of citrated blood, which may result in citrate binding with calcium
- osteoblast metastasis, which is attributed to increased calcium influx into osteoblastic lesions.

Left untreated, hypocalcemia can lead to laryngeal spasm, seizures, cardiac arrhythmias and, possibly, respiratory arrest.

Signs and symptoms

- Digital and perioral paresthesia and muscle cramps
- Twitching, carpopedal spasm, tetany, and seizures
- Cardiac arrhythmias
- Hyperactive reflexes, a positive Trousseau's sign, and a positive Chvostek's sign

The patient may have a history of risk factors, such as hypothyroidism or renal failure.

Diagnostic tests

▶ *Blood tests* reveal a total serum calcium level below 8.9 mg/dl or an ionized serum calcium level below 4.5 mg/dl.
▶ *Electrocardiography* (ECG) may show lengthened QT interval, prolonged ST segment, and arrhythmias.

Treatment

Treatment aims to correct an acute deficiency, to provide follow-up maintenance therapy, and to correct the underlying cause.

Mild hypocalcemia may require only a diet adjustment to provide adequate intake of calcium, vitamin D, and protein, possibly with oral calcium supplements. Acute hypocalcemia requires immediate correction by I.V. administration of calcium gluconate, which is usually preferable to calcium chloride. If the hypocalcemia is related to hypomagnesemia, magnesium replacement may be necessary because hypocalcemia often doesn't respond to calcium therapy alone.

Chronic hypocalcemia requires vitamin D supplements to facilitate GI calcium absorption. For a mild deficiency, the amount of vitamin D found in most multivitamin preparations is adequate. For a severe deficiency, vitamin D is used in four forms: ergocalciferol (vitamin D_2), cholecalciferol (vitamin D_3), calcitriol, and dihydrotachysterol, a synthetic form of vitamin D_2.

Key nursing diagnoses and outcomes

Imbalanced nutrition: Less than body requirements related to inadequate intake of calcium and vitamin D in diet

Treatment outcomes: The patient will identify food sources rich in calcium and vitamin D, consume a diet high in calcium and vitamin D, and develop a total serum calcium level within the normal range.

Acute pain related to hypocalcemia-induced muscle cramps

Treatment outcomes: The patient will carry out appropriate interventions for pain relief and will experience relief of muscle cramps.

Nursing interventions

▶ Calcium gluconate can be given I.V. either diluted or undiluted. Dilution is preferred, but undiluted calcium gluconate is used in emergencies. Use an infusion pump to regulate administration of the calcium solution so that the rate is no faster than 200 mg per minute.

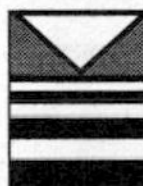

Key point Calcium gluconate is incompatible with many medications, including most of the drugs used in emergencies (such as epinephrine, bicarbonate, and dobutamine). Precipitation will occur. Never add calcium gluconate to I.V. solutions containing medications until their compatibility is confirmed.

▶ Give oral calcium supplements 1 to 1½ hours after meals, as ordered. If GI upset occurs, administer the supplements with milk.
▶ Provide a quiet, safe, stress-free environment for the patient. Observe seizure precautions for patients with severe hypocalcemia.
▶ If the patient is symptomatic, keep a tracheotomy tray and handheld resuscitation bag at the bedside in case of laryngeal spasm.
▶ Watch for hypocalcemia in patients at risk, such as those receiving massive transfusions of citrated blood and those with chronic diarrhea, severe infections, or insufficient dietary intake of calcium and protein. (See *Preventing hypocalcemia,* page 136.)
▶ Assess the patient's respiratory status, including rate, depth, pattern, and rhythm. Be alert for stridor, dyspnea, or crowing.

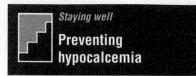

To help your patient prevent hypocalcemia, be sure to:

- advise him to eat foods rich in calcium, vitamin D, and protein (such as fortified milk and cheese)
- explain how important calcium is for normal bone formation and blood coagulation
- discourage long-term use of laxatives.

▶ Monitor serum calcium levels every 12 to 24 hours, and report any decrease.
▶ Monitor the patient for ECG changes. Notify the physician if ventricular arrhythmias or heart block develops.
▶ When giving calcium supplements, frequently check the patient's pH because a pH exceeding 7.45 (alkalosis) inhibits calcium ionization.
▶ Check for Trousseau's and Chvostek's signs, and report positive signs to the physician.
▶ When administering calcium solutions, watch for anorexia, nausea, and vomiting — possible signs of overcorrection that may result in hypercalcemia.
▶ Observe the I.V. site for signs of infiltration because calcium can cause tissue sloughing.
▶ If the patient is receiving calcium chloride, watch for abdominal discomfort.

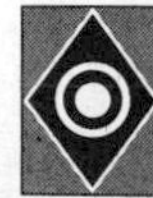

Drug alert Monitor the patient closely for a possible drug interaction if he's receiving a cardiac glycoside with large doses of oral calcium supplements; watch for signs and symptoms of digoxin toxicity (anorexia, nausea, vomiting, yellow vision, and cardiac arrhythmias).

PATIENT TEACHING

▶ If the patient requires oral calcium preparations or vitamin D supplements, make sure he understands his regimen.

CALCIUM EXCESS

Because calcium plays a critical role in blood coagulation, nerve impulse transmission, normal muscle contraction, and the formation of bones and teeth, an excess — known as hypercalcemia — can have life-threatening effects.

Hypercalcemia may result from:
▶ hyperparathyroidism, a primary cause, which increases serum calcium levels by promoting calcium absorption from the intestine, resorption from bone, and reabsorption from the kidneys
▶ hypervitaminosis D, which may increase absorption of calcium from the intestine
▶ certain cancers, such as multiple myeloma, lymphoma, squamous cell carcinoma of the lung, and breast cancer, which raise serum calcium levels by destroying bone or by releasing parathyroid hormone (PTH) or a PTH-like substance, osteoclast-activating factor, prostaglandins and, perhaps, a sterol resembling vitamin D
▶ multiple fractures and prolonged immobilization, which release bone calcium and raise the serum calcium level.

Other causes of hypercalcemia include milk-alkali syndrome, renal failure, sarcoidosis, hyperthyroidism, adrenal insufficiency, use of thiazide diuretics, and excessive administration of calcium during cardiopulmonary arrest.

Allowed to progress, hypercalcemia may cause coma and cardiac arrest. Hypercalcemia may also lead to renal calculi.

Signs and symptoms

▶ Lethargy
▶ Weakness with hyporeflexia and decreased muscle tone
▶ Anorexia

- Constipation
- Nausea
- Vomiting
- Polyuria
- Personality changes
- Confusion or, in severe cases, coma.

The patient may have a history of risk factors, such as excessive ingestion of vitamin D or prolonged immobilization.

Diagnostic tests

- *Blood tests* reveal a total serum calcium level greater than 10.5 mg/dl or an ionized serum calcium level greater than 5.3 mg/dl.
- *Sulkowitch's urine test* may reveal increased calcium precipitation.
- *Electrocardiography* (ECG) may reveal a shortened QT interval and, in severe hypercalcemia, ventricular arrhythmias.

Treatment

If hypercalcemia produces no symptoms, managing the underlying cause may be sufficient treatment. If the imbalance produces symptoms, treatment is aimed at eliminating excess serum calcium through hydration with normal saline solution, which promotes calcium excretion in urine. Loop diuretics, such as ethacrynic acid and furosemide, also promote calcium excretion.

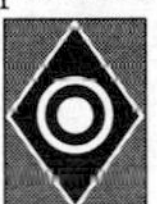

Drug alert Thiazide diuretics are contraindicated in hypercalcemia because they inhibit calcium excretion.

Corticosteroids, such as prednisone and hydrocortisone, help treat hypercalcemia associated with lymphoma, multiple myeloma, sarcoidosis, hypervitaminosis D, and certain tumors metastatic to the bone. Plicamycin can also lower serum calcium levels and is especially effective against hypercalcemia secondary to certain tumors. Calcitonin may also be helpful in certain instances. I.V. phosphates can be hazardous to the patient and are used only when other treatments prove ineffective.

Key nursing diagnoses and outcomes

Risk for imbalanced fluid volume related to hypercalcemia-induced polyuria

Treatment outcomes: The patient will have a total serum calcium level within the normal range and will maintain a normal balance between intake and output.

Impaired physical mobility related to hypercalcemia-induced muscle weakness

Treatment outcome: The patient will adhere to his treatment regimen, thus preventing or minimizing further elevations in serum calcium level.

Nursing interventions

- Increase fluid intake to dilute calcium in serum and urine and to prevent renal damage and dehydration.
- Administer loop diuretics (not thiazide diuretics), as ordered. Provide acid-ash drinks, such as cranberry juice, because calcium salts are more soluble in acid than in alkali.
- Help the patient ambulate as soon as possible. Handle the patient with chronic hypercalcemia gently to prevent pathologic fractures. If the patient is bedridden, reposition him frequently and encourage range-of-motion exercises to promote circulation and prevent urinary stasis and calcium loss from bone.
- Provide a safe environment. Keep the bed's side rails raised and the bed in the lowest position with the wheels locked.
- Orient the patient to his surroundings as needed, and assess his level of consciousness frequently.
- Watch for signs of heart failure in patients receiving diuresis therapy with normal saline solution.
- When administering loop diuretics, monitor intake and output and strain urine for renal calculi.
- If the patient is receiving a cardiac glycoside, watch for signs of toxicity, such as anorexia, nausea, vomiting, and an irregular pulse.

- Monitor serum calcium levels frequently, and report increasing levels.
- Check ECG results and vital signs frequently. Observe for arrhythmias if hypercalcemia is severe.
- Assess for signs of deep vein thrombosis, such as calf pain and swelling. Hypercalcemia increases the risk of clot formation. Encourage ambulation and leg exercises.

PATIENT TEACHING

- To prevent a recurrence of hypercalcemia, suggest a low-calcium diet with increased fluid intake.
- Review nonprescription medications that are high in calcium, and advise the patient to avoid them. Also caution him not to take megadoses of vitamin D.
- Stress the importance of increased fluid intake (up to 3 L in nonrestricted patients) to minimize the possibility of renal calculi formation.

CARDIAC CATHETERIZATION

Cardiac catheterization permits visualization of cardiac contraction and coronary artery anatomy through the insertion of a catheter into the right or left heart chamber and the injection of a contrast medium. Left-sided heart catheterization helps evaluate aortic and mitral valve function, cardiac output, and coronary artery patency. It also helps assess candidates for coronary artery bypass surgery or interventional procedures such as percutaneous transluminal coronary angioplasty, stent placement, and directional coronary atherectomy. Right-sided heart catheterization permits evaluation of pulmonic and tricuspid valve function, cardiac output, right-sided heart pressures, and pulmonary artery wedge pressure. It can demonstrate valvular efficiency or defects, assess the causes of chest pain, and detect congenital heart defects.

Supplies

- Cardiac monitor
- Pulse oximeter
- Blood pressure monitoring device
- I.V. line with dextrose 5% in water (D_5W) or normal saline solution
- Local anesthetic
- Catheterization kit

Implementation

- Administer prescribed sedatives and antihistamines 30 minutes before catheterization.
- Place the patient on a padded table in a supine position.
- Attach the patient to a continuous cardiac monitor, blood pressure monitor, and pulse oximeter.
- Make sure that an I.V. line is in place and functioning, with D_5W or normal saline solution infusing at a keep-vein-open rate.
- A local anesthetic is injected into the catheterization site. A small incision or percutaneous puncture is made in the artery or vein, depending on whether left-sided or right-sided studies are to be performed, and the catheter is passed through the sheath into the vessel. The catheter is guided to the cardiac chambers or coronary arteries using fluoroscopy. When the catheter is in place, the contrast medium is injected through it to enable visualization of the cardiac vessels and structures. (See *Understanding cardiac catheterization.*)
- Administer nitroglycerin during the procedure, if necessary, to eliminate catheter-induced spasm or to measure the drug's effect on the coronary arteries.
- Monitor heart rate and rhythm, respiratory and pulse rates, blood pressure, and oxygen saturation frequently during the procedure.
- After the procedure, the catheter is removed, and direct pressure is applied to the incision site for 30 minutes; a pressure dressing is applied when hemostasis is achieved.
- Monitor vital signs every 15 minutes for 1 hour, then every 30 minutes for

Understanding cardiac catheterization

For right-sided heart catheterization (below left), the catheter is inserted through veins to the inferior vena cava and to the right atrium and ventricle. For left-sided heart catheterization (below right), the catheter is inserted through arteries to the aorta and into the coronary artery orifices or left ventricle (or both). Note that both approaches use the antecubital and femoral vessels.

RIGHT-SIDED CATHETERIZATION

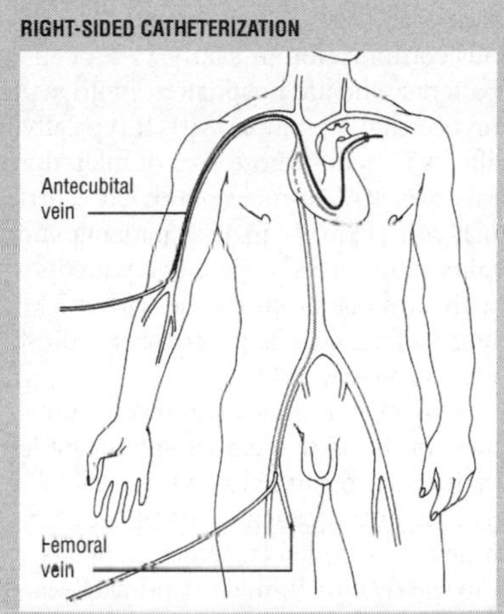

LEFT-SIDED CATHETERIZATION

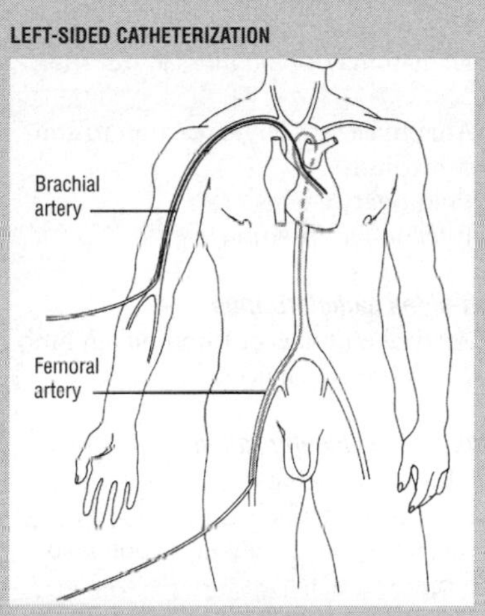

the next 2 hours, then every hour for 2 hours. If no hematoma or other problems arise, check every 4 hours. If signs are unstable, check every 5 minutes and notify the physician.

▶ Observe the insertion site for a hematoma or blood loss, and reinforce the pressure dressings as needed.

▶ Check the patient's color, skin temperature, and peripheral pulses below the puncture site.

▶ Enforce bed rest for 6 to 8 hours. If the femoral route was used for catheter insertion, keep the patient's leg extended for 6 to 8 hours; if the antecubital fossa was used, keep the arm extended for at least 3 hours.

▶ Continue I.V. therapy as ordered to enhance renal clearance of the contrast agent. Monitor intake and output.

▶ Diet is usually resumed after the test, but, at mealtimes, keep in mind that for the first 6 to 8 hours the head of the bed can be elevated only to 30 degrees.

▶ Make sure a posttest electrocardiogram is scheduled to check for possible myocardial damage.

Complications

Because cardiac catheterization is an invasive test that's usually done on high-risk patients, it poses a greater risk than most other diagnostic tests. Although complications are rare, they are potentially life-threatening and require careful observation during the procedure. Keep in mind that some complications are common to both left-sided and right-sided heart catheterization; others result only from catheterization of one side. In either case, complications require that you notify the physician and carefully document the complication and its treatment.

Left- or right-sided catheterization

- Perforation of the heart or great vessels
- Myocardial infarction
- Acute tubular necrosis (contrast medium–induced)
- Arrhythmias
- Cardiac tamponade
- Infection (systemic)
- Hypovolemia
- Hematoma or blood loss at insertion site
- Anaphylactic allergic reaction to contrast medium
- Pulmonary edema
- Infection at insertion site

Left-sided catheterization

- Arterial embolus or thrombus in limb
- Cerebrovascular accident

Right-sided catheterization

- Thrombophlebitis
- Pulmonary embolism
- Vagal response (nausea, hypotension, and bradycardia)

Patient teaching

- Explain to the patient that this test evaluates the function of the heart and its vessels. Also explain the actual procedure.
- Instruct the patient not to eat or drink anything for 6 hours before the test.
- Inform the patient that the contrast agent may produce a warm sensation.
- Instruct the patient to report any chest pain during the procedure.
- Inform him that he'll have to remain in bed for 8 hours after the test.
- Tell the patient to keep his leg extended for 6 to 8 hours if the femoral route was used, or for at least 3 hours if the antecubital fossa was used.

Documentation

Document the patient's response to the procedure, including vital signs, the condition of the insertion site, and the presence of pulses distal to the insertion site. Also document your patient teaching.

CARDIOGENIC SHOCK

Sometimes called pump failure, cardiogenic shock is diminished cardiac output that severely impairs tissue perfusion. Cardiogenic shock occurs as a serious complication in nearly 15% of all patients who are hospitalized with acute myocardial infarction (MI). It typically affects patients whose area of infarction involves 40% or more of the left ventricular muscle mass; in such patients, mortality may exceed 85%. Most patients with cardiogenic shock die within 24 hours of onset. The prognosis for those who survive is poor.

Cardiogenic shock can result from any condition that causes significant left ventricular dysfunction with reduced cardiac output, such as MI (most common), myocardial ischemia, papillary muscle dysfunction, and end-stage cardiomyopathy. Other causes include myocarditis and depressed myocardial contractility after cardiac arrest or prolonged cardiac surgery. Mechanical abnormalities of the ventricle, such as acute mitral or aortic insufficiency or an acutely acquired ventricular septal defect or ventricular aneurysm, may also result in cardiogenic shock.

Regardless of the cause, left ventricular dysfunction initiates a series of compensatory mechanisms that attempt to increase cardiac output and, in turn, maintain vital organ function. As cardiac output falls, aortic and carotid baroreceptors activate sympathetic nervous responses. These compensatory responses increase heart rate, left ventricular filling pressure, and peripheral resistance in order to enhance venous return to the heart.

The compensatory response initially stabilizes the patient but later causes deterioration with rising oxygen demands on the already compromised myocardium. These events constitute a vicious circle of low cardiac output, sympathetic compensation, myocardial ischemia, and even lower cardiac output. Death usually ensues because the vital organs can't overcome the deleterious effects of extended hypoperfusion.

Signs and symptoms

- Anginal pain due to decreased myocardial perfusion and oxygenation
- Urine output usually less than 20 ml/hour
- Pale, cold, and clammy skin (may not be apparent in older patients, who experience decreased peripheral circulation and sweat gland function as a normal consequence of aging)
- Decreased sensorium
- Rapid, shallow respirations
- Rapid, thready peripheral pulses (in older patients with arteriosclerosis, pulses possibly strong and bounding because of the artery's associated changes)
- Mean arterial pressure of less than 60 mm Hg and narrowing pulse pressure (in patients with chronic hypotension, mean pressure may fall below 50 mm Hg before signs of shock occur)
- Gallop rhythm, faint heart sounds and, possibly (if shock results from rupture of the ventricular septum or papillary muscles), a holosystolic murmur

The patient history typically includes a disorder that severely decreases left ventricular function (such as MI or cardiomyopathy). Although many of the clinical features listed above also occur in heart failure and other shock syndromes, they're usually more profound in cardiogenic shock. Patients with pericardial tamponade may have distant heart sounds.

Diagnostic tests

- *Pulmonary artery pressure monitoring* reveals increased pulmonary artery pressure (PAP) and pulmonary artery wedge pressure (PAWP), reflecting a rise in left ventricular end-diastolic pressure (preload) and heightened resistance to left ventricular emptying (afterload) caused by ineffective pumping and increased peripheral vascular resistance. Thermodilution catheterization reveals a reduced cardiac index (< 1.8 L/minute/ml).
- *Invasive arterial pressure monitoring* shows systolic arterial pressure less than 80 mm Hg due to impaired ventricular ejection.
- *Arterial blood gas (ABG) analysis* may show metabolic and respiratory acidosis and hypoxia.
- *Electrocardiography* (ECG) may demonstrate evidence of acute MI, ischemia, or ventricular aneurysm.
- *Serum enzyme measurements* display elevated levels of troponin (Tn), creatine kinase (CK), lactate dehydrogenase (LDH), aspartate aminotransferase, and alanine aminotransferase, which indicate MI or ischemia and suggest heart failure or shock. CK-MB (an isoenzyme of CK that occurs in cardiac tissue) and LDH isoenzyme levels may confirm acute MI. Elevations of troponin I (Tn I) can also confirm acute MI.
- *Cardiac catheterization* and *echocardiography* reveal other conditions that can lead to pump dysfunction and failure, such as cardiac tamponade, papillary muscle infarct or rupture, ventricular septal rupture, pulmonary emboli, venous pooling (associated with venodilators and continuous or intermittent positive-pressure breathing), and hypovolemia.

Treatment

Treatment aims to increase cardiac output, improve myocardial perfusion, and decrease cardiac workload with a combination of cardiovascular drugs and mechanical-assist techniques.

Dopamine, a vasopressor, may be used to increase cardiac output, blood pressure, and renal blood flow. The inotropic agents amrinone and dobutamine may be used to increase myocardial contractility. Norepinephrine is used when a more potent vasoconstrictor is necessary. Nitroprusside, a vasodilator, may be used with a vasopressor to further improve cardiac output by decreasing peripheral vascular resistance (afterload) and reducing left ventricular end-diastolic pressure (preload). However, the patient's blood pressure must be adequate to support nitroprusside therapy and must be monitored closely.

An intra-aortic balloon pump (IABP), a mechanical-assist device that attempts to improve coronary artery perfusion and decrease cardiac workload, may also be used. The inflatable balloon pump is inserted through the femoral artery into the descending thoracic aorta. The balloon inflates during diastole to increase coronary artery perfusion pressure and deflates before systole (before the aortic valve opens) to reduce resistance to ejection (afterload) and therefore lessen cardiac workload. Improved ventricular ejection, which significantly improves cardiac output, and a subsequent vasodilation in the peripheral vessels lead to lower preload volume.

Cultural diversity In the Ultra-Orthodox Jewish community, the patient may need to consult with his rabbi before consenting to IABP therapy to ensure that this technology is acceptable under Jewish law.

A ventricular-assist pump may be used when drug therapy and the IABP fail.

Key nursing diagnoses and outcomes

Ineffective (cardiopulmonary) tissue perfusion related to decreased cardiac output caused by left ventricular dysfunction

Treatment outcomes: The patient will have ABG values within the normal range, exhibit no cardiac arrhythmias, and remain free from chest pain.

Decreased cardiac output related to left ventricular dysfunction caused by myocardial injury

Treatment outcomes: The patient will regain and maintain normal cardiac output.

Fear related to threat of death caused by cardiogenic shock

Treatment outcome: The patient will exhibit fewer physical symptoms of fear.

Nursing interventions

- In the intensive care unit (ICU), start an I.V. infusion of normal saline solution or lactated Ringer's solution, using a large-bore (14G to 18G) catheter.
- Administer oxygen by face mask or artificial airway to ensure adequate oxygenation of tissues. Adjust the oxygen flow rate according to ABG measurements. Many patients need 100% oxygen, and some require 5 to 15 cm H_2O of positive end-expiratory or continuous positive airway pressure ventilation.
- Administer an osmotic diuretic such as mannitol, if ordered, to increase renal blood flow and urine output.

Drug alert Older patients receiving mannitol must be closely observed and may require reduced dosages. Excessive diuresis causes rapid dehydration, leading to hypovolemia, hypokalemia, and hyponatremia.

- When a patient is on the IABP, move him as little as possible. Never flex the patient's "ballooned" leg at the hip because this may displace or fracture the catheter. Never place the patient in a sitting position for any reason (including chest X-rays) while the balloon is inflated; the balloon will tear through the aorta and result in immediate death.
- During IABP use, assess pedal pulses and skin temperature and color to ensure adequate peripheral circulation. Check the dressing over the insertion site frequently for bleeding, and change it according to facility protocol. Also

check the site for hematoma or signs of infection, and culture any drainage.

- When weaning the patient from the IABP, watch for ECG changes, chest pain, and other signs of recurring cardiac ischemia as well as for shock.
- If the patient becomes hemodynamically stable, gradually reduce the frequency of balloon inflation to wean him from the IABP.
- To ease emotional stress and decrease oxygen demands, plan your care to allow frequent rest periods. Provide as much privacy as possible. Allow family members to visit and comfort the patient as much as possible.
- Allow family members to express their anger, anxiety, and fear.
- Frequently monitor and record blood pressure, pulse and respiratory rates, and peripheral pulses until the patient stabilizes. Monitor cardiac rhythm continuously. Systolic blood pressure less than 80 mm Hg usually results in inadequate coronary artery blood flow, cardiac ischemia, arrhythmias, and further complications of low cardiac output. A progressive drop in blood pressure accompanied by a thready pulse generally signals inadequate cardiac output. Notify the physician immediately.
- Using a pulmonary artery catheter, closely monitor PAP, PAWP, central venous pressure (CVP), and cardiac output. A high PAWP indicates heart failure, increased systemic vascular resistance, decreased cardiac output, and decreased cardiac index, which should be reported immediately.
- Insert an indwelling urinary catheter to measure hourly urine output. If output is less than 30 ml/hour, increase the fluid infusion rate but watch for signs of fluid overload, such as an increase in PAWP. Notify the physician if urine output doesn't improve.
- Determine how much fluid to give by checking blood pressure, urine output, CVP, and PAWP.
- Monitor ABG values, complete blood count, and electrolyte levels.
- During therapy, assess skin color and temperature and note any changes. Cold, clammy skin may be a sign of continuing peripheral vascular constriction, indicating progressive shock.

PATIENT TEACHING

- Because the patient and his family may be anxious about the ICU and special devices such as the IABP, offer explanations and reassurance.
- Prepare the patient and his family for a probable fatal outcome, and help them find effective coping strategies.
- Provide spiritual support as appropriate.

CARDIOMYOPATHY

Cardiomyopathy is the general term applied to diseases of the heart's muscle fibers. It occurs in three main forms: dilated, hypertrophic, and restrictive. (See *Three types of cardiomyopathy*, page 144.) The origin of most cardiomyopathies is unknown. However, hypertrophic cardiomyopathy is almost always inherited as a non-sex-linked autosomal dominant trait.

Signs and symptoms

Dilated cardiomyopathy

- Shortness of breath
- Orthopnea
- Chest pain
- Dyspnea on exertion
- Fatigue
- Irritating dry cough at night
- Edema
- Jugular vein distention
- S_3 and S_4 gallop
- Arrhythmias or heart block

Hypertrophic cardiomyopathy

- Angina pectoris
- Arrhythmias
- Dyspnea
- Orthopnea
- Syncope
- Heart failure

Three types of cardiomyopathy

Dilated cardiomyopathy

Dilated cardiomyopathy results from extensively damaged myocardial muscle fibers. This disorder interferes with myocardial metabolism and grossly dilates all four heart chambers, giving the heart a globular appearance. Dilated cardiomyopathy leads to intractable heart failure, arrhythmias, and emboli. Because it's usually not diagnosed until the advanced stages, this form of cardiomyopathy typically has a poor prognosis.

Hypertrophic cardiomyopathy

Hypertrophic cardiomyopathy (also known as idiopathic hypertrophic subaortic stenosis) is characterized by disproportionate asymmetrical thickening of the interventricular septum and heart walls. Cardiac output may be low, normal, or high, depending on whether stenosis is obstructive or nonobstructive. If cardiac output is normal or high, the disease may go undetected for years; however, low cardiac output may lead to potentially fatal heart failure. The disease course varies: Some patients deteriorate progressively while others remain stable for years. Eventually, left ventricular dysfunction leads to pump failure.

Restrictive cardiomyopathy

Restrictive cardiomyopathy is marked by restrictive ventricular filling and endocardial fibrosis and thickening. If severe, it's irreversible.

- Early systolic murmur
- Sudden death

Restrictive cardiomyopathy

- Fatigue
- Dyspnea
- Orthopnea
- Chest pain
- Generalized edema
- Liver engorgement
- Peripheral cyanosis
- Pallor

Diagnostic tests

Dilated cardiomyopathy

Diagnosis requires elimination of other possible causes of heart failure and arrhythmias.

- *Electrocardiography* (ECG) and *angiography* rule out ischemic heart disease; ECG may also show biventricular hypertrophy, sinus tachycardia, atrial enlargement and, in 20% of patients, atrial fibrillation and bundle-branch block.
- *Chest X-rays* reveal cardiomegaly—usually affecting all heart chambers—and may demonstrate pulmonary congestion, pleural or pericardial effusion, or pulmonary venous hypertension.
- *Echocardiography* identifies left ventricular thrombi, global hypokinesia, and the degree of left ventricular dilation.
- *Radionuclide imaging* may be used to evaluate ventricular wall motion, ventricular function, and hypertrophy.

Hypertrophic cardiomyopathy

Diagnosis depends on typical clinical findings and test results.

- *Echocardiography* (most useful) shows increased thickness of the intraventricular septum and abnormal motion of the anterior mitral leaflet during systole, occluding left ventricular outflow in obstructive disease.
- *Cardiac catheterization* reveals elevated left ventricular end-diastolic pressure (LVEDP) and, possibly, mitral insufficiency.
- *ECG* usually demonstrates left ventricular hypertrophy, T-wave inversion, left anterior hemiblock, Q waves in precordial and inferior leads, ventricular arrhythmias and, possibly, atrial fibrillation.

Restrictive cardiomyopathy

- In advanced stages of this disease, *chest X-rays* show massive cardiomegaly affecting all four chambers of the heart, pericardial effusion, and pulmonary congestion.
- *Echocardiography* rules out constrictive pericarditis as the cause of restricted filling by detecting increased left ventricular muscle mass and differences in end-diastolic pressures between the ventricles.
- *ECG* may show low-voltage complexes, hypertrophy, atrioventricular conduction defects, or arrhythmias.
- *Arterial pulsation* reveals blunt carotid upstroke with small volume.
- *Cardiac catheterization* demonstrates increased LVEDP and rules out constrictive pericarditis as the cause of restricted filling.

Treatment

Treatment varies with the type of cardiomyopathy.

Dilated cardiomyopathy

The goal of treatment is to correct the underlying cause. Specific measures include administration of digoxin to improve the heart's pumping ability; diuretics, sodium-restricted diet, and fluid restriction to help combat heart failure; oxygen to improve oxygenation; and vasodilators to reduce preload and afterload, thereby decreasing congestion and increasing cardiac output.

Acute heart failure requires vasodilation with nitroprusside or I.V. nitroglycerin. Long-term treatment may include prazosin, hydralazine, isosorbide dinitrate, angiotensin-converting enzyme inhibitors, and anticoagulants.

Heart transplantation may be an option for a patient who is otherwise healthy.

Hypertrophic cardiomyopathy

The goals of treatment are to relax the ventricle and to relieve outflow tract obstruction. A beta-adrenergic blocking agent (such as metoprolol or propranolol), slows the heart rate and increases ventricular filling by relaxing the obstructing muscle, thereby reducing angina, syncope, dyspnea, and arrhythmias. However, beta-adrenergic blockers must be used cautiously because they may aggravate symptoms of cardiac decompensation and heart failure. Calcium channel blockers such as verapamil are also used to relieve symptoms and improve exercise tolerance.

Cardioversion is used if the patient is experiencing atrial fibrillation. Because of the high risk of systemic embolism, the patient should receive anticoagulant therapy until fibrillation subsides.

Surgery, such as ventriculomyomectomy, may be used to increase the patient's exercise tolerance, which would allow the patient to do more without becoming short of breath.

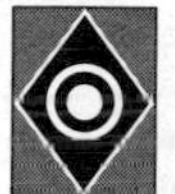

Drug alert Vasodilators, such as nitroglycerin, are contraindicated in patients with hypertrophic cardiomyopathy because they reduce venous return by permitting pooling of blood in the periphery. This action decreases ventricular volume and chamber size, which may cause further obstruction. Also contraindicated are sympathetic stimulators such as isoproterenol, which enhance cardiac contractility and myocardial oxygen demands, intensifying the obstruction.

Restrictive cardiomyopathy

Although no therapy currently exists for restricted ventricular filling, cardiac glycosides, diuretics, and sodium restriction may ease the symptoms of heart failure. Oral vasodilators — such as isosorbide dinitrate, prazosin, and hydralazine — may control intractable heart failure. Anticoagulant therapy may be necessary to prevent thrombophlebitis in patients on prolonged bed rest.

Key nursing diagnoses and outcomes

Activity intolerance related to imbalance between oxygen supply and demand

Treatment outcome: The patient will maintain his blood pressure, pulse, and respiratory rate within prescribed limits during exertion.

Decreased cardiac output related to ventricular dysfunction

Treatment outcome: The patient will remain hemodynamically stable, as evidenced by the absence of cardiac arrhythmias and chest pain and by the maintenance of blood pressure and pulse and respiratory rates within a safe range.

Nursing interventions

- Monitor the patient's vital signs and cardiovascular status frequently.
- Monitor the patient's weight and intake and output.
- Alternate periods of rest with required activities of daily living and treatments. Provide personal care as needed to prevent fatigue.
- If the patient is on bed rest, provide active or passive range-of-motion exercises to prevent muscle atrophy.
- Because therapeutic restrictions and an uncertain prognosis may cause profound anxiety and depression, offer support and let the patient and his family express their fears and concerns. As needed, help them identify effective coping strategies. Be flexible about visiting hours.
- To determine the patient's tolerance for an increased dose of a beta-adrenergic blocking agent, take his pulse to check for bradycardia and have him stand and walk around slowly to check for orthostatic hypotension (hypertrophic cardiomyopathy).

PATIENT TEACHING

- Teach the patient about his illness and treatment. Emphasize the need to avoid alcohol (because of its cardiac depressant effect), to restrict sodium intake, and to watch for weight gain.
- If the patient is taking digoxin, tell him to watch for signs of toxicity (anorexia, nausea, vomiting, yellow vision).
- If the patient is taking propranolol, inform him and his family that the drug may cause depression. Tell them to notify the physician if symptoms appear.
- Instruct the patient with hypertrophic cardiomyopathy to notify any physician caring for him that he shouldn't be given nitroglycerin, cardiac glycosides, or diuretics because they can worsen the obstruction.
- Inform the patient that he'll need antibiotic prophylaxis for subacute bacterial endocarditis before dental work or surgery.

CARDIOPULMONARY RESUSCITATION

A basic life support procedure performed on victims of cardiac arrest, cardiopulmonary resuscitation (CPR) seeks to restore and maintain the patient's respiration and circulation after his heartbeat and breathing have stopped.

Most adults in sudden cardiac arrest develop ventricular fibrillation and require defibrillation; CPR alone won't improve their chances of survival. Therefore, you must assess the patient and contact the emergency medical service (EMS) or call a code *before* starting CPR. Timing is critical. Early access to EMS, early CPR, and early defibrillation greatly improve the patient's chances of survival.

In most instances, you perform CPR to keep the patient alive until a defibrillator or automatic external defibrillator is available or advanced cardiac life support (ACLS) can begin. The basic CPR procedure consists of assessing the victim, calling for help, and then following the ABC protocol: opening the airway, restoring breathing, and then restoring circulation. After the airway has been opened and breathing and circulation have been restored, diagnosis by electrocardiogram (ECG), defibrillation, or drug therapy may follow. CPR is contraindicated in "no code" patients.

Supplies

- Hard surface on which to place the patient, such as a bed headboard, a cardiac resuscitation board, or the floor
- Gloves, if available
- One-way valve mask, if available

Implementation

One-person rescue

- Put on gloves if available.
- Determine the patient's level of consciousness. Gently shake his shoulder and shout, "Are you okay?" in both ears in case he has difficulty hearing. This simple action ensures that you don't start CPR on a conscious person.
- Quickly scan the patient for major injuries, particularly to the head or neck. Call for help. Ask the person who arrives to call a code. (If you're outside a health care facility and treating an unresponsive adult, call 911 or another local emergency number for help.)
- Place the patient in the supine position on a hard, flat surface. If the patient is in bed, use a cardiac resuscitation board or put the bed's headboard under him. If you suspect a head or neck injury, move the patient as little as possible to reduce the risk of paralysis. If you must move him, logroll him into the supine position, supporting his head and neck to keep his spinal column from twisting.
- To ensure an open airway, position yourself near the patient's shoulders, and perform the head-tilt, chin-lift maneuver (if you don't suspect a neck injury). Place one hand on the patient's forehead and the fingers of the other hand under the bony portion of his chin near the jaw. Lift the chin forward and support the jaw, helping to tilt the head back.
- If you suspect a neck injury, open the airway using the jaw-thrust maneuver. Kneel behind the patient's head with your elbows on the ground. Rest your thumbs on his lower jaw near the corners of his mouth. Your thumbs should point toward the patient's feet. Then place your fingertips around the lower jaw. With a steady, strong motion, lift the jaw upward and outward with your fingertips. This maneuver opens the airway without moving the neck.
- While keeping the patient's airway open, place your ear over his mouth and nose and look toward his feet. Look for chest movement and listen for the sound of moving air. You may feel a breath of air on your cheek. This evaluation procedure should take 3 to 5 seconds. If you detect signs of breathing, keep the patient's airway open and continue checking his breathing until help arrives.
- If the patient doesn't start breathing once you've opened his airway, begin rescue breathing. Use the one-way valve mask as directed by your facility's policy. If necessary, connect the one-way valve to the mask. Place the mask over the patient's nose and mouth.
- Seal the mask by placing the heel and thumb of each hand along the border of the mask and compressing firmly to provide a tight seal along the margin of the mask. Place your remaining fingers along the bony margin of the jaw while performing a head tilt.

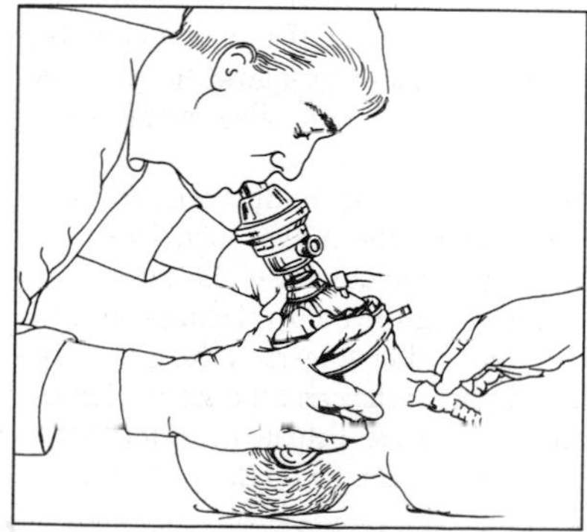

▶ Take a deep breath and seal your lips around the victim's mask, creating an airtight seal. Deliver two full ventilations, taking a deep breath after each. This allows time for the patient's chest to expand and relax and prevents gastric distention. Each ventilation should last 1.5 to 2 seconds with a tidal volume of 400 to 600 ml provided by mouth-to-mask ventilation.

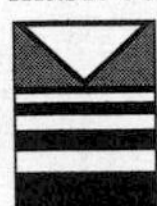

Key point Although human immunodeficiency virus isn't known to be transmitted in saliva, you may be reluctant to give mouth-to-mouth rescue breaths. For this reason, the American Heart Association (AHA) recommends that all health care professionals use airway equipment, such as the one-way valve mask.

▶ If you don't have a mask, perform mouth-to-mouth rescue breathing. Once you've opened the patient's airway, pinch his nostrils shut with the thumb and index finger of the hand you had on his forehead.

▶ Take a deep breath, and cover the patient's mouth with yours. Aim for a tight seal. Deliver two full ventilations, taking a deep breath after each to allow time for the patient's chest to expand and relax and to prevent gastric distention. Each ventilation should last 1.5 to 2 seconds with a tidal volume of 700 to 1000 ml provided by mouth-to-mouth ventilation. If this attempt fails, reposition the patient's head and try again. If the second attempt fails, suspect an airway obstruction. If a foreign body is blocking the airway, follow the basic life support procedure for clearing an obstructed airway.

▶ Keep one hand on the patient's forehead to keep the airway open. With your other hand, palpate the carotid artery closer to you by placing your index and middle fingers in the groove between the trachea and the sternocleidomastoid muscle. Palpate the artery for 5 to 10 seconds. If you detect a pulse, don't begin chest compressions. Instead, continue rescue breathing, giving 12 ventilations each minute (or one every 5 seconds). After every 12 ventilations, recheck the pulse.

▶ If you don't detect a pulse and help has not arrived yet, start chest compressions. Still kneeling, move to the patient's side. Spread your knees apart for a wide base of support. Next, using the hand closer to the patient's feet, locate the lower margin of his rib cage, as shown below.

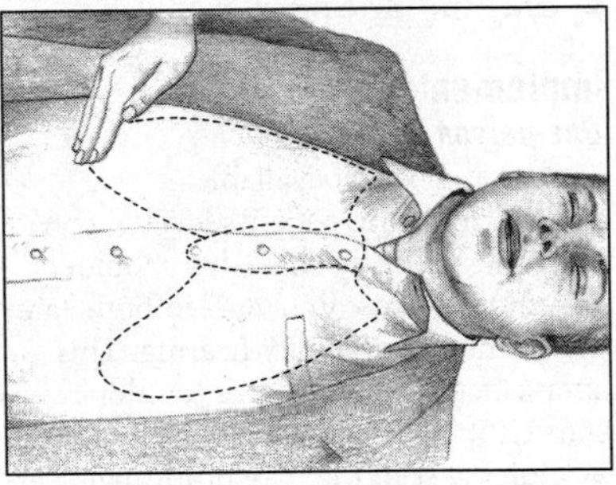

▶ Move your fingertips along the margin to the notch where the ribs meet the sternum.

▶ Place your middle finger on that notch (the xiphoid process) and your index finger next to it, as shown below. Your index finger should be on the bottom of the patient's sternum. Take care to find the correct hand position because improper placement can lead to complications.

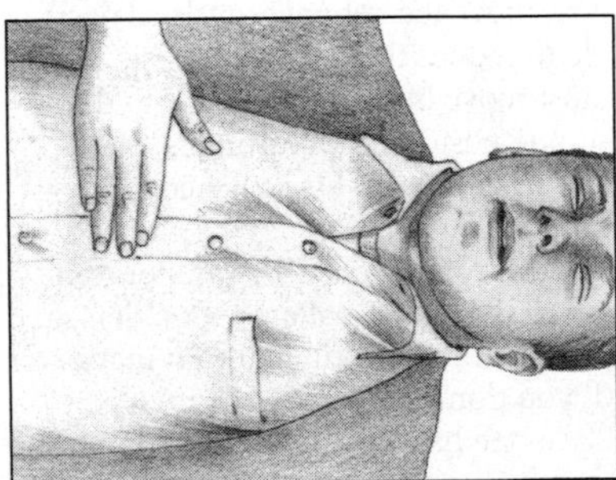

▶ Put the heel of your other hand on the lower half of the patient's sternum, next to your index finger, as shown below. The long axis of the heel of your hand should align with the long axis of the sternum.

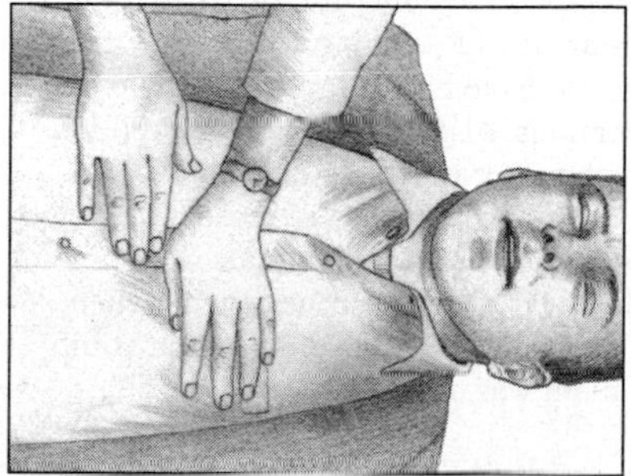

▶ Take your fingers off the notch, and place that hand directly on top of your other hand. Make sure your fingers don't rest on the patient's chest. This keeps the force of the compressions on the sternum and reduces the risk of a rib fracture, lung puncture, or liver laceration. Keep in mind that liver laceration occurs more often with improper hand placement, especially if the hands are too low.

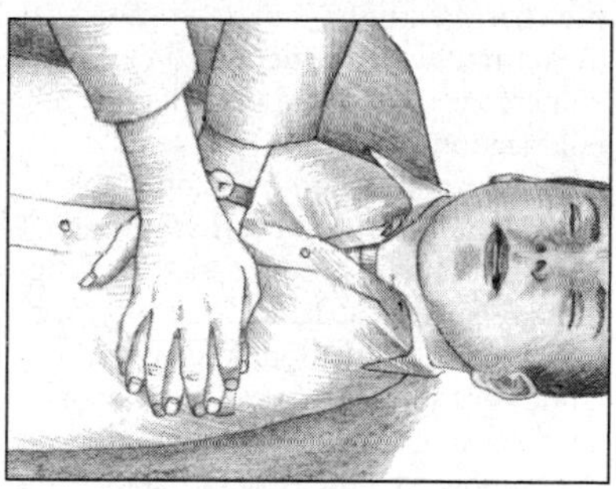

▶ With your elbows locked, arms straight, and shoulders directly over your hands, start chest compressions. Using the weight of your upper body, compress the patient's sternum 1½″ to 2″ (3.8 to 5 cm), delivering the pressure through the heels of your hands. Don't let your fingers rest on the patient's chest.

▶ After each compression, release the pressure and allow the chest to return to its normal position so the heart can fill with blood. To prevent injuries, don't change your hand position during compressions.

▶ Give 15 chest compressions at a rate that simulates 100 heartbeats/minute. Count "one and two and..." up to 15, compressing on the number and releasing on the "and." After 15 compressions, give 2 ventilations. Reposition your hands properly and deliver 15 more compressions. Continue this pattern for four full cycles.

▶ Palpate the carotid artery again. If you still don't detect a pulse, continue CPR in cycles of 15 compressions and 2 ventilations. Perform CPR for 1 more minute, check for a pulse, and then call for help again. In most health care facilities, help arrives promptly.

▶ Without help, however, continue CPR. Check for renewed respirations and a pulse. If you feel a pulse but no breath, give 12 ventilations per minute, and monitor the pulse. Don't stop CPR until the patient's breathing and pulse resume, someone takes over for you, or you become too exhausted to continue.

▶ If you detect both a pulse and respirations, position the patient on his side (turning his body as a unit), and monitor his condition. If the patient has sustained trauma or if injury is suspected, the patient should not be moved.

Two-person rescue

▶ Continue one-person CPR until the second rescuer takes the proper position (at the patient's chest) opposite you. This tells you that he knows the standard AHA procedures for CPR.

▶ The second rescuer can start assisting after you've finished a cycle of 15 compressions, 2 ventilations, and a pulse check. The second rescuer can check for a returning pulse while you perform chest compressions. If he feels a pulse, he may ask you to stop compressions for 5 seconds so that he can assess for an independent heartbeat.

- Move to the patient's head and check for a pulse while the second rescuer locates the correct hand position for delivering chest compressions.
- If you don't detect a pulse, say "No pulse; continue CPR" and give one ventilation. Meanwhile, the second rescuer starts compressions at a rate of 100/minute in a ratio of 15:2 (fifteen compressions to two ventilations). The compressor (at this point, the second rescuer) should count out loud so that you know when to give the next ventilation. Then the second rescuer should stop compressions long enough for the patient's chest to rise and fall with two ventilations.
- Periodically signal the compressor to stop for 10 seconds so you can check for breathing and a pulse.
- The compressor may grow tired and call for a change in positions. This switch should be done carefully, so as not to interrupt CPR. Give 2 ventilations and move into place to deliver chest compressions.
- Now, the second rescuer moves to the patient's head to begin ventilations. First, he checks the patient's pulse for 10 seconds. If he doesn't find a pulse, he says, "No pulse" and gives a ventilation. Then you start compressions. Both of you should continue CPR until the patient's respirations and pulse return, ACLS can begin, or you both become exhausted.
- Once the victim's pulse and respirations have returned, place him in the recovery position by turning him on his side.

Complications
CPR can cause certain complications, especially if the compressor doesn't place his hands properly on the sternum. These complications include fractured ribs, a lacerated liver, punctured lungs, regurgitation, and aspiration. Gastric distention, a common complication, results from giving too much air during ventilation.

Documentation
Whenever you perform CPR, document why you initiated it, whether the patient suffered from cardiac or respiratory arrest, when you found the patient and started CPR, and how long he received CPR. Note his response and any complications. Also include any interventions taken to correct complications.

If the victim also received ACLS, document which interventions were performed, who performed them, when they were performed, and what equipment was used.

CARDIOVERSION, SYNCHRONIZED

Used to treat tachyarrhythmias, synchronized cardioversion delivers an electric charge to the myocardium at the peak of the R wave. This causes immediate depolarization, interrupting reentry circuits and allowing the sinoatrial node to resume control. Synchronizing the electric charge with the R wave ensures that the current won't be delivered on the vulnerable T wave and thus disrupt repolarization.

Synchronized cardioversion is the treatment of choice for arrhythmias that don't respond to vagal massage or drug therapy, such as atrial tachycardia, atrial flutter, atrial fibrillation, and symptomatic ventricular tachycardia. It may be an elective or urgent procedure, depending on how well the patient tolerates the arrhythmia. For example, a hemodynamically unstable patient would require urgent cardioversion. Remember when preparing for cardioversion that the patient's condition can deteriorate quickly, necessitating immediate defibrillation.

Supplies
- Cardioverter-defibrillator
- Conductive gel

- Anterior, posterior, or transverse paddles
- Electrocardiogram (ECG) monitor with recorder
- Sedative
- Oxygen therapy equipment
- Airway, suction, and intubation equipment
- Handheld resuscitation bag
- Emergency pacing equipment
- Emergency cardiac medications
- Automatic or manual blood pressure cuff
- Pulse oximeter

Implementation

- Explain the procedure to the patient and family to reduce fear and promote cooperation.
- Make sure the patient has signed a consent form.
- Check the patient's recent serum potassium and magnesium levels, arterial blood gas results, and digoxin levels. Although digitalized patients may undergo cardioversion, they tend to require lower energy levels to convert. If the patient takes digoxin, withhold the dose on the day of the procedure.
- Withhold all food and fluids for 6 to 12 hours before the procedure.
- Obtain a 12-lead ECG to serve as a baseline.
- Check to see if the physician has ordered administration of any cardiac drugs before the procedure. Make sure the patient has a patent I.V. site in case drug administration becomes necessary.
- Connect the patient to a pulse oximeter and an automatic blood pressure cuff, if available.
- Consider administering oxygen for 5 to 10 minutes before the cardioversion to promote myocardial oxygenation.
- If the patient wears dentures, remove them.
- Place the patient in the supine position, and assess his vital signs, level of consciousness (LOC), cardiac rhythm, and peripheral pulses.
- Remove any oxygen delivery device just before cardioversion to avoid possible combustion.
- Have emergency cardiac drugs such as amiodarone, procainamide, epinephrine, lidocaine, and atropine available at the patient's bedside.

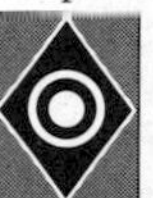

Drug alert Use lidocaine with caution in elderly patients, especially those weighing less than 110 lb (50 kg) and those with heart failure, renal disease, or hepatic disease. Such patients will require a dosage reduction.

- Administer a sedative or analgesic as ordered. The patient should be heavily sedated but still able to breathe adequately.
- Carefully monitor the patient's blood pressure, respiratory rate, and oxygen saturation until he recovers.
- If the patient is attached to a bedside or telemetry monitor, disconnect the unit before cardioversion. The electric current it generates could damage the equipment.
- Be aware that improper synchronization may result if the patient's ECG tracing contains artifact-like spikes, such as peaked T waves or bundle-branch blocks when the R′ wave may be taller than the R wave.
- Press the POWER button to turn on the defibrillator. Attach the monitor leads from the defibrillator to the patient, making sure there is a clear display of the patient's rhythm. Next, push the SYNC button to synchronize the machine with the patient's QRS complexes. Make sure the SYNC button flashes with each of the patient's QRS complexes. You should also see a bright green flag flash on the monitor.
- Turn the energy SELECT dial to the ordered amount of energy (usually 50 to 100 joules to start).
- Remove the paddles from the machine, and prepare them with conductive gel as you would if you were defibrillating the patient. Then place the paddles: one paddle to the right of the

upper sternum, just below the right clavicle, and the other over the fifth or sixth intercostal space at the left anterior axillary line.

- Although the electric shock of cardioversion won't usually damage an implanted pacemaker, avoid placing the paddles directly over the pacemaker.
- Make sure everyone stands away from the bed; then push the discharge buttons simultaneously. Hold the paddles in place, applying approximately 25 lb of pressure on both paddles, and wait for the energy to be discharged. The machine has to synchronize the discharge with the R wave.
- Check the waveform on the monitor. If the arrhythmia fails to convert, repeat the procedure two or three more times at 3-minute intervals. Be sure to reset the SYNC button after each attempt at cardioversion because most defibrillators default back to unsynchronized mode. Gradually increase the energy level with each additional countershock.
- After the cardioversion, frequently assess the patient's LOC and respiratory status, including airway patency, respiratory rate and depth, and the need for supplemental oxygen. Because the patient will be heavily sedated, he may require airway support.
- Record a postcardioversion 12-lead ECG, and monitor the patient's ECG rhythm for several hours. Check his chest for electrical burns.

Complications

Common complications following cardioversion include transient, harmless arrhythmias, such as atrial, ventricular, and junctional premature beats. Serious ventricular arrhythmias such as ventricular fibrillation may also occur. However, this type of arrhythmia is more likely to result from high amounts of electrical energy, digoxin toxicity, severe heart disease, electrolyte imbalance, or improper synchronization with the R wave.

Patient teaching

- Explain the procedure to the patient. Tell him he will be heavily sedated but may experience minor discomfort.

Documentation

Document the procedure, including the voltage delivered with each attempt, rhythm strips before and after the procedure, and how the patient tolerated the procedure. Also document your patient teaching.

CATARACT

A common cause of gradual vision loss, a cataract is an opacity of the lens or lens capsule of the eye. The clouded lens blocks light shining through the cornea, which in turn blurs the image cast onto the retina. As a result, the brain interprets a hazy image.

Cataracts commonly affect both eyes, but each cataract progresses independently. Exceptions are traumatic cataracts, which are usually unilateral, and congenital cataracts, which may remain stationary. Cataracts are most prevalent in people over age 70. Surgery restores vision in about 95% of patients. Without surgery, cataracts eventually lead to complete vision loss.

Cataracts are classified according to their cause:

- Senile cataracts develop in older people, probably because of chemical changes in lens proteins.
- Congenital cataracts occur in neonates from inborn errors of metabolism or from maternal rubella infection during the first trimester of pregnancy. These cataracts may also result from a congenital anomaly or from genetic causes. Transmission is usually autosomal dominant; however, recessive cataracts may be sex-linked.
- Traumatic cataracts develop after a foreign body injures the lens with sufficient force to allow aqueous or vitreous humor to enter the lens capsule.

▶ Complicated cataracts occur secondary to uveitis, glaucoma, retinitis pigmentosa, or retinal detachment. They can also occur with systemic diseases, such as diabetes, hypoparathyroidism, or atopic dermatitis, or from ionizing radiation or infrared rays.
▶ Toxic cataracts result from drug or chemical toxicity with ergot or phenothiazines.

Signs and symptoms

▶ Painless, gradual vision loss
▶ Poor reading vision
▶ Annoying glare and poor vision in bright sunlight
▶ Blinding glare from headlights when driving at night
▶ Possibly better vision in dim light than in bright light (with central opacity)
▶ Milky white pupil
▶ Grayish white area behind the pupil (with an advanced cataract)

Diagnostic tests

▶ *Indirect ophthalmoscopy* reveals a dark area in the normally homogeneous red reflex.
▶ *Slit-lamp examination* confirms the diagnosis of a lens opacity.
▶ *Visual acuity testing* confirms the degree of vision loss.

Treatment

Surgical lens extraction and implantation of an intraocular lens to correct the visual deficit is the accepted treatment.

Key nursing diagnoses and outcomes

Fear related to complete loss of vision caused by untreated cataracts
Treatment outcomes: The patient will state that he feels less fearful and will exhibit no signs or symptoms of fear.

Risk for injury related to decrease in vision caused by the cataract
Treatment outcome: The patient will remain free from injury.

Disturbed sensory perception (visual) related to diminishing ability to see properly as a result of the cataract
Treatment outcome: The patient will regain lost vision with treatment.

Nursing interventions

▶ Prepare the patient for cataract surgery as appropriate.
▶ Provide a safe environment. For example, keep bed rails raised and help the patient with activities as needed. Evaluate the patient's home safety.
▶ Allow the patient to express his fears and anxieties about his vision loss.
▶ Check the patient's vision regularly.

PATIENT TEACHING

▶ Explain how and why cataracts form.
▶ Stress the importance of regular ophthalmic examinations to monitor the degree of visual impairment and to determine when surgery can be performed. Encourage the patient to have the cataract removed.
▶ Caution the patient to take safety precautions until the cataract can be removed, including avoiding night driving.

CATARACT REMOVAL

Cataracts can be removed by one of two techniques. In intracapsular cataract extraction (ICCE), the entire lens is removed, usually with a cryoprobe. In extracapsular cataract extraction (ECCE), the patient's anterior capsule, cortex, and nucleus are removed, leaving the posterior capsule intact. This technique may be carried out using manual extraction, irrigation and aspiration, or phacoemulsification.

Immediately after removal of the natural lens, many patients receive an intraocular lens implant. An implant is especially well suited for older patients who are unable to use eyeglasses or contact lenses (because of arthritis or tremors, for example).

Implementation

▶ Cataract surgery is usually an outpatient procedure performed under local anesthetic. Preoperatively, the patient will receive a sedative to promote comfort. (For a description of the actual procedure, see *Comparing methods of cataract removal.*)

▶ When the cataract has been removed, the surgeon may insert a lens implant. After enlarging the incision, he'll implant the lens into the capsular sac. If he implants the lens without sutures, he'll administer a miotic agent such as pilocarpine to prevent the iris from dilating too much and causing the lens to slip.

▶ In both ICCE and ECCE, the surgeon may also perform a peripheral iridectomy to reduce intraocular pressure and may briefly instill alpha-chymotrypsin, a proteolytic enzyme, in the anterior chamber to dissolve resistant zonular fibers. After the procedure, the surgeon may administer a miotic agent to constrict the pupil. Then he'll close the sutures, instill antibiotic drops or ointment, and patch and shield the eye.

Complications

Cataract removal can cause numerous complications, most of which can be corrected. They include pupillary block, corneal decompensation, vitreous loss, hemorrhage, cystoid macular edema, lens dislocation, secondary membrane opacification, and retinal detachment.

Key nursing diagnoses and outcomes

Pain related to elevated intraocular pressure postoperatively

Treatment outcome: The patient will remain free from severe pain.

Impaired home maintenance management related to visual disturbances following cataract removal

Treatment outcome: The patient will be able to care for himself at home following cataract removal or will identify resources to help with self-care if necessary.

Disturbed sensory perception (visual) related to potential complications caused by cataract removal

Treatment outcome: The patient will demonstrate improved or normal visual acuity postoperatively.

Nursing interventions

When caring for a patient undergoing cataract removal, your main intervention will involve instructing the patient. Most patients will go home several hours after the surgery. They'll need to be instructed on recognizing postoperative complications, administering eye medications, and avoiding activities that might injure the eye.

Before surgery

▶ Explain the planned surgical technique to the patient. Tell him that he'll receive eyedrops to dilate his eye and facilitate cataract removal, antibiotics to reduce the risk of infection, and a sedative to help him relax.

▶ If the patient takes an anticoagulant, tell him he'll need to discontinue it for a few days before surgery.

▶ Inform the patient that he'll have to wear an eye shield temporarily after surgery to prevent traumatic injury and infection. Instruct him to sleep on the unaffected side to reduce intraocular pressure.

▶ Assist the patient in identifying resources for his postoperative needs. The patient may need to arrange help with transportation, medication administration, and activities of daily living.

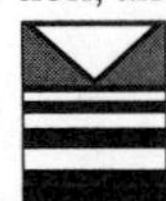

Key point Explain to the patient who doesn't have a lens implant that he'll temporarily lose his depth perception after surgery and will have reduced peripheral vision on the side that was treated.

▶ Make sure that the patient has signed a consent form.

Comparing methods of cataract removal

Cataracts can be removed by intracapsular or extracapsular techniques.

Intracapsular cataract extraction

In this technique, the surgeon makes a partial incision at the superior limbus arc. He then removes the lens using specially designed forceps or a cryoprobe, which freezes and adheres to the lens to facilitate its removal.

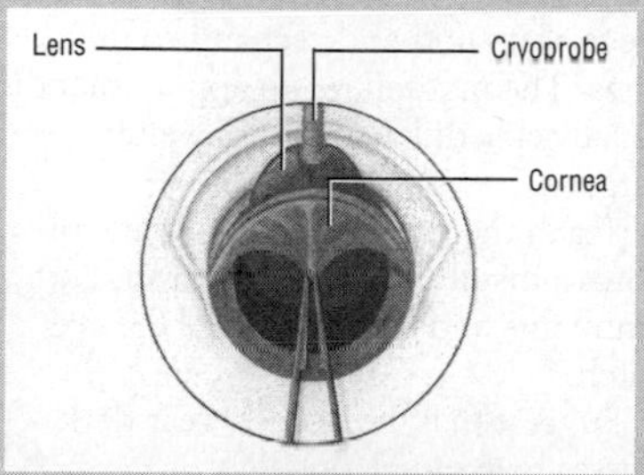

Extracapsular cataract extraction

In this technique, the surgeon may use irrigation and aspiration or phacoemulsification. In irrigation and aspiration, he makes an incision at the limbus, opens the anterior lens capsule with a cystotome, and exerts pressure from below to express the lens. He then irrigates and suctions the remaining lens cortex.

In phacoemulsification, the surgeon uses an ultrasonic probe to break the lens into minute particles, which are aspirated by the probe.

IRRIGATION AND ASPIRATION

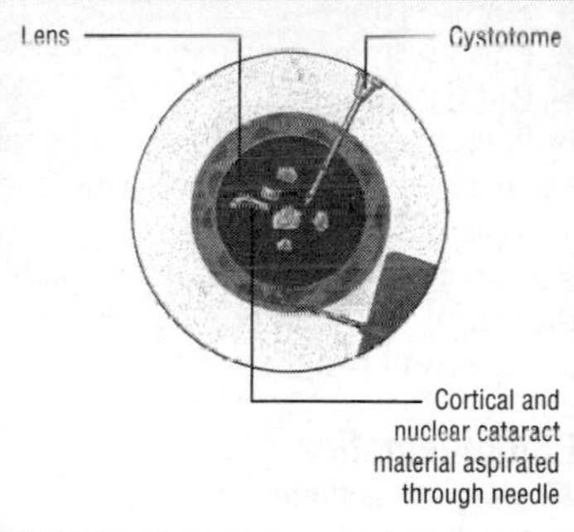

PHACOEMULSIFICATION

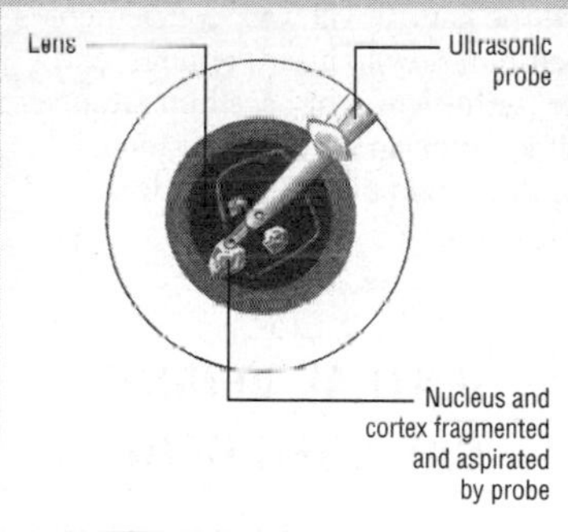

After surgery

▶ Postoperatively, monitor vital signs until stable and assess for complications. Notify the physician if the patient experiences severe pain, bleeding, increased drainage, fever, or increased intraocular pressure postoperatively.

▶ Maintain the eye patch, and have the patient wear an eye shield, especially when sleeping. Tell him to continue wearing the shield during sleep for several weeks, as ordered.

PATIENT TEACHING

▶ Warn the patient to contact the physician at once if he experiences sudden sharp eye pain, red or watery eyes, photophobia, or sudden visual changes. Instruct him to avoid activities that raise intraocular pressure, including heavy lifting, bending at the waist, straining during defecation, vigorous coughing, sneezing, and placing his head in a dependent position. Tell him not to exercise strenuously for 6 to 10 weeks.

- Explain that follow-up appointments are necessary to monitor the results of the surgery and to detect any complications. The first follow-up appointment is usually scheduled for the day after surgery.
- Teach the patient or a family member how to instill prescribed eyedrops and ointments and how to change the eye patch.
- Suggest that the patient wear dark glasses to avoid glaring light.
- If the patient will wear eyeglasses, explain that changes in his vision can present safety hazards. To compensate for loss of depth perception, show him how to use up-and-down head movements to judge distances. To overcome the loss of peripheral vision on the treated side, teach him to turn his head fully in that direction to view objects to his side.
- If the patient will wear contact lenses, teach him how to insert, remove, and care for his lenses or have him arrange to visit a physician routinely for removal, cleaning, and reinsertion of extended-wear lenses.

CENTRAL VENOUS CATHETER CARE

A central venous (CV) catheter line is a sterile catheter that is inserted through a major vein, such as the subclavian vein or, less commonly, the jugular, median basilic, or femoral vein. (See *CV catheter pathways*.)

By providing access to the central veins, CV therapy offers several benefits. It allows monitoring of CV pressure, which indicates blood volume or pump efficiency, and permits aspiration of blood samples for diagnostic tests. It also allows administration of I.V. fluids (in large amounts, if necessary) in emergencies or when decreased peripheral circulation causes peripheral veins to collapse; when prolonged I.V. therapy reduces the number of accessible peripheral veins; when solutions must be diluted (for large volumes or for irritating or hypertonic fluids, such as total parenteral nutrition solutions); and when a patient requires long-term venous access. Because repeated blood samples can be drawn through it, the CV line decreases the patient's anxiety and preserves or restores peripheral veins.

Once a CV catheter is inserted by the physician, it requires diligent maintenance that includes flushing the catheter, changing the injection cap, and performing dressing changes.

Supplies

- Gloves
- Alcohol pad
- Sterile syringe
- Flush solution
- Padded clamp
- Povidone-iodine swabs (or other antiseptic cleansing agent if the patient is allergic to iodine)
- Dressing (gauze or semipermeable dressing)
- Label and pen

Implementation

Flushing the catheter

- Flush the catheter routinely according to your facility's policy. If the system is being maintained as a heparin lock and the infusions are intermittent, the flushing procedure will vary according to the facility's policy, the medication administration schedule, and the type of catheter.
- Clean the cap of the CV catheter with an alcohol pad. Allow it to dry.
- Inject the recommended type and amount of flush solution (normal saline

CV catheter pathways

The illustrations below show several common pathways for central venous (CV) catheter insertion. Typically, a CV catheter is inserted into the subclavian or internal jugular vein. The catheter may terminate in the superior vena cava or right atrium.

Insertion: Subclavian vein
Termination: Superior vena cava

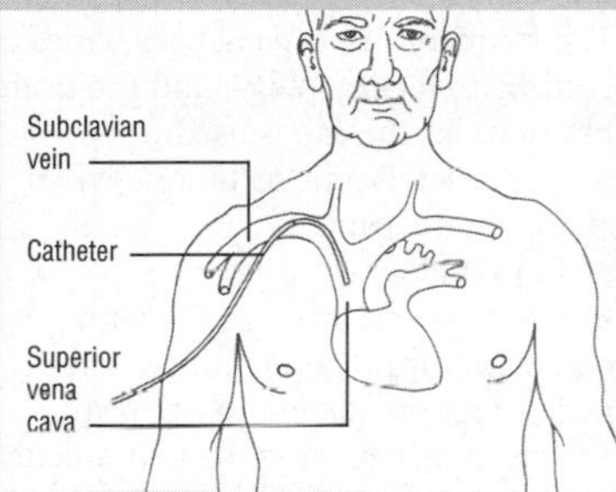

Insertion: Subclavian vein
Termination: Right atrium

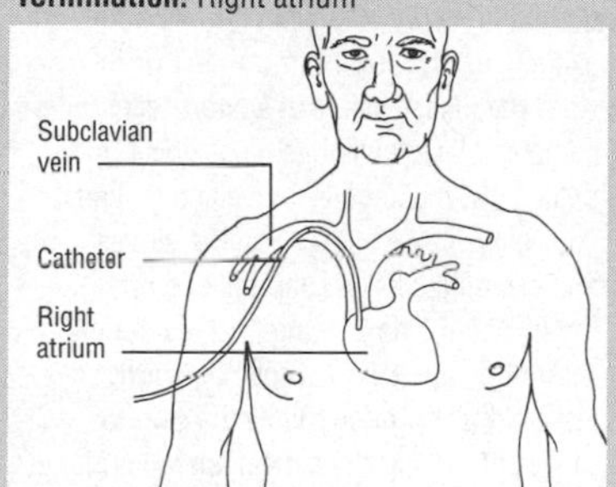

Insertion: Internal jugular vein
Termination: Superior vena cava

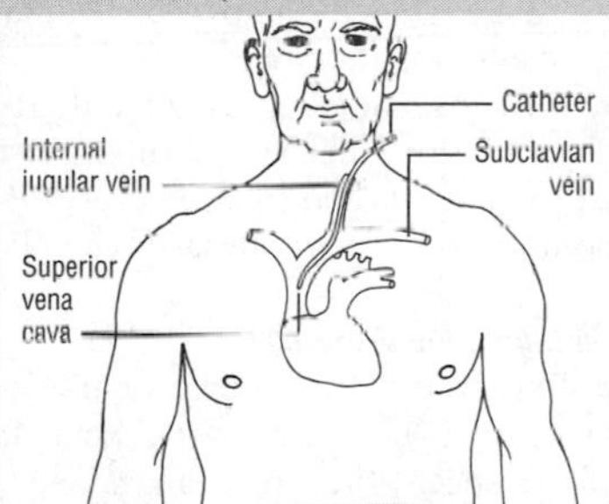

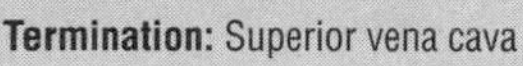

Insertion: Basilic vein
Termination: Superior vena cava

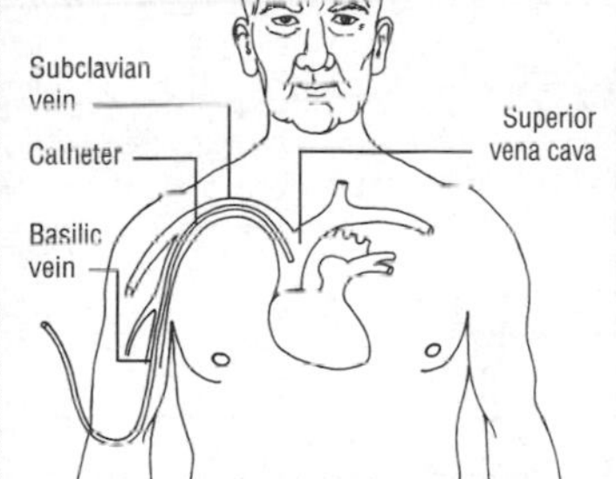

Insertion: Through a subcutaneous tunnel to the subclavian vein (Dacron cuff holds catheter in place)
Termination: Superior vena cava

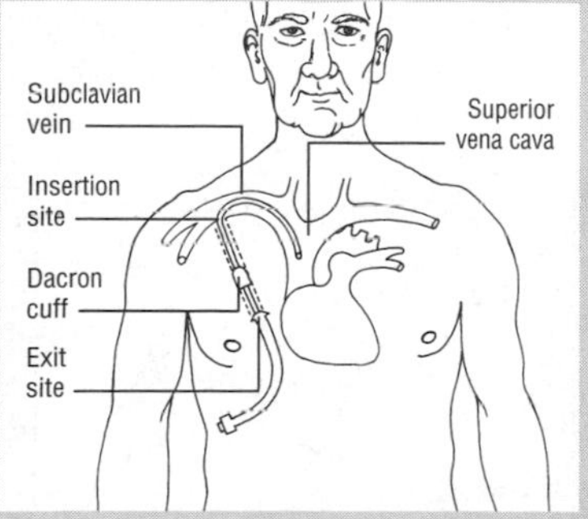

Key steps in changing a CV dressing

The following illustrations show the key steps you'll perform when changing a central venous (CV) dressing.

First, put on clean gloves and remove the old dressing by pulling it toward the exit site of the long-term catheter or toward the insertion site of a short-term catheter. (This technique helps you avoid pulling out the line.) Remove and discard your gloves. Next, put on sterile gloves and clean the skin around the site three times, using a new alcohol pad each time. Start at the center and move outward, using a circular motion. Allow the skin to dry. Confirm that the patient isn't allergic to iodine, then repeat the same cleaning procedure using three swabs soaked in povidone-iodine solution.

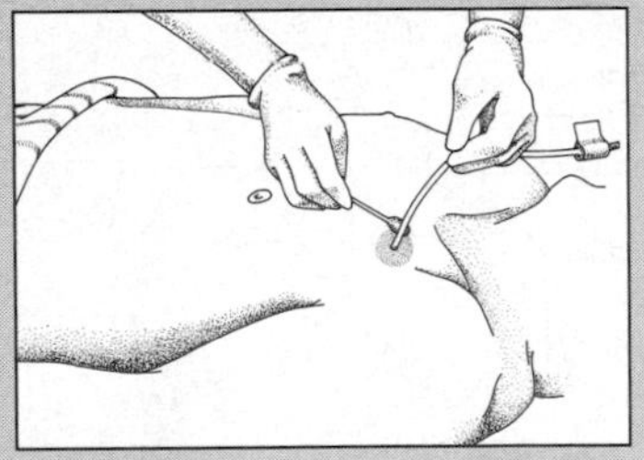

After the solution has dried, cover the site with a dressing, such as a gauze dressing or the transparent semipermeable dressing shown here. Write the time and date on the label and attach it to the dressing.

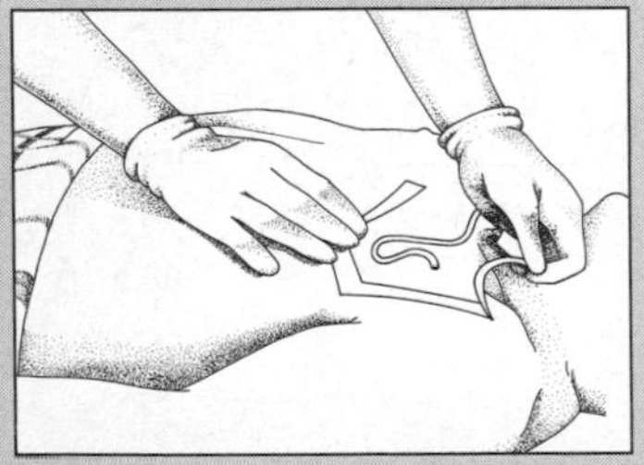

for a Groshung catheter; heparin flush solution for other types of catheters).

- After flushing the catheter, maintain positive pressure by keeping your thumb on the plunger of the syringe while withdrawing the needle. This prevents blood backflow and potential clotting in the line.

Changing the injection cap

The frequency of cap changes varies according to facility policy and the number of times the cap is used.

- Use strict aseptic technique when changing the cap.
- Put on gloves.
- Clean the connection site with an alcohol pad or povidone-iodine swab.
- Instruct the patient to perform Valsalva's maneuver while you quickly disconnect the old cap and connect the new cap, using aseptic technique. If the patient can't perform Valsalva's maneuver, use a padded clamp to prevent air from entering the catheter.
- If the patient is receiving I.V. fluids or drug infusions, change I.V. tubing every 24 to 72 hours and solution every 24 hours according to your facility's policy.

Changing the dressing

- Expect to change your patient's CV dressing at least once a week. Many facilities specify dressing changes two or three times weekly as well as whenever the dressing becomes soiled, moist, or loose. (See *Key steps in changing a CV dressing.*)

Complications

Complications can occur at any time during the infusion therapy. Traumatic complications, such as pneumothorax, typically happen as the catheter is inserted but may not be noticed until after the procedure is completed. Systemic complications, such as sepsis, typically occur later during infusion therapy. Other possible complications include phlebitis and thrombus formation.

Patient teaching

- Explain the procedure to the patient.
- Tell him to report any discomfort at the insertion site.

Documentation

Record the date and time that you provided CV care. Note the patient's response to the care as well as any complications. Also document your patient teaching.

Cerebrovascular Accident

Commonly known as a stroke, a cerebrovascular accident (CVA) occurs when impaired circulation in the brain disrupts the supply of oxygen. Recovery from a CVA depends on how quickly and completely circulation is restored. However, almost half of all patients who survive a CVA are permanently disabled and suffer a recurrent attack.

CVA is the third leading cause of death and the most common cause of neurologic disability in North America. It strikes more than 600,000 people each year, killing more than 160,000. Though a CVA can strike people of any age, it usually affects men over age 65. Blacks face an especially high risk. Improved control of hypertension, the main risk factor for CVA, and improved treatment for transient ischemic attacks (TIAs) have helped reduce the incidence of CVA over the past 30 years.

CVA results from impaired circulation in one or more blood vessels of the brain, usually due to thrombosis, embolism, or hemorrhage. The most common cause of CVA is thrombosis, which is usually related to atherosclerosis. Plaque and atheromatous deposits gradually occlude the artery. Occlusion leads to ischemia and infarction of brain tissue, followed by edema and necrosis. Thrombosis usually occurs in the extracerebral vessels but sometimes occurs in the intracerebral vessels.

With embolism, fragments usually break off from a mural thrombus in the left atrium or ventricle or from bacterial vegetations affecting heart valves. These emboli travel through the carotid artery and typically lodge in the smaller cerebral vessels, most often the left middle cerebral artery. Ischemia may occur suddenly and is often followed by necrosis and edema. However, if the embolus breaks apart, then enters and is absorbed by a smaller vessel, the person's symptoms may subside.

CVA due to hemorrhage occurs when a cerebral vessel ruptures and blood flows into brain tissue or the subarachnoid space. Hemorrhagic CVAs are usually caused by rupture of an arteriosclerotic vessel due to prolonged hypertension, a cerebral aneurysm, or an arteriovenous malformation. Effects may be severe. More than 50% of patients die of brain herniation within the first 3 days. Physical effects of a CVA vary with the part of the brain affected, the severity of the episode, and the extent that collateral circulation develops to help the brain compensate for its decreased blood supply. (See *Understanding neurologic deficits,* page 160.)

Risk factors for CVA include a history of TIAs, atherosclerosis, hypertension, arrhythmias, myocardial infarction, rheumatic heart disease, postural hypotension, cardiac hypertrophy, previous heart surgery, emboli, diabetes mellitus, gout, obesity, lack of exercise, smoking, a family history of cerebrovascular disease, and high serum cholesterol, lipoprotein, or triglyceride levels. (See *Preventing strokes,* page 161.)

Signs and symptoms

- Headache
- Vomiting
- Seizure
- Confusion
- Restlessness

Understanding neurologic deficits

A cerebrovascular accident (CVA) can cause neurologic deficits ranging from mild hand weakness to complete unilateral paralysis. Such functional loss results from damaged brain tissue normally perfused by the occluded or ruptured artery. Most CVAs affect anterior cerebral circulation and damage the middle cerebral artery, internal carotid artery, or anterior cerebral artery. Below you'll find the CVA symptoms associated with specific damage sites.

Middle cerebral artery

- Aphasia
- Reading difficulty (dyslexia)
- Writing inability (dysgraphia)
- Visual field deficits
- Contralateral hemiparesis (more severe in the face and arm than in the leg)
- Contralateral sensory deficit
- Altered level of consciousness (LOC)

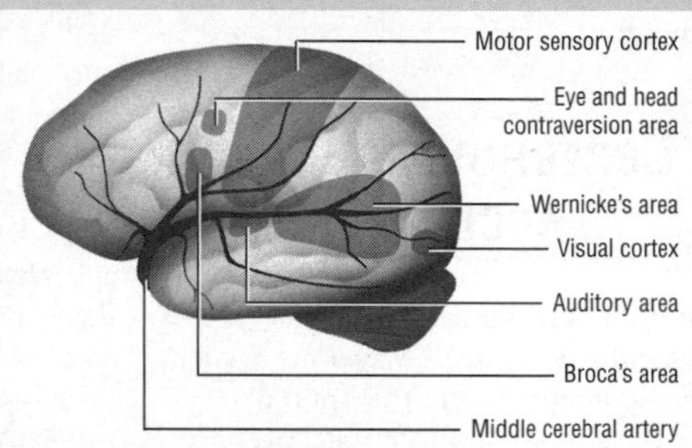

Internal carotid artery

- Headaches
- Weakness, paralysis, numbness, sensory changes, and visual deficits (such as blurring) on the affected side
- Altered LOC
- Bruits over the carotid artery
- Dysphasia
- Ptosis

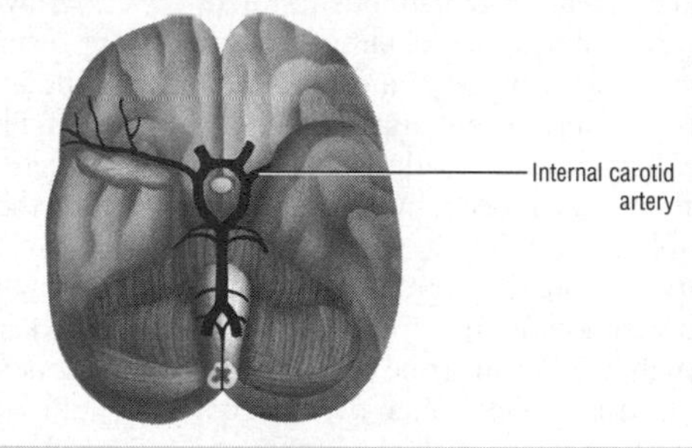

Anterior cerebral artery

- Weakness and numbness on the affected side
- Paralysis of the contralateral foot and leg
- Footdrop
- Incontinence
- Loss of coordination
- Impaired sensory functions
- Personality changes, confusion, short attention span
- Expressive aphasia

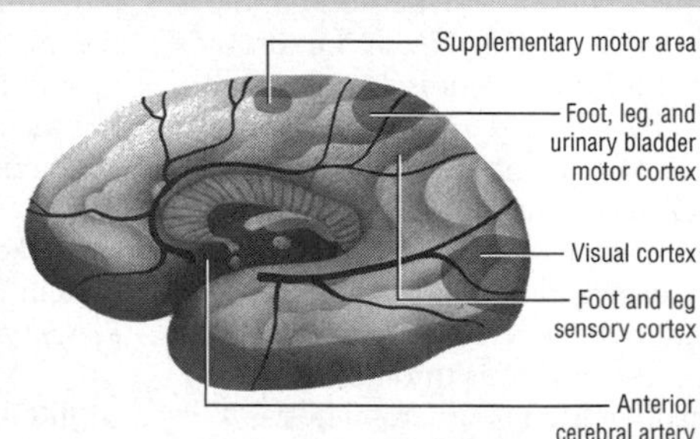

▶ Changes in sensation (may range from slight impairment of touch to inability to perceive the position and motion of body parts)
▶ Changes in motor function (may include problems with balance [ataxia] or gait, hemiparesis, or hemiplegia)
▶ Altered level of consciousness (LOC) (sudden loss of consciousness may indicate a major CVA)
▶ Cognitive problems (decreased attention span, forgetfulness, impaired judgment, lack of motivation)
▶ Anxiety
▶ Mood swings
▶ Communication problems (dysarthria or aphasia)
▶ Memory loss
▶ Bowel or bladder incontinence
▶ Vision problems (visual field deficits or diplopia)
▶ Loss of pupillary reflex
▶ Loss of corneal reflex
▶ Swallowing difficulties, causing gagging or coughing

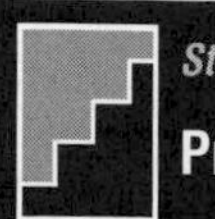

Staying well

Preventing strokes

Discuss with the older patient these guidelines for preventing strokes:

- Control high blood pressure—High blood pressure, a leading cause of stroke, can be lowered by following a physician's advice about diet, exercise, weight, and alcohol.
- Quit smoking—Smoking narrows blood vessels, making it harder for blood to get to the brain.
- Get regular checkups—The physician can help identify risk factors of stroke, such as hypertension, diabetes, and heart disease. The chance of having a stroke is reduced when these conditions are under control.
- Take medication as prescribed—Drugs can prevent or dissolve the blood clots that can cause a stroke.

Diagnostic tests

▶ *Magnetic resonance imaging* (MRI) reveals the location and size of lesions. Although not as useful as a CT scan for distinguishing among hemorrhage, tumor, and infarction, MRI is more useful for examining the cerebellum and brain stem.
▶ *Cerebral angiography* may detect disruption or displacement of cerebral circulation by occlusion or hemorrhage.
▶ *Digital subtraction angiography* allows evaluation of the patency of cerebral vessels and shows their position. It also aids detection and evaluation of lesions and other vascular abnormalities.
▶ *Computed tomography (CT) scan* may reveal structural abnormalities, edema, and lesions, such as nonhemorrhagic infarction and aneurysms.
▶ *Positron emission tomography* is used to evaluate cerebral metabolism and cerebral blood flow changes, especially in an ischemic CVA. *Single-photon emission tomography* is used to identify cerebral blood flow and cerebral infarction.
▶ *Transcranial Doppler studies* are used to evaluate the size of intracranial vessels and the direction and velocity of cerebral blood flow.
▶ *Cerebral blood flow studies* are used to measure blood flow to the brain and help detect abnormalities.
▶ *Ophthalmoscopic examination* reveals hypertension and atherosclerotic changes in retinal arteries.
▶ *Electroencephalography* is used to detect reduced electrical activity in an area of cortical infarction. It's especially useful when the CT scan is inconclusive and can be used to differentiate seizure activity from a CVA.
▶ *Neuropsychological tests* are used to evaluate mental and verbal abilities and sometimes personality traits.
▶ *Electrocardiography* reveals abnormalities caused by a cardiac-induced CVA.

Treatment

Treatment should include careful blood pressure management. Labetalol is the pressor of choice to regulate blood pressure. Blood pressure that's too low increases ischemia; blood pressure that's too high increases risk of hemorrhage. Thrombolytic agents are a consideration if there's a sign of hemorrhage on the CT scan, if there are no other contraindications, and if they're given in a timely fashion.

Acute care for a patient with a CVA may include mechanical ventilation, intracranial pressure (ICP) and cardiac monitoring, administration of I.V. fluids and electrolytes, and nasogastric intubation. If given within 3 hours of the onset of symptoms, tissue-plasminogen activator works to improve blood flow and can result in better recovery of function.

Medical management of CVA commonly includes physical rehabilitation, dietary and drug regimens to help decrease risk factors, possibly surgery, and care measures to help the patient adapt to specific deficits, such as speech impairment and paralysis.

The need for and type of surgery required for a CVA depend on its cause and extent and may include a craniotomy to remove a hematoma, an endarterectomy to remove atherosclerotic plaque from the inner arterial wall, or a bypass to circumvent an artery blocked by occlusion or stenosis. Ventricular shunts may be needed to drain cerebrospinal fluid.

Drug therapy for a CVA may include:

- stool softeners to prevent straining, which increases ICP
- anticonvulsants, such as phenytoin or phenobarbital, to treat or prevent seizures
- vasodilators to treat ischemia
- analgesics such as codeine to relieve headache
- anticoagulants to prevent thrombotic or embolic CVAs and to treat a thrombotic CVA in progress

Drug alert **Older patients metabolize and excrete phenytoin slowly, so they may require decreased dosages. Monitor them closely for toxic effects, such as drowsiness, vomiting, ataxia, hypotension, arrhythmias, respiratory depression, and coma.**

Physical rehabilitation and a special diet help decrease a person's risk factors. Other care measures may help him adapt to specific deficits, such as speech impairment and paralysis. In older adults, baseline motor and cognitive function must be taken into consideration.

Possible complications of a CVA include unstable blood pressure from loss of vasomotor control, fluid imbalances, malnutrition, depression, contractures, pulmonary emboli, and infections (such as encephalitis, brain abscess, and pneumonia). These complications may occur more readily and be more difficult to resolve in older adults.

Key nursing diagnoses and outcomes

Ineffective (cerebral) tissue perfusion related to inadequate oxygenation of cerebral tissue secondary to CVA

Treatment outcome: The patient will regain adequate tissue perfusion, as exhibited by orientation to time, person, and place.

Impaired verbal communication related to neurologic damage to speech center in brain secondary to CVA

Treatment outcomes: The patient will use adaptive equipment or take speech therapy to improve his ability to communicate his needs, thoughts, and feelings without frustration.

Risk for situational low self-esteem related to sudden devastating change in body function secondary to CVA

Treatment outcomes: The patient will verbalize his feelings about his self-esteem, engage in activities that help him achieve higher physical and emotional wellness, and express a positive self-image.

Impaired home maintenance management related to permanent neurologic deficits secondary to CVA
Treatment outcomes. The patient will identify changes needed to promote maximum health and safety at home and will remain living successfully at home.

Nursing interventions

- During the acute phase, maintain a patent airway and oxygenation. Loosen constrictive clothes. Watch for ballooning of the cheek on the affected side during respiration. If the patient is unconscious, position him on his side to allow secretions to drain and prevent aspiration; if necessary, suction the secretions. Insert an artificial airway, and start mechanical ventilation or supplemental oxygen if necessary.
- Repeatedly explain to the patient what is happening and why.
- With input from the patient, family members, and a speech therapist, help the patient develop an effective, comfortable means of communicating. Repeat yourself quietly and calmly (remember, the patient isn't deaf), and use gestures if necessary to help him understand. Make sure that the nursing staff knows of any communication problem the patient may have. Post a sign above the patient's bed to inform the health care team and visitors of alternative communication methods. Even an unresponsive patient can hear, so don't say anything in his presence you wouldn't want him to hear and remember. Involve family members in communicating with the patient. They may be able to lend insight into how the patient communicates.
- If the patient has receptive (Wernicke's) aphasia, speak slowly, using simple sentences. Use gestures or pictures when necessary. If the patient has expressive (Broca's) aphasia or dysarthria with difficulty speaking, give him enough time to speak. To help this patient, create a communication board displaying pictures of common needs, such as a bedpan and a glass of water. Or create conversation cards by printing simple messages on index cards, such as "I am thirsty" or "Please raise my bed." Punch holes in the cards, and attach them to a large key ring.
- Position the patient and align his extremities correctly. Use high-topped sneakers to prevent footdrop and contracture and a convoluted foam, flotation, or pulsating mattress to prevent pressure ulcers. To decrease the possibility of pneumonia, turn the patient at least every 2 hours. Elevate the affected hand to control dependent edema, and place it in a functional position.
- Offer the urinal or bedpan every 2 hours. The patient may need an in dwelling urinary catheter if he's incontinent, but try to avoid this because of the risk of infection.
- Ensure adequate nutrition. Check for a gag reflex before offering small oral feedings of semisolid foods. Place the food tray within the patient's visual field. Have him sit upright and tilt his head slightly forward when eating. If the patient has dysphagia or one-sided facial weakness, give him semisoft foods and tell him to chew on the unaffected side of his mouth. If oral feedings aren't possible, insert a nasogastric tube for tube feedings as ordered.
- Manage GI problems. Prevent the patient from straining during defecation because this increases ICP. Modify the patient's diet, administer stool softeners as ordered, and give laxatives if necessary. If the patient vomits (usually during the first few days), keep him positioned on his side to prevent aspiration.
- Provide careful mouth care. Clean and irrigate the patient's mouth to remove food particles, and care for his dentures as needed, if appropriate.
- Provide meticulous eye care. Remove secretions with a cotton ball and normal

saline solution. Instill eyedrops as ordered. Patch the patient's affected eye if he can't close his eyelid.

- Help the patient exercise. Perform range-of-motion exercises on both the affected and unaffected sides. Teach and encourage the patient to use his unaffected side to exercise his affected side.
- Provide psychological support, and establish rapport with the patient. Set realistic short-term goals. Spend time with him, involve his family members or friends in his care when possible, and explain his deficits and strengths. Remember that building rapport may be difficult because of the mood changes that may result from brain damage or as a reaction to being dependent.
- Consult the social services department to establish the patient's specific needs for maximum rehabilitation, such as home care and family involvement.
- Consult with the dietitian about proper nutrition and with the speech pathologist about managing the impaired swallowing and gag reflex.
- After consulting with the physical therapist, plan a rehabilitation schedule with the patient and his family.
- Encourage the patient and his family to contact a local support group and to obtain information from the National Institute of Neurological Disorders and Stroke. Refer them to a local home health care agency.

PATIENT TEACHING

- Counsel the patient and his family about lifestyle changes that may reduce the risk of another CVA, such as smoking cessation and measures to control diabetes or hypertension, if applicable. Explain the importance of increasing activity, avoiding prolonged bed rest, minimizing stress, maintaining an ideal weight, and following a low-cholesterol, low-salt diet.
- After consulting an occupational therapist and a physical therapist, teach the patient self-care skills. When describing self-care skills to patients with sensory or cognitive impairment, demonstrate each step of the activity. Then redemonstrate the complete skill. Be sure to give the patient time to understand.
- If the patient requires speech therapy, encourage him to begin it as soon as possible.
- If the patient requires a special diet, have the dietitian explain it to him.
- If appropriate, explain the danger of aspiration to the patient's family, and teach them preventive measures. Make sure that they know how to perform the abdominal thrust maneuver.
- Inform the patient and family about special glasses, cups, plates, and utensils that can make eating easier and more enjoyable.
- Explain to the patient and his family members the importance of following the prescribed exercise program, and make sure they can perform the exercises.
- Emphasize the importance of wearing slings, splints, or other prescribed devices to prevent complications.
- Teach the patient and family members about any medications that are prescribed. Explain what each is for and any possible adverse effects, both physical and psychological.

CERUMEN IMPACTION

A frequently overlooked cause of hearing loss in older people, cerumen impaction is easily treatable. However, most older adults who have the condition don't realize that their hearing is reduced and don't seek treatment. Such persons may be inappropriately labeled as "confused" or "uncooperative" when they misinterpret spoken instructions or respond improperly. In some cases, the cerumen causes sudden tinnitus and hearing loss. Impacted cerumen may be rock hard; in men, it also may contain a generous amount of exfoliated hair.

Cerumen is produced by the ceruminous glands that line the outer two-thirds of the external ear canal. It intercepts small particles that find their way into the ear canal and prevents them from reaching the tympanic membrane, where they might cause irritation. In older people, the keratin component of cerumen is increased, making it thicker and liable to form a blockage.

Signs and symptoms

- Hearing loss
- Feeling of fullness in the ear
- Visible blockage on inspection of the ear canal

Diagnostic tests

Cerumen impaction can be identified by inspection alone.

Treatment

Gentle removal of the blockage is usually all that's required. The physician may use a cerumen spoon and an aural speculum for good visualization. Because the skin of the external canal is easily traumatized and sensitive to manipulation, the physician may instead order application of a cerumen-softening agent for several days to a week, followed by irrigation. If an infection is suspected, the softening agent may contain an antibiotic solution. Irrigation is contraindicated if the tympanic membrane is perforated because it may cause an infection.

Key nursing diagnoses and outcomes

Disturbed sensory perception (auditory) related to loss of hearing

Treatment outcome: The patient will have improved hearing after the impaction has been removed.

Anxiety related to inability to hear clearly

Treatment outcomes: The patient will verbalize decreased anxiety and will exhibit no physical signs or symptoms of anxiety.

Nursing interventions

- Inspect the older person's ear canals during the initial physical examination and periodically thereafter.
- Administer eardrops, as ordered, to soften the blockage, and tell the patient to lie on his side for 5 to 10 minutes after instillation to allow the medication to travel down into the ear canal.
- Perform irrigation as ordered, taking care not to direct the stream of liquid directly at the canal.
- Encourage the patient to express his emotions over his hearing loss.
- Watch for social isolation, depression, inappropriate acting out, and paranoia in a patient with blockage-related hearing loss.

PATIENT TEACHING

- Warn your patient not to insert anything into his ear to avoid the risk of perforating the eardrum and subsequent infection.
- Encourage regular ear examinations, and tell the patient to report any changes in hearing acuity.
- Explain that although loss of hearing often occurs with advancing age, it's often treatable and not something to be ashamed of.
- Tell family members to inspect the patient's ears if he starts to display signs of decreased hearing.

CERVICAL CANCER

The third most common cancer of the female reproductive system, cervical cancer is classified as either preinvasive or invasive. Preinvasive cancer ranges from minimal cervical dysplasia, in which the lower third of the epithelium contains abnormal cells, to carcinoma in situ, in which the full thickness of epithelium contains abnormally proliferating cells (also known as cervical intraepithelial neoplasia). Preinvasive cancer is curable in 75% to 90% of patients with early detection and proper treatment. If untreated, it may progress to invasive cervical cancer.

In invasive disease, cancer cells penetrate the basement membrane and can spread directly to contiguous pelvic structures or disseminate to distant sites via lymphatic routes. Invasive cancer of the uterine cervix accounts for about 5,000 deaths annually in the United States. In 95% of cases, the histologic type is squamous cell carcinoma, which varies from well-differentiated cells to highly anaplastic spindle cells. Only 5% of cases are adenocarcinomas. Invasive cancer typically occurs between ages 30 and 50; rarely, under age 20. Women age 65 or older account for 24% of new cases and 40% of deaths. Among older women, Chinese-Americans have a higher incidence of cervical cancer.

Although the cause is unknown, several predisposing factors have been associated with cervical cancer: frequent intercourse at a young age (under 16), multiple sexual partners, multiple pregnancies, and a history of human papillomavirus or other bacterial or viral venereal infections. Other risk factors include low socioeconomic status, smoking, exposure to diethylstilbestrol, vitamin A and C deficiency and, possibly, use of oral contraceptives.

Signs and symptoms

In invasive cancer

- Abnormal vaginal bleeding (such as a persistent vaginal discharge that may be yellowish, blood-tinged, and foul-smelling), postcoital pain and bleeding
- Gradually increasing flank pain (may indicate sciatic nerve involvement)
- Leakage of urine (may point to metastasis into the bladder with formation of a fistula)
- Leakage of feces (may indicate metastasis to the rectum with fistula development)

Preinvasive cancer produces no symptoms or other clinical changes.

Diagnostic tests

- *Papanicolaou (Pap) test* identifies abnormal cells.

Cultural diversity It may be difficult to convince an older Hispanic woman to have regular gynecologic checkups if she feels no discomfort. In the Hispanic community, a person with no obvious symptoms is considered healthy and requires no medical intervention.

- *Colposcopy* determines the source of the abnormal cells seen on the Pap test.
- *Cone biopsy* is performed if endocervical curettage is positive.
- *Lymphangiography, cystography,* and *major organ and bone scans* can detect metastasis.

Treatment

Accurate clinical staging determines the type of treatment. Preinvasive lesions may be treated with total excisional biopsy, cryosurgery, laser destruction, conization (followed by frequent Pap test follow-ups) or, rarely, hysterectomy. Therapy for invasive squamous cell carcinoma may include radical hysterectomy and radiation therapy (internal, external, or both). Rarely, pelvic exenteration may be performed for recurrent cervical cancer.

Key nursing diagnoses and outcomes

Fear related to potential for cervical cancer to become invasive

Treatment outcome: The patient will experience no physical signs or symptoms of fear.

Impaired tissue integrity related to changes in cervical tissue caused by cervical cancer

Treatment outcomes: The patient will verbalize an understanding of the need for adequate fluid and nutritional intake to promote tissue healing and will exhibit healing cervical tissue on physical examination.

Pain related to invasive cervical cancer
Treatment outcomes: The patient will obtain pain relief through administered analgesics and will become free from pain through therapy.

Nursing interventions

▶ Listen to the patient's fears and concerns, and offer reassurance when appropriate. Encourage her to use relaxation techniques to promote comfort during the diagnostic procedures.
▶ If you assist with a biopsy, drape and prepare the patient as for a routine pelvic examination. Have a container of formaldehyde ready to preserve the specimen during transfer to the pathology laboratory. Assist the physician as needed, and provide support for the patient throughout the procedure.
▶ If you assist with laser therapy, drape and prepare the patient as for a routine pelvic examination. Assist the physician as necessary, and provide support for the patient throughout the procedure.
▶ Prepare the patient for surgery or internal radiation therapy, if indicated.
▶ Monitor the patient's response to therapy through frequent Pap tests and cone biopsies, as ordered.
▶ Watch for complications related to therapy by listening to and observing the patient, monitoring laboratory studies, and obtaining frequent vital signs. Institute measures to prevent or alleviate complications, as indicated.

PATIENT TEACHING

▶ Explain to the patient who's having a biopsy performed that she may feel pressure, minor abdominal cramps, or a pinch from the punch forceps. Reassure her that the pain will be minimal because the cervix has few nerve endings.
▶ Explain any surgical or therapeutic procedure to the patient, including what to expect both before and after the procedure.
▶ After excisional biopsy or laser therapy, tell the patient to expect a discharge or spotting for about 1 week. Advise her to avoid douching, using tampons, or engaging in sexual intercourse during this time. Caution her to report signs of infection. Stress the need for a follow-up Pap test and pelvic examination in 3 to 4 months and periodically thereafter.
▶ Review the possible complications of the ordered therapy. Remind the patient to watch for and report uncomfortable adverse reactions.
▶ Reassure the patient that this disease and its treatment shouldn't radically alter her lifestyle or prohibit sexual intimacy.
▶ Explain the importance of complying with follow-up visits to the gynecologist and oncologist to detect disease progression or recurrence.

CHEMOTHERAPY

Chemotherapy is the use of one or more drugs to destroy cancer cells or suppress their growth. A single drug typically prompts a limited response, but the use of two or more drugs may result in a long remission or a cure. Unfortunately, remissions and cures aren't always possible. That's because many cancers become resistant to chemotherapeutic drugs. Also, the toxic effects of some drugs may prevent dosages high enough to effectively destroy the cancer cells. (See *Chemotherapy's action in the cell cycle,* page 168.)

Various types and combinations of chemotherapeutic drugs are used to deal with the many types of cancer. Classified according to mechanism of action, these drugs include alkylating agents, antimetabolites, antibiotic antineoplastic agents, and hormonal antineoplastic agents.

Alkylating agents can inhibit cell division at any point in the cell cycle, but

Chemotherapy's action in the cell cycle

Some chemotherapeutic agents are cell-cycle specific, impairing cellular growth by causing changes in the cell during specific phases of the cell cycle. Other agents are cell-cycle nonspecific, affecting the cell at any phase during the cell cycle. The illustration below shows where the cell-cycle-specific agents work to disrupt cancer cell growth.

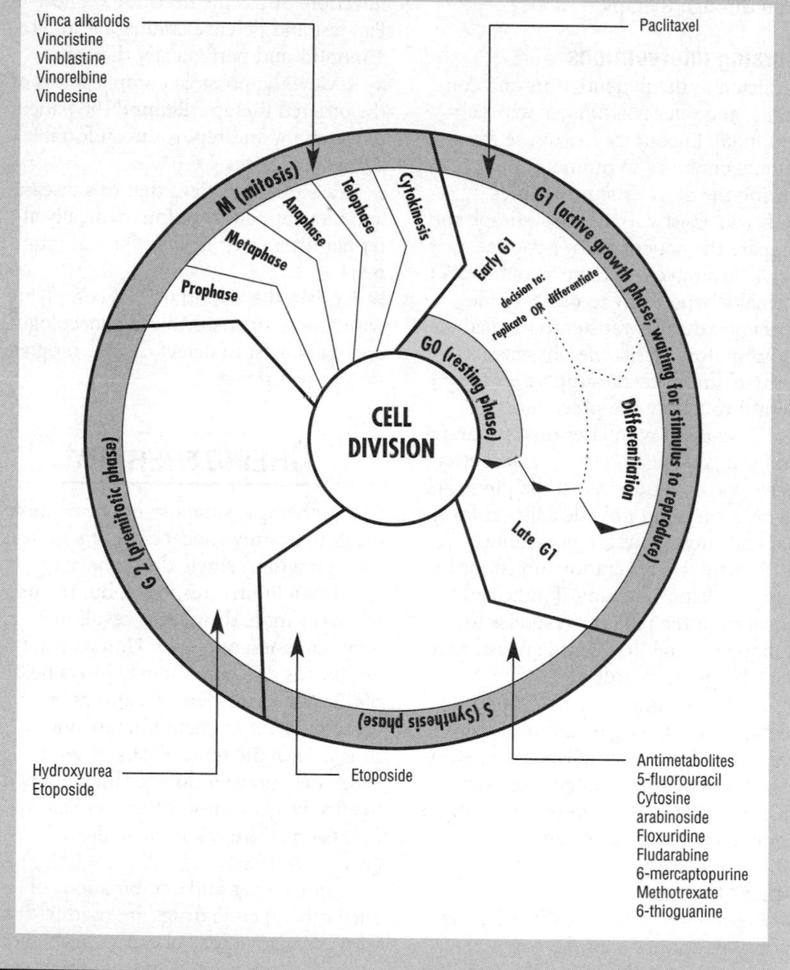

they're particularly effective in the late G_1 and S phases. Examples of alkylating agents include busulfan, carmustine (BCNU), cisplatin, ifosfamide, and mechlorethamine. Given alone or with other drugs, these drugs help treat chronic and acute leukemias, malignant lymphomas, multiple myeloma, melanoma, sarcoma, and cancers of the breast, ovaries, uterus, lung, brain, testes, bladder, prostate, and stomach.

Antimetabolites structurally resemble natural metabolites. As a result, they can become involved in processes associated with the natural metabolites — that is, the synthesis of nucleic acids and proteins. However, the antimetabolites differ sufficiently from the natural metabolites to interfere with this synthesis. Because the antimetabolites are cell-cycle specific and primarily affect cells that actively synthesize deoxyribonucleic acid (DNA), they're referred to as S-phase specific. Examples of antimetabolites include mercaptopurine and thioguanine, which inhibit purine synthesis; cytarabine, floxuridine, and fluorouracil, which inhibit pyrimidine synthesis; and methotrexate, which prevents reduction of folic acid to dihydrofolate reductase. Cancers that respond to antimetabolites include acute leukemia, breast cancer, adenocarcinomas of the GI tract, malignant lymphomas, and squamous cell carcinomas of the head, neck, and cervix.

Antibiotic antineoplastic agents achieve their effects by binding with DNA. These drugs inhibit the cellular processes of normal and malignant cells and are cell-cycle nonspecific, except for bleomycin, which causes its major effects in the G_2 phase of the cell cycle. Examples of antibiotic antineoplastics include bleomycin, dactinomycin, doxorubicin, and mitomycin, which are used mainly to treat carcinomas, sarcomas, and lymphomas; daunorubicin, which is used in acute nonlymphoblastic leukemia; and mitoxantrone, which is used to treat acute nonlymphocytic leukemia and breast cancer.

Hormonal antineoplastic agents inhibit cancer growth in specific tissues without directly causing toxicity. Although their mechanisms of action aren't completely understood, hormonal therapies are effective against hormone dependent tumors, such as cancers of the prostate, breast, and endometrium. Some examples of hormonal antineoplastic agents include estrogens (such as chlorotrianisene and diethylstilbestrol), antiestrogens (such as tamoxifen citrate), androgens (such as testolactone and testosterone), progestins (such as medroxyprogesterone acetate), corticosteroids (such as prednisone and dexamethasone), and gonadotropin-releasing hormone analogues (such as leuprolide acetate).

Tubulin-interactive agents, such as the vinca alkaloids (vincristine and vinblastine) and paclitaxel, interfere with the normal microtubule function necessary for mitosis. Vinca alkaloids are used to treat lymphomas, leukemias, and sarcomas, whereas paclitaxel is used in breast and ovarian cancers.

A chemotherapeutic regimen may consist of one or multiple drugs. Chemotherapy may be used alone or as an adjunct to surgery or radiation therapy.

Implementation

Chemotherapy may be administered in a hospital, an ambulatory care setting, or the patient's home. The drugs are typically given intermittently to allow healthy tissues time to recover and to minimize adverse reactions. Chemotherapeutic drugs are given by any one of a number of routes, including I.M., I.V., S.C, intra-arterially, orally, topically, intracavitarily, intravesically, and intrathecally.

Of these routes, the I.V. route is the most common because, whether given through a peripheral or central line, it delivers the drug directly to the body's tissues. On occasion, a patient may require continuous chemotherapy, in which case an ambulatory infusion pump may be used.

Only trained personnel, using a laminar airflow hood, should reconstitute chemotherapeutic drugs. Furthermore, only physicians or chemotherapy certified nurses should administer the drugs. The route, dose, frequency, and length of administration of each drug will vary according to the type of cancer and the patient's physical condition.

Complications

The adverse effects of chemotherapy depend on the specific drug used, its dosage and schedule, the type and extent of cancer, the patient's physical and psychological status, and his sensitivity to the drug. Some patients experience only mild or temporary reactions, whereas others experience severe or even permanent effects.

The most common and potentially most serious adverse effect is bone marrow suppression (myelosuppression). This reaction causes the number of circulating blood cells to drop, placing the patient at risk for several problems. A reduced white blood cell (WBC) count (leukopenia) increases the patient's risk of infection, especially if the granulocyte count is under 1,000/µl; a low platelet count (thrombocytopenia) increases the risk of bleeding; and a low red blood cell count can lead to anemia.

Other common adverse effects include nausea and vomiting (which can lead to fluid and electrolyte imbalances), stomatitis, and alopecia. Also, because some chemotherapeutic agents are vesicants, significant tissue damage may occur if the drug leaks outside the vein.

Some patients may also experience psychological complications, such as depression and altered body image, resulting from either the disease process or the treatment regimen.

Key nursing diagnoses and outcomes

Imbalanced nutrition: Less than body requirements related to adverse GI reactions secondary to chemotherapy

Treatment outcome: The patient will remain free from protein-calorie malnutrition.

Fatigue related to adverse reactions secondary to chemotherapy

Treatment outcomes: The patient will pace activities to avoid exacerbating fatigue and will obtain adequate sleep.

Risk for infection related to myelosuppression secondary to chemotherapy

Treatment outcomes: The patient will regain a normal WBC count after chemotherapy is completed and will not develop an infection.

Nursing interventions

When caring for a patient receiving chemotherapy, your responsibilities range from instructing and supporting the patient to observing for adverse reactions.

Before therapy

- Ensure that the patient has signed an informed consent document.
- Provide emotional support to the patient and his family.
- Gather the patient's past medical and drug history, and perform a complete physical assessment. Pay attention to the patient's laboratory test results (particularly the complete blood count), nutritional status, rehabilitation needs, and self-care ability.
- Develop a plan of care for managing the patient's symptoms, identifying both long-term and short-term needs.
- Instruct the patient to tell his physician or nurse immediately if he experiences any adverse reactions during therapy, such as burning or irritation at the treatment site, nausea, or vomiting. (See *Managing common adverse effects of chemotherapy*.)
- Examine the patient's veins, starting with the hand and proceeding to the forearm, to identify a viable route of drug administration. If you'll be administering a vesicant agent, avoid sites on the wrist or dorsum of the hand.
- Don't use an existing I.V. line to administer chemotherapy. Instead, perform

Managing common adverse effects of chemotherapy

Adverse effects	Nursing actions	Patient teaching
Bone marrow depression (leukopenia, thrombocytopenia, anemia)	■ Establish baseline white blood cell (WBC) and platelet counts, hemoglobin levels, and hematocrit before therapy begins. Monitor studies during therapy. ■ If WBC count drops suddenly or falls below 2,000/µl, stop the drug and notify the physician. Initiate reverse isolation if absolute granulocyte count falls below 1,000/µl. Report a platelet count below 100,000/µl. If necessary, assist with a transfusion. ■ Monitor oral temperature every 4 hours, and regularly inspect the skin and body orifices for signs of infection. Observe for petechiae, easy bruising, and bleeding. Check for hematuria, and monitor the patient's blood pressure. Be alert for signs of anemia. ■ Limit S.C. and I.M. injections. If they're necessary, apply pressure for 3 to 5 minutes after injection to prevent leakage or hematoma. Report unusual bleeding after injection. ■ Take precautions to prevent bleeding. Use extra care with razors, nail trimmers, dental floss, toothbrushes, and other sharp or abrasive objects. ■ Give vitamin and iron supplements, as ordered. Provide a diet high in iron.	■ Instruct the patient to immediately report fever, chills, sore throat, lethargy, unusual fatigue, or pallor. ■ Warn him to avoid exposure to persons with infections during chemotherapy and for several months after it. ■ Explain that the patient should not receive immunizations during or shortly after chemotherapy because an exaggerated reaction may occur. ■ Tell the patient to avoid activities that could cause traumatic injury and bleeding. Advise him to report any episodes of bleeding or bruising to the physician. ■ Tell him to eat high-iron foods, such as liver and spinach. ■ Stress the importance of follow-up blood studies after completion of treatment.
Anorexia	■ Assess the patient's nutritional status before and during chemotherapy. Weigh him weekly or as ordered. ■ Explain the need for adequate nutrition despite the loss of appetite.	■ Encourage the patient's family to supply favorite foods to help him maintain adequate nutrition. ■ Suggest that the patient eat small, frequent meals.
Nausea and vomiting	■ Before chemotherapy, administer antiemetics, as ordered, to reduce the severity of nausea and vomiting. ■ Monitor and record the frequency, character, and amount of vomitus. ■ Monitor serum electrolyte levels, and provide total parenteral nutrition if necessary.	■ Tell the patient to take the drug on an empty stomach, with meals, or at bedtime and to report any vomiting to the physician. GI upset indicates that the drug is working. ■ Teach the patient and his family to insert antiemetic suppositories. ■ Encourage a high-protein diet.

(continued)

Managing common adverse effects of chemotherapy *(continued)*

Adverse effects	Nursing actions	Patient teaching
Diarrhea and abdominal cramps	■ Assess the frequency, color, consistency, and amount of diarrhea. Give antidiarrheals as ordered. ■ Assess the severity of cramps, and observe for signs of dehydration and acidosis, which may indicate electrolyte imbalance. ■ Encourage fluid intake; if ordered, give I.V. fluids and potassium supplements. ■ Provide good skin care, especially to the perianal area.	■ Teach the patient how to use antidiarrheals, and instruct him to report diarrhea to the physician. ■ Encourage him to maintain adequate fluid intake and to follow a bland, low-fiber diet. ■ Explain that good perianal hygiene can help prevent skin breakdown and infection.
Stomatitis	■ Before drug administration, observe for dry mouth, erythema, and white patchy areas on the oral mucosa. Be alert for bleeding gums or complaints of a burning sensation when drinking acidic liquids. ■ Provide mouth care every 4 to 6 hours with normal saline solution or half-strength hydrogen peroxide. Coat the oral mucosa with milk of magnesia. Avoid lemon-glycerin swabs because they tend to reduce saliva and change mouth pH. ■ To make eating more comfortable, apply a topical viscous anesthetic such as lidocaine before meals. Administer special mouthwashes, as ordered. ■ Ask the dietitian to provide bland foods at medium temperatures. ■ Treat cracked or burning lips with petroleum jelly.	■ Teach the patient the importance of good mouth care. Instruct him to rinse his mouth with 1 tsp of salt dissolved in 8 oz (236 ml) of warm water or hydrogen peroxide diluted to half strength with water. ■ Advise him to avoid acidic, spicy, or extremely hot or cold foods. ■ Instruct the patient to report stomatitis to the physician, who may order a change in medication.
Alopecia	■ Reassure the patient that alopecia is usually temporary. ■ Inform him that he may experience discomfort before hair loss starts.	■ Suggest to the patient that he have his hair cut short to make thinning hair less noticeable. ■ Advise him to wash his hair with a mild shampoo and to avoid frequent brushing or combing. ■ Suggest that he wear a hat, scarf, toupee, or wig.

a new venipuncture proximal to the old site. Then test vein patency by infusing 10 to 20 ml of normal saline solution. Never test vein patency by infusing the chemotherapeutic drug.

▶ Administer any premedications, such as antiemetics, as ordered to minimize adverse effects.

During therapy

▶ Provide an environment that promotes relaxation by darkening lights, providing soothing music, and keeping out extraneous noises if possible.

▶ To protect your skin from contact with chemotherapeutic drugs, wear gloves, a nonpermeable gown, and protective eyewear whenever preparing or administering these agents.

▶ Give nonvesicant agents by I.V. push or admixed in a bag of I.V. fluid. Give vesicant agents by I.V. push through the side port of a rapidly infusing I.V. line.

▶ Monitor the patient closely for signs of a hypersensitivity reaction or extravasation. To prevent extravasation, check the I.V. catheter for blood return after injecting each 5 ml of medication or according to your facility's policy. Keep emergency medications on hand to treat a hypersensitivity reaction or extravasation.

▶ If you suspect extravasation, stop the infusion immediately. Leave the needle in place, and notify the patient's physician. Be familiar with your facility's policy for treating drug extravasation.

▶ Infuse 20 ml of normal saline solution between each chemotherapeutic drug and before discontinuing the I.V. line.

After therapy

▶ Dispose of used needles and syringes carefully. Leave the needles intact and place them in a leakproof, puncture-resistant container for incineration. Dispose of I.V. bags, bottles, gloves, and tubing in a covered trash container. Remove all chemotherapy trash for incineration.

▶ Wash your hands thoroughly after giving any chemotherapeutic drug, even though you've used gloves.

▶ Observe the patient for adverse reactions, and prepare to provide appropriate nursing care.

▶ For 48 hours after drug administration, wear gloves when handling items contaminated with the patient's excreta.

▶ Make appointments for follow-up laboratory studies and physician's visits, as indicated.

▶ Help the patient plan for his home needs. Evaluate whether his home environment is safe and whether he'll have any rehabilitation needs. Refer the patient to a home health care agency if indicated.

▶ Provide the patient and family with a list of local resources such as the American Cancer Society.

Patient teaching

Before therapy

▶ Answer all the patient's and family's questions, and provide explanations if the patient appears confused about the disease process or treatment regimen.

▶ Teach the patient the potential adverse effects of chemotherapy, and explain the interventions that can be used to treat those effects.

After therapy

▶ Teach the patient and family members how to manage the adverse effects of chemotherapy at home.

▶ Inform them that myelosuppression will be most severe 12 to 24 days after the last dose of chemotherapy. Explain that they'll need to take precautions against bleeding and infection during this time.

▶ Tell the patient to notify his physician at once if he develops unusual bleeding or signs or symptoms of infection.

▶ Make sure the patient has correct phone numbers for his physician, his nurse, and other resource personnel so that he can report adverse reactions promptly.

CHEST DRAINAGE

Insertion of a drainage tube into the pleural space helps treat pneumothorax, hemothorax, empyema, pleural effusion, or chylothorax. A drainage tube is also routinely inserted at the completion of a thoracotomy. The tube drains blood, fluid, pus, or air from the pleural space. In pneumothorax, it restores negative pressure to the pleural space by means of an underwater-seal drainage system. The water in the system prevents air from being sucked back into the pleural space during inspiration. (If the leak is through the bronchi and can't be sealed, suction applied to the underwater-seal system removes air from the pleural space faster than it can collect.) As negative pleural pressure is restored, the lung can reinflate.

Implementation

Position the patient on his unaffected side. After the physician injects the local anesthetic at the insertion site, help the patient hold still while the physician makes a small incision and tunnels the tube through the tissue into the pleural space. Usually, the physician places the tube anteriorly near the second or third intercostal space if he wants to remove air; laterally and slightly posteriorly at about the eighth intercostal space if he wants to remove fluid. He may place tubes at both locations if he wishes to remove both air and fluid.

As soon as the physician inserts the tube into the pleural space, connect the external end of the tube to the underwater-seal drainage system. The physician stabilizes the proximal end by suturing the tube into place. Apply petroleum gauze and a dry sterile dressing. As ordered, tape the tube to the patient's chest wall distal to the insertion site to help prevent accidental dislodgment. Tape all tube connections and regulate suction, as ordered.

Complications

Possible complications include lung puncture, bleeding, or additional hemothorax at the insertion site. Chest tube obstruction or blockage of the air vent in the underwater-seal drainage system may cause tension pneumothorax, a life-threatening complication. (See *Combating tension pneumothorax*.)

Key nursing diagnoses and outcomes

Ineffective breathing pattern related to thoracic pain and decreased lung expansion

Treatment outcome: The patient will exhibit increased lung expansion and easy, unlabored respirations at a rate of 12 to 28 breaths/minute.

Impaired physical mobility related to thoracic pain and discomfort

Treatment outcomes: The patient will maintain full range of motion in his affected arm and shoulder and will regain physical mobility after analgesic administration.

Fear related to pain and chest tube procedure

Treatment outcome: The patient will demonstrate no physical signs of fear related to the chest tube and chest drainage.

Nursing interventions

When caring for a patient with chest tubes, much of your care will center on monitoring for, and preventing, complications.

Before the procedure

- Explain the procedure to the patient. Tell him the chest tube will help him breathe more easily. Take his vital signs to serve as a baseline, and make sure that he has signed a consent form. Then administer a sedative, as ordered.
- Collect necessary equipment, including a thoracotomy tray and an underwater-seal drainage system. Prepare lidocaine for local anesthesia, as directed. While the physician cleans the insertion site with povidone-iodine solution, set up the underwater-seal drainage system according to the manufacturer's instructions and place it at the bedside, below

Combating tension pneumothorax

Tension pneumothorax is a life-threatening complication that may be fatal if not treated promptly. Air becomes entrapped within the pleural space, which can result from either dislodgment or obstruction of the chest tube. Either way, increasing positive pressure within the patient's chest cavity compresses the affected lung and the mediastinum, shifting them toward the opposite lung. The result is markedly impaired venous return and cardiac output, leading to cardiac arrest.

Signs and symptoms

Suspect tension pneumothorax if the patient develops cyanosis, air hunger, agitation, hypotension, tachycardia, and profuse diaphoresis. As part of your assessment, palpate the patient's face, neck, and chest wall for subcutaneous emphysema. Also check to see if his trachea has deviated from its normal midline position—a telltale sign of tension pneumothorax. Auscultate the lungs for decreased or absent breath sounds on the affected side, and percuss the chest for hyperresonance.

Emergency interventions

If you suspect a tension pneumothorax, take these steps:

- Notify the patient's physician immediately.
- Be prepared to assist with reinsertion of the chest tube or insertion of a large-bore needle to relieve air pressure in the thorax.
- Inspect the chest drainage unit for kinks in the tubing. Correct any mechanical problems immediately.
- Expect to administer a high concentration of oxygen to treat hypoxia.
- Continue to monitor vital signs and vital functions.

chest level. Stabilize the unit to avoid knocking it over.

After the procedure

- Once the patient's chest tube is stabilized, have him take several deep breaths to inflate his lungs fully and to help push pleural air out through the tube. Take his vital signs immediately after tube insertion and then every 15 minutes or as ordered until his condition is stabilized.
- Prepare the patient for a chest X-ray to verify tube placement and to assess the outcome of treatment. As ordered, arrange for daily X-rays to monitor his progress.
- Palpate the patient's chest above the tube for subcutaneous emphysema, and notify the physician of any increase.
- Routinely assess the function of the patient's chest tube. Describe and record the amount of drainage on the intake and output sheet. Once most of the air has been removed, the drainage system should bubble only during forced expiration unless the patient has a bronchopleural fistula. However, constant bubbling in the system when suction is attached may indicate a loose connection or that the tube has advanced slightly out of the patient's chest. Promptly correct any loose connections to prevent complications.
- If the chest tube becomes dislodged, cover the opening immediately with petroleum gauze and apply pressure to prevent negative inspiratory pressure from sucking air into the patient's chest. Call the physician, and have an assistant obtain the equipment necessary for tube reinsertion while you continue to keep the opening closed. Reassure the patient and monitor him closely for signs of tension pneumothorax.

▶ Change the dressing over the chest tube site daily. At the same time, clean the site and remove any drainage.
▶ The physician will remove the patient's chest tube when the lung has fully reexpanded. As soon as the tube is removed, apply an airtight, sterile petroleum dressing.

PATIENT TEACHING
▶ Typically, the patient will be discharged with a chest tube only if it's being used to drain a loculated empyema because this doesn't require an underwater-seal drainage system. Teach this patient how to care for his tube, dispose of drainage and soiled dressings properly, and perform wound care and dressing changes.
▶ Teach the patient with a recently removed chest tube how to clean the wound site and change dressings. Tell him to report any signs of infection.

CHEST PHYSIOTHERAPY

Chest physiotherapy (CPT) includes postural drainage, chest percussion and vibration, and coughing and deep-breathing exercises. Together, these techniques mobilize and eliminate secretions, reexpand lung tissue, and promote efficient use of respiratory muscles. Of critical importance to the bedridden patient, CPT helps prevent or treat atelectasis and may also help prevent pneumonia — respiratory complications that can seriously impede recovery.

Postural drainage performed in conjunction with percussion and vibration encourages peripheral pulmonary secretions to empty by gravity into the major bronchi or trachea; it's accomplished by sequential repositioning of the patient. Usually, secretions drain best with the patient positioned so that the bronchi are perpendicular to the floor. Lower and middle lobe bronchi usually empty best with the patient in the head-down position; upper lobe bronchi, in the head-up position.

Percussing the chest with mechanical percussors or with cupped hands mechanically dislodges thick, tenacious secretions from the bronchial walls. Vibration can be used with percussion or as an alternative to it in a patient who is frail, in pain, or recovering from thoracic surgery or trauma.

Candidates for CPT include patients who expectorate large amounts of sputum, such as those with bronchiectasis or cystic fibrosis. CPT hasn't proved effective in treating patients with status asthmaticus, lobar pneumonia, or acute exacerbations of chronic bronchitis when the patient has scant secretions and is being mechanically ventilated. CPT has little value in treating patients with stable, chronic bronchitis.

Contraindications may include active pulmonary bleeding with hemoptysis, the immediate posthemorrhagic stage, fractured ribs or an unstable chest wall, lung contusions, pulmonary tuberculosis, untreated pneumothorax, acute asthma or bronchospasm, lung abscess or tumor, bony metastasis, head injury, and recent myocardial infarction.

Supplies
▶ Stethoscope
▶ Pillows
▶ Tilt or postural drainage table (if available) or adjustable hospital bed
▶ Emesis basin
▶ Facial tissues
▶ Suction equipment as needed
▶ Equipment for oral care
▶ Trash bag
▶ Optional: sterile specimen container, supplemental oxygen

Implementation
▶ Gather the equipment at the patient's bedside. Set up suction equipment, if needed, and test its function.
▶ Provide privacy and wash your hands.

- Auscultate the patient's lungs to determine baseline respiratory status.
- Because chest percussion can induce bronchospasm, any adjunct treatment (for example, intermittent positive-pressure breathing or aerosol or nebulizer therapy) should precede CPT.
- Position the patient as ordered. In generalized disease, drainage usually begins with the lower lobes, continues with the middle lobes, and ends with the upper lobes. In localized disease, drainage begins with the affected lobes and then proceeds to the other lobes to avoid spreading the disease to uninvolved areas.
- Instruct the patient to remain in each position for 10 to 15 minutes. During this time, perform percussion and vibration, as ordered. (See *Performing percussion and vibration*.)
- Refrain from percussing over the spine, liver, kidneys, or spleen to avoid injury to the spine or internal organs. Also avoid performing percussion on bare skin or a female patient's breasts. Percuss over soft clothing (but not over buttons, snaps, or zippers), or place a thin towel over the chest wall. Remember to remove jewelry that might scratch or bruise the patient.
- For optimal effectiveness and safety, modify CPT according to the patient's condition. For example, initiate or increase the flow of supplemental oxygen, if indicated. Also, suction the patient who has an ineffective cough reflex. If the patient tires quickly during therapy, shorten the sessions; fatigue leads to shallow respirations and increased hypoxia.
- Maintain adequate hydration to prevent mucus dehydration and promote easier mobilization. Avoid performing postural drainage immediately before or within 1½ hours after meals to avoid nausea and aspiration of food or vomitus.
- After postural drainage, percussion, or vibration, instruct the patient to

Performing percussion and vibration

To perform percussion, instruct the patient to breathe slowly and deeply, using the diaphragm, to promote relaxation. Hold your hands in a cupped shape, with fingers flexed and thumbs pressed tightly against your index fingers. Percuss each segment for 1 to 2 minutes by alternating your hands against the patient in a rhythmic manner. Listen for a hollow sound on percussion to verify correct performance of the technique.

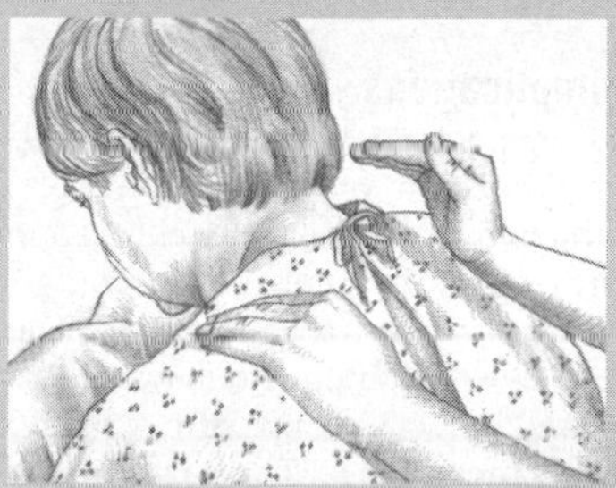

To perform vibration, ask the patient to inhale deeply and then exhale slowly through pursed lips. During exhalation, firmly press your fingers and the palms of your hands against the chest wall. Tense the muscles of your arms and shoulders in an isometric contraction to send fine vibrations through the chest wall. Vibrate during five exhalations over each chest segment.

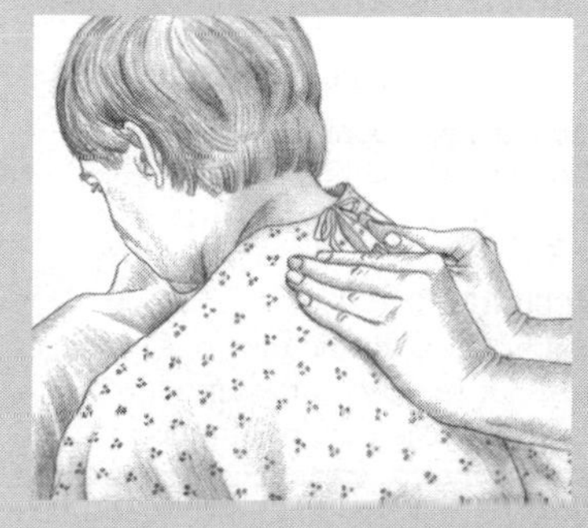

cough to remove loosened secretions. First, tell him to inhale deeply through his nose and then exhale in three short huffs. Then have him inhale deeply again and cough through a slightly open mouth. Three consecutive coughs are highly effective. An effective cough sounds deep, low, and hollow; an ineffective one, high pitched. Have the patient perform these exercises for about 1 minute and then rest for 2 minutes. Gradually progress to a 10-minute exercise period four times daily.

▶ Provide oral hygiene because secretions may taste foul or have a stale odor.

▶ Auscultate the patient's lungs to evaluate the effectiveness of therapy.

Complications

During postural drainage in the head-down position, pressure on the diaphragm by abdominal contents can impair respiratory excursion and lead to hypoxia or postural hypotension. The head-down position also may lead to increased intracranial pressure, which precludes the use of CPT in a patient with acute neurologic impairment. Vigorous percussion or vibration can cause rib fracture, especially in an older patient with osteoporosis. In an emphysematous patient with blebs, coughing can lead to pneumothorax.

Patient teaching

▶ Explain the procedure to the patient to reduce his fear and promote cooperation.

▶ Explain coughing and deep-breathing exercises preoperatively, so the patient can practice them when he's free of pain and better able to concentrate.

Documentation

Record the date and time of CPT; positions for secretion drainage and the length of time each position is maintained; chest segments percussed or vibrated; color, amount, odor, and viscosity of secretions produced and presence of any blood; any complications and nursing actions taken; and the patient's tolerance of the procedure.

CHLORIDE DEFICIENCY

Secreted by the stomach mucosa as hydrochloric acid, chloride provides an acidic medium that's conducive to digestion and the activation of enzymes. It also helps maintain acid-base and body water balances, influences the osmolality or tonicity of extracellular fluid, plays a role in oxygen and carbon dioxide exchange in red blood cells, and helps activate salivary amylase (which, in turn, activates the digestive process). A predominantly extracellular anion, chloride accounts for two-thirds of all serum anions.

A deficiency of serum chloride levels, known as hypochloremia, may result from:

▶ decreased chloride intake or absorption, as occurs in low dietary sodium intake, sodium deficiency, potassium deficiency, or metabolic alkalosis; prolonged use of mercurial diuretics; or administration of I.V. dextrose without electrolytes

▶ excessive chloride loss, resulting from prolonged diarrhea or diaphoresis; or loss of hydrochloric acid in gastric secretions due to vomiting, gastric suctioning, or gastric surgery.

Signs and symptoms

Hypochloremia associated with hyponatremia

▶ Muscle weakness and twitching

Hypochloremia due to metabolic alkalosis secondary to loss of gastric secretions

▶ Tetany

▶ Shallow, depressed breathing

▶ Muscle hypertonicity

Diagnostic tests

▶ *Serum chloride measurement* reveals levels under 95 mEq/L. Supportive values with metabolic alkalosis include serum pH over 7.45 and serum carbon dioxide levels greater than 32 mEq/L.

- *Arterial blood gas (ABG) analysis* may reveal metabolic acidosis.

Treatment

Treatment is aimed at correcting the underlying disorder. When oral therapy is possible, give an oral replacement such as salty broth. When oral therapy isn't possible or when emergency measures are necessary, treatment may include I.V. administration of normal saline solution (if hypovolemia is present) or chloride-containing drugs, such as ammonium chloride, to increase serum chloride levels and potassium chloride for metabolic alkalosis.

Key nursing diagnoses and outcomes

Risk for injury related to inability of body to maintain homeostasis without adequate chloride ions

Treatment outcomes: The patient will sustain no injury because of muscle weakness and will recover and maintain a normal serum chloride level.

Ineffective breathing pattern related to weakness of respiratory muscles caused by hypochloremia

Treatment outcome: The patient will recover and maintain a normal breathing pattern.

Nursing interventions

- Provide foods high in chloride, such as salty broth.
- Implement measures to correct the underlying cause of the chloride deficiency.
- Administer oral or I.V. chloride supplements, as ordered, if the deficiency is severe, oral intake is restricted, or dietary adjustment is not effective.
- If the patient has muscle weakness, initiate measures to prevent injury. Help the patient move about, and keep personal articles within easy reach.
- Monitor serum chloride levels frequently, particularly during I.V. therapy.
- Watch for signs of hyperchloremia, which would indicate overcorrection, or continued hypochloremia, which would indicate insufficient correction. Watch for respiratory difficulty.
- To detect hypochloremia, monitor laboratory test results (serum electrolyte levels and ABG values) and fluid intake and output of patients who are vulnerable to chloride imbalance, particularly those recovering from gastric surgery. Record and report excessive or continuous loss of gastric secretions. Also report prolonged infusion of dextrose in water without normal saline solution.

PATIENT TEACHING

- Explain all tests and procedures to the patient and family members.
- Discuss food sources of sodium, potassium, and chloride.

CHLORIDE EXCESS

An excess of chloride levels, known as hyperchloremia, may result from:

- excessive chloride intake or absorption, as occurs in hyperingestion of ammonium chloride or ureterointestinal anastomosis, allowing reabsorption of chloride by the bowel
- hemoconcentration caused by dehydration
- compensatory mechanisms for other abnormalities, as in metabolic acidosis, brain stem injury causing neurogenic hyperventilation, and hyperparathyroidism.

Signs and symptoms

Hyperchloremia associated with hypernatremia

- Agitation
- Pitting edema
- Dyspnea
- Tachycardia
- Hypertension

Hyperchloremia associated with metabolic acidosis

- Deep, rapid breathing
- Weakness
- Diminished cognitive ability
- Coma

Diagnostic tests

- *Serum chloride measurement* reveals levels greater than 106 mEq/L. With metabolic acidosis, serum pH is under 7.35 and serum carbon dioxide levels are less than 22 mEq/L.
- *Arterial blood gas analysis* may reveal metabolic acidosis.

Treatment

Treatment must correct the underlying disorder. For severe hyperchloremic acidosis, administer sodium bicarbonate I.V. to raise serum bicarbonate levels and permit renal excretion of the chloride anion (because bicarbonate and chloride compete for combination with sodium).

For mild hyperchloremia, administer lactated Ringer's solution, which converts to bicarbonate in the liver, thus increasing base bicarbonate to correct acidosis.

Key nursing diagnoses and outcomes

Disturbed thought processes related to adverse neurologic effects of hyperchloremia on cognitive function

Treatment outcome: The patient will become oriented to time, person, and place.

Excess fluid volume related to simultaneous increase in sodium caused by natural affinity of sodium for chloride

Treatment outcome: The patient will recover a normal fluid balance, as exhibited by the absence of edema, balanced intake and output, and normal serum sodium and chloride levels.

Nursing interventions

- Insert an I.V. line, and administer lactated Ringer's solution or sodium bicarbonate, as ordered.
- If the patient shows signs of altered thought processes, provide a safe environment and assess his neurologic status frequently for signs of deterioration.
- Check serum electrolyte levels every 3 to 6 hours. If the patient is receiving high doses of sodium bicarbonate, watch for signs of overcorrection (metabolic alkalosis, respiratory depression) or lingering signs of hyperchloremia, which indicate inadequate treatment.
- If sodium excess is also present, assess for signs of fluid overload.
- Assess respiratory function. Rapid, deep respirations, a compensatory mechanism, may accompany hyperchloremic acidosis.
- To detect hyperchloremia, check laboratory test results for elevated serum chloride levels (or potassium imbalance if the patient is receiving I.V. solutions containing sodium chloride), and monitor fluid intake and output. Also, watch for signs of metabolic acidosis. When administering I.V. fluids containing lactated Ringer's solution, monitor the flow rate according to the patient's age, physical condition, and bicarbonate level. Report any irregularities promptly.

Patient teaching

- Explain all tests and procedures to the patient and family members.
- Discuss dietary restrictions if ordered.
- Explain the importance of replenishing lost fluids during hot weather.

CHOLECYSTECTOMY

When drug therapy, dietary changes, and supportive treatments fail to control gallbladder or biliary duct disease, the patient's gallbladder may have to be removed. Known as a cholecystectomy, this procedure helps restore biliary flow from the liver to the small intestine. The procedure may be performed either as abdominal surgery, which uses one large abdominal incision, or as a laparoscopic procedure, which uses several small abdominal incisions (making this procedure safer for older adults).

After gallbladder resection, choledochoduodenostomy (anastomosis of the common bile duct to the duodenum) or choledochojejunostomy (anastomosis of the common bile duct to the jejunum) may be necessary to restore biliary flow.

Implementation

Both abdominal and laparoscopic cholecystectomies are performed under general anesthesia. An abdominal cholecystectomy begins with a right subcostal or paramedial incision. The surgeon then surveys the abdomen and uses laparotomy packs to isolate the gallbladder from the surrounding organs. After identifying biliary tract structures, he may use cholangiography or ultrasonography to help identify gallstones. Using a choledoscope, he directly visualizes the bile ducts and inserts a Fogarty balloon-tipped catheter to clear the ducts of stones.

The surgeon ligates and divides the cystic duct and artery and removes the entire gallbladder. Typically, he performs a choledochotomy — the insertion of a T tube into the common bile duct to decompress the biliary tree and prevent bile peritonitis during healing. He may also insert a Penrose drain into the ducts. After completion of the surgery and, if necessary, implantation of the T tube, the surgeon removes blood and debris from the abdomen, closes the incision, and applies a dressing.

For a laparoscopic cholecystectomy, the surgeon begins by making a small incision just above the umbilicus and injecting either carbon dioxide or nitrous oxide into the abdominal cavity. This inflates the abdomen and lifts the abdominal wall away from the abdominal organs, allowing the surgeon to readily identify the gallbladder. He then connects a trocar to an insufflator and inserts it through the incision. Next, he passes a thin, flexible optical instrument, called a laparoscope, through the trocar. The laparoscope allows the surgeon to view the intra-abdominal contents.

At this time, the patient is placed in Trendelenburg's position. This causes the small intestines to fall out of the pelvis, making room for the initial needle and trocar insertion. Then, while looking through the laparoscope, the surgeon makes three incisions in the patient's right upper quadrant: one 2" (5 cm) below the xiphoid process in the midline, one 1" (2 cm) below the right costal margin in the midclavicular line, and one in the anterior axillary line at the level of the umbilicus.

While continuing to look through the laparoscope, the surgeon passes instruments through the three incisions in the right upper quadrant. He uses these to clamp and then tie off the cystic duct and to excise the gallbladder. The gallbladder is then removed through the umbilical opening. After this, the surgeon sutures all four incisions and places a dressing over each one.

Complications

Although relatively rare, complications from cholecystectomy can be grave. Peritonitis, for instance, may occur from obstructed biliary drainage and resultant leakage of bile into the peritoneum.

Postcholecystectomy syndrome, marked by fever, jaundice, and pain, is possible. As in all abdominal surgeries, postoperative atelectasis may result from hampered respiratory excursion if an abdominal surgical approach was used. If a laparoscopic approach was used, bile duct or small-bowel injury may occur during introduction of the trocar.

Other possible complications include superficial wound infection, prolonged ileus, urine retention, and retained gallstones.

Key nursing diagnoses and outcomes

Ineffective breathing pattern related to guarded respirations secondary to one or more incisions in the right upper quadrant of the abdomen

Treatment outcome: The patient will regain and maintain a normal breathing pattern.

Risk for infection related to potential for leakage of biliary drainage into the abdominal cavity

Treatment outcome: The patient will experience no signs or symptoms of peritonitis, such as abdominal distention or increased abdominal pain.

Acute pain related to one or more surgical incisions

Treatment outcomes: The patient will verbalize a decrease in pain within 24 hours, express relief from pain after analgesic administration, and become pain-free after healing is complete.

Nursing interventions

With a cholecystectomy patient, your major roles include instruction and care tailored to the patient's condition.

Before surgery

- Monitor and, if necessary, help stabilize the patient's nutritional status and fluid balance. Such measures may include administering vitamin K, blood transfusions, or glucose and protein supplements. Twenty-four hours before surgery, administer only clear liquids. Then, after midnight the night before surgery or as ordered, withhold all food and fluid.
- Administer preoperative medications and assist with insertion of a nasogastric (NG) tube.
- Make sure that the patient or a responsible family member has signed a consent form.

After surgery

- When the patient returns from surgery, place him in low Fowler's position. As ordered, attach the NG tube to low intermittent suction. Monitor the amount and characteristics of drainage from the NG tube as well as from any abdominal drains. Check dressings frequently and change them as necessary.
- If the patient has a T tube in place, frequently assess the position and patency of the tube and drainage bag. The drainage bag should be level with his abdomen to prevent excessive drainage. Also note the amount and characteristics of drainage; bloody or blood-tinged bile normally occurs for only the first few hours after surgery. Provide meticulous skin care around the tube insertion site to prevent irritation.
- After a few days, expect to remove the NG tube, if present, and begin to introduce foods: first liquids and then gradually, soft solids. As ordered, clamp the T tube for an hour before and an hour after each meal to allow bile to travel to the intestine to aid digestion. If the patient has had a laparoscopic cholecystectomy, expect him to begin clear liquids when fully recovered from general anesthesia and to resume his normal diet the day of or the day after surgery.
- Be alert for signs of postcholecystectomy syndrome (fever, abdominal pain, and jaundice) and other complications involving obstructed bile drainage. For several days after surgery, monitor vital signs and record intake and output every 8 hours. If any complications occur, report them to the physician and collect urine and stool specimens for laboratory analysis of bile content.
- Assist the patient with ambulation on the first postoperative day, unless contraindicated. Have him cough, deep breathe, and perform incentive spirometry every hour; provide analgesics to ease discomfort during these exercises, as ordered. Assess respiratory status every 2 hours to detect hypoventilation and signs of atelectasis.

Patient teaching

Before surgery

▶ Explain the planned surgery to the patient using clear, simple terms and diagrams. Reassure him that the surgery will relieve his symptoms. Also reassure him that his recovery should be rapid and uneventful and that he may be allowed to resume his full range of activities within 4 to 6 weeks.

▶ If the patient is scheduled for an abdominal surgical approach, warn him that, after surgery, he may have an NG tube in place for 1 to 2 days and an abdominal drain at the incision site for 3 to 5 days. If appropriate, tell him that a T tube will be inserted in the common bile duct during surgery to drain excess bile and allow removal of retained stones. Explain that the T tube may remain in place for up to 2 weeks, depending on the surgery, and that he may be discharged with it still in place.

▶ If the patient is scheduled for a laparoscopic approach, tell him that an indwelling urinary catheter will be inserted into his bladder and an NG tube into his stomach after general anesthesia has been administered. Reassure him that these tubes will be removed in the postanesthesia room following the procedure. Explain that he'll have three small incisions in the right upper quadrant of his abdomen and one small incision in his umbilicus. Each of these incisions will be covered with a small sterile dressing postoperatively. Also inform him that he may be discharged the day of surgery or the day after.

▶ Teach the patient how to perform coughing and deep-breathing exercises to prevent postoperative atelectasis, which can lead to pneumonia. Tell him that an analgesic may be administered before these exercises to relieve discomfort.

After surgery

▶ If the patient is being discharged with a T tube in place, show him and his family how to care for it, stressing the need for meticulous tube care.

▶ Tell the patient to immediately report any signs of biliary obstruction: fever, jaundice, pruritus, pain, dark urine, and clay-colored stools.

▶ Tell the patient that, although there are typically no dietary restrictions, he may wish to avoid excessive fat intake for 4 to 6 weeks.

CHOLECYSTITIS

In cholecystitis, the gallbladder becomes acutely or chronically inflamed, usually because a gallstone is lodged in the cystic duct, causing painful gallbladder distention. Although the exact cause of gallstone formation is unknown, abnormal metabolism of cholesterol and bile salts clearly plays an important role. The acute form is most common in middle-aged adults; the chronic form, in older adults. The prognosis is good with treatment.

Gallbladder and duct diseases typically occur during middle age. Between ages 20 and 50, they're six times more common in women, but after age 50, the incidence in men and women equalizes. The incidence rises with each succeeding decade.

A number of risk factors predispose a person to calculi formation. These include:

▶ a high-calorie, high-cholesterol diet, associated with obesity

▶ elevated estrogen levels from postmenopausal hormone-replacement therapy

▶ the use of clofibrate

▶ diabetes mellitus, ileal disease, hemolytic disorders, hepatic disease, or pancreatitis.

Acute cholecystitis also may result from conditions that alter the gallbladder's ability to fill or empty, such as trauma, reduced blood supply to the gallbladder, prolonged immobility, poor nutrition, adhesions, prolonged anesthesia, and narcotic abuse.

If not treated, cholecystitis can progress to gallbladder complications, such as chronic cholecystitis, empyema, hydrops or mucocele, or gangrene. Gangrene may lead to perforation, resulting in peritonitis, fistula formation, or pancreatitis.

Signs and symptoms

Chronic cholecystitis

- Sudden onset of steady or aching pain in the midepigastric region or the right upper abdominal quadrant, possibly after eating a high-fat meal or a large meal after fasting for an extended time; may awaken the patient in the middle of the night and may last a few hours
- Pain radiating to the back, between the shoulder blades, over the right shoulder blade, or just to the shoulder area (biliary colic)
- Nausea and vomiting
- Chills
- Low-grade fever
- History of milder GI symptoms, such as indigestion, vague abdominal discomfort, belching, and flatulence after eating high-fat foods

Acute cholecystitis

- Sudden onset of severe pain in right upper quadrant or aching pain in midepigastric region; may last several days
- Pallor
- Diaphoresis
- Exhaustion
- Mild jaundice
- Dark-colored urine
- Clay-colored stools
- Tachycardia
- Tenderness over gallbladder on palpation
- Hypoactive bowel sounds

Diagnostic tests

- *Ultrasonography* detects gallstones.
- *Abdominal X-rays* identify gallstones if they contain enough calcium to be radiopaque.
- *Radionuclide imaging* of the gallbladder indicates cystic duct obstruction and acute or chronic cholecystitis if the gallbladder can't be seen.
- *Blood studies* may reveal elevated levels of serum alkaline phosphatase, lactate dehydrogenase, aspartate aminotransferase, and total bilirubin. The white blood cell count is slightly elevated during a cholecystitis attack.

Treatment

Surgery, usually elective, remains the most common treatment for gallbladder and duct disease. Surgery is usually recommended if the patient's symptoms occur frequently enough to interfere with his regular routine, if he has any complications of gallstones, or if he has had a previous attack of cholecystitis. Procedures may include cholecystectomy, cholecystectomy with operative cholangiography, choledochostomy, exploration of the common bile duct or, possibly, laparoscopic cholecystectomy.

Gallstone dissolution therapy is used if the patient's gallstones are radiolucent and consist totally or partly of cholesterol. In this treatment, oral chenodeoxycholic acid or ursodiol is used to partially or completely dissolve gallstones. However, this treatment has several limitations, including the need for prolonged treatment, the fact that it dissolves only small calculi, the high incidence of adverse reactions, and the frequency of calculus reformation after treatment ends.

Other, more direct methods of removing gallstones may be used. Insertion of a percutaneous transhepatic biliary catheter under fluoroscopic guidance permits visualization of the calculi and their removal using a basket-shaped tool called a Dormia basket. In endoscopic retrograde cholangiopancreatography (ERCP), the calculi are removed with a balloon or basketlike tool passed through an endoscope. Both of these techniques permit decompression of the biliary tree, allowing bile to flow.

Lithotripsy breaks up gallstones using ultrasonic waves. It has been used successfully in some patients with radiolucent calculi.

If the patient is asymptomatic or has recovered from a first attack of biliary colic, noninvasive treatment may be attempted. This treatment includes a low-fat diet with replacement of the fat-soluble vitamins A, D, E, and K and administration of bile salts to facilitate digestion and vitamin absorption.

During an acute attack, treatment may include narcotics for pain relief, antispasmodics and anticholinergics to relax smooth muscles and decrease ductal tone and spasm, and antiemetics to reduce nausea and vomiting. A nasogastric tube may also be inserted and connected to intermittent low-pressure suction to relieve vomiting.

In patients with severe acute cholecystitis, I.V. fluids and I.V. antibiotic therapy are usually given before surgery. Cholestyramine may be given if the patient has obstructive jaundice with severe itching from accumulation of bile salts in the skin.

Nonsuppurative cholangitis usually responds quickly to antibiotic therapy. Suppurative cholangitis requires antibiotic therapy, prompt surgical correction of the obstruction, and drainage of the infected bile.

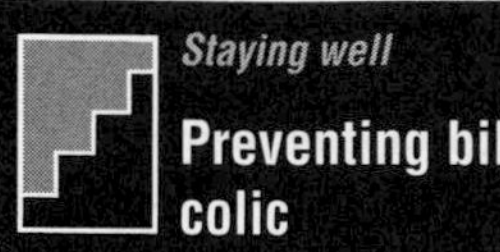

Staying well

Preventing biliary colic

If a low-fat diet is prescribed for your patient, suggest ways to implement it. The older patient may be more willing to decrease his intake of hidden fat than to eliminate butter on bread and vegetables. Suggest that the patient skim fat off soups and broths and use applesauce as a replacement for oil in baking. These measures decrease fat content without altering taste. If necessary, ask the dietitian to reinforce your instructions.

Key nursing diagnoses and outcomes

Risk for deficient fluid volume related to nausea and vomiting secondary to cholecystitis

Treatment outcome: The patient will exhibit no signs or symptoms of dehydration.

Risk for infection related to biliary obstruction secondary to one or more gallstones lodging in a duct or the small intestine

Treatment outcomes: The patient will maintain a normal temperature and white blood cell count and will exhibit no signs or symptoms of infection.

Acute pain related to inflammation of the gallbladder secondary to a gallstone lodging in the cystic duct

Treatment outcome: The patient will be free from pain.

Nursing interventions

- Administer antiemetics to relieve nausea and vomiting as ordered.
- If the patient experiences nausea or vomiting, assess his vital signs and monitor his intake and output for signs of a fluid deficit. Also, withhold food and oral fluids.
- Provide a low-fat diet and smaller, more frequent meals; replace vitamins A, D, E, and K; and administer bile salts as ordered. (See *Preventing biliary colic.*)
- Administer narcotic and anticholinergic medications, as ordered, to relieve pain, and monitor their effectiveness.
- Provide support to the patient before and after surgery, as indicated.
- After percutaneous transhepatic biliary catheterization or ERCP to remove gallstones, give the patient nothing by mouth until his gag reflex returns.

PATIENT TEACHING

▶ Teach the patient about the disease and the reasons for his symptoms.

▶ Explain scheduled diagnostic tests, reviewing pretest instructions and necessary aftercare.

▶ Review the proper use of prescribed medications, explaining their desired effects. Point out possible adverse reactions, especially those that warrant a call to the physician.

▶ Reinforce the physician's explanation of the ordered treatment, such as surgery, ERCP, or lithotripsy. Make sure the patient fully understands the possible complications, if any, associated with the treatments.

Special considerations

The older patient with a gallbladder rupture may not experience abdominal pain, which may significantly delay treatment and increase mortality.

CHRONIC OBSTRUCTIVE PULMONARY DISEASE

Also called chronic airflow limitation disease, chronic obstructive pulmonary disease (COPD) is characterized by a reduced airway lumen, caused by mucosal thickening, and increased airway compliance, caused by destruction of the lumen. In older adults, this disease most commonly takes three forms: emphysema, chronic bronchitis, and asthma.

Emphysema distends or ruptures the terminal alveoli, causing a loss of elasticity. These changes in the lung tissue interfere with expiration. Emphysema is more prevalent in men than in women; about 65% of people with well-defined emphysema are men; about 35% are women. Postmortem findings reveal few adult lungs without some degree of emphysema. Many older adults have a persistent productive cough, wheezing, recurrent respiratory infections, and shortness of breath associated with chronic bronchitis. The symptoms usually develop gradually and are often first noticed when the patient has difficulty breathing in cold or damp weather. Older adults with a combination of chronic bronchitis and emphysema usually have a long history of smoking.

Emphysema may be caused by cigarette smoking or a deficiency of alpha$_1$-antitrypsin (usually seen in younger people). Recurrent inflammation associated with the release of proteolytic enzymes from lung cells causes abnormal, irreversible enlargement of the air spaces distal to the terminal bronchioles. This leads to the destruction of alveolar walls, which results in a breakdown of elasticity. (See *Air trapping in chronic obstructive pulmonary disease.*)

Chronic bronchitis is marked by excessive production of tracheobronchial mucus sufficient to cause a cough for at least 3 months each year for 2 consecutive years. It results in hypertrophy and hyperplasia of the bronchial mucous glands, increased goblet cells, ciliary damage, squamous metaplasia of the columnar epithelium, and chronic leukocytic and lymphocytic infiltration of bronchial walls. Additional effects include widespread inflammation, airway narrowing, and mucus within the airways — all producing resistance in the small airways and, in turn, a severe ventilation-perfusion mismatch. The severity of the disease is linked to the amount of cigarette smoke or other pollutants inhaled and the duration of the inhalation. A respiratory tract infection typically exacerbates the cough and related symptoms.

The most common cause of chronic bronchitis is cigarette smoking, although some studies suggest a genetic predisposition to the disease as well. The disease is directly correlated with heavy pollution and is more prevalent in people exposed to certain types of dust (such as sawdust and plaster dust) and noxious gases.

Air trapping in chronic obstructive pulmonary disease

In chronic obstructive pulmonary disease, mucus plugs and narrowed airways trap air (also called *ball valving*). During inspiration, the airways enlarge and gas enters; on expiration, the airways narrow and air can't escape. This commonly occurs in asthma and chronic bronchitis.

INSPIRATION: Air is allowed to flow freely in

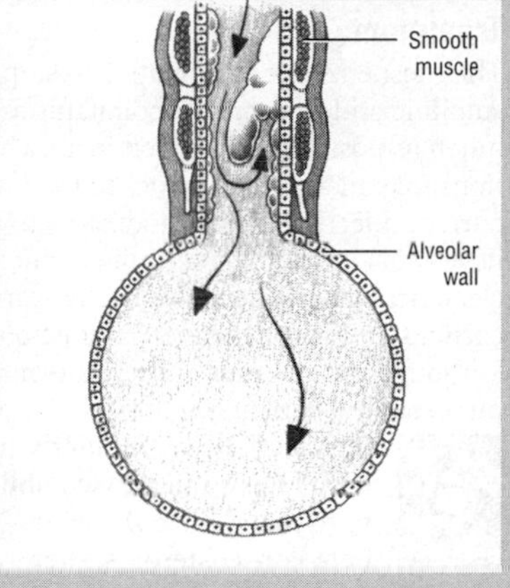

EXPIRATION: Air is trapped

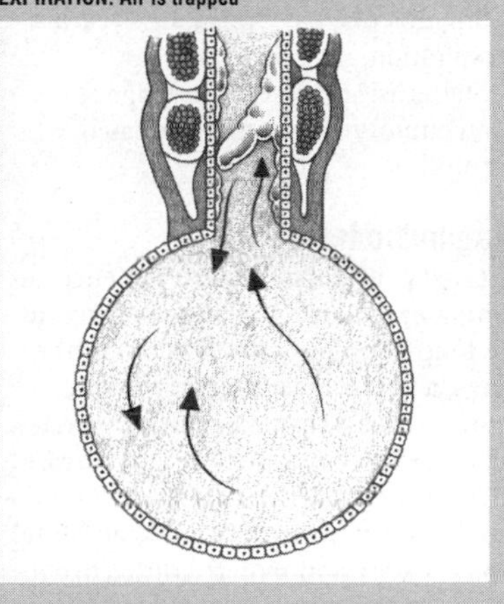

Asthma is characterized by an increase in bronchial reactivity to a variety of stimuli, which produces episodic bronchospasm and airway obstruction in conjunction with airway inflammation. Some older patients have had asthma throughout their lives, and others first develop it later in life.

Complications of COPD may include recurrent respiratory tract infections, cor pulmonale, right ventricular hypertrophy, and respiratory failure. Peptic ulcer disease strikes between 20% and 25% of people with COPD. Additionally, alveolar blebs and bullae may rupture, leading to spontaneous pneumothorax or pneumomediastinum.

Signs and symptoms

Emphysema

- Dyspnea (predominant symptom)
- Anorexia, weight loss, malaise, barrel chest, use of accessory muscles of respiration, prolonged expiratory period with grunting, pursed-lip breathing, tachypnea
- Hyperresonance on percussion
- Decreased breath sounds and quiet heart sounds on auscultation

Chronic bronchitis

- Productive cough and exertional dyspnea (predominant symptoms)
- Colds associated with increased sputum production and worsening dyspnea, which take progressively longer to resolve; copious sputum (gray, white, or yellow); weight gain due to edema; cyanosis; tachypnea; wheezing; prolonged expiratory time; use of accessory muscles of respiration
- Rhonchi and wheezing on auscultation
- Neck vein distention

Asthma

- History of intermittent attacks of dyspnea and wheezing

- Mild wheezing progressing to severe dyspnea, audible wheezing, chest tightness (a feeling of being unable to breathe), and cough producing thick mucus
- Prolonged expiration, intercostal and supraclavicular retraction on inspiration, use of accessory muscles of respiration, flaring nostrils, tachypnea, tachycardia, perspiration, flushing
- Status asthmaticus (can progress to respiratory failure unless treated promptly)

Diagnostic tests

- *Chest X-rays* may show a flattened diaphragm, reduced vascular markings at the lung periphery, overaeration of the lungs, a vertical heart, enlarged anteroposterior chest diameter, and large retrosternal air space (in advanced disease).
- *Pulmonary function tests* typically indicate increased residual volume and total lung capacity and reduced diffusing capacity. In emphysema, inspiratory flow is increased and diffusing capacity is decreased. In chronic bronchitis, static compliance and diffusion capacity are normal, and expiratory flow is decreased. In asthma, forced expiratory volumes are decreased and improve significantly after bronchodilator inhalation; residual volume is increased.
- *Arterial blood gas* (ABG) *analysis* usually shows reduced partial pressure of arterial oxygen ($Pa{O_2}$) and normal partial pressure of arterial carbon dioxide ($Pa{CO_2}$) until late in the disease.
- In chronic bronchitis and emphysema, *electrocardiography* (ECG) may reveal tall, symmetrical P waves in leads II, III, and aV_F; vertical QRS axis; and signs of right ventricular hypertrophy late in the disease. In asthma, the ECG may reveal sinus tachycardia and, during a severe attack, signs of cor pulmonale (right axis deviation, peaked P waves) that resolve after the attack.
- *Red blood cell* (RBC) *count* usually demonstrates an increased hemoglobin level late in the disease when the patient has persistent severe hypoxia.
- *Sputum specimen* may reveal many microorganisms and neutrophils in chronic bronchitis. Sputum may exhibit Curschmann's spirals (casts of airways), Charcot-Leyden crystals, and eosinophils in asthma.

Treatment

The most effective treatment is to stop smoking and to avoid air pollutants as much as possible. Prescribed medications may include antibiotics to treat recurrent infections, bronchodilators to relieve bronchospasm and facilitate mucus clearance, diuretics to treat edema, and corticosteroids to relieve inflammation (although the risks for older adults may outweigh the benefits).

Drug alert Because elderly patients have a decreased ability to metabolize and eliminate corticosteroids, they may have higher plasma drug levels and a higher incidence of adverse reactions. Monitor older patients closely for adverse reactions.

Adequate fluid intake (2 to 3 L/day) is essential. Chest physiotherapy may be needed to mobilize secretions, and ultrasonic or mechanical nebulizer treatments may help to loosen and mobilize secretions. Some older patients may require oxygen therapy (limited to 2 to 3 L/minute) to correct hypoxia. COPD patients may require transtracheal catheterization to receive oxygen at home.

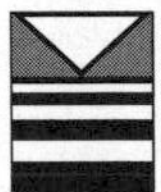

Key point Remember that respirations in people with severe COPD are stimulated by low oxygen levels, not high carbon dioxide levels.

Most older adults should be immunized to prevent influenza and pneumococcal pneumonia.

Key nursing diagnoses and outcomes

Activity intolerance related to fatigue secondary to chronic tissue hypoxia

Treatment outcomes: The patient will skillfully conserve energy while performing daily activities at a tolerable level and will seek assistance when necessary to complete an activity.

Impaired gas exchange related to lung tissue changes secondary to recurrent inflammation

Treatment outcome: The patient will have adequate ventilation.

Ineffective airway clearance related to increased bronchial secretions secondary to recurrent lung inflammation

Treatment outcome: The patient will skillfully perform bronchial hygiene to clear secretions from the airway.

Nursing interventions

- Assess respiratory status and monitor ABG levels and pulmonary function studies when ordered.
- Monitor the patient's RBC count for increases (a warning sign of increasing lung and vascular congestion).
- Watch for complications, such as respiratory tract infections, cor pulmonale, spontaneous pneumothorax, respiratory failure, and peptic ulcer disease.
- Provide a high-calorie, protein-rich diet to promote health and healing. Give small, frequent meals to conserve the patient's energy and prevent fatigue.
- Encourage daily activity, and provide diversionary activities as appropriate. To conserve energy and prevent fatigue, have the patient alternate rest and activity periods.
- Perform chest physiotherapy, including postural drainage and chest percussion and vibration, several times daily.
- Schedule respiratory treatments at least 1 hour before or after meals. Provide the patient with mouth care after bronchodilator therapy.
- Make sure the patient receives adequate fluids (2 to 3 L/day) to loosen secretions.
- Provide supportive care, and help the patient adjust to lifestyle changes imposed by a chronic illness.
- Answer the patient's questions about his illness honestly. Encourage him to express his fears and concerns, and stay with him during periods of extreme stress and anxiety.
- Include the patient and his family in care-related decisions. Refer them to appropriate support services as needed to help the patient maintain as much independence as possible.

PATIENT TEACHING

- Review the patient's medications and explain the rationale, dosage, and adverse effects of prescribed drugs. Instruct him to report adverse reactions to the physician immediately. Show him how to use an inhaler correctly, if appropriate.
- Advise the patient to avoid crowds and people with known infections. Also tell him to obtain influenza and pneumococcal pneumonia immunizations.
- If the patient is receiving home oxygen therapy, explain the treatment rationales and proper use of equipment.
- If the patient requires a transtracheal catheter, teach him about catheter care, precautions, and follow-up care
- If the patient smokes, urge him to stop. Provide him with smoking cessation resources or counseling, if necessary.
- Urge the patient to avoid respiratory irritants, such as automobile exhaust fumes, aerosol sprays, and industrial pollutants.
- Teach the patient the signs and symptoms of ruptured alveolar blebs and bullae. Explain the seriousness of possible spontaneous pneumothorax. Urge him to notify the physician if he feels sudden, sharp pleuritic pain that's exacer-

bated by chest movement, breathing, or coughing.

- Teach the patient and family members how to perform postural drainage and chest percussion. Tell them that the patient should maintain each position for about 10 minutes. During this time, a family member should perform percussion and direct the patient to cough.
- Teach the patient coughing and deep-breathing techniques to promote good ventilation and mobilize secretions.
- Encourage the patient to eat high-calorie, protein-rich foods. Urge him to drink plenty of fluids to prevent dehydration and to help loosen secretions.
- Warn the patient that exposure to blasts of cold air may precipitate bronchospasm. Tell him to avoid cold, windy weather and to cover his mouth and nose with a scarf or mask if he must go outside.

CHRONIC RENAL FAILURE

Usually the end result of a gradually progressive loss of renal function, chronic renal failure is also occasionally caused by a rapidly progressive disease of sudden onset that gradually destroys the nephrons and eventually causes irreversible renal damage. Few symptoms develop until after more than 75% of glomerular filtration is lost; then, the remaining normal parenchyma deteriorates progressively, and symptoms worsen as renal function decreases.

Causes of chronic renal failure in older adults include chronic glomerular disease (such as glomerulonephritis), chronic infections (such as chronic pyelonephritis or tuberculosis), vascular diseases (such as renal nephrosclerosis or hypertension), obstructive processes (such as calculi), nephrotoxic agents (such as long-term aminoglycoside therapy), and endocrine diseases (such as diabetic neuropathy).

Chronic renal failure may progress through the following stages:

- reduced renal reserve (glomerular filtration rate [GFR] 35% to 50% of normal)
- renal insufficiency (GFR 25% to 35% of normal)
- renal failure (GFR 20% to 25% of normal)
- end-stage renal disease (GFR less than 20% of normal).

If chronic renal failure continues unchecked, uremic toxins accumulate and produce potentially fatal physiologic changes in all major organ systems. This syndrome is fatal without treatment, but maintenance dialysis can sustain life. Some older patients decide not to go through the rigors of dialysis and choose hospice care at home instead.

Even if the patient can tolerate life-sustaining maintenance dialysis, he may still have anemia, peripheral neuropathy, cardiopulmonary and GI complications, sexual dysfunction, and skeletal defects. The prognosis is poor in older patients because of the risk of concomitant diseases, such as diabetes mellitus, cardiac disease, and cancer.

Signs and symptoms

- Dry mouth
- Fatigue
- Hypotension
- Listlessness progressing to somnolence and confusion
- Decreased urine output
- Very dilute urine, with casts and crystals
- Muscle irritability and then muscle weakness
- Irregular pulses and life-threatening cardiac arrhythmias
- Fluid overload and palpable edema
- Pericardial friction rub, distant heart sounds
- Pleuritic pain, bibasilar crackles
- Kussmaul's respirations in metabolic acidosis
- Gum ulceration, bleeding, and parotitis
- Hiccups, metallic taste in the mouth, anorexia, nausea, and vomiting

- Uremic fetor (ammonia smell to the breath)
- Pallid, yellowish-bronze skin
- Brittle fingernails with characteristic lines
- Severe itching
- Apathy, drowsiness, and irritability
- Restless legs syndrome
- Decreased libido or impotence (in men)
- Easy bruising, ecchymoses, and petechiae caused by thrombocytopenia and platelet defects
- Pathologic fractures and complaints of bone and muscle pain
- Gait abnormalities

Diagnostic tests

- *Blood studies* show elevated blood urea nitrogen, serum creatinine, sodium, and potassium levels; low hemoglobin and hematocrit; decreased red blood cell (RBC) survival time; mild thrombocytopenia; platelet defects; increased aldosterone secretion and blood glucose levels; hypertriglyceridemia; and decreased high-density lipoprotein levels.
- *Arterial blood gas analysis* reveals decreased pH and bicarbonate levels, indicating metabolic acidosis.
- *Urine specific gravity* becomes fixed at 1.010.
- *Urinalysis* may show proteinuria, glycosuria, RBCs, leukocytes, and casts and crystals.
- *Renal biopsy* allows histologic identification of the underlying pathology.
- *X-ray studies*, including kidney-ureter-bladder radiography, excretory urography, nephrotomography, renal scan, and renal arteriography, show reduced kidney size.
- *EEG* may show metabolic encephalopathy.

Treatment

Conservative treatment aims to correct specific symptoms. A low-protein diet reduces the production of end products of protein metabolism that the kidneys can't excrete. (However, a patient receiving continuous peritoneal dialysis should have a high-protein diet.) A high-calorie diet prevents ketoacidosis and the negative nitrogen balance that results in catabolism and tissue atrophy. The diet also should restrict sodium and potassium.

Cultural diversity **Asian Americans consume high amounts of sodium. Encourage an Asian patient to substitute fresh vegetables, herbs, and spices for monosodium glutamate, soy sauce, and canned foods.**

Fluid retention can be reduced with loop diuretics such as furosemide (if some renal function remains) and with fluid restriction. Cardiac glycosides in small doses may be used to mobilize the fluids causing the edema; antihypertensives may be used to control blood pressure and associated edema.

Antiemetics taken before meals may relieve nausea and vomiting, and ranitidine or famotidine may decrease gastric irritation. Methylcellulose or docusate can help prevent constipation.

Anemia necessitates iron and folate supplements; severe anemia requires infusion of packed RBCs or leukocyte-poor packed cells. Transfusions relieve anemia only temporarily. Synthetic erythropoietin (epoetin alfa) stimulates the division and differentiation of cells with in the bone marrow to produce RBCs.

Drug therapy commonly relieves associated symptoms. For example, an antipruritic, such as trimeprazine or diphenhydramine, can relieve itching, and aluminum hydroxide gel can lower serum phosphate levels. The patient also may benefit from vitamin supplements (particularly B vitamins and vitamin D) and essential amino acids.

Careful monitoring of serum potassium levels is necessary to detect hyperkalemia. Emergency treatment for severe hyperkalemia includes dialysis therapy and administration of 50% hypertonic glucose I.V., regular insulin, calcium gluconate I.V., sodium bicarbonate I.V., and cation exchange resins such as sodium polystyrene sulfonate. Cardiac tamponade resulting from pericardial effusion may require emergency pericardial tap or surgery.

Intensive dialysis and thoracentesis can relieve pulmonary edema and pleural effusion. Hemodialysis or peritoneal dialysis (particularly the newer techniques — continuous ambulatory peritoneal dialysis and continuous cyclic peritoneal dialysis) can help control most manifestations of end-stage renal disease. Altering the dialysate can correct fluid and electrolyte disturbances. However, maintenance dialysis itself may produce complications, including serum hepatitis (hepatitis B) from numerous blood transfusions, protein wasting, refractory ascites, and dialysis dementia.

Key nursing diagnoses and outcomes

Imbalanced nutrition: Less than body requirements related to adverse GI effects

Treatment outcome: The patient will not develop malnutrition.

Excess fluid volume related to inability of the kidneys to regulate water balance

Treatment outcome: The patient will exhibit no signs or symptoms of excessive fluid retention.

Risk for injury related to adverse effects of chronic renal failure on all major organ systems

Treatment outcome: The patient will take precautions in daily life to minimize or prevent injury caused by organ dysfunction.

Nursing interventions

▶ Provide good oral hygiene. Brush the patient's teeth often with a soft-bristled toothbrush or sponge tip to reduce breath odor. Hard candy and mouthwash minimize metallic taste in the mouth and alleviate thirst.

▶ Offer small, palatable, nutritious meals. Try to provide favorite foods within dietary restrictions, and encourage intake of high-calorie foods.

▶ Schedule medication administration carefully. Give iron before meals, aluminum hydroxide gels after meals, and antiemetics (as necessary) a half hour before meals.

▶ Measure daily intake and output, including all drainage, vomitus, diarrhea, and blood loss. Record daily weight, presence or absence of thirst, axillary sweat, tongue dryness, hypertension, and peripheral edema.

▶ Administer loop diuretics and restrict fluid and sodium intake to alleviate excess fluid retention, as ordered.

▶ Prepare the patient for hemodialysis or peritoneal dialysis, as indicated.

▶ Carefully assess the patient's hydration status. Check for jugular vein distention, and auscultate the lungs for crackles, rhonchi, and decreased breath sounds. Be alert for clinical signs of pulmonary edema (such as dyspnea and restlessness).

▶ Provide good skin care. Bathe the patient daily, using superfatted soaps or oatmeal baths, and apply skin lotion to ease pruritus. Give good perineal care, using mild soap and water. Pad side rails to guard against ecchymoses. Turn the patient often, and use a convoluted foam or low-pressure mattress to prevent skin breakdown.

▶ Prevent pathologic fractures by turning the patient carefully and ensuring his safety. Perform passive range-of-motion exercises for the bedridden patient.

▶ Encourage deep-breathing and coughing exercises to prevent pulmonary congestion.

▶ Maintain strict aseptic technique. Use a micropore filter during I.V. therapy. Warn the outpatient to avoid contact with infected people during the cold and flu season.

▶ Infuse sodium bicarbonate for acidosis and sedatives or anticonvulsants for seizures, as ordered. Keep an oral airway and suction setup at the bedside.

▶ Administer antihypertensives at appropriate intervals. If the patient requires a rectal infusion of sodium polystyrene sulfonate for dangerously high potassium levels, apply an emollient to soothe the perianal area.

▶ Watch for signs of hyperkalemia. Observe for cramping of the legs and abdomen and for diarrhea. As potassium levels rise, watch for muscle irritability and a weak pulse rate. Monitor the ECG for tall, peaked T waves; a widening QRS complex; a prolonged PR interval; and the disappearance of P waves.

▶ Watch for signs of infection, such as listlessness, confusion, high fever (may or may not be present in the older patient), and leukocytosis.

▶ Carefully observe and document seizure activity. Periodically assess neurologic status, and check for Chvostek's and Trousseau's signs, indicators of low serum calcium levels.

▶ Observe for signs of bleeding. Watch for prolonged bleeding at puncture sites and at the vascular access site used for hemodialysis. Monitor hemoglobin and hematocrit, and check stool, urine, and vomitus for blood.

▶ Report signs of pericarditis, such as a pericardial friction rub and chest pain. Also watch for the disappearance of friction rub, with a drop of 15 to 20 mm Hg in blood pressure during inspiration (paradoxical pulse), an early sign of pericardial tamponade.

PATIENT TEACHING

▶ Teach the patient how to take his medications and what adverse effects to watch for. Suggest that he take diuretics in the morning so his sleep won't be disturbed.

▶ Instruct the anemic patient to conserve energy by resting frequently.

▶ Tell the patient to report leg cramps or excessive muscle twitching. Stress the importance of keeping follow-up appointments to have his electrolyte levels monitored.

▶ Tell the patient to avoid high-sodium and high-potassium foods, and encourage him to follow fluid and protein restrictions. To prevent constipation, stress the need for exercise and sufficient dietary fiber.

▶ If the patient is having dialysis, remember that he and his family are under extreme stress. If your facility doesn't offer a course on dialysis, teach them about the process to help decrease their anxiety.

▶ Refer the patient and his family for counseling if they need help coping with chronic renal failure.

▶ Suggest that the patient wear a medical identification bracelet or carry pertinent information with him.

COCHLEAR IMPLANT

Older adults who have become profoundly deaf because of sensorineural hearing loss may benefit from a cochlear implant. This auditory prosthetic device improves auditory awareness. In some individuals, it improves hearing enough so that the patient can understand conversation. Sensorineural hearing loss is caused by damage to or loss of hair cells in the cochlea. The implant works by directly stimulating the auditory nerve transmitting impulses to the brain's hearing center.

A cochlear implant is most successful in patients who have not been deaf for long and who have a strong desire to hear. (See *Cochlear implant: A closer look,* page 194.)

Implementation

The cochlear implant is surgically inserted during an operating room procedure. The surgeon implants the internal component of the device, complete with one or more electrodes, into the cochlea of the ear and then implants a receiver behind the top of the auricle. The receiver

Cochlear implant: A closer look

The illustration below shows a patient with a cochlear implant in place.

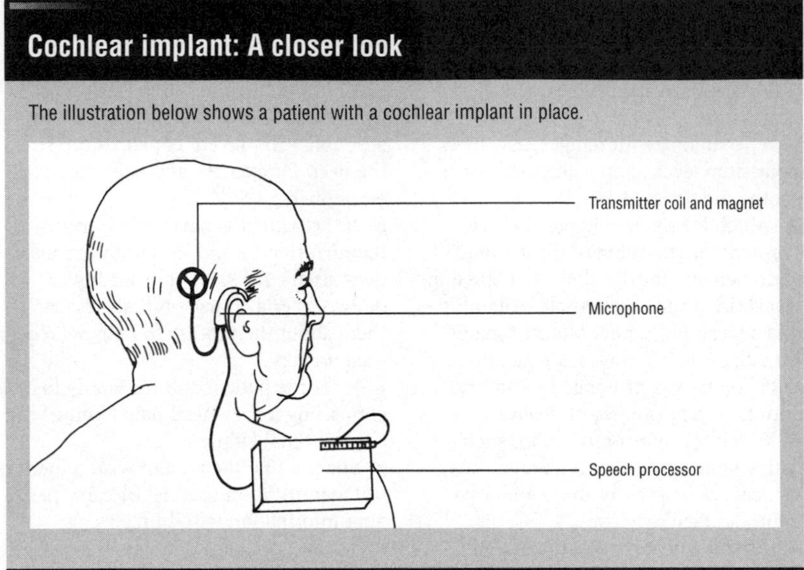

transmits the electrical signal to the electrode.

The cochlear device also has an external component that consists of a small microphone with an ear hook that is worn over the ear and is connected to a speech processor and to a transmitter coil with a magnet that keeps it in place over the receiver stimulator. These devices are put in place 10 to 15 days postoperatively when wound healing is complete. The device then picks up sound through the microphone and sends it to the processor, where it's broken down and stored. The converted sound information is transferred to the external device, further processed, and sent through any surviving nerve cells to the hearing center of the brain. After this chain of events, the patient is able to hear.

Complications

As with any surgical procedure, there is a risk of infection with a cochlear implant. The patient may also be at risk for depression if his expectations exceed the limitations of the implant.

Key nursing diagnoses and outcomes

Disturbed sensory perception (auditory) related to sensorineural hearing loss requiring a cochlear implant

Treatment outcome: The patient will verbalize that hearing is improved after insertion of cochlear implant.

Anxiety related to the need for a cochlear implant and rehabilitation

Treatment outcomes: The patient will verbalize a decrease in anxiety and will show no physical signs of anxiety.

Nursing interventions

- When addressing the patient, speak in a clear, loud voice. Speak slowly and allow him to process the information. Give him enough time to respond.
- Provide support to the patient and his family. Reassure them that the patient's hearing may not improve until he undergoes rehabilitation.

- Monitor the incision site, and report any redness, swelling, or drainage.

PATIENT TEACHING

- Teach the patient and his family about sensorineural hearing loss and treatment options.
- Make sure the patient understands that his hearing won't return to his preloss level. Also, explain that he'll need rehabilitation to learn how to interpret the sounds produced by the device.
- Teach the patient an alternative method of communication.

COLD APPLICATION

The application of cold constricts blood vessels; inhibits local circulation, suppuration, and tissue metabolism; relieves vascular congestion; slows bacterial activity in infections; reduces body temperature; and may act as a temporary anesthetic during brief painful procedures. Because treatment with cold also relieves inflammation and slows bleeding, it may be effective in initial treatment of eye injuries, strains, sprains, bruises, muscle spasms, and burns. Cold doesn't reduce existing edema, however, because it inhibits reabsorption of excess fluid.

Cold may be applied in dry or moist forms. Moist application of cold is more penetrating than dry because moisture aids conduction. Devices for applying dry cold include ice bags or collars, K pads (which can produce cold or heat), and chemical cold packs. Devices for applying moist cold include cold compresses for small body areas and cold packs for large areas.

Supplies

For all types

- Patient thermometer
- Towel
- Adhesive tape or roller gauze
- Gloves (if necessary)

For an ice bag or collar

- Tap water
- Ice chips
- Absorbent, protective cloth covering

For a K pad

- Distilled water
- Temperature-adjustment key
- Absorbent, protective cloth covering

For a chemical cold pack

- Single-use cold packs or reusable, sealed cold packs

For a cold compress or pack

- Basin of ice chips
- Container of tap water
- Bath (utility) thermometer
- Compress material (4″ × 4″ gauze pads or washcloths) or pack material (towels or flannel)
- Linen-saver pad
- Waterproof covering

Preparation of equipment

Ice bag or collar

- Select a device of the correct size, fill it with cold tap water, and check for leaks.
- Empty the device and fill it about halfway with crushed ice. (Using small pieces of ice keeps the device flexible enough to mold to the patient's body.)
- Squeeze the device to expel air, which could interfere with conduction.
- Fasten the cap and wipe any moisture from the outside of the device.
- Wrap the bag or collar in a cloth covering, and secure it with tape or roller gauze.

K pad

- Check the cord for frayed or damaged insulation.
- Fill the control unit two-thirds full with distilled water. (Tap water leaves mineral deposits in the unit.)
- After checking for leaks, tilt the unit several times to clear the pad's tubing of air.

▶ Tighten the cap and ensure that the hoses between the control unit and pad are free of tangles.
▶ Place the unit on the bedside table, slightly above the patient, so that gravity can assist water flow.
▶ Use the key provided to adjust the unit to the lowest temperature.
▶ Cover the pad with an absorbent, protective cloth, and secure it with tape or roller gauze.
▶ Plug in the unit and turn it on. Allow the pad to cool for 2 minutes before placing it on the patient.

Chemical cold pack

▶ Select a pack of the appropriate size, and follow the manufacturer's directions (strike, squeeze, or knead) to activate the cold-producing chemicals.
▶ Make certain that the container isn't broken during activation; such damage could allow the chemicals to leak.
▶ Wrap the pack in a cloth cover, and secure the cover with tape or roller gauze.

Cold compress or pack

▶ Cool the tap water by placing the container of water in a basin of ice or by adding ice to the water.
▶ Adjust the water temperature to 59° F (15° C) or as ordered (using a bath thermometer).
▶ Immerse the compress or pack in the water.

Implementation

▶ Check the physician's order and assess the patient's condition.
▶ Explain the procedure to the patient, and provide privacy.
▶ Make sure the patient's room is warm and free of drafts.
▶ Wash your hands thoroughly.
▶ Record the patient's temperature, pulse, and respirations to serve as a baseline.
▶ Expose only the treatment site to avoid chilling the patient.

Ice bag or collar, K pad, or chemical cold pack

▶ Place the covered device on the treatment site.
▶ Begin timing the application.
▶ Observe the site frequently for signs of tissue intolerance: blanching, mottling, graying, cyanosis, maceration, or blisters.
▶ Be alert for shivering and complaints of burning or numbness. If any of these signs or symptoms develop, discontinue the treatment and notify the physician.
▶ Refill or replace the cold device as necessary to maintain the correct temperature.
▶ Change the protective cover if it becomes wet.
▶ Remove the device after the prescribed treatment period (usually 30 minutes).

Cold compress or pack

▶ Place a linen-saver pad under the treatment area.
▶ Remove the compress or pack from the water, and wring it out to prevent dripping. Apply it to the treatment site, and begin timing the application.
▶ Cover the compress or pack with a waterproof covering to provide insulation and to keep the surrounding area dry.
▶ Secure the covering with paper tape or roller gauze to prevent it from slipping and injuring the older patient's friable skin.
▶ Check the application site frequently for signs of tissue intolerance. Also note any complaints of burning or numbness. If any of these signs or symptoms develop, discontinue the treatment and notify the physician.
▶ Change the compress or pack as necessary to maintain the correct temperature.
▶ Remove the compress or pack after the prescribed treatment period (usually 20 minutes).

Final steps

- Dry the patient's skin, and redress the treatment site according to the physician's orders.
- Position the patient comfortably.
- Record temperature, pulse, and respirations for comparison with baseline values.
- Dispose of liquids and soiled materials properly. If treatment is to be repeated, clean and store the equipment in the patient's room, out of his reach; otherwise, return it to storage.

Complications

Older persons, especially those with impaired circulation or arthritis, are at risk for ischemic tissue damage from cold application. Extreme cold may cause burns, and placing ice directly on the skin may exacerbate tissue damage. Hemoconcentration may result in thrombi. Intense cold may cause pain, burning, or numbness.

Patient teaching

- Explain the procedure to the patient.
- Instruct the patient to notify you immediately if he experiences any pain, burning, or numbness.

Special considerations

- Apply cold immediately after an injury to minimize edema. Although colder temperatures can be tolerated for a longer time when the treatment site is small, don't continue any application for longer than 1 hour to prevent reflexive vasodilation. Application of temperatures below 59° F (15° C) will also cause local reflex vasodilation.
- Use sterile technique when applying cold to an open wound or to a lesion that may open during treatment. Also maintain sterile technique during eye treatment, and use separate sterile equipment for each eye to prevent cross-contamination.
- Avoid securing cooling devices with pins because an accidental puncture could allow extremely cold fluids to leak out and burn the patient's skin.
- If the patient is unconscious, anesthetized, neurologically impaired, irrational, or otherwise insensitive to cold, stay with him throughout the treatment and check the application site frequently for signs of complications.

Documentation

Record the time, date, and duration of cold application; the type of device used; the application site; the temperature or temperature setting; the patient's temperature, pulse, and respirations before and after application; the skin's appearance before, during, and after application; any signs of complications; and the patient's tolerance of the treatment.

COLORECTAL CANCER

The second most common visceral neoplasm in the United States and Europe, colorectal cancer affects men and women equally but is more common in those over age 40. The risk of developing colorectal cancer doubles every decade after age 55 and peaks at age 75. Malignant tumors of the colon or rectum are almost always adenocarcinomas. About half of them are sessile lesions of the rectosigmoid area; the rest, polypoid lesions.

Colorectal cancer progresses slowly, remaining localized for a long time. Unless the tumor has metastasized, the 5-year survival rate is 50%. If left untreated, the disease is invariably fatal.

Although the exact cause of colorectal cancer is unknown, studies show a greater incidence in areas of higher economic development, suggesting a relation to diet (excess animal fat, particularly beef, and low fiber). Other risk factors include diseases of the digestive tract, a history of ulcerative colitis (in which case cancer usually starts in 11 to 17 years) or familial polyposis (in which case cancer almost always develops by

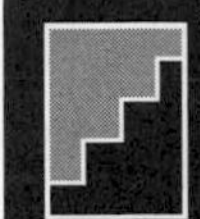

Staying well

Reducing the risk of colorectal cancer

Express to your patient the importance of screening and early detection as keys to reducing the risk of colorectal cancer. Be sure to cover these points:

- Annual fecal occult blood testing is recommended in combination with flexible sigmoidoscopy every 5 years in normal-risk adults beginning at age 50. The American Cancer Society further advises that a digital rectal examination be performed along with endoscopic or radiologic procedures.
- It's important to intake an adequate amount of fiber in the diet. Fiber protects against colorectal cancer by increasing stool bulk, shortening intestinal transit time, and altering the flora of the colon.

age 50), and a family history of the disease (first-degree relative) (*See Reducing the risk of colorectal cancer.*)

Signs and symptoms

With tumor on right side

▶ Usually no signs or symptoms in the early stages because stool is still liquid in this part of colon

▶ Possibly black, tarry stools, anemia, abdominal aching, pressure, and dull cramps

▶ As disease progresses, weakness, diarrhea, constipation, anorexia, weight loss, and vomiting

With tumor on left side

▶ Symptoms of obstruction even in early disease stages because stools are more completely formed when they reach this part of the colon

▶ Possibly rectal bleeding (often ascribed to hemorrhoids), intermittent abdominal fullness or cramping, and rectal pressure

▶ As disease progresses, constipation, diarrhea, or ribbon- or pencil-shaped stools; pain relief from passage of flatus or stool; possibly obvious blood or mucus in feces

Rectal tumor

▶ Change in bowel habits, beginning with an urgent need to defecate on arising ("morning diarrhea") or constipation alternating with diarrhea

▶ Possible blood or mucus in the stools and sensation of incomplete evacuation

▶ Late in disease, feeling of rectal fullness that progresses to a dull, sometimes constant ache confined to the rectum or sacral region

All types

▶ Distention or visible masses on inspection

▶ Enlarged abdominal veins

▶ Abnormal bowel sounds on abdominal auscultation

▶ Abdominal mass on palpation

Diagnostic tests

▶ *Digital rectal examination* can detect almost 15% of colorectal cancers, including suspicious rectal and perianal lesions.

▶ *Fecal occult blood test* can detect blood in stools, a warning sign of rectal cancer.

▶ *Proctoscopy* or *sigmoidoscopy* can detect up to 66% of colorectal cancers.

▶ *Colonoscopy* provides access for biopsies of suspected lesions.

▶ *Excretory urography* verifies bilateral renal function and allows inspection for displacement of the kidneys, ureters, or bladder by a tumor pressing against these structures.

▶ *Barium enema studies* help locate lesions that aren't detectable manually or visually. (Barium examination shouldn't precede colonoscopy or excretory urography because barium sulfate interferes with these tests.)

▶ *Computed tomography scan* allows better visualization if a barium enema yields inconclusive results or if metastasis to the pelvic lymph nodes is suspected.
▶ *Carcinoembryonic antigen level* permits patient monitoring before and after treatment to detect metastasis or recurrence.

Treatment

The most effective treatment for colorectal cancer is surgery to remove the malignant tumor and adjacent tissues, along with any lymph nodes that may contain cancer cells. After surgery, treatment continues with chemotherapy, radiation therapy, or both.

The type of surgery depends on the tumor's location. Tumors in the cecum and ascending colon require a right hemicolectomy (for advanced disease), which may include resection of the terminal segment of the ileum, cecum, ascending colon, and right half of the transverse colon with corresponding mesentery. Tumors in the proximal and middle transverse colon require a right colectomy, which includes the transverse colon and mesentery corresponding to midcolic vessels or segmental resection of the transverse colon and associated midcolic vessels. Surgery for sigmoid colon tumors usually is limited to the sigmoid colon and mesentery.

For tumors in the upper rectum, surgery usually involves anterior or low anterior resection. A newer method, using a stapler, allows for much lower resections than were previously possible. Tumors in the lower rectum require abdominoperineal resection and permanent sigmoid colostomy.

If metastasis has occurred, or if the patient has residual disease or a recurrent inoperable tumor, he needs chemotherapy. The drug regimen most commonly used consists of fluorouracil combined with levamisole or leucovorin. Researchers are evaluating the effectiveness of fluorouracil with recombinant interferon alfa-2a.

Radiation therapy, used before or after surgery, induces tumor regression.

Key nursing diagnoses and outcomes

Constipation related to presence of a cancerous tumor in the colon or rectal area

Treatment outcomes: The patient will have no constipation and will regain a normal bowel pattern.

Diarrhea related to presence of a cancerous tumor in the colon or rectal area

Treatment outcomes: The patient will exhibit no signs of fluid or electrolyte imbalance and will develop a normal elimination pattern.

Fear related to potential for colorectal cancer to recur or metastasize

Treatment outcomes: The patient will express his fears about being diagnosed with colorectal cancer and will exhibit a reduction in physical and psychological symptoms of fear.

Deficient fluid volume related to chemotherapy or radiation

Treatment outcome: The patient will have adequate fluid volume balance.

Nursing interventions

▶ Prepare the patient for surgery, as indicated.
▶ Monitor the patient's bowel patterns.
▶ Monitor the patient's diet modifications, and assess the adequacy of his nutritional intake.
▶ If the patient is receiving radiation therapy, watch for adverse reactions, such as nausea, vomiting, hair loss, and malaise. Also provide comfort measures and reassurance.
▶ If he's receiving chemotherapy, be prepared for common adverse reactions while watching for complications such

as infection. Prepare the patient for adverse effects, and take steps to minimize them. For example, offer the patient a normal saline solution mouthwash to help prevent mouth ulcers.

▶ To help prevent infection, use strict aseptic technique when caring for I.V. catheters. Change I.V. tubing and sites as directed by your facility's policy. Have the patient wash his hands before and after meals and after going to the bathroom.

▶ Listen to the patient's fears and concerns, and stay with him during periods of severe stress and anxiety.

▶ Encourage the patient to identify actions and care measures that will promote his comfort and relaxation. Try to perform these measures, and encourage the patient and his family members to do likewise.

▶ Include the patient and his family members in care decisions.

▶ A colostomy may threaten a patient's self-concept and pose major adjustment problems, such as isolation, fear of socializing, and fear of embarrassing episodes. Provide reassurance to the patient as needed. Other health problems, such as arthritis, poor eyesight, and reduced energy, may hinder the older patient's ability to care for a colostomy, leaving him feeling a significant loss of independence. If your patient has such problems, refer him to a home health care agency that can check on his physical care at home.

PATIENT TEACHING

▶ Throughout the treatment regimen, answer the patient's questions and tell him what to expect from surgery and other therapies. Explain to the patient's family that their positive reactions will foster the patient's adjustment.

▶ Instruct the patient to follow a high-fiber diet. Teach him which foods to eat and which to avoid.

▶ Caution the patient to take laxatives and antidiarrheal medications only as prescribed by his physician.

▶ Stress the need for regular check-ups because of the patient's increased risk of developing another primary cancer. Annual screening and follow-up testing are strongly recommended.

▶ Explain radiation therapy or chemotherapy, as appropriate. Make sure the patient understands the adverse reactions that usually occur and the measures he can take to prevent them or decrease their severity.

COMPLIANCE

Getting an older person to follow medication instructions can be a challenge. Older patients may have many reasons for noncompliance, such as poor vision or hearing, physical disability, or failure to understand the importance of taking prescribed medications. Problems with specific drugs—such as adverse reactions, drug interactions, or inconvenient dosage times or methods—can also foster noncompliance. The danger is that noncompliance may lead to unsuccessful treatment and an apparent lack of therapeutic response. Furthermore, the physician may misinterpret the inadequate response and increase the drug dosage or prescribe a second drug, compounding the patient's problems.

To avoid such dangers, make sure your older patient understands why and how to take all his medications correctly. Make sure he understands that when a new drug is added to his regimen, that doesn't mean that he should stop taking any of his previously prescribed drugs unless specifically told to. To promote compliance in an older adult, first determine his ability to comply; then intervene to prevent noncompliance.

Assessing compliance ability

▶ Learn your patient's health and drug history. Determine his previous success in adhering to treatment plans.

▶ List all drugs, prescription and nonprescription, that the patient currently takes and those he has taken in the past. (If possible, encourage the patient to bring his medications to his practitioner's office.) Have the patient name each drug and tell you why, when, how much, and how often he takes it. Find out if he has drugs that are prescribed by more than one physician. Also, ask if he's taking any drugs originally prescribed for another person or family member (this is common).

- Evaluate the patient's cognitive and psychomotor skills.
- Assess the patient's beliefs about drug use. For example, he may believe that long-term medication use implies that he's sick or weak and, therefore, may take medications erratically.
- Identify possibly harmful food or drug interactions that may interfere with compliance (such as those caused by alcohol or caffeine).
- Assess the older person's lifestyle. Does he live with family or friends? Does he live alone or with a debilitated spouse?

Preventing noncompliance

- Help your patient evaluate misguided beliefs about sickness and the use of medications. Emphasize the medication's ability to enhance his health.

Drug Alert Collaborate with the patient's pharmacist to help prevent drug interactions. The patient may be taking multiple medications that were prescribed by different physicians, over-the-counter medications, or other remedies that may not be compatible.

- Review the findings about potential interactions with the patient, and give him the list. If he knows what to expect, he's more likely to comply with treatment. Advise him about specific food-drug interactions, and provide a list of foods and beverages to avoid. As your patient receives drugs (new or familiar), name them, explain their intended effect, and describe possible adverse effects to watch for and report.
- Encourage the patient to purchase drugs from only one pharmacy, preferably one that maintains a drug profile for each customer. Advise him to consult the pharmacist, who can warn him about potentially harmful drug or food interactions before they occur.
- If the patient's forgetfulness interferes with compliance, devise a system to help him remember to take his drugs properly. Suggest that he purchase or make a scheduling aid, such as a calendar, a checklist, an alarm wristwatch, or a compartmentalized drug container or blister packs that can be prepared by a pharmacist. (See *Using compliance aids*, pages 202 and 203.)
- If the patient simply can't remember to take his drugs on time and in the right amounts, or can't remember where he stored them, explore his family's ability to help. If he lives alone or with a debilitated spouse, he may need continuing support from a visiting nurse or another caregiver. Refer him to appropriate community resources for supervision to avoid drug misuse.
- To circumvent noncompliance caused by visual impairment, provide dosage instructions in large print, if necessary.
- To correct problems related to dosage form and administration, help the patient find easier ways to take the drug. For example, if he can't swallow tablets or capsules, find out if he can switch to a liquid or powdered form of the drug. Or suggest that he slide the tablet down with soft foods such as applesauce. Keep in mind that some drug forms — for example, enteric-coated tablets, timed-release capsules, or sublingual or buccal tablets — should not be crushed because doing so might affect their absorption and effectiveness. Also, some crushed drugs taste bitter or can stain teeth or irritate oral mucosa.
- To alter eating habits that lead to noncompliance, emphasize which drugs the patient must take with food and

Using compliance aids

To help your patient safely comply with oral or injectable drug therapy, you or a family member can premeasure doses for him, using compliance aids such as those shown below or ones you create yourself. Most pharmacies or community service agencies can supply similar aids.

One-day pill pack

A plastic box with four lidded medication compartments marked "breakfast," "lunch," "dinner," and "bedtime" helps the older person see whether he's taken all the medications prescribed for one day. The lids may also be embossed with braille characters if needed.

The patient, caregiver, or visiting nurse must remember to fill the device each day because it doesn't hold many tablets or capsules.

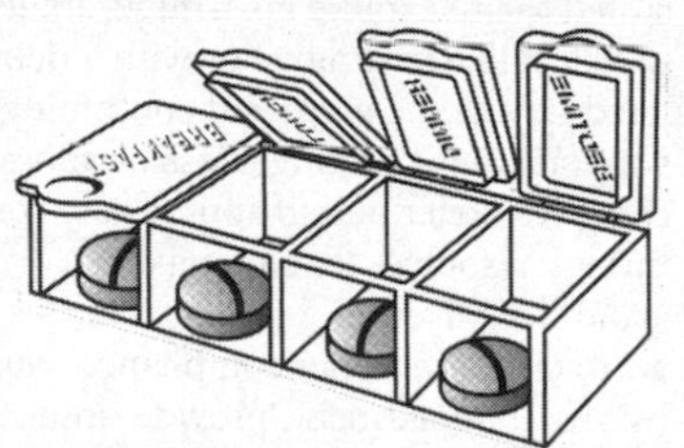

Seven-day pill reminder

The boxes shown here can help the patient remember if he has taken all the tablets and capsules prescribed for each day of the week. Each box has seven medication compartments marked with the initials for each day of the week (in both braille characters and printed letters).

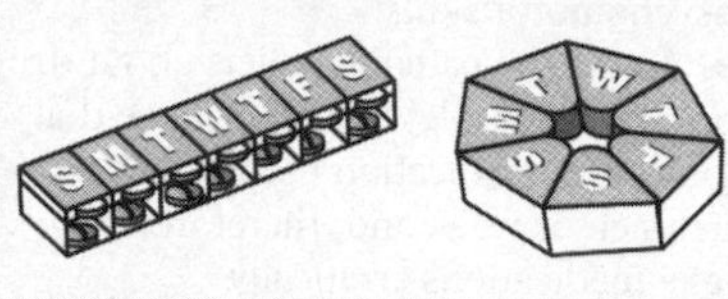

Like the one-day pill container, this device is inappropriate for large numbers of tablets or capsules, or for tablets and capsules that must be taken at different times each day.

Blister pack

A blister pack is prepared by the pharmacist and consists of bubbled compartments with foil backs that contain pills. Each compartment is labeled with the day of the week and "morning" or "night." In this way, the patient can locate "Monday morning" on the blister pack and find in that compartment all of the

which he must take on an empty stomach. Explain that taking some drugs on an empty stomach may cause nausea, whereas taking some drugs on a full stomach may interfere with absorption. Also, find out whether the patient eats regularly or skips meals. If he skips meals, he may be skipping drug doses too. As needed, help him coordinate his drug administration schedule with his eating habits.

▶ If mobility or transportation deters compliance, help the patient locate a pharmacy that delivers or suggest that he consider using a mail-order pharmacy.

▶ If financial considerations prevent compliance, help the older adult explore new ways to manage. Perhaps he's trying to save money by not having prescriptions filled or by taking fewer doses than ordered to make the drug last longer. Suggest that he ask his physician if he can use less expensive generic equivalents of name-brand drugs whenever possible. Some drugs may also be available over the counter and are less expensive than if purchased by prescription. Encourage the patient to speak with the pharmacist if his physician doesn't know about the generic option. Also, explore ways that family members

prescribed drugs he needs to take that day and time.

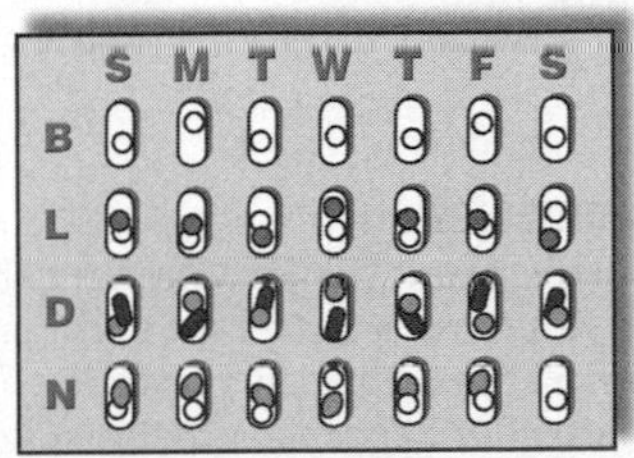

Homemade dosing aids

Show the patient and his caregivers how to make their own compliance aids by labeling clean empty jars, extra prescription bottles (obtainable from the pharmacist), or envelopes with the drug name, the time of day, and the day of the week to take the medication. Recommend that the patient use a separate container for each time and fill this container every morning with the correct dose of each medication.

Syringe scale magnifier

This device helps a visually impaired diabetic patient read syringe markings, thereby enabling him to fill his own syringe. The plastic magnifier snaps onto the syringe barrel. This device may be impractical for a patient with arthritis who can't easily attach the magnifier to the syringe.

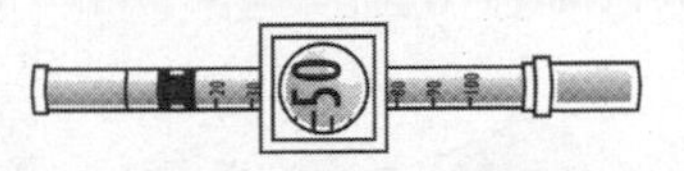

Syringe-filling device

This device precisely measures insulin doses for a visually impaired diabetic patient. Designed for use with a disposable U-100 syringe and an insulin bottle, the device is set by the caregiver to accommodate the syringe's width. She then positions the plunger at the point determined by the dose and tightens the stop. When the device is set, the patient can draw up the precise dose ordered for each injection.

There are several drawbacks to this device: It can't be used if insulin needs to be mixed or if doses vary; the settings must be checked and adjusted whenever the syringe size or type is changed; and the screws must be checked regularly because they loosen with repeated use.

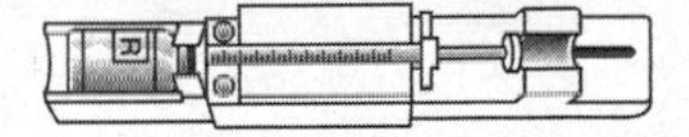

can help, or refer the patient to the social services department and appropriate community agencies. For example, many states have programs to help low-income elderly people buy needed drugs.

Special considerations

The abilities and needs of older adults differ from those of younger people. Therefore, tailor your style of teaching to take into account older patients' learning, motivational, and social differences. To teach successfully, keep in mind how the individual's intelligence and disease process may affect his mental capacity, sensory perception, and psychomotor function. Also, enlist the help of family members, the patient's pharmacist, and other caregivers to tailor supervision and teaching to fit the patient's needs.

CONDOM CATHETER APPLICATION

Not all patients require an indwelling urinary catheter to manage incontinence. For male patients, an incontinence device reduces the risk of urinary

Applying a condom catheter

Apply an adhesive strip to the shaft of the penis about 1″ (2.5 cm) from the scrotal area.

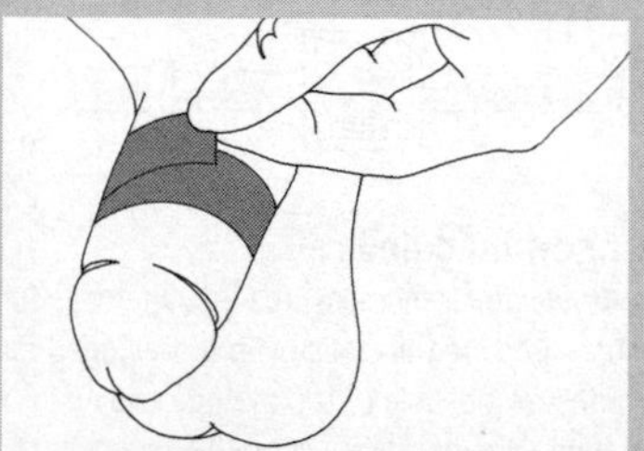

Then roll the condom catheter onto the penis past the adhesive strip, leaving about 1⁄2″ (1.3 cm) of clearance at the end. Press the sheath gently against the strip until it adheres.

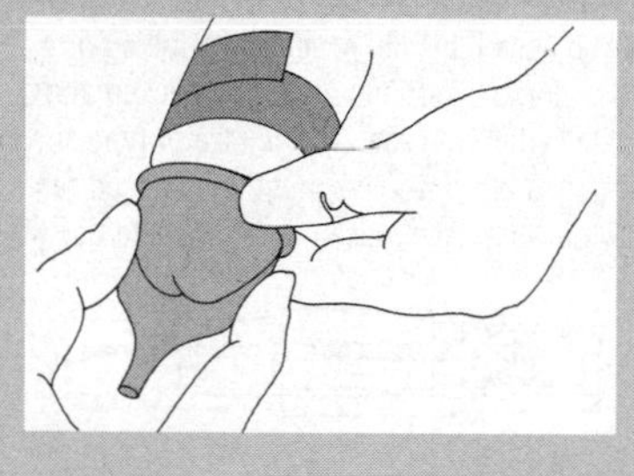

tract infection from catheterization, promotes bladder retraining when possible, helps prevent skin breakdown, and improves the patient's self-image. This device consists of a condom catheter secured to the shaft of the penis and connected to a leg bag or drainage bag. It has no contraindications.

Supplies

- Condom catheter
- Drainage bag
- Extension tubing
- Hypoallergenic tape or incontinence sheath holder
- Commercial adhesive strip or skin-bond cement
- Elastic adhesive or Velcro, if needed
- Gloves
- Razor, if needed
- Basin
- Soap
- Washcloth
- Towel

Implementation

- Fill the basin with lukewarm water. Then carry the basin and the remaining equipment to the patient's bedside.
- Wash your hands thoroughly and put on gloves.
- Provide privacy.

Applying the device

- If the patient is circumcised, wash the penis with soap and water, rinse well, and pat dry with a towel. If the patient is uncircumcised, gently retract the foreskin and clean beneath it. Rinse well but don't dry (because moisture provides lubrication and prevents friction during foreskin replacement). Replace the foreskin to avoid penile constriction. Then, if necessary, shave the base and shaft of the penis to prevent the adhesive strip or skin-bond cement from pulling pubic hair.
- If you're using a precut commercial adhesive strip, insert the glans penis through its opening, and position the strip 1″ (2.5 cm) from the scrotal area. If you're using uncut adhesive, cut a strip to fit around the shaft of the penis. Remove the protective covering from one side of the adhesive strip, and press this side firmly to the penis to enhance adhesion. Then remove the covering from the other side of the strip. If a commercial adhesive strip isn't available, apply skin-bond cement and let it dry for a few minutes.
- Position the rolled condom catheter at the tip of the penis, with its drainage opening at the urinary meatus.

▶ Unroll the catheter upward, past the adhesive strip on the shaft of the penis. Then gently press the sheath against the strip until it adheres. (See *Applying a condom catheter*.)
▶ After the condom catheter is in place, secure it with hypoallergenic tape or an incontinence sheath holder.
▶ Using extension tubing, connect the condom catheter to the leg bag or drainage bag. Attach the leg bag or drainage bag to the patient's leg, using elastic adhesive or Velcro.
▶ Inspect the condom catheter for twists and the extension tubing for kinks to prevent obstruction of urine flow, which could cause the condom to balloon, eventually dislodging it.
▶ Remove and discard your gloves.

Removing the device

▶ Put on gloves and simultaneously roll the condom catheter and adhesive strip off the penis and discard them. If you've used skin-bond cement rather than an adhesive strip, remove it with solvent. Also remove and discard the hypoallergenic tape or incontinence sheath holder.
▶ Clean the penis with lukewarm water, rinse thoroughly, and dry. Check for swelling or signs of skin breakdown.
▶ Remove the leg bag by closing the drain clamp, unlatching the leg straps, and disconnecting the extension tubing at the top of the bag.
▶ Discard your gloves.

Complications

Condom catheters can cause skin irritation, edema, infection, and penile circulatory impairment.

Patient teaching

▶ Explain the procedure to the patient to reduce fear and promote cooperation.
▶ If the patient is sent home with this device, instruct him on proper application and removal.

Documentation

Record the date and time of application and removal of the incontinence device. Also note skin condition and the patient's response to the device, including voiding pattern, to assist with bladder retraining.

CONSTIPATION

With advancing years and normal physiologic changes, constipation is common in older adults. Characterized by a decrease in the frequency of bowel movements, constipation is exacerbated by poor nutrition, low fluid intake, and immobility. Individuals who complain of constipation experience prolonged periods of time between bowel movements and a sensation of incomplete evacuation after having one. Constipation occurs because of a decrease in colonic peristalsis and slower neural impulses that sense the need to defecate. With age, the internal anal sphincter loses its tone, and defecation is postponed. A sedentary lifestyle and misuse of laxatives increase the risk of constipation. (About 30% of people over age 60 take a laxative at least once a week.) If not treated, constipation can lead to fecal impaction and megacolon.

Signs and symptoms

▶ Prolonged period of time between bowel movements
▶ Abdominal cramping and bloating
▶ Firm abdomen
▶ Straining during defecation
▶ Small, hard feces
▶ Distant or muffled bowel sounds
▶ Backache
▶ Headache
▶ Reduced activity level (sluggishness)

Diagnostic tests

▶ *Digital rectal examination* can confirm or rule out a physiologic problem.

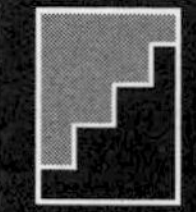

Staying well

Avoiding constipation

If your older patient complains of constipation, first make sure he's aware that a daily bowel movement is not necessarily the norm for every person. Inform him that every individual has his own pattern of regularity, which may vary from three times per day to once every 3 to 5 days, depending on his bowel muscle tone, activity level, and food intake.

Then teach him steps he can take to help prevent this problem, such as:

- increasing the amount of high-fiber foods (fresh, uncooked fruits and vegetables, bran, and other whole grain products) in his daily diet (may result in temporary bloating or flatulence)
- drinking at least 10 glasses of liquids, such as water and fruit juice, each day
- avoiding laxatives and enemas, if possible, but using a bulk-forming laxative to help maintain bowel regularity if necessary (this type is least likely to cause problems, especially if he drinks enough liquids)
- never ignoring the urge to defecate (trying to respond as soon as he gets the urge)
- trying to exercise regularly (increases bowel activity).

Treatment

Short-term treatment may consist of a powerful laxative to empty the entire bowel. Long-term treatments include a high-fiber diet, adequate fluid intake, reduced use of laxatives, and providing enough time to completely evacuate the bowel on a routine basis.

For fecal impaction, manual removal of the stools is followed by a warm oil-retention enema and a cleansing soapsuds enema. After 3 days, the patient receives a stool softener and a bowel stimulant.

Key nursing diagnosis and outcome

Constipation related to neuromuscular impairment, intestinal obstruction, megacolon, painful defecation, drug adverse effects, immobility, inadequate intake of fluids and fiber, or other metabolic conditions

Treatment outcome: The patient will have adequate bowel movements on a regular basis.

Nursing interventions

- Ask the patient about his dietary intake. Encourage increased fluid intake and a high-fiber diet.
- Provide stool softeners as prescribed.
- Encourage an immediate response to the urge to defecate.
- Encourage an increase in activity and exercise.

PATIENT TEACHING

Teach an older patient methods to reduce constipation, including:

- a high-fiber diet
- increased fluid intake
- more physical activity
- making adjustments for physical limitations that may interfere with the ability to get to the bathroom before the urge to defecate leaves. (See *Avoiding constipation.*)

Special considerations

Have a physician determine any underlying cause for constipation before you suggest that an older patient alter his dietary pattern. Once intestinal obstructions or neoplasms have been ruled out, the appropriate interventions can help your patient reduce episodes of constipation.

CORONARY ARTERY BYPASS GRAFTING

Coronary artery bypass grafting (CABG) circumvents one or more occluded coronary arteries with an autogenous graft (usually a segment of the saphenous vein from the leg or internal mammarian artery), thereby restoring blood flow to the myocardium. Performed to prevent a myocardial infarction (MI) in a patient with acute or chronic myocardial ischemia, CABG is one of the most commonly performed surgeries in the United States.

The need for CABG is determined by evaluating the results of cardiac catheterization and the patient's signs and symptoms. Prime candidates for CABG include people with any of the following conditions:

- medically uncontrolled angina interfering with the patient's lifestyle
- left main coronary artery stenosis
- severe proximal left anterior descending coronary artery stenosis
- three-vessel disease with proximal stenoses or left ventricular dysfunction
- three-vessel disease with normal left ventricular function at rest but with inducible ischemia and poor exercise capacity.

Successful CABG can relieve anginal pain, improve cardiac function, and possibly enhance the patient's quality of life. CABG techniques vary according to the patient's condition and the number of arteries being bypassed. (See *Mini-CABG.*)

Mini CABG

Two new surgical procedures can decrease the risk of cerebral complications and accelerate recovery for selected patients: mini-CABG (minimally invasive coronary artery bypass grafting), which uses a thoracotomy incision rather than a sternotomy, and direct coronary artery bypass, in which grafts are sewn directly to the stabilized, yet beating, heart. Both techniques are used for grafts of only one or two coronary arteries. Long-term information on these procedures is not yet available; however, nursing care guidelines are the same as for CABG.

Implementation

After the patient has received general anesthesia, surgery begins with graft harvesting; the surgeon makes a series of incisions in the patient's thigh or calf and removes a saphenous vein segment for grafting. Some surgeons prefer using a segment of the internal mammarian artery because this provides an artery to do the job of an artery.

Once the graft is obtained, the surgeon performs a medial sternotomy and exposes the heart. He then initiates cardiopulmonary bypass. (See *Understanding cardiopulmonary bypass*, page 208.) To reduce myocardial oxygen demands during surgery and to protect the heart, the surgeon induces cardiac hypothermia and standstill by injecting a cold cardioplegic solution (potassium-enriched saline solution) into the aortic root.

After the patient is fully prepared, the surgeon sutures one end of the venous graft to the ascending aorta and the other end to a patent coronary artery distal to the occlusion. He sutures the graft in a reverse position to promote proper blood flow. He then repeats this procedure for each artery he bypasses.

Once the grafts are in place, the surgeon flushes the cardioplegic solution from the heart and discontinues cardiopulmonary bypass. He then implants epicardial pacing electrodes, inserts a chest tube, closes the incision, and applies a sterile dressing.

Understanding cardiopulmonary bypass

Open-heart surgery commonly involves a technique known as cardiopulmonary bypass to divert blood from the heart and lungs to an extracorporeal circuit with a minimum of hemolysis and trauma. As shown in this simplified diagram, the cardiopulmonary bypass (or "heart-lung") machine uses a mechanical pump to provide ventricular pumping action, an oxygenator to perform gas exchange, and a heat exchanger to cool the blood and lower the metabolic rate during surgery.

To perform this procedure, the surgeon inserts catheters into the right atrium or the inferior or superior vena cava for blood removal and into the ascending aorta for blood return. After heparinizing the patient and priming the pump with fluid to replace diverted venous blood, he turns on the machine. The pump draws blood from the vena cava catheters into the machine, where it passes through a filter, oxygenator, heat exchanger, and another filter and bubble trap before being returned to arterial circulation. During cardiopulmonary bypass, an anesthesiologist or perfusionist maintains mean arterial pressure by adjusting the rate of perfusion or by infusing fluids or vasopressor drugs.

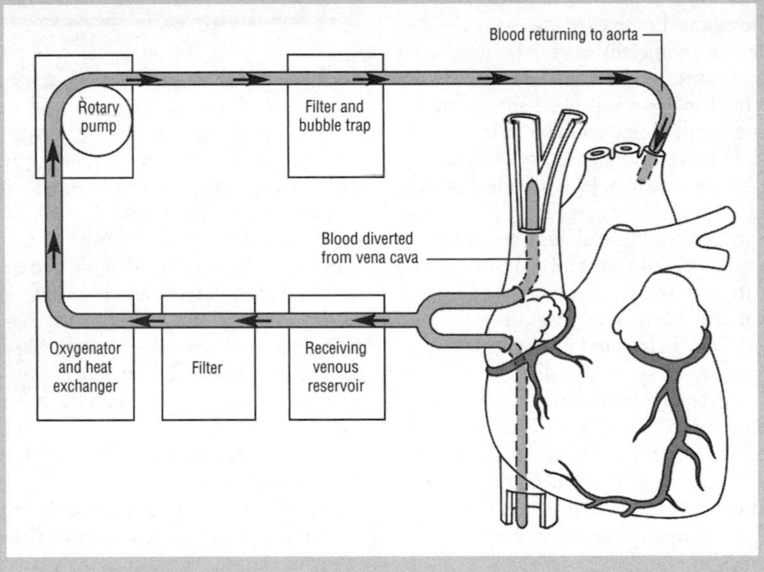

A newer surgical technique available as an alternative to traditional CABG surgery is minimally invasive coronary artery bypass surgery, also known as "keyhole" surgery. This procedure requires a shorter recovery period and has fewer postoperative complications. Instead of sawing open the patient's sternum and spreading the ribs apart, the surgeon makes several small cuts in the torso, through which small surgical instruments and fiber-optic cameras are inserted. All procedures are done without the use of cardiopulmonary bypass. This procedure was originally designed to correct blockages in just one or two easily reached arteries; it may not be suitable for more complicated cases.

Newer equipment, such as stabilization devices, can also drastically cut surgical time by allowing surgery to be performed on a beating heart, thus eliminating the need for heart-lung equipment.

Complications

CABG can cause many postoperative complications, including arrhythmias, hypertension or hypotension, cardiac tamponade, thromboembolism, hemorrhage, postpericardiotomy syndrome, and MI. Noncardiac complications include cerebrovascular accident (CVA), postoperative depression or emotional instability, pulmonary embolism, decreased renal function, and infection. Certain complications, such as graft rupture or closure or the development of atherosclerosis in other coronary arteries, may prompt repeat surgery.

With the minimally invasive CABG, such complications as MI, CVA, hemorrhage, infection, renal failure, and respiratory distress occur less often.

Key nursing diagnoses and outcomes

Decreased cardiac output related to hypothermia, recovery from general anesthesia, and complications such as arrhythmias, fluid and electrolyte imbalances, and pericardial tamponade

Treatment outcomes: The patient will maintain adequate cardiac output, as evidenced by normal blood pressure and pulse rate, and adequate tissue perfusion, as evidenced by urine output of at least 30 ml/hour and orientation to time, person, and place.

Risk for injury related to fluid and electrolyte imbalances secondary to the use of cardiopulmonary bypass

Treatment outcomes: The patient will suffer no injuries because of a fluid or electrolyte imbalance and will maintain serum electrolyte levels within normal limits.

Hypothermia related to cooling procedures used during CABG

Treatment outcomes: The patient will regain and maintain a normal temperature and will not shiver (which increases heart rate, blood pressure, and myocardial oxygen requirement) during the postoperative rewarming process.

Nursing interventions

When caring for a CABG patient, your major roles include caring for the patient's changing cardiovascular needs and patient teaching.

Before surgery

- Begin by reinforcing the physician's explanation of the surgery. Next, explain the complex equipment and procedures used in the intensive care unit or postanesthesia room. If possible, arrange for a tour of the unit for the patient and his family. Tell him that he'll awaken from surgery with an endotracheal tube in place and connected to a mechanical ventilator. He'll also be connected to a cardiac monitor and have in place a nasogastric tube, a chest tube, an indwelling urinary catheter, arterial lines, epicardial pacing wires and, possibly, a pulmonary artery catheter. Tell him that he'll feel some discomfort and that the equipment will be removed as soon as possible.
- Ensure that the patient or a responsible family member has signed a consent form.
- The evening before surgery, have the patient shower with antiseptic soap. Restrict food and fluids after midnight, and provide a sedative if ordered. On the morning of surgery, provide another sedative, as ordered, to help him relax.
- Immediately before surgery, assist with pulmonary artery catheterization and insertion of arterial lines. Then begin cardiac monitoring.

After surgery

- Look for signs of hemodynamic compromise, such as severe hypotension, decreased cardiac output, and shock. Check and record vital signs every 5 to 15 minutes until the patient's condition stabilizes. Monitor the electrocardiogram for disturbances in heart rate and rhythm. If you detect serious abnormalities, notify the physician and prepare to assist with epicardial pacing or, if necessary, cardioversion or defibrillation.

▶ To ensure adequate myocardial perfusion, keep arterial pressure within the limits set by the physician. Usually, mean arterial pressure below 70 mm Hg results in inadequate tissue perfusion; pressure above 110 mm Hg can cause hemorrhage and graft rupture. Monitor pulmonary artery, central venous, and left atrial pressures, as ordered.

▶ Frequently evaluate the patient's peripheral pulses, capillary refill time, and skin temperature and color, and auscultate for heart sounds; report any abnormalities. Also evaluate tissue oxygenation by assessing breath sounds, chest excursion, and symmetry of chest expansion. Check arterial blood gas (ABG) results every 2 to 4 hours, and adjust ventilator settings to keep ABG values within ordered limits. Monitor the patient's intake and output, and assess him for electrolyte imbalances, especially hypokalemia.

▶ Maintain chest tube drainage at the ordered negative pressure (usually −10 to −40 cm H_2O), and assess regularly for hemorrhage, excessive drainage (more than 200 ml/hour), and a sudden decrease in or cessation of drainage.

▶ As the patient's incisional pain increases, give him an analgesic, as ordered, as well as other prescribed drugs.

▶ Throughout the recovery period, assess for symptoms of CVA, pulmonary embolism, and impaired renal perfusion.

▶ After you wean the patient from the ventilator and remove the endotracheal tube, arrange for chest physiotherapy. Start him on incentive spirometry, and encourage him to cough, turn frequently, and deep breathe. Assist him with range-of-motion exercises, as ordered, to enhance peripheral circulation and prevent thrombus formation.

▶ Monitor the older patient closely for complications.

PATIENT TEACHING

▶ Instruct the patient to watch for and notify the physician of any signs of infection (fever, confusion, sore throat, or redness, swelling, or drainage at the leg or chest incision) or possible arterial reocclusion (angina, dizziness, dyspnea, rapid or irregular pulse, or prolonged recovery time from exercise).

▶ Explain that postpericardiotomy syndrome commonly develops after open-heart surgery. Tell the patient to call his physician if he experiences such symptoms as fever, muscle and joint pain, weakness, or chest discomfort.

▶ Prepare the patient for the possibility of postoperative depression, which may not develop until weeks after discharge. Reassure him that this symptom is normal and should pass quickly.

▶ Encourage the patient to express his feelings. Some patients may focus on physical needs and ignore emotional needs; they may be reluctant to discuss psychological problems, such as depression, with outsiders.

▶ Make sure the patient understands the dose, frequency of administration, and possible adverse effects of all prescribed medications.

▶ Encourage him to follow his prescribed diet, especially noting any sodium and cholesterol restrictions. Explain that this diet can help reduce the risk of recurrent arterial occlusion.

▶ Instruct the patient to maintain a balance between activity and rest. Tell him to try to sleep at least 8 hours a night, to schedule a short rest period each afternoon, and to rest frequently when engaging in tiring physical activity. As appropriate, tell him he can climb stairs, engage in sexual activity, take baths and showers, and do light chores. Tell him to avoid lifting heavy objects (more than 20 lb [9 kg]), driving a car, or doing strenuous work (such as lawn mowing or vacuuming) until his physician grants permission. If the physician has prescribed an exercise program, encourage the patient to follow it.

- Refer the patient to a local chapter of the Mended Hearts Club and the American Heart Association for information and support.

CORONARY ARTERY DISEASE

In coronary artery disease (CAD), fatty fibrous plaques or calcium-plaque deposits (or a combination of both) narrow the lumina of coronary arteries, reducing the volume of blood that can flow through them. The diminished coronary blood flow leads to a loss of oxygen and nutrients to myocardial tissue. CAD is nearly epidemic in the Western world. It's most prevalent in middle-aged and older white males; however, nonwhite women are more susceptible than white women.

Atherosclerosis, the most common cause of CAD, has been linked to many risk factors. Some risk factors, such as advanced age, sex, and heredity, can't be controlled. However, the patient can modify other risk factors, such as high blood pressure, high cholesterol level, cigarette smoking, obesity, sedentary lifestyle, and stress, with good medical care and appropriate lifestyle changes.

Signs and symptoms

- Angina (burning, squeezing, or crushing tightness in substernal or precordial area of chest that may radiate to left arm, neck, jaw, or shoulder blade)
- Nausea
- Vomiting
- Fainting
- Sweating
- Cool extremities
- Xanthelasma (yellowish, slightly raised tumor usually found on eyelids)
- Increased light reflexes and arteriovenous nicking on ophthalmoscopic inspection, suggesting hypertension
- Thickened or absent peripheral arteries
- Signs of cardiac enlargement and abnormal contraction of the cardiac impulse, such as left ventricular akinesia or dyskinesia
- Bruits, S_3, S_4 (not a reliable indicator of CAD in older adults because it's a normal change of aging), or a late systolic murmur (if mitral insufficiency is present) on auscultation

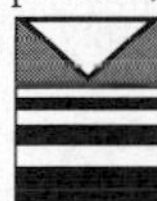

Key point **CAD may be asymptomatic in the older adult because of a decrease in sympathetic response. Dyspnea and fatigue are two key signals of ischemia in an active older adult.**

Diagnostic tests

- *Electrocardiography* (ECG) is the chief diagnostic test. During an angina attack, the ECG shows ischemia, as demonstrated by T-wave inversion or ST-segment depression and, possibly, arrhythmias, such as premature ventricular contractions. ECG results may be normal during pain-free periods. Arrhythmias may occur without infarction, secondary to ischemia.
- *Exercise stress tests* may provoke chest pain and show signs of myocardial ischemia in response to physical exertion. Monitoring of electrical rhythm may demonstrate T-wave inversion or ST-segment depression in the ischemic areas.
- *Coronary angiography* reveals coronary artery stenosis or obstruction, collateral circulation, and the arteries' condition beyond the narrowing.
- *Myocardial perfusion imaging* with thallium-201 during treadmill exercise detects ischemic areas of the myocardium, visualized as "cold spots."
- *Pharmacological myocardial perfusion imaging* can be done in combination with stress testing. A patent coronary

artery vasodilator, usually dipyridamole, is administered and the patient's response is tested. In normal arteries, coronary blood flow is increased to 3 to 4 times baseline. In arteries with stenosis, the decrease in blood flow is proportional to the percentage of occlusion.

▶ *Multiple gated acquisition scanning* demonstrates cardiac wall motion and reflects injury to cardiac tissue.

Treatment

The goal of treatment in patients with angina is to reduce myocardial oxygen demand or increase the oxygen supply and reduce pain. Activity restrictions may be required to prevent the onset of pain. Rather than eliminating activities, performing them more slowly often averts pain. Stress reduction techniques are essential, especially if known stressors precipitate pain.

Nitrates, such as nitroglycerin or isosorbide dinitrate, or beta-adrenergic blockers may be administered to reduce myocardial oxygen consumption. Long-acting nitrates aren't usually prescribed for older adults.

Obstructive lesions may require atherectomy or coronary artery bypass graft (CABG) surgery, using vein grafts. Percutaneous transluminal coronary angioplasty (PTCA) may be performed during cardiac catheterization to compress fatty deposits and relieve occlusion. In patients with calcification, PTCA may reduce the obstruction by fracturing the plaque.

PTCA may be done in combination with coronary stenting, or stents may be placed alone. Stents provide a framework to hold an artery open by securing flaps of tunica media against an artery wall. Intravascular coronary stenting is done to reduce the incidence of restenosis. Prosthetic intravascular cylindrical stents are positioned at the site of the occlusion. To be eligible for this procedure, the patient must be able to tolerate anticoagulant therapy and the blood vessel to be stented must be at least 3 mm in diameter.

Laser angioplasty corrects occlusion by vaporizing fatty deposits with an excimer or hot-tip laser device. Rotational ablation (or rotational atherectomy) removes atheromatous plaque with a high-speed, rotating burr covered with diamond crystals.

Key nursing diagnoses and outcomes

Ineffective (cardiopulmonary) tissue perfusion related to reduced blood flow to the myocardium caused by coronary artery spasm or occlusion

Treatment outcome: The patient will maintain adequate myocardial tissue perfusion, as exhibited by a normal heart rate and rhythm and the absence of ischemic ECG changes.

Acute pain related to inadequate oxygen flow to the myocardium as a result of reduced myocardial blood flow

Treatment outcome: The patient will experience a reduction in the severity and frequency of anginal pain by complying with medical or surgical therapy.

Activity intolerance related to an imbalance between myocardial oxygen supply and demand

Treatment outcome: The patient will identify activities he needs to avoid and activities for which he must obtain assistance.

Nursing interventions

▶ During anginal episodes, monitor the patient's blood pressure and heart rate. Take a 12-lead ECG before administering nitroglycerin or other nitrates.

▶ Record the duration, location, and intensity of pain; the amount of medication required to relieve it; and accompanying symptoms. Ask the patient to grade the severity of his pain on a scale of 1 to 10. This allows him to assess his own pain as well as the effectiveness of pain-relieving medications. Keep nitroglycerin available for immediate use. Instruct the patient to call immediately whenever he feels chest, arm, or neck pain and before taking nitroglycerin.

▶ During cardiac catheterization, monitor the patient for adverse reactions to the dye. If he has such symptoms as falling blood pressure, bradycardia, diaphoresis, and light-headedness, increase parenteral fluids as ordered, administer nasal oxygen, place the patient in Trendelenburg's position, and administer I.V. atropine if necessary.

▶ After catheterization, review the expected course of treatment with the patient and his family. Monitor the catheter site for bleeding. Also check for distal pulses. To counter the diuretic effect of the dye, increase I.V. fluids and make sure the patient drinks plenty of fluids. Assess potassium levels, and add potassium to the I.V. fluid, if necessary.

▶ After PTCA, maintain heparin therapy, observe for bleeding systemically and at the site, and keep the affected leg immobile. After rotational ablation, monitor the patient for chest pain, hypotension, coronary artery spasm, and bleeding from the catheter site. Provide heparin and antibiotic therapy for 24 to 48 hours, as ordered.

▶ After CABG, provide care for the I.V. site, pulmonary artery catheter, and endotracheal tube. Monitor blood pressure, intake and output, breath sounds, chest tube drainage, and cardiac rhythm, watching for signs of ischemia and arrhythmias. I.V. administration of epinephrine, nitroprusside, dopamine, albumin, potassium, and blood products may be necessary. The patient may also need temporary epicardial pacing, especially if the surgery included replacement of the aortic valve.

▶ Insertion of an intra-aortic balloon pump may be necessary until the patient's condition stabilizes. Also observe for and treat chest pain.

▶ Perform vigorous chest physiotherapy and guide the patient in pulmonary toilet practices.

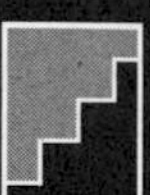

Staying well

Reducing the risk of coronary artery disease

To reduce the patient's risk of coronary artery disease, certain lifestyle factors may need to be altered. Teach the patient about:

- stress reduction techniques
- diets low in fat and cholesterol
- exercise and weight reduction programs
- smoking cessation
- caffeine intake reduction
- alcohol limitations or restrictions
- medical follow-up for such disorders as diabetes and hypertension.

PATIENT TEACHING

▶ Teach the patient what he needs to know about CAD, its treatment, and any prescribed lifestyle and diet modifications.

▶ Before cardiac catheterization, explain the procedure to the patient. Make sure he knows why it's necessary, understands the risks, and realizes that it may indicate a need for interventional therapies, such as PTCA, rotational ablation, CABG, atherectomy, and laser angioplasty.

▶ If the patient is scheduled for surgery, explain the procedure, provide a tour of the intensive care unit, introduce him to the staff, and discuss postoperative care.

▶ Help the patient determine which activities precipitate episodes of angina. Help him select coping mechanisms to deal with stress.

▶ Emphasize the need to follow the prescribed drug regimen. Teach the patient how to use nitroglycerin.

▶ Encourage the patient to maintain the prescribed low-sodium diet and to start a low-calorie, low-cholesterol diet as well. (See *Reducing the risk of coronary artery disease.*)

▶ If the patient smokes, refer him to a program to stop smoking. Acknowledge that this will be difficult, but that he should make every attempt to stop smoking immediately and never restart.

- Encourage regular, moderate exercise. Teach the patient how to exercise safely and to personalize his exercise program. Help him find his target heart rate and heart rate range for aerobic exercise. Urge other family members or a friend to join in the physical activity to encourage the patient's commitment to the exercise program.
- Reassure the patient that he can resume sexual activity without fear of overexertion, pain, or reocclusion.
- Tell him that if angina symptoms recur after PTCA or rotational ablation, he should call the physician immediately; such pain may signal reobstruction.

CYSTECTOMY

Partial or total removal of the urinary bladder and surrounding structures, cystectomy may be necessary to treat advanced bladder cancer or, rarely, other bladder disorders such as interstitial cystitis. Cystectomy may be partial, simple, or radical. (See *Types of cystectomy*.)

Implementation

In a partial cystectomy, the surgeon makes a midline incision from the umbilicus to the symphysis pubis. He then opens the bladder and removes the tumor along with a small portion of healthy tissue. To complete the procedure, he closes the wound, leaving a Penrose drain and a suprapubic catheter in place.

In a simple cystectomy, the surgeon first makes a midline abdominal incision, then removes the entire bladder, leaving only a portion of the urethra.

In a radical cystectomy, the surgeon removes the bladder, the seminal vesicles and prostate in male patients, and the uterus, ovaries, fallopian tubes, and anterior vagina in female patients. Depending on the extent of the cancer, the surgeon may also remove the urethra and surrounding lymph nodes.

To complete either a simple or radical cystectomy, the surgeon provides for urinary diversion by attaching the ureters to an external collection device, such as a cutaneous ureterostomy, an ileal conduit, or a continent urinary neobladder.

Complications

Immediately after surgery, potential complications include bleeding, hypotension, and nerve injury (such as to the genitofemoral or peroneal nerve). Later complications include anuria, stoma stenosis, urinary tract infection, pouch leakage, electrolyte imbalance, stenosis of the ureteroileal junction, and vascular compromise. Radical and simple cystectomy may also cause psychological problems relating to changes in the patient's body image and loss of sexual or reproductive function.

Key nursing diagnoses and outcomes

Impaired urinary elimination related to removal of bladder

Treatment outcome: The patient will demonstrate an ability to manage the altered route of urinary elimination.

Risk for infection related to manipulation of bowel and instrumentation in the abdominal cavity

Treatment outcome: The patient will exhibit no signs or symptoms of infection.

Acute pain related to extensive abdominal surgery needed to perform a cystectomy

Treatment outcome: The patient will be free from pain after healing is complete.

Nursing interventions

When caring for a cystectomy patient, you'll typically focus on instructing the patient and monitoring for complications.

Before surgery

- Review the surgery with the patient and his family, if appropriate. If possible, have an enterostomal therapist meet with the patient. Pay special attention to the patient's emotional state, since he'll probably be anxious. Help allay his fears by listening to his concerns and answering his questions. If the patient is undergoing a simple or radical cystectomy, he'll also worry about the effects of a urinary diversion on his lifestyle. Reassure him that such diversion need not interfere with his normal activities, and arrange for a visit by an enterostomal therapist, who can provide additional information.
- If the patient is scheduled for a radical cystectomy, address his concerns about the inevitable loss of sexual and reproductive function.
- Explain to the patient that he'll awaken in the intensive care unit (ICU) after a radical cystectomy. He'll return to his own hospital room following a partial cystectomy unless complications occur in the perioperative period. Mention that he'll have a nasogastric (NG) tube, a central venous catheter, and an indwelling urinary catheter in place and a drain at the surgical site. Tell him that he'll be unable to eat or drink until bowel function returns and that he'll be given I.V. fluids during this period. After that, he can resume oral fluids and eventually progress to solids. If possible, arrange for the patient and family to visit the ICU before surgery to familiarize themselves with the unit and meet the staff.
- Perform a standard bowel preparation as ordered. Antibiotics administered orally (such as neomycin) or parenterally (such as cefazolin) are used prophylactically to reduce colonic microbial flora. To further clean the bowel, a high colonic enema or oral polyethylene glycol (PEG) electrolyte solution, a nonabsorbable osmotic agent, is given. Large amounts of PEG electrolyte solution (4 L) are administered over 3 to 4 hours; diarrhea begins within 1 hour.

Types of cystectomy

In cystectomy, the surgery may be partial, simple, or radical.

Partial cystectomy involves resection of a portion of the bladder wall. Usually preserving bladder function, this surgery is commonly indicated for a single, easily accessible bladder tumor.

Simple cystectomy, which involves resection of the entire bladder, is indicated for benign conditions limited to the bladder. It may also be performed as a palliative measure—for example, to stop bleeding—when cancer isn't curable.

Radical cystectomy is generally indicated for muscle-invasive primary bladder carcinoma. This procedure entails removing the bladder and several surrounding structures. Because this surgery is so extensive, it typically produces impotence in men.

Whenever the entire bladder is removed, the patient will require a permanent urinary diversion, such as an ileal conduit or a continent urinary neobladder.

After surgery

- Monitor the amount and character of urine drainage every hour. Each ureter may have a stent and drain into a separate urine drainage bag. Output from each ureter is recorded separately.Report output of less than 30 ml/hour, which may indicate retention. (Other signs of retention include bladder distention and spasms in a partial cystectomy.) If output is low, check the patency of the indwelling urinary catheter or stoma, as appropriate, and irrigate as ordered.
- Monitor vital signs closely. Watch especially for signs of hypovolemic shock: increased pulse and respiratory rates, hypotension, diaphoresis, and pallor. (Be especially alert for hemorrhage if the

physician has ordered anticoagulant therapy to reduce the risk of pulmonary embolism.)

▶ Periodically inspect the stoma (if present) and incision site for bleeding, and observe urine drainage for frank hematuria and clots. Slight hematuria normally occurs for several days after surgery but should clear thereafter. Test all drainage from the NG tube, abdominal drains, indwelling urinary catheter, and urine collection appliance for blood, and notify the physician of positive findings.

▶ Observe the wound site and all drainage for signs of infection. Change abdominal dressings frequently, using sterile technique.

▶ Periodically ask the patient about incisional pain and, if he's had a partial cystectomy, about bladder spasms as well. Provide analgesics as ordered.

▶ To prevent pulmonary complications associated with prolonged immobility, encourage frequent position changes, coughing, deep breathing and, if possible, early ambulation. Assess respiratory status regularly.

▶ Provide care for the type of urinary diversion present.

▶ Continue to offer the patient emotional support throughout the recovery period to help him accept changes in body image and, if appropriate, sexual function. If possible, refer the patient and his family for psychological and sexual counseling to further aid in this adjustment.

PATIENT TEACHING

▶ Explain to the patient that incisional pain and fatigue will probably last for several weeks after discharge. Tell him to notify the physician if these effects persist or worsen.

▶ Instruct the patient and family members to watch for and report any signs of urinary tract infection (confusion, chills, flank pain, decreased urine volume, and possibly fever) or wound infection (redness, swelling, and purulent drainage at the incision site). Also tell them to report persistent hematuria.

▶ Make sure the patient or a family member understands how to care for his type of urinary diversion and where to obtain needed supplies. If needed, arrange for visits by a home care nurse, who can reinforce urinary diversion care measures and provide emotional support. If the patient has a stoma, refer him to a support group, such as a local chapter of the United Ostomy Association.

▶ Stress the importance of follow-up examinations to evaluate healing and recurrence of cancer.

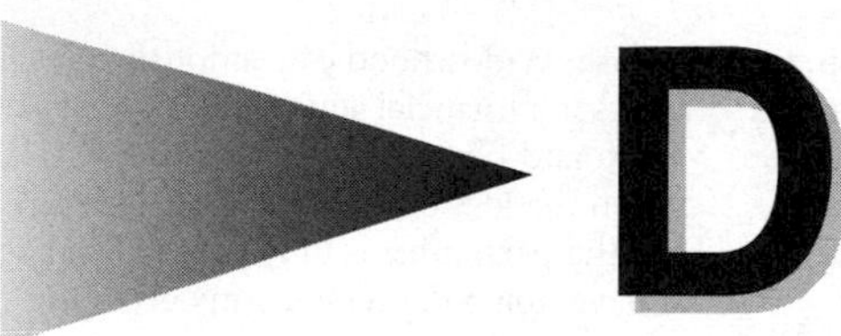

Dance therapy

Also known as *dance movement therapy,* dance therapy capitalizes on the direct relationship between body movement and the mind. Specific aspects of dance therapy, such as music, rhythm, and synchronous movement, alter mood states, reawaken old memories and feelings, and reduce isolation. In addition, dance therapy organizes thoughts and actions and assists in establishing relationships. Used in a group setting, dance therapy is believed to create the emotional intensity necessary for behavioral change.

Dance therapy is used in a wide variety of settings. It's used to help emotionally disturbed patients express their feelings, gain insight, and develop relationships. With physically disabled people, dance therapy increases movement and self-esteem while providing an enjoyable, creative outlet. In other groups of older people, dance therapy is used to maintain physical function, enhance self-worth, develop relationships, and help them express fear and grief.

A wide variety of disorders and disabilities can be treated using dance therapy. Typically, the target patient has social, emotional, cognitive, or physical problems. Dance therapy is even being used as a method of disease prevention and health promotion among healthy patients. In addition, it's used for stress reduction by caregivers and patients with cancer, acquired immunodeficiency syndrome, and Alzheimer's disease.

Dance therapy promotes flexibility, strengthens muscles, improves cardiovascular function, and improves pulmonary function. In addition, it provides touch, socialization, and a sense of connectedness.

Group dance, probably the most common form of dance therapy, allows people of all different physical abilities to participate. By simply tapping their toes or patting their thighs in time to the music, patients can feel a part of the session. Dance routines range from simple clapping and swaying to intricate aerobic sessions.

The music should be appropriate to the group, both in its pace and aesthetic appeal. Fast-moving rock and roll music probably is less enjoyable for a group of agile senior citizens than a fast polka would be. Use faster music to stimulate the group, and slower music for a calming effect.

Implementation

- Arrange the space to accommodate free movement of the participants.
- Arrange chairs around the periphery for those who can't stand or become tired during the session.
- Assess the group for risk factors. The presence of one or more risk factors does not preclude group members from participating but may influence the type of dance and the length of the session. Risk factors to consider include poor cardiovascular status, a history of chronic obstructive pulmonary disease, or degenerative musculoskeletal problems.

- Explain the purpose of the session, and encourage everyone to participate to the degree they feel able.
- When the group is ready, start the music and position yourself so you're facing the group.
- If a structured routine is being used, demonstrate the movements you're seeking and encourage the group to mimic your movements.
- If free expression is sought, circulate through the group, providing encouragement and motivation to those who are hesitant.
- Praise the participants' efforts, and encourage them to discuss the feelings they experienced while dancing.
- After the session, document the type of activity and the group's response.

Special considerations

Because dancing is an aerobic activity, watch for signs of cardiovascular compromise, such as dizziness, flushing, profuse sweating, and disorientation.

Rapid motion may result in dizziness. Help a person who becomes dizzy to a seat as needed, and check his vital signs.

DEATH AND DYING

Aging is associated with major physical, psychological, and sociological losses as well as reduced ability to adapt and compensate for stressors. Older adults may lose a sense of control because of such factors as physical decline, status and role changes, negative cultural attitudes, negative mass media portrayals, and crime victimization. Loss of loved ones can increase the older adult's sense of vulnerability, stir up fears and anxiety about facing his own death, and deplete coping resources.

Death of a spouse

One of the most profound losses a person can experience is the death of a spouse. Widowhood can seriously affect a person's financial status, social network, and physical and mental health. When the loss of a spouse occurs late in life, the person has a much greater risk of developing depression, anxiety, and substance abuse than a younger person because of decreased resilience, a higher incidence of chronic illness, and the breakdown of social support networks. Older men have an even greater risk of developing physical and mental disorders than older women.

In addition to the loss of marital companionship, unsettled issues may remain for years after the death of a spouse. A long marriage doesn't necessarily mean a happy one. Unresolved guilt feelings related to infidelity, physical or substance abuse, and financial problems after widowhood are a few examples of issues that can fester and lead to serious mental illness — sometimes decades after the death of a spouse. Family and spousal caregivers, especially, may have unresolved issues.

Death of an adult child

Adult children are an important part of the older adult's social support network. The death of an adult child can be even more devastating to an elderly person than the death of a spouse because parents expect their children to outlive them and be a support in old age.

Special considerations

Make your patient aware of counseling services, support groups, and other resources that are available to help him cope with the loss of a spouse.

Refer a patient who must cope with the loss of an adult child to an appropriate community resource, such as Interfaith, a clergyman, or a grief therapist.

Encourage the patient to verbalize his fears and concerns about his own death. Preparing for death can be a positive experience and a major developmental task of adulthood.

DELIRIUM

Also called *acute confusional state, acute encephalopathy,* and *altered mental status,* delirium isn't a disease but a symptom of an underlying problem. It can develop from infection, blood glucose imbalance, pain, or head injury; after a surgical procedure, anesthesia, or a sudden change in physical surroundings; or from a drug interaction or drug withdrawal.

If your patient develops a sudden change in mental status, assess him for cardiovascular problems, such as fluid shift or arrhythmias; infections, including urinary tract and pulmonary infections; unrelieved pain; electrolyte imbalance; and drug toxicity. Delirium may be the first symptom of these disorders in the older adult.

Signs and symptoms

Symptoms that may duplicate those of depression and psychosis, such as decreased attention span, diminished alertness, and altered sleep patterns (delirium, though, has a sudden onset, whereas depression and psychosis are marked by a slower onset).

Treatment

The goal of treatment is to identify and treat the underlying cause. The process begins with a thorough physical assessment, including vital signs and an assessment for pain and sensory deprivation. It includes ruling out drug toxicity as the cause by obtaining blood tests of any patient who takes drugs with an overdose potential, such as alcohol, salicylates, theophylline, digoxin, thyroid hormone, and benzodiazepines.

Key nursing diagnoses and outcomes

Disturbed thought processes related to neurologic dysfunction

Treatment outcome: The patient will regain and maintain orientation to time, place, and person.

Risk for injury related to altered mental status

Treatment outcome: The patient will remain free from injury.

Nursing interventions

- Have someone stay with the patient while you notify the physician of his change in mental status.
- Obtain the most recent laboratory test results and specimens for any newly ordered tests. Review the patient's current medications with the pharmacist for possible delirium-inducing interactions.
- Reassure the patient by speaking in a calm voice, moving slowly and deliberately, and explaining your actions.
- Be consistent. Have the same caregiver tend to the patient whenever possible.
- Reorient the patient. Decrease noise, light, and other environmental stimuli.
- Use restraints only if other safety measures have failed.
- Medicate only if other measures to reduce the patient's agitation have failed.

PATIENT TEACHING

- Tell family members or friends that measures are being taken to determine the source of the delirium and to correct the cause.
- Educate the patient and his family about the cause of his delirium to prevent future episodes.

DEMENTIA

Dementia, or cognitive loss, can take many forms. Alzheimer's disease is one form, although it's not considered a psychiatric disorder according to the

Alzheimer's Association. Many types of dementia are reversible, such as the dementia that occurs with pernicious anemia and responds to vitamin B_{12} therapy. Other types are not reversible. These include vascular dementia that results from underlying cerebrovascular disease, or dementia that results from other underlying medical conditions, such as human immunodeficiency virus infection, Creutzfeldt-Jakob disease, Pick's disease, Huntington's disease, or head trauma.

Between 60% and 75% of nursing home residents have some form of dementia, and a sizable portion of them are receiving psychotropic drugs inappropriately or excessively. As a result of the Omnibus Budget Reconciliation Act of 1987, efforts have been made to reduce the use of such chemical restraints. This act regulates the use of neuroleptics and benzodiazepines in long-term care facilities. Several research studies have indicated that about one-third of these patients could do without neuroleptics and would benefit instead from nursing, environmental, and other multidisciplinary interventions.

Signs and symptoms

- Decreased intellectual function
- Personality changes
- Impaired judgment
- Change in affect
- Impaired memory, especially short-term
- Impaired physical coordination

Treatment

Treatment aims to correct the underlying cause, while keeping the patient as independent and functional as possible.

Key nursing diagnosis and outcome

Disturbed thought processes related to organic mental disorder

Treatment outcome: The patient will maintain stability to the extent of his mental capability.

Nursing interventions

- Administer vitamin B_{12} if pernicious anemia is the underlying cause.
- Decrease environmental stimuli, such as noise, excessive artificial light, and television use.
- Speak to your patient in a soft, calm, low-pitched voice.
- Redirect him to appropriate activities when behavior problems occur. For example, if the patient wanders, walk after him, engage him in conversation to distract him, and lead him back to his room or other appropriate location.
- Avoid placing him in large rooms with large numbers of people, such as dining rooms or group activity rooms; small, private gathering places are less overwhelming.
- Thoroughly assess the patient's behavior for underlying causes. For example, agitation may be a result of constipation.

PATIENT TEACHING

- Suggest that family members consult a mental health professional for help in coping with caregiver stress, financial pressures, and other related issues. Also refer them to other community resources as appropriate.
- Teach family members or friends to encourage independent activity to the extent possible.

DEPRESSION

Although depression is the most common psychiatric illness affecting older adults, it's often underdiagnosed and untreated in this age-group. The term *depression* is used to describe a mood, a symptom, or a disease. Despite its high incidence in the elderly, depression should not be regarded as a normal response to aging. Physical, hormonal, psychological, and social factors play a major role in its development in older people.

The first episode of a major depressive disorder in people over age 50 usually has a specific medical cause requiring a thorough diagnostic evaluation. For example, Parkinson's disease is strongly associated with depression because of the imbalance in brain chemicals it causes. Urinary tract infections also are strongly associated with depression, because they may recur often, wearing the patient down with discomfort of urinary frequency, urgency, and dysuria. Several nonpsychotropic drugs may produce depression as an adverse effect, including beta-adrenergic blockers (such as propranolol and atenolol), methyldopa, and corticosteroids. Stress, too, is strongly associated with the development of depression in older people.

If you suspect your patient is depressed, evaluate his symptoms carefully.

Signs and symptoms

Major depression

- Persistent depressed mood
- Diminished interest or pleasure in daily activities
- Sleep disturbances
- Inappropriate guilt
- Loss of energy
- Poor concentration
- Changes in appetite
- Psychomotor retardation or agitation
- Passive wish for death
- Suicidal thoughts or attempts

Minor depression

- Short-term memory loss
- Irritability
- Short attention span

Suicidal thinking

- Sudden hoarding of medications
- Giving away possessions
- Sudden interest in guns
- Despondent comments

Treatment

Be aware that suicide among older adults is a serious problem. If your patient exhibits any signs of suicidal thinking, obtain an immediate assessment by a mental health professional. A thorough assessment helps to rule out possible underlying causes of depression, such as adverse reactions to medications, hypothyroidism, and other disorders. Depression also should be differentiated from dementia, although they may coexist.

Treatment initially consists of therapy with a mental health care provider, who may prescribe antidepressant medication. Drug therapy may include tricyclic antidepressants (TCAs), such as imipramine or doxepin, or a subclass of the TCAs known as *secondary amines*, including nortriptyline, protriptyline, and desipramine. The secondary amines have fewer adverse effects than the TCAs and may be preferred for older patients. Electroconvulsive therapy may be necessary if drug treatment fails.

Key nursing diagnoses and outcomes

Impaired social interaction related to altered thought processes

Treatment outcome: The patient will demonstrate effective social interaction skills in both one-on-one and group settings.

Ineffective coping related to depression

Treatment outcome: The patient will identify at least two new coping mechanisms.

Nursing interventions

- Encourage the patient to verbalize his feelings.
- Monitor the patient's potential for suicide.
- Investigate coping abilities that the patient has used successfully in the past.
- Express positive reinforcement for the patient's coping skills.
- Administer antidepressant medications, as ordered, and monitor their effectiveness.

▶ Refer the patient to a support group or counselor, if appropriate.

PATIENT TEACHING

▶ Explain the patient's state of mind to his family.

▶ Encourage the patient to try exercise, such as walking and swimming, as a natural means of treating depression. Explain that exercise helps replace certain depleted brain chemicals, such as serotonin and norepinephrine.

▶ Teach the patient about his depression. Emphasize that effective methods are available to relieve his symptoms. Help him to recognize distorted perceptions and link them to his depression. Once the patient learns to recognize depressive thought patterns, he can consciously begin to substitute self-affirming thoughts.

▶ If the patient has been prescribed an antidepressant, stress the need for compliance and review adverse reactions. For drugs that produce anticholinergic effects, such as nortriptyline, suggest sugarless gum or hard candy to relieve dry mouth. Many antidepressants (such as doxepin and imipramine) are sedating. Warn the patient to avoid activities that require alertness, including driving and operating mechanical equipment.

▶ Caution the patient taking a TCA to avoid drinking alcoholic beverages or taking other central nervous system depressants during therapy.

Special considerations

Depressed older adults at highest risk for suicide are at least age 85, have high self-esteem, and have a need to control life. Even a frail nursing home resident with these characteristics may have the strength required to kill himself.

DIABETES MELLITUS

A chronic disease of insulin deficiency or resistance, diabetes mellitus is characterized by disturbances in carbohydrate, protein, and fat metabolism. Insulin's role in the body is to transport glucose into the cells for fuel or for storage as glycogen. Insulin also stimulates protein synthesis and free fatty acid storage in the adipose tissues. A deficiency of insulin compromises the body's ability to access essential nutrients for fuel and storage. Because the incidence of diabetes increases with age, health care professionals who care for older people must have a thorough understanding of this common disease.

Diabetes may occur in two primary forms: type 1, insulin-dependent diabetes mellitus, and the more prevalent type 2, non-insulin-dependent diabetes mellitus. Among older adults, type 2 diabetes accounts for 90% of cases.

Type 2 diabetes mellitus

As the body ages, the cells become more resistant to insulin, reducing the older adult's ability to metabolize glucose. In addition, the release of insulin from the pancreatic beta cells is reduced and delayed. The result of these combined processes is hyperglycemia. In the older patient, sudden concentrations of glucose cause increased and more prolonged hyperglycemia.

Diabetes affects almost one in five people ages 65 and over. Because symptoms are vague, researchers believe many more older people probably have undiagnosed type 2 diabetes. In addition, over 40% of people this age have some form of glucose intolerance.

Type 2 diabetes in older persons is caused by abnormal insulin secretion, resistance to insulin action in target tissues, and faulty hepatic gluconeogenesis. The primary cause of hyperglycemia in older adults is increased insulin resistance in the peripheral tissues. Although the actual number of insulin receptors decreases slightly with age, resistance is believed to occur after insulin binds with the receptor. In addition, the beta cells in the islets of Langerhans are less sensitive to high glucose levels, delaying the production of insulin. Some older adults are also unable to inhibit glucose production in the liver. (See *Reducing the risk of diabetes*.)

Complications

Hypoglycemia is a potential complication for diabetics who are treated with insulin or oral antidiabetic drugs. It may be caused by excessive insulin administration, inadequate caloric intake, alcohol consumption, or excessive exercise. Older adults are more sensitive to low blood glucose levels than younger adults. Their hypoglycemic symptoms may range from mild to severe and may go unrecognized until the condition is life-threatening.

You may encounter two other metabolic complications of diabetes: Diabetic ketoacidosis, characterized by severe hyperglycemia, is a life-threatening condition. It usually occurs in people with type 1 diabetes, but may occasionally affect people with type 2 diabetes who are under extreme physical or emotional stress. Hyperosmolar hyperglycemic nonketotic syndrome (HHNS), also known as *hyperosmolar coma,* is the most common acute metabolic complication seen in older patients with diabetes. A medical emergency, HHNS is characterized by severe hyperglycemia (blood glucose level above 800 mg/dl), hyperosmolarity (above 280 mOsm/L), and severe dehydration from osmotic diuresis. Signs and symptoms include seizures and hemiparesis (which are often misdiagnosed as a cerebrovascular accident) and impaired level of consciousness (typically coma or near coma).

People with diabetes mellitus also have a greater risk of developing various chronic illnesses affecting virtually all body systems. In the older population, macrovascular and microvascular complications are accelerated because of preexisting cardiovascular effects of aging. The most common chronic complications include peripheral and autonomic neuropathy, peripheral vascular disease, cardiovascular disease, retinopathy, nephropathy, and diabetic dermopathy.

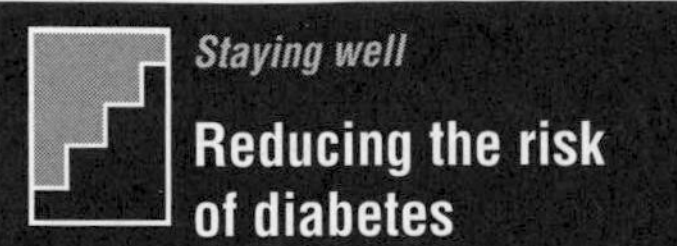

Obesity, reduced physical activity, coexisting illnesses, and poor eating habits increase the risk of type 2 diabetes in older adults. The geriatric patient can reduce his risk of developing diabetes by:

- keeping his body weight within the ideal range for his height, age, and sex
- limiting fat to 20% to 30% of his diet
- exercising regularly
- keeping other disorders that he may have (such as hypertension and heart disease) under control.

Peripheral neuropathy usually affects the hands and feet and may cause numbness or pain and possibly skin lesions. Autonomic neuropathy manifests itself in several ways, including gastroparesis (delayed gastric emptying which leads to a feeling of nausea and fullness after meals), nocturnal diarrhea, impotence, and orthostatic hypotension.

Older patients who have diabetes have 10 times the incidence of hypertension found in nondiabetic older adults. This results in a greatly increased risk of transient ischemic attacks and cerebrovascular accident, coronary artery disease and myocardial infarction, cerebral atherosclerosis, progression of retinopathy and neuropathy, cognitive impairment, and central nervous system depression.

Hyperglycemia impairs an older adult's resistance to infection because the glucose content of the epidermis and urine encourages bacterial growth. This makes the older person susceptible to skin and urinary tract infections and vaginitis.

Signs and symptoms

- Weight loss and fatigue (classic signs and symptoms in older patients)
- Loss of appetite
- Incontinence
- Decreased vision
- Confusion or even delirium
- Constipation or abdominal bloating (from gastric hypotonicity)
- Retinopathy or cataract formation
- Skin changes, especially on the legs and feet, due to impaired peripheral circulation; possibly a chronic skin condition, such as cellulitis or a nonhealing wound; poor skin turgor and dry mucous membranes due to dehydration
- Decreased peripheral pulses, cool skin, decreased reflexes, and possibly peripheral pain or numbness
- Orthostatic hypotension

Key point Older adults may not experience polydipsia, a hallmark of diabetes in younger adults, because their thirst mechanism functions less effectively.

Diagnostic tests

- *Fasting serum glucose levels* and the *glucose tolerance test* provide the definitive diagnosis for diabetes. However, in older adults, the *2-hour postprandial serum glucose test* and the *oral glucose tolerance test* are more helpful in diagnosing diabetes because older adults may have a near-normal fasting glucose level but prolonged hyperglycemia after eating.

  Diagnosis is usually made when one of the following three criteria is met:
  –Random plasma glucose concentrations are 200 mg/dl or higher.
  –Fasting blood glucose concentrations are 126 mg/dl or higher.
  –Fasting blood glucose levels after oral glucose intake are 200 mg/dl or higher.
- *Glycosylated hemoglobin (hemoglobin* A or *HbA_{1C}) test,* which reflects the average level of serum glucose within the previous 3 months, is usually performed to monitor the effectiveness of antidiabetic therapy. This test is useful, but elevated results have been found in some older adults with normal glucose tolerance.
- *Serum fructosamine,* which reflects the average serum glucose level over the preceding 2 to 3 weeks, is a better indicator in older adults because it's less prone to error.

Treatment

Patients with type 1 diabetes need insulin replacement and close monitoring of serum glucose levels as well as diet and exercise regimens. Patients with type 2 diabetes may require oral antidiabetic drugs to stimulate endogenous insulin production, increase insulin sensitivity at the cellular level, suppress hepatic gluconeogenesis, and delay GI absorption of carboyhydrates. For some patients, blood glucose levels may be controlled by diet and lifestyle changes alone.

There are several drug classes for type 2 diabetes mellitus that may be helpful. They include the second-generation sulfonylureas (such as glyburide and glipizide), alpha-glucosidase inhibitors (such as acarbose and maglitol), biguanides (such as metformin), glitazones (such as rosiglitazone) and meglitinide (repaglinide).

A dietitian can develop an individualized diet to meet the patient's needs. The diet should meet nutritional guidelines, control blood glucose levels, and maintain appropriate body weight.

Exercise is an important tool in managing type 2 diabetes. Physical activity increases insulin sensitivity, improves glucose tolerance, and promotes weight control. Research also suggests that moderate exercise can delay or prevent the onset of type 2 diabetes in high-risk groups. When you plan an exercise program for an older person, make sure the level of exertion matches his level of fitness. Preferred exercises for the older adult include walking, swimming, and cycling.

Key nursing diagnoses and outcomes

Risk for injury related to complications of diabetes mellitus

Treatment outcome: The patient will experience no injuries from diabetes.

Deficient knowledge related to diabetes mellitus and the complex treatment regimen

Treatment outcomes: The patient will express an understanding of his prescribed regimen and will demonstrate skill in managing it.

Nursing interventions

- Keep in mind that older people are likely to resist drastic lifestyle changes. You may need to adapt your interventions to the individual and compromise to achieve treatment goals.
- Initially, you'll need precise records of vital signs, weight, fluid intake, urine output, and caloric intake.
- Administer insulin or an oral antidiabetic drug as prescribed.
- When a therapeutic regimen has been established, monitor serum glucose or glycosylated hemoglobin levels every 6 to 8 weeks.
- Monitor for acute complications of diabetic therapy, especially hypoglycemia (slow cerebration, dizziness, weakness, pallor, tachycardia, diaphoresis, seizures, and coma), which requires that you give the patient carbohydrates immediately in the form of fruit juice, hard candy, honey or, if he's unconscious, glucagon or I.V. dextrose. Also be alert for signs of HHNS (urinary incontinence, abdominal discomfort, neurologic abnormalities, and stupor).
- Watch for signs of diabetic neuropathy (numbness or pain in the hands and feet, footdrop, gastroparesis, diarrhea, constipation, erectile dysfunction, and neurogenic bladder). Also watch for signs of urinary tract and vaginal infections.
- Provide meticulous skin care, especially to the feet and legs. Treat all injuries, cuts, and blisters promptly. Avoid constricting hose, slippers, or bed linens. Refer the older adult to a podiatrist for regular foot and nail care, if needed.
- Encourage the patient to verbalize his feelings about diabetes and its effects on his lifestyle and life expectancy.
- Help the patient develop new coping strategies. Refer him and his family members to a counselor, or encourage them to join a support group, if appropriate.

PATIENT TEACHING

- Teach the patient about the disease process, and stress the importance of carefully following the prescribed treatment plan. Tailor your teaching to the patient's needs and abilities. Discuss diet, medications (including administration techniques), exercise, monitoring techniques, hygiene, and how to prevent, recognize, and treat hypoglycemia and hyperglycemia.
- Encourage the patient to keep all physician and laboratory test appointments and to maintain a log of blood glucose results. Explain that he can still do the activities he enjoys, including traveling and eating out.
- To encourage compliance with necessary lifestyle changes, explain how blood glucose control affects the patient's long-term health. Tell him about assistive devices that may make compliance easier, such as magnifying attachments for the syringe and nonslip pads and holders for people with weak arms.
- Instruct the patient in foot care. Tell him to wash his feet daily, carefully dry between his toes, and inspect for corns, calluses, redness, swelling, bruises, and breaks in the skin. Urge him to report any skin changes to the physician. Advise him to wear comfortable, nonconstricting shoes and never to walk barefoot.
- Describe the signs and symptoms of diabetic neuropathy, and emphasize the

need for precautions because decreased sensation can mask injuries.

- Urge the patient to have annual eye examinations for early detection of diabetic retinopathy.
- Teach the patient how to manage his diabetes when he has a minor illness, such as a cold, the flu, or an upset stomach.
- Teach the patient and family members how to monitor his diet and use food exchange lists. Make sure the exchange lists contain ethnic-appropriate foods. Show them how to read labels in the supermarket to identify fat, carbohydrate, protein, and sugar content.
- Teach the patient and family members to use a home glucose monitor, if prescribed. Then have them give a return demonstration of the procedure. Arrange for a visiting nurse to check on the patient's technique after discharge.
- Encourage the patient and family members to contact the American Association of Diabetes Educators and the American Diabetes Association for additional information.

DIARRHEA

Defined as an increase in volume, frequency, or fluidity of stools, diarrhea is common in older adults. Causes include fecal impaction, bacterial or viral infections, overindulging in food, and the use of certain medications. Chronic diarrhea is seen in diverticular disease, thyrotoxicosis, diabetes mellitus, steatorrhea, gastric disease, hepatic disease, and sometimes ulcerative colitis.

In any older patient with diarrhea who has been on a broad-spectrum antibiotic, pseudomembranous colitis must be considered a possible cause. This disease is caused by an overgrowth of *Clostridium difficile*. This bacterium releases a toxin causing necrosis of the colon's epithelium, which results in fever, cramping, and profuse, watery diarrhea. With treatment (usually oral vancomycin or parenteral metronidazole), symptoms usually subside in 3 to 5 days.

Signs and symptoms

- Loose liquid stools
- Increased frequency of bowel movements
- Abdominal cramps or pain (unless the diarrhea is a result of diabetes mellitus)
- Signs of potassium depletion (muscle weakness, confusion, shallow irregular respirations, and cardiac arrhythmias)
- Signs of volume depletion (tachycardia, postural hypotension, poor skin turgor, and increased blood urea nitrogen [BUN] and hematocrit)

Diagnostic tests

- *Stool culture* can rule out the possibility of an infectious organism as the cause.
- *Stool specimen analysis* can rule out steatorrhea or blood in stools.

Treatment

Treatment for diarrhea focuses on providing support, relieving symptoms, preventing skin breakdown, and treating the underlying condition. Depending on the cause, medications such as antimicrobials, steroids, or enzyme preparations may be indicated.

Key nursing diagnoses and outcomes

Diarrhea related to GI disorders, infectious processes, or adverse effects of laxatives or other drugs

Treatment outcome: The patient will have fewer and less fluid bowel movements.

Risk for deficient fluid volume related to an abnormal loss of volume caused by diarrhea

Treatment outcome: The patient will have a normal fluid volume.

Risk for impaired skin integrity related to frequent bowel movements
Treatment outcome: The patient will have intact perianal skin.

Nursing interventions

▶ Assess the patient to ensure that leaking, loose, or liquid stools aren't a result of fecal impaction.
▶ Provide antidiarrheals as prescribed. Make sure that pseudomembranous colitis has been ruled out before administering antidiarrheals because these drugs put the patient at risk for developing toxic megacolon.
▶ Encourage a diet high in fiber.
▶ Monitor the frequency and characteristics of bowel movements.
▶ Monitor intake and output. Replace excessive output with I.V. or by mouth fluids as ordered.
▶ Assess the abdomen for distention and the presence of bowel sounds.
▶ Weigh the patient daily, and assess his vital signs.
▶ Evaluate serum electrolyte, BUN, creatinine, and hematocrit levels.
▶ Provide electrolyte supplements as ordered. If I.V. potassium is ordered, the infusion rate shouldn't exceed 10 mEq/hour and the patient should be attached to a continuous cardiac monitor. Monitor the patient for arrhythmias.
▶ Assist with hygiene after every diarrheal episode. Help the patient to change soiled clothing.
▶ Encourage good hand washing.
▶ Apply moisture-repellent salves or ointments as prescribed.

PATIENT TEACHING

▶ To minimize orthostatic changes due to diarrhea, encourage the patient to change positions slowly and to stand for a few seconds after changing positions and before beginning to walk.
▶ Teach the patient and his family the importance of using good hand-washing technique.
▶ Teach the patient and his family the importance of a high-fiber diet. Tell him to include foods, such as whole-grain cereals and breads, raw fruits, leafy vegetables, and legumes.

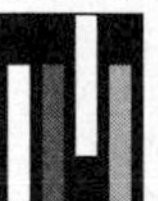

Cultural diversity **Diarrhea caused by lactose intolerance is prevalent in Asian Americans, Native Americans, Blacks, and Hispanics. Suggest that these patients substitute nondairy sources of calcium in their diet.**

DIVERTICULAR DISEASE

In this disorder, bulging pouches (diverticula) in the GI wall push the mucosal lining through the surrounding muscle. Diverticula usually occur in the sigmoid colon, but they may develop anywhere, from the proximal end of the pharynx to the anus. Other typical sites are the duodenum, near the pancreatic border or the ampulla of Vater, and the jejunum.

Diverticular disease has two clinical forms. In diverticulosis, diverticula are present but don't cause symptoms. In diverticulitis, a far more serious disorder, diverticula become inflamed and may cause obstruction, infection, and hemorrhage. Approximately 15% of patients with diverticulosis develop diverticulitis.

Most common in adults ages 45 and older, diverticular disease affects about 30% of adults over age 60. Diverticulosis is less common in nations where traditional diets contain abundant natural fiber.

A diverticulum develops when high intraluminal pressure is exerted on weaker areas — for example, points where blood vessels enter the intestine — causing a break in the muscular continuity of the GI wall. The pressure in the intestinal lumen forces the intestine out, creating a pouch (diverticulum).

Dietary elements, especially highly refined foods, may be a contributing factor. Lack of fiber reduces fecal residue, narrows the bowel lumen, and leads to higher intra-abdominal pressure during defecation.

Diverticulitis occurs when retained undigested food mixed with bacteria accumulates in the diverticulum, forming a hard mass (fecalith). This substance cuts off the blood supply to the diverticulum's thin walls, increasing its susceptibility to attack by colonic bacteria. Inflammation follows bacterial infection. The patient may report that he recently ate foods containing seeds or kernels, such as tomatoes, nuts, popcorn, or strawberries, or indigestible fiber, such as celery or corn.

Diverticulitis may lead to intestinal obstruction, resulting from edema or spasm related to inflammation or, in chronic diverticulitis, from fibrosis and adhesions that narrow and seal the bowel lumen. In severe diverticulitis, the diverticula can rupture, producing abscesses or peritonitis. Diverticular rupture occurs in up to 20% of such patients.

Other complications include rectal hemorrhage or portal pyemia (generalized septicemia with abscess formation) from arterial or venous erosion. Occasionally, the inflamed colon segment may produce a fistula by adhering to the bladder or other organs.

In older patients, a rare complication of diverticulosis (without diverticulitis) is hemorrhage from colonic diverticula, usually in the right colon. Such hemorrhage is usually mild to moderate and easily controlled. Occasionally, bleeding is life-threatening.

Signs and symptoms

Diverticulosis

- Usually no symptoms
- Occasionally, intermittent pain in the left lower abdominal quadrant relieved by defecation or the passage of flatus
- Possibly alternating bouts of constipation and diarrhea
- Possibly abdominal tenderness in the left lower quadrant on palpation

Diverticulitis

- History of diverticulosis
- Moderate pain in the left lower abdominal quadrant, described as dull or steady and aggravated by straining, lifting, or coughing
- Mild nausea, flatus, and intermittent bouts of constipation, sometimes accompanied by rectal bleeding
- Low-grade fever
- Diarrhea (rare)

Diagnostic tests

- *Barium studies* confirm the diagnosis. An *upper GI series* confirms or rules out diverticulosis of the esophagus and upper bowel; a *barium enema* confirms or rules out diverticulosis of the lower bowel.
- *Abdominal X-rays* may reveal colonic spasm if irritable bowel syndrome accompanies diverticular disease.
- *Biopsy* rules out cancer; however, a colonoscopic biopsy isn't recommended during acute diverticulitis because of the strenuous bowel preparation it requires.
- *Blood studies* may show leukocytosis and elevated erythrocyte sedimentation rate in diverticulitis, especially if the diverticula are infected.
- *Stool tests* detect occult blood in 20% of patients with diverticulitis.

Treatment

Patient management depends on the type of diverticular disease and the severity of symptoms. Asymptomatic diverticulosis generally requires no treatment. Intestinal diverticulosis that causes pain, mild GI distress, constipation, or difficult defecation may respond to a liquid or bland diet, stool softeners, and occasional doses of mineral oil. These measures relieve symptoms, minimize irritation, and decrease the risk of progression to diverticulitis. After the pain subsides, patients also benefit from a high-residue diet and a bulk medication such as psyllium.

Treatment of mild diverticulitis without signs of perforation aims to prevent constipation and combat infection. Therapy may include bed rest, a liquid diet, stool softeners, a broad-spectrum antibiotic, morphine to control pain and relax smooth muscle, and an antispasmodic such as propantheline to control muscle spasms.

For more severe diverticulitis, treatment consists of the above measures and I.V. therapy. A nasogastric (NG) tube to relieve intra-abdominal pressure is usually required.

Patients who hemorrhage need blood replacement and careful monitoring of fluid and electrolyte balance. Such bleeding usually stops spontaneously. If it continues, angiography for catheter replacement and infusion of vasopressin into the bleeding vessel is effective. Surgery is rarely required.

A colon resection to remove a diseased segment of intestine may be required to treat diverticulitis that fails to respond to medical treatment or that causes severe recurrent attacks in the same area. The surgeon may create a temporary colostomy to allow the inflamed bowel to rest.

Key nursing diagnoses and outcomes

Constipation related to changes in the intestinal tract

Treatment outcome: The patient will regain and maintain a normal elimination pattern.

Risk for infection related to the diverticulum's susceptibility to bacterial activity

Treatment outcomes: The patient will maintain a normal temperature and white blood cell count and will exhibit no signs or symptoms of an intestinal infection, such as abdominal distention or pain, diarrhea, or nausea and vomiting.

Acute pain related to inflammation

Treatment outcome: The patient will have no pain when diverticulitis resolves.

Nursing interventions

- Administer stool softeners, antispasmodics, and antibiotics, as ordered. For severe pain, administer analgesics such as morphine as ordered.
- Maintain the diet as ordered. The patient having an acute attack is usually on a liquid diet. If symptoms are severe or if he has nausea and vomiting or abdominal distention, insert an NG tube and attach it to intermittent suction as ordered. Make sure the patient receives nothing by mouth, and administer ordered I.V. fluids. As symptoms subside, gradually advance the diet.
- Inspect all stools carefully for color and consistency. Note the frequency of bowel movements.
- Monitor the patient for signs and symptoms of complications. Watch for temperature elevation (often minor in the older patient), increasing abdominal pain, blood in stools, and leukocytosis. Behavioral changes (such as agitation or confusion) may be the only indicators
- Maintain bed rest for the patient with acute diverticulitis. Caution the patient not to lift, strain, bend, cough, or perform any other actions that increase intra-abdominal pressure.
- If the patient is to undergo surgery, provide routine preoperative care. Also perform any special required procedures, such as administering antibiotics or providing a specific diet for several days preoperatively.

PATIENT TEACHING

- In uncomplicated diverticulosis, focus your patient teaching on bowel and dietary habits. Explain what diverticula are and how they form. Teach the patient about necessary diagnostic tests and prescribed treatments.
- Make sure the patient understands the desired actions and possible adverse effects of prescribed medications.

Key point Tell the patient to notify the physician if he has signs of complications, such as a temperature above

100° F (37.8° C), abdominal pain that's severe or lasts for more than 3 days, or blood in his stools.

▶ Review recommended dietary changes. Encourage the patient to drink 2 to 3 qt (2 to 3 L) of fluid daily. Emphasize the importance of dietary fiber and the harmful effects of constipation and straining during a bowel movement. Advise him to gradually increase his intake of foods high in undigestible fiber, such as fresh fruits and vegetables, whole grain breads, and wheat or bran cereals. Warn that a fiber-rich diet may cause temporary flatulence.

▶ Advise the patient to relieve constipation with stool softeners or bulk-forming cathartics. Instruct him to take bulk-forming cathartics with plenty of water; if swallowed dry, they may absorb enough moisture in the mouth and throat to swell and obstruct the esophagus or trachea.

▶ Provide preoperative teaching as appropriate. Reinforce the physician's explanation of the surgery, and discuss possible complications.

▶ If a colostomy is constructed during surgery, teach the patient how to care for it. Arrange for a visit with an enterostomal therapist.

DRUG ABUSE AND MISUSE

Substance abuse is a widespread but often hidden problem in the geriatric population. Its magnitude is unknown because older people typically deny it and caregivers often fail to recognize it. Yet it's likely to increase as the number of elderly adults in the United States increases.

A 1979 federal government study defined drug abuse as the "nontherapeutic use of any psychoactive substance, including alcohol, in such a manner as to adversely affect some aspect of the user's life. The use pattern may be habitual or occasional. The user may obtain the substance from legitimate prescriptions, friends, nonprescription preparations, or illegal channels."

Drug misuse, defined as the "inappropriate use of drugs for therapeutic purposes," may include inappropriately prescribing drugs for oneself, taking medications prescribed for other people, or failing or forgetting to take drugs according to the physician's instructions (noncompliance).

The incidence of drug dependence in older adults isn't as well documented as that of alcohol abuse. However, we know that only about 60% of older people take their prescribed medications properly and that approximately 30% of all medications they take are nonprescription preparations.

Very few older adults are reported to use illegal substances (such as marijuana, heroin, cocaine, or LSD). This may be because older adults simply "outgrow" the desire to take such drugs or because addicts tend to die before reaching old age. Or the problem may simply be underreported because elderly drug abusers have escaped treatment or contact with law enforcement. Studies indicate that older men tend to misuse psychoactive substances more than women, except for psychotropic drugs such as haloperidol.

Information overload, self-medication, polypharmacy, and misinterpretation of symptoms are among the many factors that can contribute to drug abuse or misuse in older adults. (See *Risk factors for substance abuse in older adults*.)

Older adults typically suffer from several chronic disorders — some of which require lifelong drug therapy. This translates to frequent physician's visits and extensive information to learn about prescribed medications. Older people take longer to process new information because of age-related sensory deficits and changes in short-term memory. They also may be poorly educated and hard to teach. Furthermore, people who live alone make more medication errors, which can lead to more drug interac-

Risk factors for substance abuse in older adults

Older people may become dependent on drugs for many reasons. Look for the following risk factors when assessing your patient for substance abuse.

Predisposing factors

- Family history (alcohol abuse)
- Previous substance abuse
- Previous pattern of substance consumption (alone or with others)
- Personality traits (anxiety, insomnia)

Factors that may increase substance exposure and consumption

- Gender (men: alcohol and illicit drugs; women: sedative-hypnotics and anxiolytics)
- Chronic illness with pain (opioid analgesics); insomnia (hypnotic drugs); anxiety (anxiolytics)
- Excessive administration of "as-needed" drugs by caregivers, for example, for sleep or pain (institutionalized older people)
- Life stressors, losses, and social isolation (alcohol used to numb self and deal with emotional pain)

Factors that may increase the effects and abuse potential of substances

- Age-associated drug sensitivity (pharmacokinetic and pharmacodynamic factors)
- Chronic medical illnesses
- Other medications (alcohol-drug or drug-drug interactions)

tions. This is especially true in the rapidly growing home care population.

Cultural diversity **Many older people have cultural attitudes and beliefs that increase their risk of noncompliance. For example, patients from Asian cultures may prefer alternative therapies, such as herbal remedies, over conventional drug therapy to treat various disorders.**

An older person may stop taking a drug when his symptoms subside even though the drug has been prescribed for long-term use. In addition, he may suspect that any symptom that occurs after he takes the medication was caused by it.

Other factors affecting drug compliance are whether the older person can afford the treatment and has access to a physician. If money and accessibility of medical care are significant obstacles, the patient may be drawn by necessity or convenience to self-medication with nonprescription preparations.

Symptoms for which an older person might seek nonprescription drugs are pain, insomnia, indigestion, and constipation.

Eventually, the older person's medicine cabinet or bedside table may contain dozens of containers filled with prescription and nonprescription drugs (some of which may have been prescribed originally for a spouse or another family member), setting the stage for a pattern of inappropriate or excessive drug use known as polypharmacy. This tendency puts the older patient, especially a cognitively impaired patient, at risk for drug interactions and adverse reactions.

Special considerations

Encourage a responsible family member to look through the patient's medicine cabinet and discard any prescription drugs that are no longer being used and any drugs that are past the expiration date.

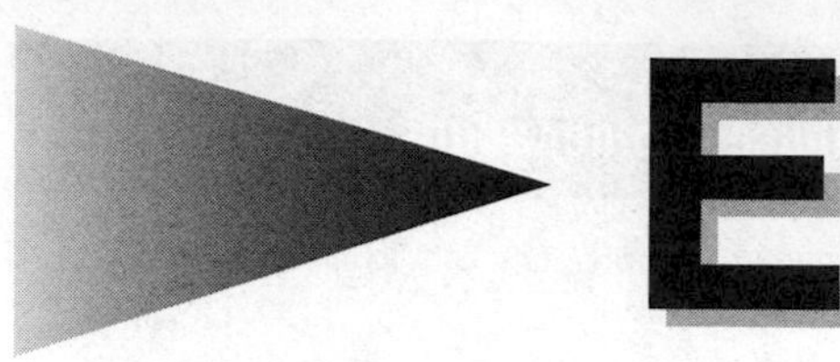

Ear medication administration

Eardrops may be given to treat infection and inflammation, to soften cerumen for later removal, to produce local anesthesia, or to help remove an insect trapped in the ear by immobilizing and smothering it. Instillation of eardrops is usually contraindicated if the patient has a perforated eardrum; however, it may be permitted with certain medications and adherence to sterile technique. Other conditions may also prohibit putting certain medications into the ear. For instance, drops containing hydrocortisone are contraindicated if the patient has herpes, another viral infection, or a fungal infection.

Supplies

- Prescribed eardrops
- Patient's medication record and chart
- Light source
- Facial tissue or cotton-tipped applicator
- Optional: cotton ball, bowl of warm water

Implementation

- Confirm the patient's identity by asking his name and checking the name, room number, and bed number on his wristband.
- Verify the order on the patient's medication record by checking it against the physician's order.
- Compare the label on the eardrops with the order on the patient's medication record and chart. Check the label again while drawing the medication into the dropper. Check the label for the final time before returning the eardrops to the shelf or drawer.
- To avoid adverse effects (such as vertigo, nausea, and pain) caused by eardrops that are too cold, warm the medication to body temperature in the bowl of warm water or carry the container in your pocket for 30 minutes before you give drops to the patient. If necessary, test the temperature of the medication by placing a drop on your wrist. (Drops that are too hot may burn the patient's eardrum.) Before using a glass dropper, make sure it isn't chipped to avoid injuring the ear canal.
- Wash your hands.
- Provide privacy, if possible. Have the patient lie on the side opposite the affected ear.
- Remember that some conditions make the normally tender ear canal even more sensitive, so be especially gentle when performing this procedure.
- Straighten the patient's ear canal by pulling the auricle of the ear up and back. (See *Positioning the patient for eardrop instillation*.)
- Using a light source, examine the ear canal for drainage. If you find any, clean the canal with the tissue or the cotton-tipped applicator because drainage can reduce the effect of the drops.
- To avoid damaging the ear canal with the dropper, gently support the hand holding the dropper against the patient's head. Straighten the patient's ear canal once again and instill the ordered num-

ber of drops. To avoid patient discomfort, aim the dropper so that the drops fall against the sides of the ear canal, not on the eardrum. Hold the ear canal in position until you see the medication disappear down the canal. Then release the ear.

- Instruct the patient to remain on his side for 5 to 10 minutes to allow the medication to run down into the ear canal.
- If ordered, tuck the cotton ball loosely into the opening of the ear canal to keep the medication from leaking out. Take care not to insert it too deeply into the canal, because this would prevent drainage of secretions and increase pressure on the eardrum.
- To prevent injury to the eardrum, never insert a cotton-tipped applicator into the ear canal past the point where you can no longer see the tip. After applying eardrops to soften cerumen, irrigate the ear as ordered.
- Clean and dry the outer ear.
- Wash your hands.
- If ordered, repeat the procedure in the other ear after 5 to 10 minutes.
- Help the patient into a comfortable position.

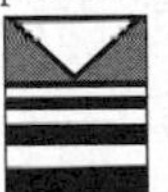

Key point If the patient has vertigo, keep the side rails of his bed up and help him move during the procedure as necessary. Also, move slowly to avoid exacerbating his vertigo.

Complications

As with the administration of any drug, adverse effects may occur. Improper instillation can lead to eardrum injury.

Patient teaching

- Explain the need for treatment and any adverse effects.
- Teach the older adult or his significant other to instill the eardrops correctly so that he can continue treatment at home, if necessary

Positioning the patient for eardrop instillation

Before instilling eardrops, have the patient lie on his side with the affected ear facing up. Then straighten the patient's ear canal to help the medication reach the eardrum. Do this by gently pulling the auricle up and back, as shown below.

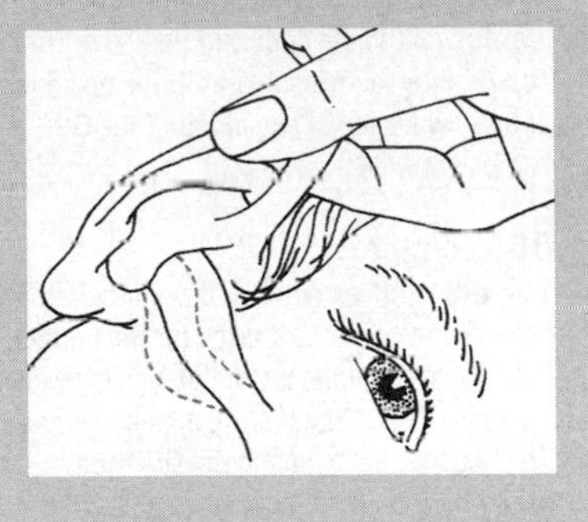

- Review the procedure, and allow the person administering the drops to try it himself while you observe.

Documentation

Record the medication, the ear treated, and the date, time, and number of eardrops instilled. Also, note any signs or symptoms that arise during the procedure, such as drainage, redness, vertigo, nausea, or pain. Document your patient teaching measures and their effect.

ELECTROCARDIOGRAPHY

One of the most valuable and commonly used diagnostic tools, electrocardiography (ECG) measures the heart's electrical activity as waveforms. Impulses moving through the heart's conduction system create electric currents that can be monitored on the body's surface. Electrodes attached to the skin can detect these electric currents and transmit

Reviewing ECG waveform components

An electrocardiogram (ECG) waveform has three basic components: P wave, QRS complex, and T wave. These elements can be further divided into a PR interval, J point, ST segment, U wave, and QT interval.

P wave and PR interval

The P wave represents atrial depolarization. The PR interval represents the time it takes an impulse to travel from the atria through the atrioventricular node and bundle of His. The PR interval measures from the beginning of the P wave to the beginning of the QRS complex.

QRS complex

The QRS complex represents ventricular depolarization (the time it takes for the impulse to travel through the bundle branches to the Purkinje fibers). The Q wave appears as the first negative deflection in the QRS complex; the R wave, as the first positive deflection. The S wave appears as the second negative deflection or the first negative deflection after the R wave.

J point and ST segment

Marking the end of the QRS complex, the J point also indicates the beginning of the ST segment. The ST segment represents part of ventricular repolarization.

T wave and U wave

Usually following the same deflection pattern as the P wave, the T wave represents ventricular repolarization. The U wave follows the T wave but isn't always seen.

QT interval

The QT interval represents ventricular depolarization and repolarization. It extends from the beginning of the QRS complex to the end of the T wave.

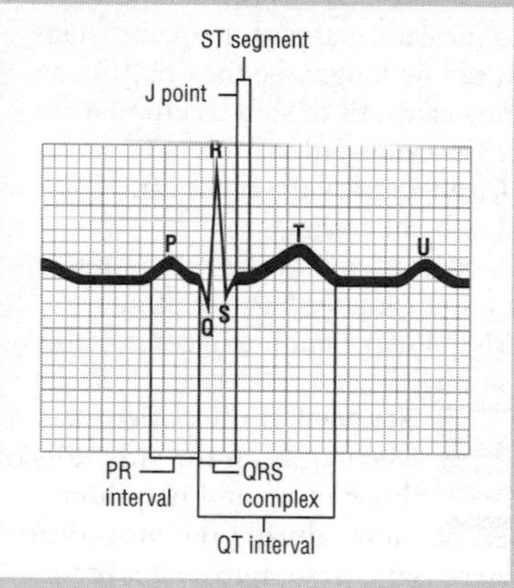

them to an instrument that produces a record (the electrocardiogram) of cardiac activity.

ECG can be used to identify myocardial infarction (MI) and ischemia, rhythm and conduction disturbances, chamber enlargement, electrolyte imbalances, cor pulmonale, and drug toxicity.

The standard 12-lead ECG uses a series of electrodes placed on the extremities and the chest wall to assess the heart from 12 different views (leads). The 12 leads consist of three standard bipolar limb leads (designated I, II, III), three unipolar augmented leads (aV_R, aV_L, aV_F), and six unipolar precordial leads (V_1 to V_6). The limb leads and augmented leads show the heart from the frontal plane. The precordial leads show the heart from the horizontal plane.

The ECG device measures and averages the differences between the electrical potential of the electrode sites for each lead and graphs them over time.

This creates the standard ECG complex, called *P-QRS-T.* The P wave represents atrial depolarization; the QRS complex, ventricular depolarization; and the T wave, ventricular repolarization. (See *Reviewing ECG waveform components.*)

Variations on the standard ECG include exercise ECG (stress ECG) and ambulatory ECG (Holter monitoring). Exercise ECG monitors heart rate, blood pressure, and ECG waveforms as the patient walks on a treadmill or pedals a stationary bicycle. For ambulatory ECG, the patient wears a portable Holter monitor to record heart activity continuously over 24 hours.

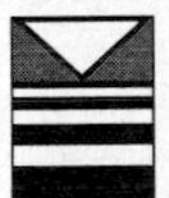

Key point In the older patient, a negative study at a lower workload level may be clinically significant if the workload is similar to the patient's daily level of activity. Other patients may have a greater frequency of resting ECG abnormalities, an increase in intraventricular conduction delays, and prior MIs that could interfere with the interpretation of exercise-induced ST segment changes. The type of testing that will yield the most useful data will depend on the patient and the benefits of the particular test.

ECG may be accomplished using a multichannel or a single-channel method. For the multichannel method, all electrodes are attached to the patient at once and the machine prints a simultaneous view of all leads. The single-channel method requires systematic attachment and removal of selected electrodes and stopping and starting the tracing each time.

Supplies

- ECG machine
- Recording paper
- Test request form
- Pregelled disposable electrodes
- Optional: shaving supplies

Implementation

- Check the patient's history for cardiac medications, and note any current therapy on the test request form.
- Place the patient in the supine position. If he can't tolerate lying flat, help him assume semi-Fowler's position.
- Provide privacy for the procedure.
- Expose the patient's chest, arms, and legs, and drape appropriately.
- Select flat, fleshy areas to place electrodes. Small areas of hair on the patient's chest or extremities may be shaved, if necessary. Clean excess oil or other substances from the skin to enhance electrode contact.
- Place the disposable electrodes on the inner aspect of the wrists, the medial aspect of the lower legs, and the chest. If your geriatric patient is a woman, place the chest electrodes below the breast tissue. In a large-breasted woman, you may need to displace the breast tissue laterally. (See *Positioning chest electrodes,* page 236.) Then connect the leadwires after all electrodes are in place.
- Set the paper speed to 25 mm/second or as ordered. Enter patient identification data. Press the start button and the machine will produce a printout showing all 12 leads simultaneously on recording paper.
- As the machine records the ECG, check to make sure that all leads are represented in the tracing. If not, determine which one has come loose, reattach it, and restart the tracing. Check for any artifact in the tracing.
- Also, make sure that the wave doesn't peak beyond the top edge of the recording grid. If it does, adjust the machine to bring the wave inside the boundaries.
- When the machine finishes the tracing, remove the electrodes and reposition the patient's gown and bed covers.

Patient teaching

- Explain the procedure to the patient and his family members to reduce the patient's fear and promote cooperation.

Positioning chest electrodes

To ensure accurate test results, position chest electrodes as follows:

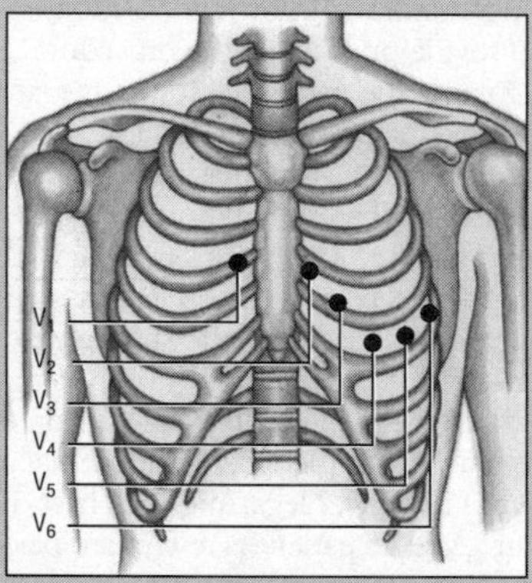

V_1: Fourth intercostal space at right border of sternum
V_2: Fourth intercostal space at left border of sternum
V_3: Halfway between V_2 and V_4
V_4: Fifth intercostal space at midclavicular line
V_5: Fifth intercostal space at anterior axillary line (halfway between V_4 and V_6)
V_6: Fifth intercostal space at midaxillary line, level with V_4

▶ Inform the patient that no special preparation is required and that the procedure takes no longer than 15 minutes.
▶ Urge him to relax, lie still, and breathe normally.
▶ Advise him not to talk during the procedure because the movement of his muscles may distort the ECG tracing.

Documentation

Record the test's date and time. Note any appropriate clinical information on the ECG. Document your patient teaching measures and their effect.

ELECTROPHYSIOLOGY STUDIES

Electrophysiology studies (also known as *His bundle electrography*) of the heart's function measure discrete conduction intervals and diagnose serious arrhythmias by recording electrical conduction during the slow withdrawal of a bipolar or tripolar electrode catheter from the right ventricle through the bundle of His to the sinoatrial node. A catheter is introduced into the femoral vein and passed through the right atrium and across the septal leaflet of the tricuspid valve.

These studies can localize disturbances within the atrioventricular conduction system. When an ectopic site takes over as pacemaker for the heart, the tests can help pinpoint its origin. The tests also aid in the diagnosis of syncope, help evaluate a candidate for permanent pacemaker implantation, and help select or evaluate antiarrhythmic drugs.

Supplies

▶ X-ray table
▶ ECG monitor (continuous)
▶ Shave and preparation kit
▶ Local anesthetic
▶ Electrophysiologic catheter
▶ Dressings

Implementation

▶ Place the patient in a supine position on a special X-ray table.
▶ Apply limb electrodes and precordial leads for electrocardiogram (ECG) recording.
▶ Ensure that the insertion site is shaved, scrubbed, and sterilized.
▶ The physician injects a local anesthetic and introduces the electrophysiologic catheter into the femoral vein (occasionally, into a vein in the antecubital fossa).

Guided by fluoroscopy, the catheter is advanced until it crosses the tricuspid

Catheter placement in electrophysiology studies

In this schematic view, a multipolar electrode catheter is inserted through the superior vena cava, right atrium, and tricuspid valve. When the catheter is withdrawn, the tip moves downward along the ventricle wall; as it passes the bundle of His—located in the septum—a characteristic spike appears on the electrocardiogram.

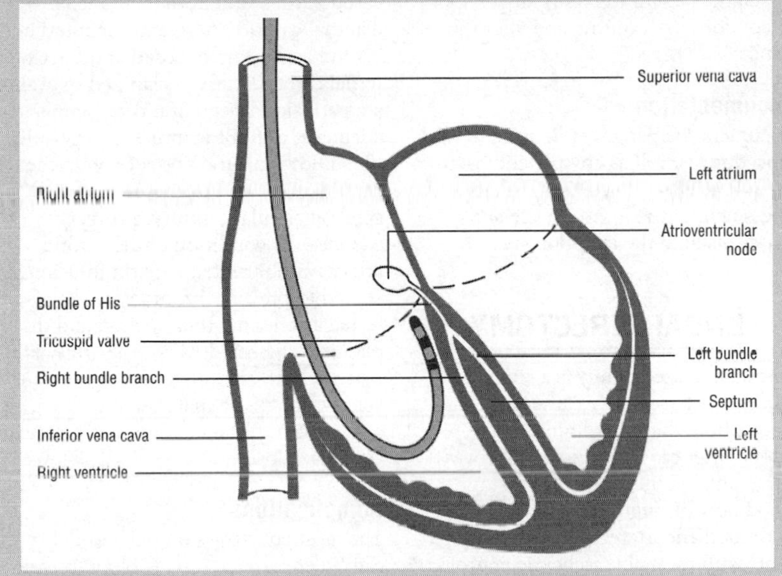

valve and enters the right ventricle. Then the catheter is slowly withdrawn from the tricuspid area, and recordings of conduction intervals are made from each pole of the catheter, either simultaneously or sequentially.

▶ After recordings and measurements are completed, the catheter is removed and a pressure dressing is applied to the site. (See *Catheter placement in electrophysiology studies*.)

▶ Monitor the patient's vital signs, as ordered—usually every 15 minutes for 1 hour, and then every hour for 4 hours. If they're unstable, check every 15 minutes and notify the physician. Observe for shortness of breath, chest pain, pallor, or changes in pulse rate or blood pressure. Enforce bed rest for 4 to 6 hours.

▶ Check the catheter insertion site for bleeding as ordered—usually every 30 minutes for 8 hours; apply a pressure dressing until the bleeding stops.

▶ Advise the patient that he may resume his usual diet.

▶ Make sure a 12-lead resting ECG is scheduled to assess for changes.

Complications

The following complications may occur as a result of electrophysiology studies: arrhythmias, phlebitis, pulmonary emboli, thromboemboli, or catheter-site hemorrhage.

Patient teaching

- Explain the procedure to the patient and tell him the procedure may take from 1 to 3 hours to complete.
- Inform the patient that he will need to stay on bed rest for 4 to 6 hours after the procedure, with the insertion site (typically the leg) kept straight.
- Tell the patient to report any pain or discomfort, both during and after the test.

Documentation

Document the patient's tolerance to the procedure as well as any patient teaching and its effect. Record vital signs and assessment of the insertion site and pulses distal to the insertion site.

ENDARTERECTOMY

Carotid endarterectomy is a surgical procedure that removes atheromatous plaque from the inner lining of the carotid arteries. The surgery improves intracranial perfusion by increasing blood flow through the carotid arteries.

Carotid endarterectomy may help patients with reversible ischemic neurologic deficit or a completed cerebrovascular accident (CVA). Patients who experience transient ischemic attacks, syncope, and dizziness and those who have high-grade asymptomatic or ulcerative lesions may also profit from this procedure.

Because carotid lesions commonly lead to CVA in both symptomatic and asymptomatic patients, some surgeons consider this operation a prophylactic treatment for CVA. However, many intraoperative and postoperative risks are associated with the procedure, making it unsuitable for some patients. (See *Risk levels in carotid endarterectomy*.)

Implementation

Cervical block anesthesia and sedatives are commonly used, allowing you to closely monitor the patient. Alternatively, the patient may be given a light general anesthetic during a carotid endarterectomy so that his brain waves can be assessed.

An incision is made along the anterior border of the sternocleidomastoid muscle or transversely in a skin crease in the neck. Once the incision is made, the carotid artery and both its branches (the external carotid artery and the internal carotid artery) are exposed and the external carotid artery is clamped to evaluate perfusion. If cerebral perfusion is inadequate, a shunt is inserted to permit blood flow past the obstruction in the carotid artery and to ensure adequate cerebral circulation during surgery.

Once the condition of the carotid artery is stabilized, a heparin infusion is started to prevent thrombosis. The affected arteries are then incised and the plaque is dissected. Next, the artery is patched with an autogenous saphenous vein or prosthetic material and closed. If a shunt is in place, it's removed before complete closure.

Complications

The most common complication of carotid endarterectomy is blood pressure lability. Transient hypertension is also common from manipulation of the carotid body.

Perioperative CVA, the most serious complication, may be caused by embolization of debris during dissection. Rethrombosis may occur.

Temporary or permanent loss of carotid body function is a potential problem. Blood pressure and ventilation normally increase in response to hypoxia; however, with the loss of carotid body function, blood pressure and ventilation decrease in response to hypoxia.

Postoperative respiratory distress sometimes is caused by tracheal compression from a hematoma, and wound infection may occur at the surgical site.

A sudden increase in cerebral blood flow can lead to ipsilateral vascular headaches, seizures, and intracerebral

Risk levels in carotid endarterectomy

Is your patient a good candidate for a carotid endarterectomy? One tool for evaluating the patient's chances for a good outcome is the risk-benefit guide below.

Grade 1 patients have the least risk of surgical failure and may benefit the most from carotid endarterectomy. Grade 4 patients have the highest risk and may benefit the least.

Grade 1

Patients classified as grade 1 are under age 70. Medical risk factors, such as diabetes or hyperlipidemia, and lifestyle risk factors, such as alcohol abuse or cigarette smoking, may make patients appear older physiologically than their stated age. Grade 1 patients have bilateral or unilateral focal carotid stenosis and no fixed neurologic deficits. They're considered neurologically stable.

Grade 2

These patients appear clinically equal to patients in grade 1. However, in grade 2, angiographic findings are more extensive; for example, coexisting stenosis of the internal carotid artery in the siphon area, extensive involvement of the vessel to be operated on, or occlusion of the opposite internal carotid artery.

Grade 3

These patients have angiographic evidence of significant lesions similar to that of patients in grade 2. However, grade 3 patients also have significant medical risk factors that will complicate surgery, such as coronary artery disease, myocardial infarction (within 6 months), blood pressure above 180/110 mm Hg, chronic obstructive pulmonary disease, severe obesity, or a physiologic age over 70.

Grade 4

Patients in this classification are neurologically unstable and represent the greatest surgical risk. Neurologic instability includes a cerebrovascular accident in progress, frequent uncontrolled transient ischemic attacks, or multiple neurologic deficits from previous cerebral infarctions.

hemorrhage, which is rare. Also rare, vocal cord paralysis may arise from manipulation of the vagus nerve.

Key nursing diagnoses and outcomes

Risk for injury related to possible complications of surgery

Treatment outcome: The patient will have unchanged or improved neurologic, cardiac, and respiratory function.

Risk for suffocation related to potential tracheal compression from a hematoma at the surgical site

Treatment outcome: The patient will maintain a patent airway.

Ineffective protection related to temporary or permanent loss of carotid body function

Treatment outcome: The patient will be aware of the signs and symptoms of hypoxia, so he'll know when to seek medical attention. He'll wear or carry medical identification. In an emergency, this alerts health care professionals to look for deviations in the signs of hypoxia the patient may exhibit.

Nursing interventions

When preparing the patient for carotid endarterectomy or caring for him afterward, implement these interventions.

Before surgery

▶ To reduce their anxiety, teach the patient and his family members about the procedure and answer their questions.

▶ Discuss the location of the lesion. Also, describe the atherosclerotic process so that after surgery the patient can modify risk factors through diet, medication, and exercise.

▶ Explain all preoperative diagnostic tests used to evaluate carotid disease, including periorbital ultrasonography, ocular pneumoplethysmography, carotid phonoangiography, computed tomography scan, electroencephalography (EEG), and cerebral angiography. If the patient has concurrent coronary artery disease (CAD), also explain electrocardiography (ECG), coronary angiography, and the treadmill exercise stress test.

▶ Give the patient and family members a tour of the intensive care unit to help prepare them for the postoperative stay.

▶ Explain postoperative care, and warn the patient and family members that I.V. lines, hemodynamic measuring devices, tubes, and machinery will be connected to the patient.

▶ Tell the patient that he'll have some postoperative discomfort or pain but that pain medication will be available.

▶ Inform the patient that a nurse will check his neurologic status, including level of consciousness (LOC), orientation, extremity strength, speech, and fine hand movements, every hour after surgery. Explain that this is routine, not an indication that he isn't doing well.

▶ Help the physician insert a radial arterial catheter to monitor arterial blood gas levels and blood pressure.

▶ Ensure that a baseline EEG is done before the patient is anesthetized.

After surgery

▶ Monitor vital signs every 15 minutes for the 1st hour until the patient is stable. Lowered blood pressure and elevated heart rate and respirations could indicate cerebral ischemia.

▶ Perform a neurologic assessment every hour for the first 24 hours. Check extremity strength, fine hand movements, speech, LOC, and orientation.

▶ Monitor intake and output hourly for the first 24 hours.

▶ Perform continuous cardiac monitoring for the first 24 hours. Take an ECG if the patient has any chest pain or arrhythmias. Many patients undergoing this procedure also have CAD.

PATIENT TEACHING

▶ Teach the patient and a family member or friend surgical wound care. Review the signs and symptoms of infection (fever, sore throat, or redness, swelling or drainage from the wound), and tell them to call the physician immediately if these occur.

▶ Encourage the patient to stop smoking, reduce lipid levels, lose weight, and lower any other risk factors.

▶ Make sure that the patient understands the dosage and possible adverse effects of all prescribed medications.

▶ If the patient has had a CVA and needs follow-up care, refer him and his family member to a home health care agency.

Cultural diversity **Among black Americans, extended family is very important, and relatives are generally involved in the treatment process. Remember to include these individuals in the treatment plan, when possible.**

▶ Teach the patient how to manage any neurologic, sensory, or motor deficits that occurred during surgery.

▶ Tell the patient to contact the physician immediately if any new neurologic signs or symptoms occur.

▶ Emphasize the importance of regular checkups.

END-OF-LIFE CARE

Death may be difficult to face, but it's common to all humans and is a natural part of life. Many people are reluctant to accept their own mortality. Nurses, too, may be reluctant to face the death of their patient. Many nurses have had little education on caring for dying patients and may feel uncomfortable caring for them. In addition, the causes of death have changed over the years with the shift from acute to chronic disease. These chronically ill patients face the prospect of dying slowly in old age with some of these patients needing support ive, palliative care. Goals of nursing care at the end-of-life include helping the older patient to maintain dignity, be comfortable, and control symptoms, and addressing spiritual concerns.

End-of-life care settings

Elderly patients and their families have choices about the setting in which they would like to receive end-of-life care.. Most people die in a health care facility, followed by long-term care facilities. However, an increasing number of people are choosing to die at home. Only a small percentage of people die under the care of a hospice program and most of these people have cancer. Health insurance benefits may also mandate where a person receives care.

An elderly person may choose to receive end-of-life care in a health care facility for several reasons. The person may have had a long-term relationship with a health care team that he trusts. He may also want to relieve his family of the burden of providing increasingly time-consuming and difficult care to a dying person. Many families feel overwhelmed and exhausted caring for their older family member at home and prefer hospitalization for end-of-life care.

Many elderly patients spend their end-of-life in a long-term care facility. Their deaths may be imminent or years away. Long-term care facilities differ in their ability to provide palliative care. The high nurse-to-patient ratio reduces the ability to provide palliative care. Many facilities care for their dying residents while others transfer them to a health care facility to die in an unfamiliar environment among strangers.

An older adult may choose to die at home instead of a health care facility or long-term care facility because the surroundings are familiar. The home setting also provides more privacy, allows greater flexibility for visiting with family and friends, and the patient can remain involved in family life. A dying patient may also feel more secure that unwanted procedures and life-saving therapies can be better avoided at home. Several types of care are available to those older adults who choose to die at home, including hospice and home health care.

Hospice care is a method of providing palliative and supportive care when the older adult no longer wants active medical treatment. Hospice care focuses on providing the individual with comfort and dignity using a multidisciplinary team approach. Reimbursement for hospice care may be limited to those elderly patients with a predictable prognosis. Although hospice care typically takes place in the home, the elderly patient may also receive hospice care in an inpatient hospice unit or in a long-term care facility.

Home health care, in contrast, provides care in the home and eases the burden that family members may feel. Among the services provided is skilled nursing care, including administering medications and performing treatments. Typically the nurse coordinates the multidisciplinary health care team, including home health aides. Aides can provide assistance with self-care activities, such as feeding, bathing, and dressing. They may also perform light household chores, laundry, and shopping. Not all health insurance policies cover home health care. Some home health agencies adjust their fees based on ability to pay.

Nursing care of the dying patient

The dying older adult may experience a variety of physical and emotional symptoms. Recognizing and treating these symptoms can ease the suffering of the dying patient.

Nursing care of physical symptoms

PAIN

Older adults experience and express pain based on their past experiences, culture, gender, emotional status, medical diagnosis, and cognitive function. Some patients verbalize pain and discomfort, while others don't. If a patient doesn't verbalize pain, don't assume he isn't in pain. Observe for nonverbal clues.

Encourage the patient to report his pain as soon as possible and to openly discuss his concerns about pain. The goal of pain management for the dying patient is to manage the pain so that it's prevented from occurring rather than treating it when it does occur.

In the home, provide the patient and his family with guidelines for obtaining pain relief. Make sure they have the name and telephone number of the person to call if pain control is inadequate.

RESPIRATORY DISTRESS

Respiratory distress produces physical discomfort, feelings of helplessness, anxiety, and fear that result from the thought of suffocation. In addition to treating the underlying cause, position your patient to improve his breathing (such as in semi-Fowler's position), provide supplemental oxygen administration, morphine, or benzodiazepines to improve breathing. Your calm presence and soothing words can also help the patient stay calm and slow his respirations. Relaxation techniques, massage, and other alternative therapies may also relieve an elderly patient's respiratory distress.

ANOREXIA

Anorexia may be the result of several factors, including nausea, weakness, inactivity, adverse effects of medications, difficulty swallowing, and pain. Offer the patient smaller, more frequent meals, special foods or favorite meals brought from home. Sips of water or other beverages, soft foods, ice chips and providing good oral hygiene can help. Explain to the family that the patient may be more comfortable without artificial nutrition and hydration.

NAUSEA AND VOMITING

Nausea and vomiting may be due to a variety of causes, such as effects of medications, slowed gastric emptying, constipation, uremia, or bowel obstruction. Medications may be given to alleviate nausea and vomiting. Just as for pain medications, antiemetics should be administered around-the-clock rather than "as needed" for more effective control of nausea and vomiting.

BOWEL PROBLEMS

Constipation may be the result of inactivity, dehydration, lack of dietary fiber, and adverse effects of medications. Assess and record bowel elimination patterns and administer laxatives and stool softeners regularly to prevent constipation.

If the dying patient experiences diarrhea, offer clear liquids and bland carbohydrates, and administer medications to control diarrhea, in addition to treating the underlying cause. Provide good perianal hygiene, and use a protective skin barrier to prevent skin irritation and breakdown.

Nursing care of emotional symptoms

CONFUSION

The dying patient may be confused as a result of medications, hypoxia, his disease process, pain, and metabolic disturbances. Assist in treating the cause and administer sedatives to calm an agitated patient. Drugs such as haloperidol may reduce threatening hallucinations or disturbing dreams.

DEPRESSION AND ANXIETY

Antidepressants may be appropriate for some patients with depression. Use therapeutic communication skills in communicating with the patient, and let him know that you're there to listen. Allow the patient sufficient time to verbalize feelings. Refer the patient to a social worker, mental health professional, or chaplain.

Provide opportunities for the patient to discuss his anxieties. Encourage the patient to be involved in care-related decisions, if the patient wishes, and offer the patient choices. Teach stress-reduction strategies, and administer antianxiety agents, if indicated.

SLEEP DISTURBANCES

The dying patient may experience sleep disturbances as a result of anxiety, depression, pain, inactivity, or adverse effects of medications. Provide interventions to correct the cause of insomnia, teach relaxation strategies, and administer hypnotics, if needed.

SPIRITUAL DISTRESS

Many dying patients have spiritual concerns that may include the meaning of life, God's existence, or the afterlife. Spiritual distress may result in despair and hopelessness. Listen to your patient and show that you care, and allow him to speak with a chaplain or the support of a family member or friend to help resolve his distress.

Special considerations

- Educate your patient and his family on the differences between active, therapeutic treatment, and palliative care (symptomatic treatment). Explain that the goal of palliative care is to provide the best quality of life for the critically or terminally ill patient by ensuring his comfort and dignity. In addition to these physical needs, palliative care also attempts to meet the psychosocial, emotional, cultural, and spiritual needs of the patient.
- Keep the environment quiet and comfortable for the patient, and instruct the family on care of the patient, if the family desires this.
- Initiate conversation about the past, and inquire about the patient's life to facilate a life review.
- Engage the patient or family in comforting conversation and provide companionship if the family or friends aren't available.
- Respond to requests for prayers, rituals, a religious reading or service from the patient or family. Contact the facility's chaplain or the patient's own priest, minister, or rabbi.
- Listen carefully for clues to feelings and anxieties. Act as a patient advocate in decisions about death and dying.

Cultural diversity Ask about the dying patient's cultural beliefs and practices and incorporate them into the care plan. Determine whether the patient or his family wants a member of the clergy present. Be aware of and respect cultural, ethnic, and religious practices that families may engage in before and after death.

- Allow family and friends to visit and remain nearby as indicated.

ENDOSCOPY

Endoscopy is used to inspect either the upper GI tract or the intestine. Upper GI endoscopy, called *esophagogastroduodenoscopy* (EGD), is the visual inspection of the lining of the esophagus, the stomach, and the upper duodenum using a flexible fiber-optic endoscope. It's indicated for patients with hematemesis, melena, or substernal or epigastric pain and in postoperative patients with recurrent or new signs and symptoms. It's also indicated for suspected esophagitis, hiatal hernia, esophageal stenosis or varices, gastritis, gastric ulcers or varices, duodenitis, duodenal ulcer, diverticula or neoplasm.

EGD, which can detect small or surface lesions missed by radiography, eliminates the need for extensive exploratory surgery. It also permits laboratory evaluation of abnormalities first detected by radiography because the scope provides a channel for biopsy forceps or a cytology brush. Similarly, it allows removal of foreign bodies by suction (for small, soft objects) or by electrocautery snare or forceps (for large, hard objects).

Colonoscopy is the visual examination of the lining of the large intestine with a flexible fiber-optic endoscope. This test is indicated for patients with a strong family history of rectal or colon cancer. It's also indicated if there's a history of constipation and diarrhea, persistent rectal bleeding, or lower abdominal pain when results of proctosigmoidoscopy and a barium enema test prove negative or inconclusive. Biopsy of the tissue or polyp can be obtained through the scope, and polyps can be removed or cauterized during the colonoscopy. Because the risk of colorectal cancer increases with age, some health care practitioners recommend that the older adult patient receive a colonoscopy at least once every 3 years.

The colonoscope is available in 42″ to 72″ (106.5- to 183-cm) lengths and contains a bundle of glass fibers that transmit light. It's inserted anally and advanced through the large intestine under direct vision, using the scope's optical system. Fluoroscopy and abdominal palpation may facilitate passage of the endoscope through the bends in the large intestine.

Supplies

- Endoscope
- Sedation and other preprocedure medications as needed (such as anticholinergics and antibiotics)
- Local anesthetic (for EGD)
- Mouthguard (for EGD)
- Biopsy forceps
- Cytology brush
- Electrocautery snare
- Tongue blade
- Pulse oximeter
- Continuous cardiac monitor
- Blood pressure monitoring supplies
- Emergency resuscitation equipment
- Gloves
- Suction equipment
- Lubricant (for colonoscopy)
- Drape (for colonoscopy)

Implementation

Esophagogastroduodenoscopy

- Make sure the patient or a responsible family member has signed a consent form.
- Check the patient's history for hypersensitivity to the medications and anesthetic ordered for the test.
- Just prior to the procedure, instruct the patient to remove eyeglasses, necklaces, hairpins, combs, and constricting undergarments.
- Obtain baseline vital signs, and leave the blood pressure cuff in place for monitoring throughout the procedure.
- Attach pulse oximeter and continuous cardiac monitor and record readings.
- Have emergency resuscitation equipment readily available.
- Ask the patient to hold his breath while his mouth and throat are sprayed with a local anesthetic.
- Place the patient in a left lateral position with his head bent forward.
- With the patient's mouth open, the examiner guides the tip of the endoscope to the back of the throat. The rubber tip is deflected downward with the left index finger to the back of the throat.
- As the endoscope passes through the posterior pharynx and the cricopharyngeal sphincter, the patient's head is slowly extended to aid advancement of the scope. The patient's chin must be kept at midline.

▶ The endoscope is then passed along the esophagus under direct vision. When the endoscope is well into the esophagus (about 12″ [30.5 cm]), the patient's head is positioned with his chin toward the table so that saliva can drain out of his mouth.

▶ When the examination of the esophagus and the cardiac sphincter is completed, the endoscope is rotated clockwise — with the tip angled upward — and advanced into the stomach. After the lining of the stomach is examined completely, including the gastric side of the cardiac and pyloric sphincters, the endoscope is advanced into the duodenum.

▶ Following this examination, the endoscope is slowly withdrawn, and suspicious areas of the gastric and esophageal lining are reexamined. Biopsy forceps (to obtain a tissue specimen) or a cytology brush (to obtain cells) may also be passed through the scope.

Colonoscopy

▶ Make sure the patient or a responsible family member has signed a consent form.

▶ Place the patient on his left side, with his knees flexed, and drape him.

▶ Instruct him to breathe deeply and slowly through his mouth as the physician inserts his gloved, lubricated index finger into the anus and rectum and palpates the mucosa. After a water-soluble lubricant has been applied to the patient's anus and to the tip of the colonoscope, tell the patient the colonoscope is ready to be inserted.

▶ After the colonoscope is inserted through the patient's anus, a small amount of air is insufflated to locate the bowel lumen.

▶ The scope is advanced through the rectum into the sigmoid colon under direct vision. When the instrument reaches the descending sigmoid junction, assist the patient to a supine position to aid the scope's advance, if necessary; this position may also be assumed to negotiate the splenic flexure.

▶ After the scope has passed the splenic flexure, it's advanced through the transverse colon and hepatic flexure, into the ascending colon and cecum.

▶ Biopsy forceps or a cytology brush may be passed through a channel in the colonoscope to obtain specimens for histologic and cytologic examinations, respectively; an electrocautery snare may be used to remove polyps.

Following the endoscopic examination

▶ Monitor the patient's vital signs every 15 minutes until stable. Increase to every 4 hours as the patient's condition warrants.

▶ Provide a safe environment for the patient until he has recovered from the sedative. Keep bed side rails up.

▶ Following an EGD, withhold food and fluids until the gag reflex returns. Test the gag reflex by touching the back of the throat with a tongue blade. When the gag reflex returns — usually within 1 hour — allow fluids and a light meal as ordered.

Complications

Complications of EGD include perforation of the esophagus, stomach, duodenum, or diaphragm and accidental aspiration of stomach materials. The patient also may suffer adverse reactions to sedation, such as hypotension, respiratory depression, apnea, diaphoresis, bradycardia, and laryngospasm.

Bowel perforation is a potential complication of colonoscopy. Bleeding may be an adverse effect of a biopsy or polypectomy. Some patients may have adverse reactions to sedation, such as hypotension, respiratory depression, apnea, diaphoresis, bradycardia, and confusion.

Patient teaching

Before esophagogastroduodenoscopy

▶ Explain the procedure to the patient.

▶ Instruct the patient to fast for 6 to 12 hours before the procedure. (If an emergency EGD is performed, tell the patient that stomach contents will be aspirated through a nasogastric tube.)

▶ Inform the patient that a bitter-tasting local anesthetic will be sprayed into his mouth and throat to calm the gag reflex, and that his tongue and throat may feel swollen, making swallowing difficult. Advise him to let the saliva drain from the side of his mouth; a suction machine may be used to remove saliva, if necessary.

▶ Tell the patient that an I.V. line will be started to allow infusion of a sedative or I.V. fluids.

▶ Tell him that a mouthguard will be inserted to protect his teeth and the endoscope; assure him that the mouthguard won't obstruct his breathing. If the patient wears dentures, instruct him to remove and store them before the test.

▶ Inform him that he'll receive a sedative before the endoscope is inserted to help him relax but that he'll remain conscious.

Before colonoscopy

▶ Inform the patient that he may need to maintain a clear liquid diet for up to 48 hours before the test and to take nothing by mouth after midnight the evening before the procedure.

▶ Explain the procedure, and tell him that it usually takes 30 to 60 minutes.

▶ Tell the patient that the large intestine must be thoroughly cleaned to be clearly visible. Give him a laxative, such as 10 oz (296 ml) of magnesium citrate, 3 tbs (44 ml) of castor oil, or a gallon of GoLYTELY solution in the evening. If you're using GoLYTELY, instruct the patient to drink the preparation quickly (8 oz [237 ml] every 10 minutes until the entire gallon is consumed). This laxative produces watery diarrhea in 30 to 60 minutes and clears the bowel in 4 to 5 hours. If fecal results are still not clear, the patient will receive a laxative, suppository, or tap water enema. (You won't use a soap and water enema because this irritates the mucosa and stimulates mucous secretions that may hinder examination.)

▶ Inform the patient that he will receive a sedative to help him relax.

▶ Instruct the patient to rest for 2 to 6 hours following the procedure.

Documentation

Document the patient's vital signs and any medications given during the procedure. Record the patient's response to the procedure as well as any complications he may experience. Note your patient teaching measures and their effect.

ENEMA ADMINISTRATION

The enema procedure involves instilling a solution into the rectum and the colon. In a retention enema, the patient holds the solution within the rectum or colon for 30 minutes to 1 hour. In an irrigating enema, the patient expels the solution almost completely within 15 minutes. Both types of enema stimulate peristalsis by mechanically distending the colon and stimulating rectal wall nerves.

Enemas are used to clean the lower bowel in preparation for diagnostic or surgical procedures, to relieve distention and promote expulsion of flatus, to lubricate the rectum and colon, and to soften hardened stool for removal. They're contraindicated, however, after recent colon or rectal surgery or myocardial infarction, and in the patient with an acute abdominal condition of unknown origin, such as suspected appendicitis. They should be administered cautiously to a patient with arrhythmia.

Remember that enema solutions and methods vary to suit your patient's condition or treatment requirements and may include:

▶ A small-volume enema is used when the patient is constipated but doesn't need the higher portion of the colon cleaned. It may also be used for the older adult who can't retain a large amount of fluid.

▶ A prepackaged disposable enema is used to clean the bowel in preparation for tests. These solutions are hypertonic—they draw fluid into the bowel, softening fecal material. Because they draw fluid from the tissues, they can't be given to a dehydrated patient.

▶ A return flow enema is used to stimulate peristalsis and remove intestinal gas. A large volume of fluid is given in small increments, then the enema is allowed to return, bringing gas with it.

▶ Emollient and oil-retention enemas contain a small amount of fluid that softens the stool.

▶ Anthelmintic (medicinal) enemas contain a medicated solution that destroys helminthes—parasitic worms that infect humans.

▶ Hypotonic enema solutions (tap water is the most common) cause water to move out of the bowel into the tissues. This flow of fluid occurs slowly, so defecation usually takes place before too much fluid is absorbed into the tissues. If defecation doesn't occur in a timely fashion, the patient may be at risk for fluid overload.

Supplies

▶ Prescribed solution
▶ Bath (utility) thermometer
▶ Enema administration bag with attached rectal tube and clamp
▶ I.V. pole
▶ Gloves
▶ Linen-saver pads
▶ Bath blanket
▶ Two bedpans with covers, or bedside commode
▶ Water-soluble lubricant
▶ Toilet tissue
▶ Bulb syringe or funnel
▶ Plastic bag for equipment
▶ Water
▶ Gown
▶ Washcloth
▶ Soap and water
▶ Optional: prepackaged disposable enema set or small-volume enema solutions in both irrigating and retention types
▶ For patients who can't retain solution: plastic rectal tube guard, indwelling urinary catheter or indwelling rectal catheter with 30-ml balloon and syringe

Implementation

▶ Prepare the prescribed type and amount of solution as indicated. Standard volumes are 750 to 1,000 ml for an irrigating enema and 50 to 250 ml for a retention enema. Very thin or frail older patients may require smaller amounts of solution. Older adult patients who receive an irrigating enema of high volume may develop colon distention and mild shock.

▶ Administer less solution when giving a hypertonic enema because osmotic pull moves fluid into the colon from body tissues, increasing the volume of colon contents.

▶ Because some ingredients may be mucosal irritants, be sure the proportions are correct and the agents are thoroughly mixed to avoid localized irritation.

▶ Warm the solution to reduce patient discomfort. Administer an enema at 100° to 105° F (37.8° to 40.6° C) to avoid burning rectal tissues. Test the solution's temperature with the bath thermometer. Note that some enemas such as milk and molasses must be heated to high temperatures for proper mixing and then cooled to proper administration temperature.

▶ Clamp the tubing and fill the solution bag with the prescribed solution. Unclamp the tubing, flush the solution through the tubing, and then reclamp it. Flushing detects leaks and removes air that could cause discomfort if introduced into the colon.

▶ Hang the solution container on the I.V. pole, and take all supplies to the patient's bedside. If you're using an in-

Giving an enema

Unless contraindicated, help the patient into the left-lateral Sims' position. After lubricating the end of the tube, separate the patient's buttocks and push the tube gently into the anus, aiming it toward the umbilicus. Insert the tube 2" to 4" (5 to 10 cm). To prevent rectal wall trauma, avoid forcing the tube. If it doesn't advance easily, let a little solution flow in to relax the inner sphincter enough to allow passage.

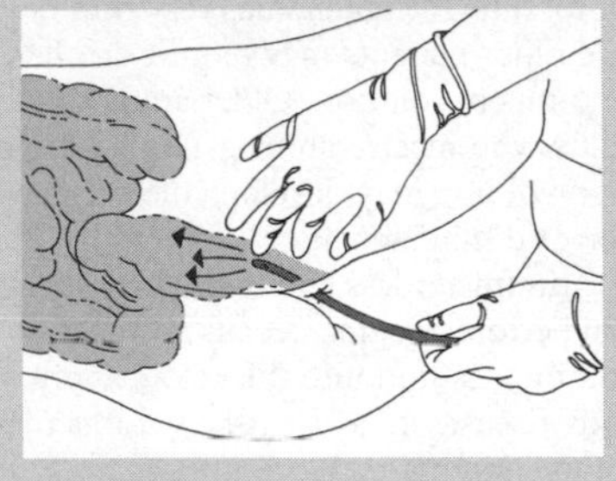

dwelling rectal catheter, fill the bulb syringe with 30 ml of water.

- Check the physician's order and assess the patient's condition.
- Provide privacy.
- Ask the patient if he has had previous difficulty retaining an enema to determine whether you need to use a rectal tube guard or a catheter.
- Wash your hands and put on gloves.
- Help the patient put on a gown, if necessary. The gown makes enema administration easier, and the patient worries less about soiling it.
- Assist the patient into left-lateral Sims' position with the right knee flexed. This will help the solution flow by gravity into the descending colon. (See *Giving an enema.*) If contraindicated or if the patient reports discomfort, reposition him on his back or right side.
- For the patient who can't tolerate a flat position (for example, a patient with shortness of breath), administer the enema with the head of the bed in the lowest position he can safely and comfortably maintain.
- Don't give an enema to a patient who's in a sitting position, unless absolutely necessary; the solution won't flow high enough into the colon and will only distend the rectum and trigger rapid expulsion.
- Place linen-saver pads under the patient's buttocks to prevent soiling the linens. Replace the top bed linens with a bath blanket to provide privacy and warmth.
- Have a bedpan or commode nearby for the patient to use. If the patient may use the bathroom, make sure that it will be available when he needs it. Have toilet tissue within his reach.

Administering the enema

- Lubricate the distal tip of the rectal catheter with water-soluble lubricant to ease rectal insertion and reduce irritation.
- If the patient has hemorrhoids, instruct him to bear down gently during tube insertion. This causes the anus to open and helps with insertion.
- Separate the patient's buttocks and touch the anal sphincter with the rectal tube to stimulate contraction. Then, as the sphincter relaxes, tell the patient to breathe deeply through his mouth as you gently advance the tube.
- If the patient feels pain or the tube meets continued resistance, notify the physician. This may signal an unknown stricture or abscess. If the patient has poor sphincter control, use a plastic rectal tube guard.
- Alternate means of instilling the solution include using a bulb syringe or a funnel with the rectal tube.
- You can also use an indwelling rectal catheter as a rectal tube if your facility's policy permits. Insert the lubricated catheter as you would a rectal tube. Then gently inflate the catheter's balloon with 20 to 30 ml of water. Gently pull

the catheter back against the patient's internal anal sphincter to seal off the rectum. If leakage still occurs with the balloon in place, add more water to the balloon in small amounts.

▶ When using an indwelling catheter, avoid inflating the balloon above 45 ml because overinflation can compromise blood flow to the rectal tissues and cause possible necrosis from pressure on the rectal mucosa.

▶ If you're using a rectal tube, hold it in place throughout the procedure because bowel contractions and the pressure of the tube against the anal sphincter can promote tube displacement.

▶ Hold the solution container slightly above bed level and release the tubing clamp. Then raise the container gradually to start the flow, usually at a rate of 75 to 100 ml/minute for an irrigating enema, but at the slowest possible rate for a retention enema to avoid stimulating peristalsis and to promote retention. Adjust the flow rate of an irrigating enema by raising or lowering the solution container according to the patient's retention ability and comfort. However, don't raise it higher than 18″ (45.5 cm) because excessive pressure can force colon bacteria into the small intestine or rupture the colon.

▶ Assess the patient's tolerance frequently during instillation. If he complains of discomfort, cramps, or the need to defecate, stop the flow by pinching or clamping the tubing. Then hold the patient's buttocks together or firmly press toilet tissue against the anus. Instruct him to gently massage his abdomen and to breathe slowly and deeply through his mouth to help relax abdominal muscles and promote retention. Resume administration at a slower flow rate after a few minutes when discomfort passes, but interrupt the flow any time the patient feels uncomfortable.

▶ If the flow slows or stops, the catheter tip may be clogged with feces or pressed against the rectal wall. Gently turn the catheter slightly to free it without stimulating defecation. If the catheter tip remains clogged, withdraw the catheter, flush with solution, and reinsert.

▶ After administering most of the prescribed amount of solution, clamp the tubing. Stop the flow before the container empties completely to avoid introducing air into the bowel.

▶ To administer a commercially prepared disposable enema, first remove the cap from the rectal tube. The tube is prelubricated. Insert the rectal tube into the rectum, and squeeze the bottle to deposit the contents in the rectum. As contents are deposited, roll up the bottle starting at the distal end. Remove the rectal tube, replace the used enema unit in its original container, and discard.

▶ For a return-flow enema, stop the flow by lowering the solution container below bed level and allowing gravity to siphon the enema from the colon. Continue to raise and lower the container until gas bubbles cease or the patient feels more comfortable and abdominal distention subsides. Don't allow the solution container to empty completely before lowering it because this may introduce air into the bowel.

▶ For an irrigating enema, instruct the patient to retain the solution for 15 minutes, if possible.

▶ For a retention enema, instruct the patient to avoid defecation for the prescribed time or as follows: 30 minutes or longer for oil-retention and milk and molasses enemas; and 15 to 30 minutes for anthelmintic and emollient enemas. If you're using an indwelling catheter, leave the catheter in place to promote retention.

▶ Schedule a retention enema before meals because a full stomach may stimulate peristalsis and make retention difficult. Follow an oil-retention enema with a soap and water enema 1 hour later to help expel the softened feces completely.

▶ If the patient is apprehensive, position him on the bedpan and allow him to hold toilet tissue or a rolled washcloth against his anus. Place the call button within his reach. If he will be using the bathroom or the commode, instruct him to call for help before attempting to get out of bed because the procedure may make him feel weak or faint. Also, instruct him to call you if he feels weak at any time.

▶ For a bedridden patient who needs to expel the enema into a bedpan, raise the head of the bed to approximate a sitting or squatting position.

▶ When the solution has remained in the colon for the recommended time or for as long as the patient can tolerate it, assist the patient onto a bedpan or to the commode or bathroom, as required.

▶ If an indwelling catheter is in place, deflate the balloon and remove the catheter, if applicable.

▶ Provide privacy while the patient expels the solution. Instruct the patient not to flush the toilet so the results can be documented.

▶ While the patient uses the bathroom, remove and discard any soiled linen and linen-saver pads.

After enema administration

▶ Assist the patient with cleaning, if necessary, and help him to bed. Make sure he feels clean and comfortable and can easily reach the call button. Place a clean linen-saver pad under him to absorb rectal drainage, and tell him that he may need to expel additional stool or flatus later. Encourage him to rest for a while because the procedure may be tiring.

▶ Cover the bedpan or commode and take it to the utility room for observation, or observe the contents of the toilet, as applicable. Carefully note fecal color, consistency, amount (minimal, moderate, or generous), and foreign matter, such as blood, rectal tissue, worms, pus, mucus, or other unusual matter.

▶ In patients with fluid and electrolyte disturbances, measure the amount of expelled solution to assess for retention of enema fluid.

▶ Send specimens to the laboratory, if ordered.

▶ If the patient fails to expel the solution within 1 hour because of diminished neuromuscular response, you may need to remove the enema solution. First, review your facility's policy because you may need a physician's order. Inform the physician when a patient can't expel an enema spontaneously because of possible bowel perforation or electrolyte imbalance. To siphon the enema solution from the patient's rectum, help him move to a side-lying position on the bed. Place a bedpan on a bedside chair so it rests below mattress level. Disconnect the tubing from the solution container, place the distal end in the bedpan, and reinsert the rectal end into the patient's anus. If gravity fails to drain the solution into the bedpan, instill 30 to 50 ml of warm water (105° F [40.6° C]) through the tube. Then quickly direct the distal end of the tube into the bedpan. In both cases, measure the return to make sure that all the solution has drained.

▶ Rinse the bedpan or commode with cold water; then wash it in hot, soapy water. Return it to the patient's bedside.

▶ Properly dispose of the enema equipment. If additional enemas are scheduled, store clean, reusable equipment in a closed plastic bag in the patient's bathroom. Discard your gloves and wash your hands.

▶ Ventilate the room or use an air freshener, if necessary.

If the physician orders enemas until the return is clear, give no more than three to avoid excessive irritation of the rectal mucosa. Notify the physician if the returned fluid isn't clear after three administrations.

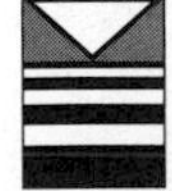

Key point Because a patient with a salt-retention disorders such as heart failure may absorb sodium from the saline enema solution, give him the solution cautiously and monitor his electrolyte status.

Complications

Enemas may produce dizziness or faintness, excessive irritation of the colonic mucosa caused by repeated administration or from sensitivity to the enema ingredients, hyponatremia or hypokalemia from repeated administration of hypotonic solutions, and cardiac arrhythmias caused by vasovagal reflex stimulation after insertion of the rectal catheter. Colonic water absorption may follow prolonged retention of hypotonic solutions, which may, in turn, cause hypervolemia or water intoxication. In addition, advancing the rectal tube too far may perforate the rectum or intestinal wall, or rupture polyps.

Patient teaching

- Describe the procedure to the patient and his family members to reduce fear and promote cooperation. Emphasize that administering an enema to a person in a sitting position or on the toilet could injure the rectal wall.
- Review measures for preventing constipation, including regular exercise, dietary modifications, and adequate fluid intake.

Documentation

Record the date and time of enema administration; special equipment used; type and amount of solution; retention time; approximate amount returned; color, consistency, and amount of the return; abnormalities within the return; any complications that occurred; and the patient's tolerance of the treatment. Document your patient teaching measures and their effects.

ENTERAL NUTRITION

Enteral nutrition is a procedure to deliver a liquid feeding formula directly to the stomach, duodenum, or jejunum. Liquid feeding typically is indicated for a patient who can't eat normally because of dysphagia or oral or esophageal obstruction or injury. It also may be appropriate for an unconscious or intubated patient or a patient recovering from GI tract surgery who can't ingest food orally.

Duodenal or jejunal feedings decrease the risk of aspiration because the formula bypasses the pylorus. Jejunal feedings reduce pancreatic stimulation; thus, the patient may require an elemental diet.

Patients may receive gastric feedings on an intermittent or a continuous schedule. For duodenal or jejunal feedings, however, most patients seem to better tolerate a continuous slow drip.

Liquid nutrient solutions come in various formulas for administration through a nasogastric tube, small-bore feeding tube, gastrostomy or jejunostomy tube, percutaneous endoscopic gastrostomy or jejunostomy tube, or gastrostomy feeding button. Tube feeding of any type is contraindicated in patients who have no bowel sounds or suspected intestinal obstruction.

Supplies

For gastric feedings

- Feeding formula
- Graduated container
- Water
- Gavage bag with tubing and flow regulator clamp
- Towel or linen-saver pad
- 60-ml bulb syringe
- Stethoscope
- Optional: infusion controller and tubing set (for continuous administration), and adapter to connect gavage tubing to feeding tube

For duodenal or jejunal feedings

- Feeding formula
- Enteral administration set containing a gavage container, drip chamber, roller clamp or flow regulator, and tube connector wih feeding tubing
- I.V. pole
- 60-ml bulb syringe with adapter tip
- Water

▶ Optional: pump administration set (for an enteral infusion pump) and Y-connector

Implementation

▶ Verify orders for enteral nutrition on the medication record and chart.

▶ Refrigerate formulas prepared in the dietary department or pharmacy. Date and refrigerate commercial formulas only after opening them.

▶ Check the date on every formula container. Discard expired commercial formula. Use powdered formula within 24 hours of mixing. Always shake the container well to mix the solution thoroughly.

▶ Allow the formula to warm to room temperature before administration. Never warm it over direct heat or in a microwave, because heat may curdle the formula or change its chemical composition. Also, hot formula may injure the patient.

▶ Pour 60 ml of water into the graduated container. After closing the flow clamp on the administration set, pour 60 ml of water into the gavage bag. Open the flow clamp and allow the water to displace the air in the tubing. Close the flow clamp and pour the appropriate amount of formula into the gavage bag. Hang no more than a 4- to 6-hour supply at one time to prevent bacterial growth.

▶ Provide privacy and wash your hands.

▶ If the patient has a nasal or oral tube, cover his chest with a towel or linen-saver pad to protect him and the bed linens from spills.

▶ Assess the patient's abdomen for bowel sounds and distention.

Gastric feeding

▶ Elevate the bed to semi-Fowler's or high Fowler's position to prevent aspiration by gastroesophageal reflux and to promote digestion. (See *Managing tube feeding problems*.)

▶ Check placement of the feeding tube to confirm it hasn't slipped out since the last feeding. Never give a tube feeding until you're sure the tube is properly positioned in the patient's stomach. Administering a feeding through a misplaced tube can cause formula to enter the patient's lungs.

▶ To check tube patency and position, remove the cap or plug from the feeding tube and use the syringe to inject 5 to 10 cc of air through the tube. At the same time, auscultate the patient's stomach with the stethoscope. Listen for a whooshing sound to confirm tube positioning in the stomach. Also, aspirate stomach contents to confirm tube patency and placement.

▶ To assess gastric emptying, aspirate and measure residual gastric contents. Reinstill any aspirate obtained.

▶ Connect the gavage bag tubing to the feeding tube. Depending on the type of tube used, you may need to use an adapter to connect the two.

▶ If you're using a bulb or catheter-tip syringe, remove the bulb or plunger and attach the syringe to the pinched-off feeding tube to prevent excess air from entering the patient's stomach, causing distention. If you're using an infusion controller, thread the tube from the formula container through the controller according to the manufacturer's directions. Purge the tubing of air and attach it to the feeding tube.

▶ Open the regulator clamp on the gavage bag tubing, and adjust the flow rate appropriately. When using a bulb syringe, fill the syringe with formula and release the feeding tube to allow formula to flow through it. The height at which you hold the syringe will determine flow rate. When the syringe is three-quarters empty, pour more formula into it.

▶ If the feeding solution doesn't initially flow through a bulb syringe, attach the bulb and squeeze it gently to start the flow. Then remove the bulb. Never use the bulb to force the formula through the tube.

Managing tube feeding problems

Complications	Interventions
Aspiration of gastric secretions	■ Discontinue feeding immediately. ■ Perform tracheal suction of aspirated contents if possible. ■ Notify the physician. Prophylactic antibiotics and chest physiotherapy may be ordered. ■ Check tube placement before feeding to prevent complication.
Tube obstruction	■ Flush the tube with warm water. If necessary, replace the tube. ■ Flush the tube with 60 ml of water after each feeding to remove excess sticky formula, which could occlude the tube.
Nasal or pharyngeal irritation or necrosis	■ Provide frequent oral hygiene using mouthwash or lemon-glycerin swabs. ■ Use petroleum jelly on cracked lips. ■ Change the tube's position. If necessary, replace the tube.
Vomiting, bloating, diarrhea, or cramps	■ Reduce the flow rate. ■ Administer metoclopramide to increase GI motility. ■ Warm the formula. ■ For 30 minutes after feeding, position the patient on his right side with his head elevated to facilitate gastric emptying. ■ Notify the physician. He may want to reduce the amount of formula being given during each feeding.
Constipation	■ Provide additional fluids if the patient can tolerate them. ■ Administer a bulk-forming laxative. ■ Increase fruit, vegetable, or sugar content of the feeding.
Electrolyte imbalance	■ Monitor serum electrolyte levels. ■ Notify the physician. He may want to adjust the formula content to correct the deficiency.
Hyperglycemia	■ Monitor blood glucose levels. ■ Notify the physician of elevated levels. ■ Administer insulin if ordered. ■ The physician may adjust the sugar content of the formula.

▶ Small-bore feeding tubes may kink, making instillation impossible. If you suspect this problem, try changing the patient's position, or withdraw the tube a few inches and restart. Never use a guide wire to reposition the tube.

▶ If the patient becomes nauseated or vomits, stop the feeding immediately. The patient may vomit if his stomach becomes distended from overfeeding or delayed gastric emptying.

▶ To prevent air from entering the tube and the patient's stomach, never allow the syringe to empty completely. If you're using an infusion controller, set the flow rate according to the manufacturer's directions. Always give a tube feeding slowly—typically 200 to 350 ml over 15 to 30 minutes, depending on the patient's tolerance and the physician's order. The slower pace is to prevent sudden stomach distention, which can cause nausea, vomiting, cramps, or diarrhea.

▶ After you give the patient the appropriate amount of formula, flush the tubing by adding about 60 ml of water to the gavage bag or bulb syringe, or manually flush it using a barrel syringe. This maintains the tube's patency by removing excess formula, which could occlude the tube. The physician may order an additional 100 to 200 ml of water instilled twice per day (b.i.d.) or three times per day (t.i.d.) (depending on the patient's hydration status) to supplement enteral formulas which only deliver about 75% to 85% of the daily fluid requirements. Water will also be used to flush the tubing after the administration of medications.

▶ If you're administering a continuous feeding, flush the feeding tube every 4 hours to help prevent tube occlusion. Monitor gastric emptying every 4 hours.

▶ To discontinue gastric feeding (depending on the equipment you're using), close the regulator clamp on the gavage bag tubing, disconnect the syringe from the feeding tube, or turn off the infusion controller.

▶ Cover the end of the feeding tube with its plug or cap to prevent leakage and contamination of the tube.

▶ Leave the patient in semi-Fowler's or high Fowler's position for at least 30 minutes.

▶ Rinse all reusable equipment with warm water. Dry the equipment and store it in a convenient place for the next feeding. Change equipment every 24 hours or according to facility policy.

▶ Monitor serum electrolyte studies, blood urea nitrogen levels, serum glucose levels serum osmolality, and other pertinent findings to determine the patient's response to therapy and assess his hydration status.

Duodenal or jejunal feeding

▶ Elevate the head of the bed and place the patient in low Fowler's position.

▶ Open the enteral administration set, and hang the gavage container on the I.V. pole.

▶ If you're using a nasoduodenal tube, measure its external length to check tube placement. Remember that you may not get any residual when you aspirate the tube.

▶ Open the flow clamp and regulate the flow to the desired rate. To regulate the rate using a volumetric infusion pump, follow the manufacturer's directions for setting up the equipment. Most patients receive small amounts initially, with volumes increasing gradually once tolerance is established.

▶ Until the patient acquires a tolerance for the formula, you may need to dilute it to half or three-quarters strength to start, and increase it gradually.

▶ Flush the tube every 4 hours with water to maintain patency and provide hydration. A needle catheter jejunostomy tube may require flushing every 2 hours to prevent formula buildup inside the tube. A Y-connector may be useful for frequent flushing. Attach the continuous feeding to the main port and use the side port for flushes.

▶ During continuous feedings, assess the patient frequently for abdominal distention. Flush the tubing by adding about 50 ml of water to the gavage bag or bulb syringe. This maintains the tube's patency by removing excess formula, which could occlude the tube. Water will also be used to flush the tubing following the administration of medications through the tube. The physician may order an additional amount of water (100 to 300 ml) instilled b.i.d. or t.i.d. according to the hydration status of the client to supplement enteral formulas, which most only deliver about 75% to 85% of the daily fluid requirements.

▶ Check the flow rate hourly to ensure correct infusion. Constantly monitor the flow rate of a blended or high-residue formula to determine if the formula is clogging the tubing as it settles. To prevent such clogging, squeeze the bag frequently to agitate the solution.

- Monitor serum electrolyte studies, blood urea nitrogen levels, serum glucose levels, serum osmolality, and other pertinent findings to determine the patient's response to therapy and assess his hydration status.

Complications

Aspiration is a very serious complication of enteral nutrition and usually results in regurgitation of the enteral formula. Aspiration can occur because of improper positioning of the feeding tube or a delay in gastric emptying. To help prevent aspiration be sure to check the placement of the tube, check residuals, and raise the head of the patient's bed whenever possible.

Erosion of esophageal, tracheal, nasal, and oropharyngeal mucosa can result if tubes are left in place for a long time. If possible, use smaller-lumen tubes to prevent such irritation. Check facility policy regarding the frequency of changing feeding tubes to prevent complications.

Using the gastric route, frequent or large-volume feedings can cause bloating and retention. Dehydration, diarrhea, and vomiting can cause metabolic disturbances. Glycosuria, cramping, and abdominal distention usually indicate intolerance.

Tube displacement can also occur. Tubes may migrate or dislodge. Gastrostomy or jejunostomy tubes can migrate up or down the GI tract. Tubes that leak onto the surface of the skin will cause excoriation and eventual erosion. Keep traction on the tube at the skin surface to prevent the stomach contents from leaking. If a leak does occur and excoriation ensues, protect the skin surface with barrier creams or stoma devices.

A clogged feeding tube is a common problem when you use the duodenal or jejunal route. The patient may experience metabolic, fluid, and electrolyte abnormalities including hyperglycemia, glycosuria, hyperosmolar dehydration, coma, edema, hypernatremia, and essential fatty acid deficiency. Occlusion can be prevented by frequent flushing of the feeding tube.

The patient also may experience dumping syndrome, in which a large amount of hyperosmotic solution in the duodenum causes excessive diffusion of fluid through the semipermeable membrane and results in diarrhea. In a patient with low serum albumin levels, these signs may be caused by low oncotic pressure in the duodenal mucosa.

Patient teaching

- Tell the patient that he'll get nourishment through a tube, and explain the procedure to him. If possible, give him a schedule of subsequent feedings.
- If he'll receive home tube feeding, teach him how to use an infusion control device to maintain accuracy, how to use the syringe or bag and tubing, how to care for the tube and insertion site, and how to mix formula. Tell him that formula may be mixed in an electric blender according to package directions. Tell him to discard any mixed formula not used within 24 hours. If the formula must hang for more than 8 hours, advise the patient to use a gavage or pump administration set with an ice pouch to decrease the incidence of bacterial growth. Instruct him to use a new bag daily.
- Explain to the patient the importance of maintaining accurate records of his weight, feeding formula, water, bowel patterns, flatulence, and emesis and residuals. These records can be shown to the physician or health care provider during follow-up appointments.
- Teach family members the signs and symptoms of complications to report to the physician or home care nurse as well as measures to take in an emergency.

Documentation

On the intake and output sheet, record the date, volume of formula, and volume of water. In your notes, include abdominal assessment (including tube exit site, if appropriate); amount of residuals; verification of tube placement; amount, type, and time of feeding; and tube patency. Discuss the patient's tolerance to the feeding, including nausea, vomiting, cramping, diarrhea, and distention. Note the result of blood and urine tests, hydration status, and any drugs given through the tube. Include the date and time of administration set changes, oral and nasal hygiene, and results of specimen collections. Document your patient teaching measures and their effects.

ENTERAL TUBE MEDICATION ADMINISTRATION

Medication may be given through a nasogastric tube, a gastrostomy tube or, in certain cases, a gastrostomy feeding button. Besides providing an alternative means of nourishment, the enteric tube allows direct instillation of medication into the GI system of a patient who can't ingest it orally. Before instillation, carefully check the patency and positioning of the tube because this procedure is contraindicated if the tube is obstructed or improperly positioned, if the patient is vomiting, or if his bowel sounds are absent.

Oily medications and enteric-coated or sustained-release tablets are contraindicated for instillation through an enteric tube. Oily medications cling to the sides of the tube and resist mixing with the irrigating solution. Also, crushing enteric-coated or sustained-release tablets to facilitate transport through the tube destroys their intended effect.

Supplies

- Patient's medication record and chart
- Prescribed medication
- Towel or linen-saver pad
- 50- or 60-ml piston type catheter-tip syringe
- Feeding tubing
- Rubber band
- Two 4″ × 4″ gauze pads
- Stethoscope
- Gloves
- Diluent
- Cup for mixing medication and fluid
- Spoon
- Water
- Gastrostomy tube and funnel (if needed)
- Mild soap
- Optional: pill-crushing equipment (mortar and pestle, for example) and a clamp (if not already attached to tube)

Implementation

- For maximum control of suction, use a piston syringe instead of a bulb syringe. The liquid for diluting the medication can be juice, water, or a nutritional supplement. Check for incompatibilities before choosing the diluent.
- Gather the necessary equipment for use at the patient's bedside. Liquids should be at room temperature. Administering cold liquid through the enteric tube can cause abdominal cramping. Although this is not a sterile procedure, make sure the cup, syringe, spoon, and gauze are clean.
- If the prescribed medication is in tablet form, crush the tablets to ready them for mixing in a cup with the diluting liquid.
- Put on gloves.
- Detach the tube from the patient's gown. To avoid soiling the sheets during the procedure, fold back the bed linens to the patient's waist and drape his chest with a towel or linen-saver pad.
- Elevate the head of the bed so that the patient is in Fowler's position, as tolerated.

▶ Inspect the tube at the nare. When the tube is first inserted and placement is checked by X-ray, document the length of the external segment. Compare the length of the external segment now with that of the initial insertion. Note whether the tape securing the tube to the patient's face is in position. If the length of the external segment of the tube has increased, the tube may be out of place. If this happens, notify the physician.

▶ If the length of the external segment is accurate, unclamp the tube, then take the 50- or 60-ml syringe and create a 10-cc air space in its chamber. Finally, attach the syringe to the end of the tube.

▶ Auscultate the patient's abdomen about 3″ (7.5 cm) below the sternum with the stethoscope. Then gently insert the 10 cc of air into the tube. You should hear the air bubble entering the stomach. If you hear this sound, gently draw back on the piston of the syringe. The appearance of gastric contents implies that the tube is patent and in the stomach. (However, only an X-ray positively confirms the tube's position.) If no gastric contents appear when you draw back on the piston, the tube may have risen into the patient's esophagus, in which case you'll have to advance it before proceeding.

▶ If you meet resistance as you aspirate for stomach contents, stop the procedure. Resistance may indicate a nonpatent tube or improper tube placement. (Keep in mind that some smaller enteric tubes can collapse when aspiration is attempted.) If the tube seems to be in the stomach, resistance probably means the tube is lying against the stomach wall. To relieve resistance, withdraw the tube slightly or turn the patient.

▶ After you establish that the tube is patent and in the correct position, clamp the tube, detach the syringe, and place the end of the tube on the 4″ × 4″ gauze pad.

▶ Mix the crushed tablets with the diluent. If the medication is in capsule form, open the capsules and empty their contents into the liquid. Pour liquid medications directly into the diluting liquid. Stir well with the spoon. (If the medication was in tablet form, make sure the particles are small enough to pass through the eyes at the distal end of the tube.) Keep in mind that you need enough diluent to dissolve the medication, but not too much, which could result in fluid overload in the older patient.

▶ Reattach the syringe, without the piston, to the end of the tube and open the clamp.

▶ Deliver the medication slowly and steadily. Don't allow it to flow in too quickly; because of age-related changes in the GI tract, older patients are at risk for cramping.

▶ If the medication flows smoothly, slowly add more until the entire dose has been given. If the medication doesn't flow properly, don't force it. It may be too thick to flow through the tube. If so, dilute it with water, being careful not to overload the patient with fluid. If you suspect tube placement is inhibiting flow, stop the procedure and reevaluate the placement.

▶ Watch the patient's reaction throughout the procedure. If he shows any signs of discomfort, stop the procedure immediately.

▶ As the last of the medication flows out of the syringe, start to irrigate the tube by adding 30 to 50 ml of water. Irrigation clears medication from the sides of the tube and from the distal end, reducing the risk of clogging.

▶ When the water stops flowing, quickly clamp the tube. Detach the syringe and dispose of it properly.

▶ Fasten the enteric tube to the patient's gown.

▶ Remove the towel or linen-saver pad and replace the bed linens.

▶ Leave the patient in Fowler's position, or have him lie on his right side with the head of the bed partially elevated. Have him maintain this position for at least 30 minutes after the procedure to facilitate the downward flow of medication into his stomach and to prevent esophageal reflux.

▶ If you're asked to deliver medications through a gastrostomy tube or gastrostomy feeding button, see *Giving medications through a gastrostomy tube*.

Key point If the feeding button pops out during the procedure, reinsert it, estimate the amount of medication already delivered, and resume. Be aware of your facility's policy regarding reinsertion. Some facilities allow only specially trained personnel to reinsert a feeding button.

▶ Once daily, clean the peristomal skin with mild soap and water and let the skin air-dry for 20 minutes, to avoid skin irritation. Also, clean the site whenever spillage occurs.

▶ To prevent instillation of too much fluid (more than 400 ml of liquid at one time for an adult), plan the medication instillation so that it doesn't coincide with the patient's regular enteric tube feeding, if possible. Make sure that you calculate the patient's fluid needs based on his condition. Take into consideration the amount of fluid used for irrigation.

▶ When you must schedule a tube feeding and medication instillation simultaneously, administer the medication first to ensure that the patient receives the full prescribed drug therapy, even if he can't tolerate an entire feeding. Remember to avoid giving him foods that may interact adversely with the medication.

▶ If the patient receives continuous tube feedings, stop the feeding and check the quantity of residual stomach contents. Although older people have decreased gastric emptying, the amount of residual that would alert you to withhold medications and feedings is usually 100 ml. However, check your facility's policy for the exact standard. An excessive amount of residual contents might indicate intestinal obstruction or paralytic ileus.

▶ If the enteric tube is attached to suction, be sure to turn off the suction for 20 to 30 minutes after administering the medication.

Complications

Aspiration of stomach contents and adverse drug reactions are potential problems with enteral tube medication administration. If medication is given in conjunction with a continuous enteral feeding, be alert for delayed or impaired drug absorption.

Patient teaching

▶ Explain the procedure to the patient and his family members to reduce their fear and promote cooperation.

▶ If possible, teach the patient who requires long-term treatment to instill the medication himself. Have him observe you as you perform the procedure several times before you allow him to try it himself.

▶ Make sure that you remain with the patient when he performs the procedure for the first few times so that you can provide assistance and answer any questions. As the patient performs the procedure, give him positive reinforcement and correct any errors in his technique as necessary.

Documentation

Note the drug administered, the dose, the date and time, and the patient's reaction, if any. If the patient refuses a drug, document the refusal and notify the patient's physician as needed. Also note if a drug was omitted or withheld for other reasons. Document your patient teaching measures and their effects.

Giving medications through a gastrostomy tube

Surgically inserted into the stomach, a gastrostomy tube reduces the risk of fluid aspiration into the lungs, a constant danger with a nasogastric (NG) tube.

To administer medication by this route, prepare the patient and medication as you would for an NG tube. Then gently lift the dressing around the tube to assess the skin for irritation caused by gastric secretions. Report any redness or irritation to the physician. If there is no irritation, follow these steps:

- Remove the dressing that covers the tube. Then remove the dressing or plug at the tip of the tube and attach the syringe or funnel to the tip.
- Release the clamp and instill about 10 ml of water into the tube through the syringe to check for patency. If the water flows in easily, the tube is patent. If it flows in slowly, raise the funnel to increase pressure. If the water still doesn't flow properly, stop the procedure and notify the physician.
- Pour up to 30 ml of medication into the syringe or funnel. Tilt the tube to allow air to escape as the fluid flows downward. Just before the syringe empties, add medication as needed.
- After giving the medication, pour in about 30 ml of water to flush the tube.
- Tighten the clamp, place a 4″ × 4″ gauze pad on the end of the tube, and secure it with a rubber band.
- Cover the tube with two more 4″ × 4″ gauze pads, and secure them firmly with tape.
- Keep the head of the bed elevated for at least 30 minutes after the procedure to aid digestion.

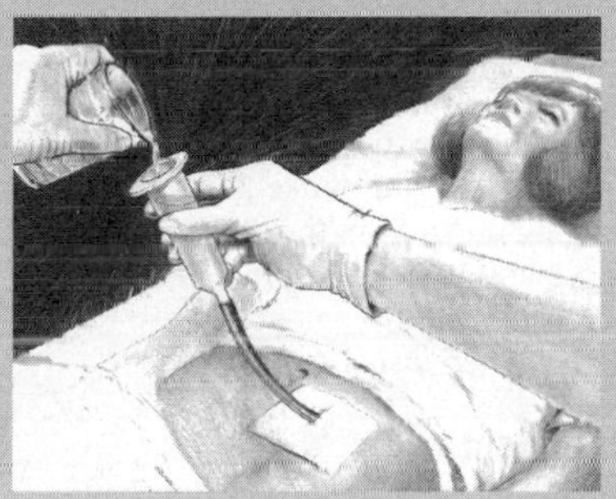

ENTROPION AND ECTROPION

An older adult's eyes sometimes appear sunken and the eyelid turned inward (entropion). In other older people, the eyelid sometimes falls away, taking on the appearance of turning outward (ectropion). Although these conditions are commonly seen, they aren't a problem unless they cause eye irritation.

Entropion is caused by a spasm in the lower orbicular muscle of the eyelid margin. This is more common in the lower lid, causing the lid to turn inward and abrade its margin against the eyeball. The lashes rub against the cornea with each blink and can cause chronic irritation.

In entropion, the fat cushion behind the eye shrinks, causing the eyes to recess into the sockets. Thus, in an older patient, sunken eyes may not always indicate dehydration.

Ectropion is caused by a loss of strength of the orbicular muscle — the muscle that squeezes the eyelids shut. Other causes include old age, relaxation of the skin, a cicatrix following trauma, infection, and palsy of the facial nerve. When the margin of the lower lid no longer touches the eye, the punctum of the medial lower lid doesn't touch it either, and tears can't drain from the conjunctival sac into the lacrimal sac. Corneal dryness and decreased visual acuity can occur if untreated.

Signs and symptoms

Entropion

- Constant sensation that something is lodged in the eye
- Margin of the eyelid turned inward
- Lashes stroking the eyeball as the patient blinks
- Photophobia
- Corneal trauma
- Decreased visual acuity

Ectropion

- Excessive tears and tears draining down the patient's face
- Eyelids not closing when the patient sleeps
- Dry eyes upon awakening
- Eyes appearing sunken, with the lid hanging down from the margin of the eye (that is, where the pink conjunctiva meets the white)
- Decreased visual acuity

Treatment

Entropion is usually treated surgically. Treatment of ectropion usually focuses on relieving signs and symptoms; if the patient's cornea becomes dry, the physician may recommend surgery.

Key nursing diagnoses and outcomes

Disturbed sensory perception (visual) related to diminishing ability to see properly as a result of entropion or ectropion

Treatment outcome: The patient will resume a functional lifestyle.

Risk for injury related to decrease in vision caused by entropion or ectropion

Treatment outcomes: The patient will take precautions to protect himself from injury and won't sustain injury.

Nursing interventions

- Instruct the patient not to rub his eyes.
- Use warm compresses to relieve irritation.

PATIENT TEACHING

- Tell the patient about the importance of having regular eye checkups.
- Advise the patient who has excessive tears to carry tissues and blot his eyes, not rub them.
- Instruct him to report any persistent dryness or itching of the eyes to the physician.

EPIDURAL ANALGESIA ADMINISTRATION

To administer epidural analgesia, the physician injects or infuses medication into the epidural space, which lies just outside the subarachnoid space where cerebrospinal fluid (CSF) flows. The drug diffuses slowly into the subarachnoid space of the spinal canal and then into the CSF, which carries it directly into the spinal area — bypassing the blood-brain barrier. In some cases, the physician injects drugs directly into the subarachnoid space.

Epidural analgesia helps manage acute or chronic pain, including moderate to severe postoperative pain, and prevents narcotic-induced hypertension. It's especially useful in patients with cancer or degenerative joint disease. This procedure works well because opiate receptors are located along the entire spinal cord. Narcotic drugs act directly on the receptors of the dorsal horn to produce localized analgesia without motor blockade.

Narcotics, such as morphine, fentanyl, and hydromorphone, are administered by a bolus dose or continuous infusion and alone or in combination with bupivacaine (a local anesthetic). The infusion, given through an epidural cath-

Placement of a permanent epidural catheter

An epidural catheter is implanted beneath the patient's skin and inserted near the spinal cord at the first lumbar (L1) interspace.

For temporary analgesic therapy (less than 1 week), the catheter may exit directly over the spine and be taped up the patient's back to the shoulder. However, for prolonged therapy, the catheter may be tunneled subcutaneously to an exit site on the patient's side or abdomen or over his shoulder.

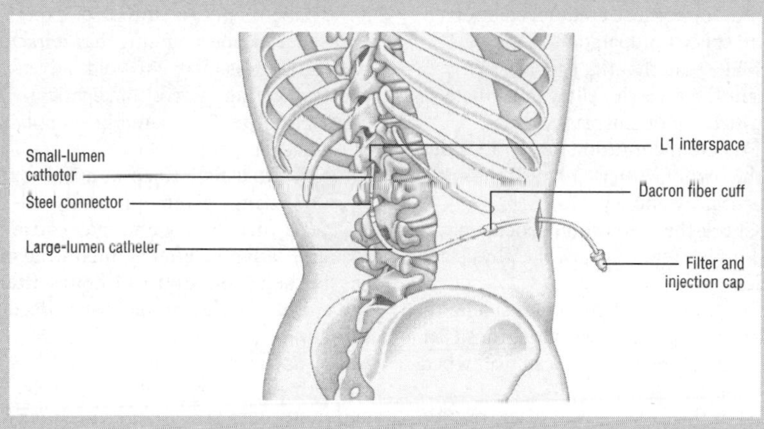

eter, is preferable because it delivers a smaller drug dose continuously. The epidural catheter, inserted near the spinal cord, eliminates the risks of multiple I.M. injections, minimizes adverse cerebral and systemic effects, and eliminates the analgesic peaks and valleys that usually occur with intermittent I.M. injections. (See *Placement of a permanent epidural catheter.*)

Typically, epidural catheter insertion is performed by an anesthesiologist using aseptic technique. Once the catheter has been inserted, the nurse is responsible for monitoring the infusion and assessing the patient.

Epidural analgesia is contraindicated in patients who have local or systemic infection, neurologic disease, anticoagulant therapy, coagulopathy, spinal arthritis or deformity, hypotension, severe hypertension, or allergy to the prescribed drug.

Supplies

- Volume infusion device and epidural infusion tubing (depending on facility policy)
- Patient's medication record
- Prescribed epidural solutions
- Transparent dressing or sterile gauze pads
- Epidural supply tray with epidural catheter
- Labels for epidural infusion line
- Silk tape
- Emergency drugs and equipment, such as naloxone and ephedrine, oxygen intubation equipment, and a handheld resuscitation bag
- Optional: monitoring equipment for blood pressure and pulse and apnea monitor

Implementation

Use of an epidural catheter

▶ Explain the procedure to the patient, and inform him that he may experience some pain with insertion.

▶ Make sure a consent form has been properly signed.

▶ Make sure the pharmacy has been notified in advance about the medication order because epidural solutions require special preparation.

▶ Make sure that the patient has a patent I.V. access to allow immediate administration of emergency drugs.

▶ Prepare the infusion device according to the manufacturer's instructions and your facility's policy.

▶ Check the medication concentration and infusion rate against the physician's order.

▶ Position the patient on his side in the knee-chest position, or have him sit on the edge of the bed and lean over a bedside table.

▶ After the catheter is in place, prime the infusion device, confirm the appropriate medication and infusion rate, and then adjust the device for the correct rate.

▶ Help the anesthesiologist connect the infusion tubing to the epidural catheter. Then connect the tubing to the infusion pump.

▶ Secure all connection sites with silk tape, and label the catheter, infusion tubing, and infusion pump with EPIDURAL INFUSION to prevent accidental infusion of other drugs into the epidural lines. Then start the infusion.

▶ Tell the patient to report immediately any feeling of pain. A pain scale from 0 to 10 is often difficult for the older patient to use. It's easier to ask him if he has no pain, or mild, moderate, severe, or the worst possible pain. If the patient reports pain that's intolerable, the infusion rate may need to be increased. Call the physician or change the rate within prescribed limits.

▶ Assess the patient's respiratory rate and blood pressure every hour, initially. Notify the physician if the patient's respiratory rate is less than 10 breaths/minute or if his systolic blood pressure is less than 90 mm Hg.

▶ Assess the patient's sedation level, mental status, and pain-relief status every hour for the first 24 hours, then every 2 to 4 hours, until adequate pain control is achieved. Notify the physician if the patient appears drowsy or experiences nausea and vomiting, has refractory itching, or is unable to void (adverse effects of certain narcotic analgesics). Also notify the physician if he complains of unrelieved pain.

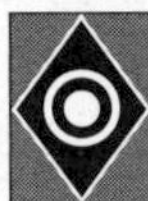

Drug alert Keep in mind that drugs given epidurally diffuse slowly and may cause adverse effects, including excessive sedation, up to 12 hours after the epidural infusion has been discontinued.

▶ Assess lower-extremity motor strength every 2 to 4 hours. If sensory and motor loss occur, large motor-nerve fibers have been affected and dosage may need to be decreased.

▶ If ordered, place the patient on an apnea monitor for the first 24 hours after beginning the infusion.

▶ Change the dressing over the catheter's exit site every 24 to 48 hours, or as needed. The dressing is usually transparent to allow inspection of drainage and commonly appears moist or slightly blood-tinged.

▶ Change the epidural infusion tubing every 48 hours, or as specified by facility policy.

Removal of an epidural catheter

▶ Typically, the anesthesiologist orders analgesics and removes the catheter. However, your facility's policy may allow a specially trained nurse to remove the catheter.

▶ If you're removing the catheter and feel resistance, stop and call the physician for further orders.

▶ The physician will examine the catheter tip to rule out any damage during removal, so be sure to save the catheter.

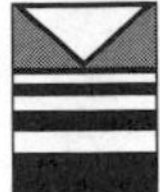

Key point If CSF leaks into the dura mater during removal of an epidural catheter, the patient usually experiences a headache. The postanalgesia headache worsens with postural changes, such as standing or sitting. The headache can be treated with a procedure called a *blood patch,* in which the patient's own blood (about 10 ml) is withdrawn from a peripheral vein and then injected into the epidural space. When the epidural needle is withdrawn, the patient is instructed to sit up. Because the blood clots seal off the leaking area, the blood patch should relieve the patient's headache immediately. The patient need not restrict his activity after this procedure.

Complications

Numbness and leg weakness may occur after the first 24 hours and is drug- and concentration-dependent. Identifying the dosage level that provides adequate pain control without causing excessive numbness and weakness requires titration of the dosage.

Respiratory depression usually occurs during the first 24 hours (treated with I.V. naloxone). Pruritus may appear (treated with I.V. nalbuphine or I.V. diphenhydramine), and nausea and vomiting (treated with I.V. prochlorperazine or I.V. metoclopramide) are possible.

Patient teaching

- Explain the procedure to the patient and his family members.
- Tell the patient to report any pain or numbness, weakness, or tingling in his extremities.
- Explain that home use of epidural analgesia is possible only if the patient or his family members are willing and able to learn the care needed.
- Tell the home-use patient that he must abstain from alcohol and street drugs, because these substances potentiate opiate action.
- Teach the patient and his family members how to administer epidural analgesia and how to identify complications and treat them.

Documentation

Record the patient's response to treatment, catheter patency, condition of the dressing and insertion site, vital signs, and assessment results. Also, document dressing changes, infusion bag changes, the need for additional analgesics, if any, and the patient's response to the additional analgesia. Also document your patient teaching measures and their effects.

ESOPHAGEAL CANCER

Most common in men over age 60, esophageal cancer is nearly always fatal. Because the patient is usually asymptomatic during the early stages of esophageal cancer, diagnosis is commonly delayed until the cancer has spread or is unresectable. The disease occurs worldwide, but incidence varies geographically. It's most commonly found in Japan, Russia, China, the Middle East, and the Transkei region of South Africa.

Esophageal tumors are usually fungating and infiltrating. In most cases, the tumor partially constricts the lumen of the esophagus. Regional metastasis occurs early by way of submucosal lymphatics, in many cases fatally invading adjacent vital intrathoracic organs. If the patient survives primary extension, the liver and lungs are the usual sites of distant metastases. Unusual metastasis sites include the bone, kidneys, and adrenal glands.

Most cases (98%) arise in squamous cell epithelium, although a few are adenocarcinomas and fewer still, melanomas and sarcomas. About half the squamous cell cancers occur in the lower portion of the esophagus, 40% in the midportion, and the remaining 10% in the upper or cervical esophagus. Regardless of cell type, the prognosis for esophageal cancer is grim: 5-year survival rates are less than 5%, and most patients die within 6 months of diagnosis.

Although the cause of esophageal cancer is unknown, several predisposing factors have been identified. These include chronic irritation from heavy smoking or excessive use of alcohol; stasis-induced inflammation, as in achalasia or stricture; previous head and neck tumors; and nutritional deficiency, as in untreated sprue and Plummer-Vinson syndrome.

Signs and symptoms

- Early complaints of mild dysphagia (commonly mistaken for a normal change of aging)
- Feeling of fullness, pressure, indigestion, or substernal burning
- Complaints of needing antacids to relieve GI upset
- Weight loss
- Hoarseness
- Chronic cough (possibly from aspiration)
- Anorexia
- Vomiting
- Regurgitation of food
- Pain that radiates to the back
- Appearance changes in late stages (thin, cachectic, and dehydrated)

Diagnostic tests

- *X-rays of the esophagus,* with *barium swallow* and *motility studies,* delineate structural and filling defects and reduced peristalsis.
- *Esophagoscopy,* punch and brush *biopsies*, and exfoliative *cytologic tests* confirm esophageal tumors.
- *Bronchoscopy* (usually performed after an esophagoscopy) may reveal tumor growth in the tracheobronchial tree.
- *Endoscopic ultrasonography* of the esophagus combines endoscopy and ultrasound technology to measure the tumor's depth of penetration.
- *Computed tomography scan* may help diagnose and monitor esophageal lesions.
- *Magnetic resonance imaging* permits evaluation of the esophagus and adjacent structures.

Treatment

Esophageal cancer usually is advanced when diagnosed, so surgery and other treatments can only relieve disease effects. Palliative therapy consists of treatment to keep the esophagus open, including esophageal dilation, laser therapy, radiation therapy, and installation of prosthetic tubes (such as a Celestin's tube) to bridge the tumor.

The surgeon may use radical surgery to excise the tumor and resect either the esophagus alone or the stomach and the esophagus. Either the stomach (gastric pull-up) or a portion of the colon (colon interposition) may be used to replace the esophagus. Other treatment choices are chemotherapy and radiation therapy to slow the growth of the tumor and gastrostomy or jejunostomy to help provide adequate nutrition.

Your patient may have a prosthesis to seal any fistula that develops. He may be given endoscopic laser treatment and bipolar electrocoagulation to help restore swallowing by vaporizing cancerous tissue. If the tumor is in the upper esophagus, however, the laser can't be positioned properly. He'll probably be given analgesics for pain control.

Key nursing diagnoses and outcomes

Imbalanced nutrition: Less than body requirements related to impaired swallowing

Treatment outcome: The patient will have no signs or symptoms of malnutrition.

Risk for aspiration related to esophageal blockage

Treatment outcomes: The patient will expectorate secretions without aspiration and won't develop aspiration pneumonia.

Impaired swallowing related to obstruction

Treatment outcomes: The patient will consent to treatments that improve swallowing such as periodic dilatation of the esophagus and won't develop malnutrition, aspiration pneumonia, or other complications of impaired swallowing.

Nursing interventions

- Monitor the patient's food and fluid intake.
- Provide rest periods before meals.
- Provide high-calorie, high-protein foods. Thicken liquids with thickening agents before offering them to the patient. Begin by giving the patient cold liquids and progressing to hot liquids. As you introduce solid foods, begin with pureed foods progressing to soft foods that are cut into bite-sized pieces.
- As ordered, provide tube feedings and prepare the patient for supplementary parenteral nutrition.
- To prevent food aspiration, place the patient in Fowler's position for meals and allow plenty of time to eat. If he regurgitates food after eating, provide mouth care.
- Prepare the patient for a gastrostomy as indicated. When using a gastrostomy tube for nutritional support, give food slowly, by gravity, in prescribed amounts (usually 200 to 500 ml). Offer the patient something to chew before each feeding. This promotes gastric secretions and provides some semblance of normal eating.
- Administer ordered analgesics for pain relief as necessary. Provide comfort measures, such as repositioning, and distractions to help decrease discomfort.
- Protect the patient from infection.
- Make sure the patient is referred to a speech therapist to help with his swallowing disorder.
- Prepare the patient for surgery to treat esophageal cancer as indicated. Answer any questions and let him know what to expect after surgery.
- After surgery, monitor vital signs, fluid and electrolyte balance, and intake and output. Immediately report any unexpected changes in the patient's condition. Also monitor for complications, such as infection, fistula formation, pneumonia, empyema, and malnutrition.
- If an anastomosis to the esophagus was performed, watch for signs of an anastomotic leak.
- If the patient had a prosthetic tube inserted, monitor for signs and symptoms of blockage or dislodgment. This can cause perforation of the mediastinum or precipitate tumor erosion.
- After radiation therapy, monitor the patient for complications, such as esophageal perforation, pneumonitis and fibrosis of the lungs, and myelitis of the spinal cord.
- After chemotherapy, monitor for complications, such as bone marrow suppression and GI reactions.
- After chemotherapy, take steps to decrease adverse effects such as providing normal saline mouthwash to help prevent mouth ulcers. Allow the patient plenty of rest, and administer medications as ordered to reduce adverse effects.
- Throughout therapy, answer the patient's questions, and tell him what to expect from surgery and other therapies. Listen to his fears and concerns, and stay with him during periods of severe anxiety.
- Encourage the patient to identify actions and care measures that will promote his comfort and relaxation. Try to perform these measures, and encourage the patient and his family members to do so, too.

▶ Whenever possible, include the patient in care decisions.
▶ Anticipate referral to home care to assist with follow-up, teaching, patient care, and support.
▶ If all other treatments have failed, concentrate on keeping the patient comfortable and free from pain, providing as much psychological support as possible.

PATIENT TEACHING

▶ If appropriate, teach a family member or friend gastrostomy tube care. This includes checking tube patency before each feeding, providing skin care around the tube, and keeping the patient upright during and after feedings.
▶ Stress the importance of adequate nutrition. Ask a dietitian to instruct the patient and his family members. If the patient has difficulty swallowing solids, instruct him to puree or liquefy his food and to follow a high-calorie, high-protein diet to minimize weight loss. Also, recommend that he add a commercially available, high-calorie supplement to his diet.
▶ If surgery is scheduled, explain the procedures the patient will undergo afterward: closed chest drainage, nasogastric suctioning, and placement of gastrostomy tubes.
▶ Encourage the patient to follow as normal a routine as possible after recovery from surgery and during radiation therapy and chemotherapy. This will help him maintain a sense of control and reduce complications associated with immobility.
▶ Advise the patient to rest between activities and to stop any activity that tires him or causes pain.
▶ Refer the patient and his family members to appropriate organizations such as the American Cancer Society.

ESOPHAGEAL DIVERTICULA

Occurring as hollow outpouchings of the esophageal wall, esophageal diverticula develop in three main areas: just above the upper esophageal sphincter (Zenker's or pulsion diverticulum, the most common type), near the midpoint of the esophagus (midesophageal diverticulum), and just above the lower esophageal sphincter (epiphrenic diverticulum, the rarest type). Diverticula may involve one or more layers of the mucosa.

Generally, esophageal diverticula occur later in life, but they can also affect infants and children. The disorder is three times more common in men than in women. Epiphrenic diverticula usually appear in middle-aged men. Zenker's diverticulum usually strikes men over age 60.

Esophageal diverticula are due to either primary muscular abnormalities that may be congenital or to inflammatory processes adjacent to the esophagus. Zenker's diverticulum is caused by developmental muscle weakness of the posterior pharynx above the border of the cricopharyngeal muscle. The pressure of swallowing aggravates this weakness, as does contraction of the pharynx before relaxation of the sphincter, resulting in the development of diverticula.

A midesophageal diverticulum may be a response to scarring and pulling on esophageal walls by an external inflammatory process such as tuberculosis or by traction from old adhesions. Another cause may be propulsion associated with esophageal motor abnormalities such as diffuse esophageal spasm. An epiphrenic diverticulum probably results from traction and pulsation or from esophageal motor disturbances, such as diffuse esophageal spasm and achalasia.

Regurgitation of saliva or food particles may lead to aspiration, causing pulmonary complications, such as bronchitis, bronchiectasis, and lung abscess. The disorder may also lead to esophageal perforation.

Signs and symptoms

- Recent weight loss
- Difficulty eating
- Throat irritation
- Heartburn
- Dysphagia and regurgitation of saliva and food particles soon after eating
- Gurgling sounds in the neck when swallowing liquids
- Nocturnal coughing
- Bad taste in the mouth
- Halitosis
- Swelling at the side of the neck caused by food trapped in the diverticulum

Diagnostic tests

- *Barium swallow* usually confirms the diagnosis by showing a characteristic outpouching.
- *Esophagoscopy* may rule out another lesion as the cause of the problem.

Treatment

For Zenker's diverticulum, treatment is usually palliative, including a bland diet, thoroughly chewed food, and water drunk after eating to flush out the sac. However, severe signs and symptoms or a large diverticulum require surgery to remove the sac or facilitate drainage. An esophagomyotomy may be necessary to prevent recurrence.

A midesophageal or an epiphrenic diverticulum typically requires no therapy because it usually produces no signs or symptoms or complications. If signs and symptoms occur, treatment includes antacids and an antireflux regimen. If the diverticulum becomes very large and causes signs and symptoms, surgical removal may be indicated. Distal myotomy is usually performed if the diverticulum is associated with esophageal motor abnormalities.

If surgery is necessary, then, depending on the patient's nutritional status, treatment may also include insertion of a nasogastric tube (passed carefully to prevent perforation) and tube feedings to prepare for the stress of surgery.

Key nursing diagnoses and outcomes

Impaired nutrition: Less than body requirements related to dysphagia

Treatment outcomes: The patient will consume a nutritionally balanced diet in a form that he can swallow and won't exhibit signs and symptoms of malnutrition.

Risk for aspiration related to regurgitation of food particles and saliva

Treatment outcomes: The patient will employ measures to prevent aspiration, such as keeping his head elevated for at least 2 hours after eating and using massage or postural drainage to empty any visible outpouching in the neck before lying down, and won't exhibit signs and symptoms of aspiration.

Impaired swallowing related to muscular abnormalities

Treatment outcome: The patient won't develop complications of dysphagia, such as malnutrition and aspiration pneumonia.

Chronic pain related to dysphagia and feelings of fullness and pressure in the sternal region.

Treatment outcome: The patient will report relief or reduction in pain.

Nursing interventions

- If the patient regurgitates food and mucus, protect him from aspiration by positioning him with his head elevated or turned to one side.
- If the patient has dysphagia, record well-tolerated foods and note circumstances that ease swallowing. If neces

sary, provide a "blenderized" diet, with vitamin or protein supplements.

▶ If the patient with a midesophageal or an epiphrenic diverticulum has discomfort, administer ordered antacids and provide antireflux care: Keep his head elevated; maintain him in an upright position for 2 hours after eating; provide small, frequent meals; control chronic coughing by administering antitussives, if ordered; and avoid constrictive clothing.

▶ If surgery is scheduled, perform required preoperative and postoperative care.

▶ Support the patient emotionally, especially if he's upset and concerned about his signs and symptoms.

▶ Regularly assess the patient's nutritional status (weight, caloric intake, physical appearance).

▶ Monitor the patient's degree of discomfort and the effectiveness of treatment.

▶ Monitor for respiratory signs and symptoms that suggest aspiration.

PATIENT TEACHING

▶ Teach the patient about his disorder. Explain necessary diagnostic tests and treatments.

▶ Emphasize the need to chew food thoroughly to prevent food particles from becoming trapped in the diverticulum.

▶ Teach the patient how to perform massage or postural drainage to prevent aspiration. He should use these techniques to empty any visible outpouching in the neck before lying down. Also teach the patient to prevent aspiration by elevating the head of the bed or turning his head to the side. Instruct him to not eat food within 2 to 4 hours of going to bed.

▶ If surgery is necessary, provide complete preoperative teaching. Make sure the patient understands the surgical approach, its desired effects, and possible complications.

EXERCISE

The value of lifelong exercise in maintaining good health has become evident to health care professionals. The benefits of exercise include increased energy and independence, a sense of well-being and relaxation, reduced stress and fatigue and, in some cases, weight loss and improved patterns of sleep.

Key point Exercise helps to prevent heart disease, type 2 diabetes, hypertension, and colon cancer. It can help lower serum triglycerides and cholesterol, decrease anxiety and depression, reduce body fat, increase bone density and lean muscle mass, increase strength and flexibility, decrease effects of arthritis, improve gait and balance, increase energy and improve mobility.

Notably, experts have singled out aerobic exercise — physical exertion that's sustained long enough to cause a marked temporary increase in respiratory and heart rates — as the key factor in healthy aging.

Studies have shown that, to be effective, exercise must be performed at regular intervals over time. Most experts believe fitness results are negligible if a person exercises fewer than three times a week. Conversely, a person seems to gain no additional benefit if he exercises more than five times per week. For a time, a regimen of 20 to 30 minutes of continuous activity per day was deemed necessary to obtain an aerobic benefit. However, more recent research that's especially germane to older adults has found that three 10-minute exercise sessions per day confer the same fitness benefits as one 30-minute session. Furthermore, people who haven't exercised at all appear to gain most significantly in reduced risk of cardiovascular problems by achieving small increases in activity.

Implementation

Many community-dwelling older people can reach an aerobic fitness level. Frail older persons who are institutionalized can also do well by maintaining or increasing minimal levels of activity.

You'll need a physician's endorsement before you plan and introduce an exercise program for an older person. The scope of this evaluation is determined by the primary care provider and may include a history and physical examination (focusing on the cardiovascular, pulmonary, musculoskeletal, and neurologic systems), diagnostic tests of renal and liver function, an electrocardiogram and, possibly, an exercise stress test. The stress test provides valuable information on maximum aerobic capacity, which can then be used to tailor an exercise program to the individual. The evaluation is less thorough for frail older people, whose exercise goals are more modest.

The individualized exercise program aims to maintain or increase flexibility, strength, endurance, range of motion, balance, and coordination. It should include a 10-minute warm-up of stretching exercises, followed by the actual conditioning activity, and end with a 10-minute cool-down session of slow walking and stretching. To ensure success and compliance, involve the individual in planning realistic and enjoyable exercises and explain their specific health benefits.

Other factors that encourage compliance include a convenient or on-site exercise location, group participation, scheduling that fits into the patient's current lifestyle, low cost, and absence of special equipment requirements. In addition, some managed care insurance plans provide financial incentives for participating in ongoing exercise programs.

Before your patient begins an exercise program, remember to document his baseline functional status, resting blood pressure, and resting pulse rate. A patient who has been sedentary most of his life must attain a minimum level of exercise intensity before he'll derive any aerobic benefit. (See *Starting an exercise program*.)

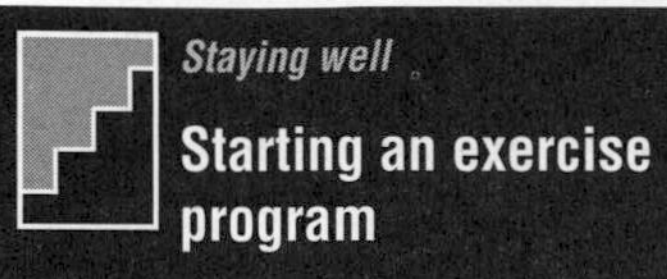

Staying well

Starting an exercise program

Exercise programs for older adults should start slowly and increase according to the individual's tolerance levels. Most programs begin with the patient exercising for 5 minutes or until he reaches his tolerance level. The patient should take frequent rest periods during exercise until he can endure 20 to 30 minutes of sustained activity. Make sure the patient consults with his physician before starting any exercise program.

The American College of Sports Medicine has identified three levels of exercise intensity: low intensity, categorized as less than 50% of maximum aerobic intensity; moderate intensity, 50% to 70%; and high intensity, greater than 70%. The minimum exercise level required for cardiovascular benefit is 40% to 50% of maximum aerobic capacity.

You can calculate maximum aerobic capacity by using the results of the exercise stress test or by using this formula:

220 − (age) = maximum predicted heart rate.

Then calculate the target heart rate by multiplying the maximum predicted heart rate by the percentage of the maximum rate desired for the particular patient. For example, for a 70-year-old sedentary patient who'll be exercising at 55% of maximum aerobic capacity (moderate intensity), calculate the target heart rate as follows:

220 − 70 = 150 (maximum predicted heart rate)
150 × 0.55 = 82 (target heart rate).

Teach the individual to monitor his pulse rate during exercise to avoid exceeding the target heart rate and overstressing the heart. Advise him to monitor his pulse rate during the cool-down phase for return to the resting heart rate.

This monitoring method is contraindicated for those who are taking medications that alter the resting heart rate. A practical safe alternative (if concurrent cardiovascular monitoring is unavailable) is to institute a low-intensity exercise program that includes normal everyday activities, such as walking, gentle stretching, and gardening.

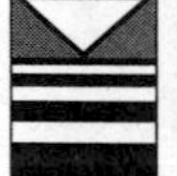

Key point Because older adults have reduced thirst perception, they're at increased risk for dehydration. Monitoring hydration status and replacing fluids are critical before, during, and after exercise.

Special considerations

Regardless of the setting in which you work, you can take steps to see that your patient becomes—and stays—physically active.

Community-based settings

If you work in a senior, adult day-care center or community health center, you can create exercise programs for individuals or groups. Check community resources. Many YMCAs and fitness centers offer programs tailored to older people. Some programs include patients with special needs, such as those who have arthritis or are physically challenged. Many shopping malls open early for senior walkers, thereby providing a safe, comfortable environment for walking at all times of the year. Hospitals are also beginning to reach out to community-dwelling older people who have fragile support systems.

If your patient says he can't exercise because of lack of time, fear of injury, or fatigue, provide encouragement to motivate him.

Institutional settings

If you're working with frail older people in a long-term care setting, you can intervene on several levels to maintain and enhance residents' physical activity. At the administrative or staff development level, you can emphasize functional mobility as a priority for staff members and educate them in specific measures to facilitate this. Staff nurses need to establish a baseline functional assessment for each patient and implement a program to maintain or improve this level, including periodic reassessment.

For independently mobile patients, offer a group exercise program three to five times per week, and provide opportunities for independent or supervised walking, which may be combined with physical, occupational, or recreational therapy (for example, group outings to a park, nature center, or mall). Another option is a therapeutic aquatic program, either on-site or at the local YMCA (with transportation provided). Individuals who use wheelchairs but are physically active can also be included in group exercises for upper-extremity strengthening—such as working out on pulleys in the physical therapy department.

Frail older people who need help to ambulate can participate in a daily walking program to improve mobility, maintain or improve endurance, and prevent falls. For example, the patient can walk to and from the dining room or the bathroom with the help of nursing assistants. Staff members also benefit because their physical care burden is decreased and the potential for back injury is reduced. Studies show patient benefits (improved mobility, decreased falls) from such activities as tai chi (an ancient Chinese system of exercises), yoga, flexibility exercises, and endurance and resistance exercises.

Ambulatory patients with dementia tend to wander. To include them in exercise activities, provide a safe area for such patients to move about, and make sure they don't physically exhaust themselves. Also, monitor their nutritional and hydration status.

If you're working with older patients in an acute care facility, perform an admission assessment to determine preadmission functional levels, current level of performance, and postdischarge goals to promote physical activity and independence. Because dramatic and rapid changes can occur in this population, evaluate activities of daily living capabilities and mobility daily. If the treatment plan calls for bed rest, continuously reassess the need for the immobility.

Early discharge planning and rehabilitation therapies can help the patient regain functional ground. Teaching patients bed exercises, such as quadriceps strengthening and preventive measures for footdrop, contribute to improvement. Carrying out or supervising patient transfers and ambulation orders is also critical. A restorative nursing program, tailored to the patient's needs, may also be indicated.

Recommend follow-up measures that promote a return to optimal functioning and create a supportive environment, such as home health services with physical or occupational therapy, specific instructions for exercises for the patient to perform at home, or an outpatient rehabilitation program (such as cardiac rehabilitation).

EYE MEDICATION ADMINISTRATION

Eye medications — drops, ointments, and disks — serve diagnostic and therapeutic purposes. During an eye examination, eyedrops can be used to anesthetize the eye, dilate the pupil to facilitate examination, and stain the cornea to identify corneal abrasions, scars, or other anomalies. Eye medications can also be used to lubricate the eye, treat certain eye conditions (such as glaucoma and infections), protect the vision of neonates, and lubricate the eye socket for insertion of a prosthetic eye.

Understanding the ocular effects of medications is important because certain drugs may cause eye disorders or have serious ocular effects. For example, anticholinergics, which are commonly used during eye examinations, can precipitate acute glaucoma in patients with a predisposition to the disorder.

Supplies

- Prescribed eye medication
- Patient's medication record and chart
- Gloves
- Warm water or normal saline solution
- Sterile gauze pads
- Facial tissues
- Optional: ocular dressing

Implementation

- Verify the order on the patient's medication record by checking it against the physician's order in his chart.
- Make sure the medication is labeled for ophthalmic use. Then check the expiration date. Remember to date the container the first time you use the medication.
- Inspect ocular solutions for cloudiness, discoloration, and precipitation, but remember that some eye medications are suspensions and normally appear cloudy. Don't use any solution that appears abnormal. If the tip of an eye ointment tube has crusted, turn the tip on a sterile gauze pad to remove the crust.
- Wash your hands.
- Check the medication label against the medication.
- Make sure you know which eye to treat because different medications or doses may be ordered for each eye.

Instilling eye medication

To instill eyedrops, pull the lower lid down to expose the conjunctival sac. Have the patient look up and away as you squeeze the prescribed number of drops into the sac. Release the patient's eyelid and have him blink to distribute the medication.

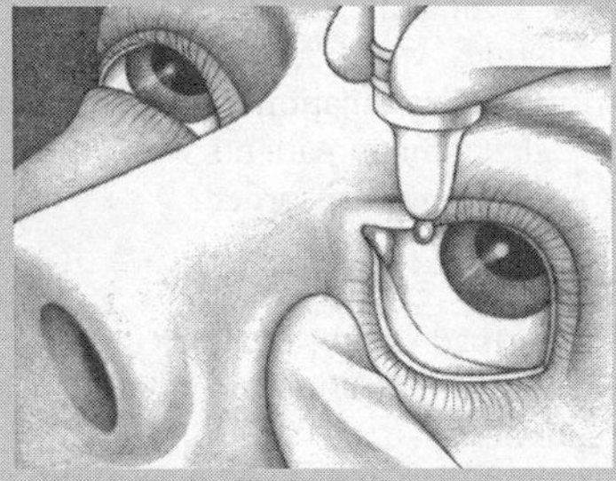

To apply an ointment, gently place a thin strip of the medication along the conjunctival sac from the inner canthus to the outer canthus. Avoid touching the tip of the tube to the patient's eye. Then release the eyelid and have the patient roll his eye behind closed lids to distribute the medication.

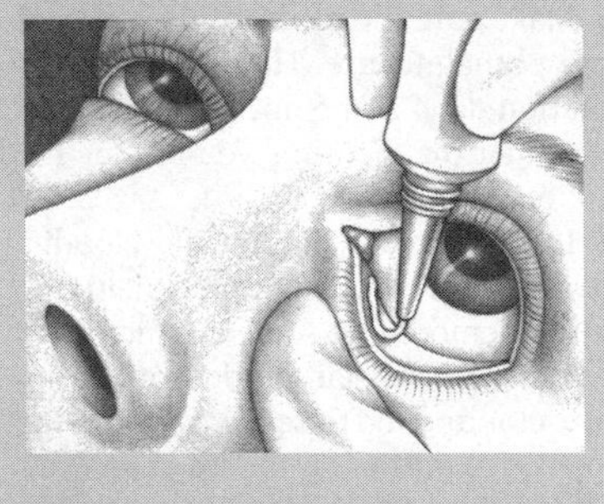

Drug alert Many geriatric patients require more than one type of eye medication in the same eye. Some eyedrops are compatible and may be given together; others aren't. When multiple eye drops are prescribed to be given at the same time, 5 minutes should elapse between drops to allow for adequate ocular absorption, to allow tearing to diminish, and to prevent washout of the first medication by the second.

▶ Confirm the patient's identity by asking his name and checking the name, room number, and bed number on his wristband.

▶ Put on gloves.

▶ If the patient is wearing an eye dressing, remove it by gently pulling it down and away from his forehead. Take care not to contaminate your hands.

▶ Remove any discharge by cleaning around the eye with sterile gauze pads moistened with warm water or normal saline solution. With the patient's eye closed, clean from the inner to the outer canthus, using a fresh sterile gauze pad for each stroke.

▶ To remove crusted secretions around the eye, moisten a gauze pad with warm water or normal saline solution. Ask the patient to close the eye, and then place the gauze pad over it for 1 to 2 minutes. Remove the pad, and then reapply moist sterile gauze pads, as necessary, until the secretions are soft enough to be removed without traumatizing the mucosa.

Instilling eyedrops

▶ Remove the dropper cap from the medication container, if necessary, and draw the medication into it. Be careful to avoid contaminating the dropper tip or bottle top.

▶ To maintain the drug container's sterility, never touch the tip of the bottle or dropper to the patient's eyeball, lids, or lashes. If the dropper or bottle tip has become contaminated, discard it and obtain another sterile dropper. To avoid cross-contamination, never use a container of eye medication for more than one patient.

▶ Before instilling the eyedrops, instruct the patient to look up and away. This moves the cornea away from the lower lid and minimizes the risk of touching the cornea with the dropper if the patient blinks.

▶ You may steady the hand in which you're holding the dropper by resting it against the patient's forehead. Then, with your other hand, gently pull down the lower lid of the affected eye and instill the drops in the conjunctival sac. Try to avoid placing the drops directly on the eyeball. (See *Instilling eye medication.*)

▶ Discard any solution remaining in the dropper before returning the dropper to the bottle.

Applying eye ointment

▶ Squeeze a small ribbon of medication on the edge of the conjunctival sac from the inner to the outer canthus. Cut off the ribbon by turning the tube. If you wish, you can steady the hand holding the medication tube by bracing it against the patient's forehead or cheek.

Using a medication disk

▶ Inserted into the conjunctival sac, a medication disk diffuses a drug into the eye in a controlled manner. The disk can release medication for up to 1 week. Pilocarpine, for example, can be administered this way to treat glaucoma.

After administration

▶ Instruct the patient to close his eyes gently, without squeezing the lids shut. If you instilled drops, tell the patient to blink. If you applied ointment, tell him to roll his eyes behind closed lids to help distribute the medication over the surface of the eyeball.

▶ Use a clean tissue to remove any excess solution or ointment leaking from the eye. Use a fresh tissue for each eye to prevent cross-contamination.

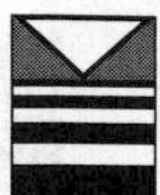

Key point Use the following method as you administer an eye medication that may be absorbed systemically (such as atropine): With the patient's eyes closed, gently press your thumb on the inner canthus for 1 to 2 minutes. The pressure helps keep eyedrops from flowing into the tear duct.

▶ Apply a new ocular dressing, if necessary.

▶ Return the medication to the storage area. Make sure you store it according to the label's instructions.

▶ Wash your hands.

Complications

Instillation of some eye medications may cause transient burning, itching, and redness. Rarely, systemic effects may also occur.

Patient teaching

▶ Explain the procedure to the patient to reduce his fear and promote cooperation.

▶ Instruct the patient not to rub the eye to minimize injury.

▶ Teach the patient to instill eye medications so that he can continue treatment at home, if necessary. Review the procedure, and ask for a return demonstration.

Documentation

Record the date and time of administration, the medication administered and the dose, and the eye or eyes treated. Note any adverse effects and the patient's response. Document your patient teaching measures.

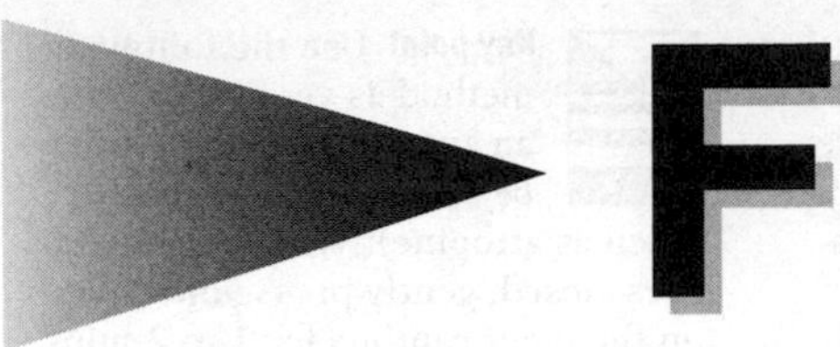

FALLS AND FALL PREVENTION

One of the primary goals of those who care for older adults is to help their patients maintain as much independence as possible, for as long as possible, in a safe environment. According to Maslow's Hierarchy of Needs, a safe environment is one that offers stability, protection, order, and freedom from fear, anxiety, and chaos. For older patients, safety and security are as important as basic physiologic needs, such as food and water.

An older adult's feelings of danger or insecurity may be based on real or perceived threats. Those fears can affect the person's behavior and responses to attempted health care interventions. For example, a person who feels threatened may impose limitations on himself and become rigid and isolated, refusing help from others. Many older people become immobilized by the fear of falling or of being the victim of a crime. For such people, providing basic physiologic needs can be a challenge. On the other hand, a perceived threat can motivate a person to adopt behaviors that promote safety and wellness, such as walking only on well-lit streets if he's afraid of falling or of crime.

In addition to physical threats, older people often face multiple losses that compromise their ability to maintain their independence and self-determination. By looking at the situation through the eyes of the older person, you'll be better able to provide interventions that increase the patient's safety.

As a person ages, his likelihood of suffering an injury from an accident and becoming disabled increases. Physiologic changes of aging, underlying disease processes, and psychological, social, and economic stresses all can increase a person's risk of accidents and injury. Among people over age 65, injuries from accidents are the fifth leading cause of death. Accidents are more common in extended-care facilities because residents have disabling conditions and are more dependent on others for care. Yet, as with accidents in other age-groups, most accidents that older adults suffer are preventable.

Incidence and impact

Falls are a leading predictor of morbidity and mortality among older people, accounting for about two-thirds of all accidents in this age-group. Nearly one-third of older adults who live outside a long-term care facility fall at least once per year, and an estimated one-half of those fall more than once. The incidence of falls is about 25% for persons age 70; it increases to 35% for those age 75 and older. About 85% of falls occur in the home, usually in the afternoon or evening. Twenty percent of hospital admissions and 40% of long-term care facility admissions are fall-related.

In all settings, most falls take place in the bedroom or bathroom and are related to going to or from the bathroom, transferring to or from the bed, or leaning out of chairs. More active people fall than inactive people, but those who are frail and have difficulty with activities of daily living (ADLs) have more repeated falls.

Falls, especially patterns of repeated falls, are one of the leading causes of institutionalization for older people. Hip fractures are a common result of a fall. People with hip fractures often suffer functional losses leading to increased dependence. Other common injuries resulting from falls include bruises, lacerations, and subdural hematomas. Acute or chronic pain is another consequence of injuries that shouldn't be overlooked or minimized. Fall-related mortality increased with age.

In addition to causing physical injuries, falls may take a psychological toll. For example, an older person may become more worried about the future, specifically, about his ability to remain independent, because of cognitive or functional losses suffered during hospitalization. The person may experience a loss of self-esteem or a fear of falling again, of being unable to perform ADLs, or of social rejection, which in turn can lead to depression and withdrawal. The result is decreased activity, a further decline in functional abilities, and an increased risk for falls.

The reactions of family members after a fall can also affect an older person's outlook. For example, they may become overprotective, trying to limit the older person's activities or making decisions for him. Such actions only increase the person's feelings of incompetence and fear of becoming dependent.

Falls also have a direct impact on health care resources by increasing the use of emergency department services for the diagnosis and treatment of injuries and by increasing hospital admissions and the length of hospital stays to treat injuries from falls and resulting complications.

Fall prevention

By focusing your efforts on preventing falls, you can make tremendous gains in preserving life; helping your patients maintain their functional abilities, independence, and quality of life; and conserving health care dollars. To be effective, a prevention program must consist of an accurate analysis of the problem, clearly stated goals, practical and efficient interventions, and a strong commitment by all participants to make it work.

By learning the causes of falls and assessing an older person for risk factors, you can predict and thus prevent falls in many instances. (See *Risk assessment for falls,* page 276.) Whether you practice in the community, a clinic or physician's office, or an acute, subacute, or long-term care setting, you'll need to compile and analyze data on the incidence of falls and any information related to those falls for the specific patient population involved. Individual data should always be a part of the older patient's record and should be updated frequently. This information is critical in detecting trends and patterns and in providing a basis for setting reasonable and measurable goals for both patients and the facility. Your assessment of the individual older patient must be comprehensive because it will provide baseline information, help you assess the patient's present status, and identify risk factors.

Document the patient's history of falls or near falls, including the specific activity the patient was engaged in at the time of the fall, any signs or symptoms he experienced at the time of or just before the fall, the time and location of the fall, and any injuries sustained. Many people will minimize or forget falls if no injuries resulted. They may also be reluctant to share this information if they perceive a threat to their independence or the possibility of having to undergo uncomfortable or costly diagnostic procedures or treatments.

Risk assessment for falls

This standardized assessment tool can help you evaluate your patient's risk for falls and plan preventive measures, if needed. A patient score above 4 indicates the need for interventions.

Parameters	4	3	2	1	Patient Score
Age		80+	70 to 79		2
Mental status	Intermittent confusion or disorientation		Confused or disoriented at all times		4
Elimination	Independent and incontinent	Needs assistance		Indwelling catheter or ostomy	3
History of falling	History of multiple falls (3 or more)		Has fallen 1 or 2 times		2
Activity level	Confined to bed or chair	Out of bed with assistance		Bathroom privileges	3
Gait and balance	Unsteady, poor balance standing or walking	Orthostatic hypotension	Spastic or jerky gait		4
Medications (current or in the past 7 days)	3 or more medications	2 medications	1 medication		4
				Total Risk Score	22

MEDICATIONS
__ Anesthetic
✓ Antidiabetic
__ Antihistamine
✓ Antihypertensive
__ Anticonvulsant
__ Benzodiazepine
✓ Cathartic
✓ Diuretic
__ Narcotic
__ Psychotropic
__ Sedative
__ Hypnotic
__ Other (specify)

PATIENT SCORES
11 to 24 = extremely high risk
5 to 10 = high risk
0 to 4 = low risk

If score is > 4, patient is at high risk for falling and fall-prevention protocol must be implemented.

Courtesy of Abington Memorial Hospital Department of Nursing, Abington, Pa.

Find out which medications the patient is taking, either from the patient himself or, if that's not possible, from his caregiver. (See *Medications associated with falls.*) Some people consider medications to be only drugs that are prescribed by a physician, so make sure that you ask about over-the-counter drugs, homeopathic remedies, and drugs borrowed from others. Also, determine the reason for taking the medication, the dosage, and the frequency. Find out if the patient is taking prescribed medications as often as he should and in the correct dosages. Socioeconomic factors, such as a limited budget or limited access to a pharmacy, can cause older people to cut down on their drug dosage or take the drug less often than they should.

Risk identification

Identification of risk factors, followed by timely and appropriate interventions, is the key to a successful fall prevention program. Whenever you perform an assessment, be alert for risk factors—such as shaky balance and gait — that should warn you about potential problems. (See *Tinetti balance and gait evaluation,* pages 278 and 279.) Also see "Minimum Data Set" in chapter 4, pages 63 to 82, for evaluating the patient.) By anticipating problems before they occur, you can take preventive action and avoid negative outcomes.

Risk assessment tools can help quantify the patient's risk for falls and serve as a basis for interventions. However, such tools should never be used instead of a full assessment.

Risk factors for falls are usually classified as intrinsic (physiologic, or within the body), extrinsic (external, or outside the body), or iatrogenic (resulting from medical care or treatment). Unclassified or idiopathic falls are those with no identifiable cause. Among older people, falls usually result not from a single risk factor but from a combination. Although the categories overlap, they help to identify which factors can be eliminated or reduced and which can only be managed.

Intrinsic factors

The following physiologic factors increase the risk of falls:

- age, with markedly increased incidences at age 75; people ages 80 to 89 at the highest risk
- sex—women at higher risk than men
- sensory deficits—vision and hearing problems
- medical conditions—neurologic, cerebrovascular, cardiovascular, or mus-

Medications associated with falls

This chart highlights some classes of drugs that are commonly prescribed for older patients and the possible adverse effects of each that may increase a patient's risk of falling. In addition, polypharmacy, or using multiple medications, can increase the risk due to a concomitant effect.

Drug class	Adverse effects
Diuretics	Hypovolemia Orthostatic hypotension Electrolyte imbalance Urinary incontinence
Antihypertensives	Hypotension
Tricyclic antidepressants	Orthostatic hypotension
Antipsychotics	Orthostatic hypotension Muscle rigidity Sedation
Benzodiazepines and antihistamines	Excessive sedation Confusion Paradoxical agitation Loss of balance
Narcotics	Hypotension Sedation Motor incoordination Agitation
Hypnotics	Excessive sedation Ataxia Poor balance Confusion Paradoxical agitation
Antidiabetic drugs	Acute hypoglycemia
Alcohol	Intoxication Motor incoordination Agitation Sedation Confusion

Tinetti balance and gait evaluation

This tool can be used to evaluate how successfully a patient remains at rest or moves about in ordinary activities. It takes 5 to 15 minutes to administer. To prepare, you'll need an armless upholstered chair, a walking space (such as a large room or a hallway), and any of the patient's walking aids (such as a cane or a walker).

Observe the patient during each of the maneuvers listed below, and select the number that best describes his performance. The maximum score is 28; the lowest is 0. The higher the score, the better the patient's gait and balance. You can assess any deterioration in his condition by periodically repeating the evaluation and comparing later scores to the baseline score.

BALANCE

Instructions: Seat the patient in a hard, armless chair and test the following maneuvers:

1. Sitting balance
0 = Leans or slides in chair
1 = Steady, safe

2. Arising
0 = Unable without help
1 = Able but uses arm to help
2 = Able without use of arms

3. Attempts to arise
0 = Unable without help
1 = Able but requires more than one attempt
2 = Able to arise with one attempt

4. Immediate standing balance
(first 5 seconds)
0 = Unsteady (staggers, moves feet, marked trunk sway)
1 = Steady but uses walker or cane or grabs other object for support
2 = Steady without walker, cane, or other support

5. Standing balance
0 = Unsteady
1 = Steady but wide stance (medial heels more than 4" [10 cm] apart) or uses walker, cane, or other support
2 = Narrow stance without support

6. Nudge
(Patient at maximum position with feet as close together as possible. Examiner pushes lightly on patient's sternum with palm of hand three times.)
0 = Begins to fall
1 = Staggers, grabs, but catches self
2 = Steady

7. Eyes closed
(at maximum position, as in number 6)
0 = Unsteady
1 = Steady

8. Turn 360 degrees
0 = Discontinuous steps
1 = Continuous steps
0 = Unsteady (grabs, staggers)
1 = Steady

9. Sit down
0 = Unsafe (misjudged distance, falls into chair)
1 = Uses arms or not a smooth motion
2 = Safe, smooth motion

0 /16 **BALANCE SCORE**

Tinetti balance and gait evaluation *(continued)*

GAIT

Instructions: Patient stands with examiner. He then walks down hallway or across room, first at his usual pace and then back at a rapid but safe pace (using usual walking aid, such as walker or cane).

10. Initiation of gait
(immediately after told to go)
0 = Any hesitancy or multiple attempts to start
1 = No hesitancy

11. Step length and height
(right foot swing)
0 = Does not pass left stance foot with step
1 = Passes left stance foot
0 = Right foot does not clear floor completely with step
1 = Right foot completely clears floor

12. Step length and height
(left foot swing)
0 = Does not pass right stance foot with step
1 = Passes right stance foot
0 = Left foot does not clear floor completely with step
1 = Left foot completely clears floor

13. Step symmetry
0 = Right and left step length not equal (estimate)
1 = Right and left step length appear equal

14. Step continuity
0 = Stopping or discontinuity between steps
1 = Steps appear continuous

15. Path
(estimated in relation to floor tiles 12″ [30.5 cm] wide; observe excursion of one foot over about 10″ [25.5 cm] of course)
0 = Marked deviation
1 = Mild to moderate deviation or uses a walking aid
2 = Straight without walking aid

16. Trunk
0 = Marked sway or uses walking aid
1 = No sway but flexes knees or back or spreads arms out while walking
2 = No sway, no flexion, no use of arms, and no walking aid

17. Walk stance
0 = Heels apart
1 = Heels almost touching while walking

0 /12 **GAIT SCORE**

0 /28 **TOTAL MOBILITY SCORE (Balance and gait)**

Adapted from Galindo, D.J., et al. "Gait Training and Falls in the Elderly," *Journal of Gerontological Nursing* 21(6):15-16, June 1995, with permission of the publisher.

culoskeletal conditions; cancer or other progressive, debilitating diseases; multiple or chronic conditions; psychiatric conditions; or cognitive losses
- gait and balance changes
- fear of falling.

Extrinsic factors

The following external factors increase the risk of falls:
- environmental traps, such as objects or barriers in the person's surroundings, wet surfaces, poor lighting, clothing

- environmental barriers, such as bed rails
- assistive devices, such as canes and walkers that are improperly used or adjusted
- inappropriate footwear
- alcohol abuse.

Iatrogenic factors

The following iatrogenic factors increase the risk of falls:

- medications
- medical devices, such as indwelling urinary catheters, I.V. tubes and poles, and feeding tubes
- restraints
- delirium.

Special considerations

You'll be able to determine the effectiveness of your fall-prevention program primarily by monitoring the incidence of falls and noting trends and patterns through a review of incident reports. The reports will reveal areas that need to be reviewed or improved. Also, encourage primary caregivers to evaluate the effectiveness of prevention measures and to continually look for ways to further reduce or eliminate risks.

Keep in mind that the benefits of a fall-prevention program, for patients, their family members, staff members, and the health care system as a whole, far outweigh the costs in money, time, and effort.

FECAL DISIMPACTION

Fecal impaction, a large, hard, dry mass of stool in the folds of the rectum and, at times, in the sigmoid colon, is caused by prolonged retention and accumulation of stool. Fecal impaction is a common cause of fecal incontinence in older persons and may result from poor bowel habits, inactivity, dehydration, improper diet (especially inadequate fluid intake), constipation-inducing drugs, and incomplete bowel cleaning after a barium enema or barium swallow. Manual removal of fecal impaction may require a health care provider's order. Prior to disimpaction, soften the stool with an oil retention enema.

This procedure is contraindicated after rectal, genitourinary, abdominal, perineal, or gynecologic reconstructive surgery; in patients with myocardial infarction, coronary insufficiency, pulmonary embolus, heart failure, heart block, or Stokes-Adams syndrome (without pacemaker treatment); and in patients with GI or vaginal bleeding, hemorrhoids, rectal polyps, or blood dyscrasias.

Supplies

- Gloves (2 pairs)
- Linen-saver pad
- Bedpan
- Plastic disposal bag
- Soap
- Water-filled basin
- Towel
- Water-soluble lubricant or lidocaine jelly (depending on your facility)
- Washcloth
- Drape

Implementation

- Provide privacy.
- Position the patient on his left side and flex his knees to allow easier access to the sigmoid colon and rectum. Drape the patient, and place a linen-saver pad beneath his buttocks to protect the bed linens.
- Put on gloves, and moisten an index finger with water-soluble lubricant to reduce friction during insertion, thereby avoiding injury to sensitive tissue.
- Instruct the patient to breathe deeply to promote relaxation. Then gently insert the lubricated index finger beyond the anal sphincter until you touch the impaction.
- Rotate your finger gently around the stool to dislodge and break it into small

fragments. Then work the fragments downward to the end of the rectum, and remove each one separately.

▶ Manipulate the blockage gently to avoid injuring the rectal lining, which is fragile in older adults. Multiple sessions over a period of several days may be required to accomplish complete evacuation.

▶ Before removing your finger, gently stimulate the anal sphincter with a circular motion two or three times to increase peristalsis and encourage evacuation.

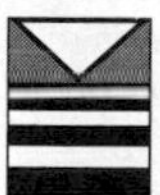

Key point If the patient experiences pain, nausea, rectal bleeding, changes in pulse rate or skin color, diaphoresis, or syncope, stop immediately and notify the physician.

▶ Remove your finger and change your gloves. Then clean the anal area with soap and a basin of water and lightly pat dry with a towel.

▶ Offer the patient the bedpan or commode because digital manipulation stimulates the urge to defecate.

▶ Place disposable items in the plastic bag and discard properly. If necessary, clean the bedpan and return it to the bedside stand.

▶ Wash your hands.

Complications

Digital removal of fecal impaction can stimulate the vagus nerve and may decrease heart rate and cause syncope.

Patient teaching

▶ Explain the procedure to the patient.

▶ Tell him to immediately report any discomfort or dizziness during the procedure.

▶ Review with the patient methods to prevent impaction from occurring in the future, such as adequate fluid intake and increasing dietary fiber.

Documentation

Record the time and date of the procedure, the patient's response, and stool color, consistency, and odor. Document your patient teaching measures and their effects.

FECAL INCONTINENCE

Although not usually a sign of a major illness, fecal incontinence can seriously impair an older person's physical and psychological well-being.

Fecal incontinence may develop gradually (as in dementia) or suddenly (as in spinal cord injury). It usually results from fecal stasis and impaction accompanying reduced activity, inappropriate diet, untreated painful anal conditions, or chronic constipation. Fecal incontinence also may be caused by chronic laxative use; reduced fluid intake; neurologic deficits; and pelvic, prostatic, or rectal surgery as well as medications, such as antihistamines, psychotropics, and iron preparations.

A person with fecal incontinence may not be aware of the need to defecate. If he can't get to the bathroom or use a commode or bedpan on his own, he may lose rectal sensitivity from having to suppress the urge while waiting for help. Musculoskeletal changes also can affect a person's ability to assume a comfortable position, interfering with the frequency and effectiveness of bowel elimination.

Signs and symptoms

▶ Ongoing seepage of stool from the rectum

▶ Inability to recognize need to move bowels

▶ Abdominal cramping and distention

▶ Possible fecal impaction

Diagnostic tests

▶ *Digital rectal examination* can rule out the possibility of fecal impaction.

Correcting fecal incontinence with bowel retraining

Numerous regimens can be used to promote successful bowel elimination and control fecal incontinence. The key to any program is time and patience. Some examples of bowel retraining programs are listed below.

For fecal incontinence caused by impaction

- Irrigate the lower bowel with daily enemas.
- Administer a suppository every morning or evening.
- Remove the impaction manually, if necessary.
- Prevent recurrence by providing the following: adequate fluid intake of 2 qt (2 L)/day; adequate dietary fiber; stool softeners or bulk laxatives (if necessary); response to the urge to defecate; activity and exercise regimen.

For fecal incontinence caused by neurologic disorders

- Provide adequate fluid intake.
- Provide a high-fiber diet.
- Initiate an activity and exercise program.
- Institute habit training, including scheduled toileting such as after breakfast; increase awareness of defecation reflex; and give a suppository or enema to stimulate the bowel if there is no bowel movement for 2 consecutive days.
- If neurologic impairment is severe, induce constipation with an antidiarrheal and low-bulk diet, alternating with planned evacuation using enemas or suppositories.

▶ *Colonoscopy* may be necessary to detect other bowel disorders.

Treatment

Patients with fecal incontinence should be carefully assessed for underlying causes. Bowel retraining is the treatment of choice. If the problem is poor anal sphincter tone, pelvic muscle exercises can help correct it. A person can be taught to contract and relax the anal sphincter in a regular program of exercise to strengthen the muscle.

Biofeedback may be helpful for patients who have incontinence that is related to sensory or motor dysfunction of the rectal sphincters. Candidates for biofeedback must be motivated and able to follow direction.

If fecal incontinence is caused by impaction, the blockage should be removed with an enema or manually. Enemas and suppositories may be used concurrently to obtain complete bowel evacuation. Failure to evacuate the entire bowel increases the chance of fecal reaccumulation. If incontinence is caused by proctitis, corticosteroid enemas as prescribed may be helpful.

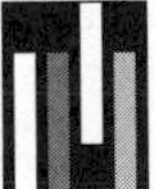

Cultural diversity In the Asian and Indian cultures, rectal examinations are regarded as offensive and enemas may be forbidden.

Key nursing diagnoses and outcomes

Bowel incontinence related to neuromuscular impairment, diarrhea, fecal impaction, or cognitive impairment

Treatment outcome: The patient will have controlled bowel movements after bowel retraining.

Anxiety related to fecal incontinence

Treatment outcomes: The patient will express his feelings of anxiety and learn coping mechanisms.

Risk for impaired skin integrity related to fecal incontinence
Treatment outcome: The patient will maintain skin integrity.

Nursing interventions

- Schedule extra time to encourage and provide support for the patient and to mitigate any feelings of shame, embarrassment, or powerlessness from loss of control. Praise the patient's successful efforts.
- Begin a bowel retraining program. (See *Correcting fecal incontinence with bowel retraining*.)
- Begin a scheduled toileting program by assessing the patient to learn what time he usually moves his bowels (for example, after breakfast or after a morning cup of coffee or other warm beverage). Remind or help the patient to use the toilet or commode 15 to 20 minutes before his habitual time. Make sure he knows where the toilet is, and stay with him to make sure he has a complete bowel movement. Encourage him to sway back and forth while on the toilet to promote peristalsis, and stay with patients with late stage Alzheimer's disease or other neurologic illnesses.
- Maintain effective hygiene care to increase the patient's comfort and prevent skin breakdown and infection; clean the perineal area frequently, and apply a moisture barrier cream; control foul odors.
- Patients with fecal incontinence are vulnerable to skin breakdown and infection. Be alert for these physiologic complications in addition to psychological problems caused by social isolation, loss of independence, decreased self-esteem, and depression.
- Encourage the patient to eat a fiber-rich diet with raw leafy vegetables (such as carrots and lettuce), unpeeled fruits (apples), and whole grains (such as wheat or rye breads and cereals); bran provides the best source of fiber.
- Encourage adequate fluid intake (8 to 10 8-oz [237-ml] glasses of water per day, if the patient's condition allows).
- Promote regular exercise by explaining how it helps to regulate bowel motility; even a nonambulatory patient can perform some exercises while sitting or lying in bed.

PATIENT TEACHING

- Teach the patient to gradually eliminate laxative use, if necessary. Point out that using over-the-counter laxatives to promote regular bowel movements can have the opposite effect and cause either constipation or incontinence over time.
- Suggest using natural laxatives, such as prunes or prune juice, instead.

FOLIC ACID DEFICIENCY

A common, slowly progressive megaloblastic anemia, folic acid deficiency anemia is most prevalent in infants, adolescents, pregnant and breast-feeding women, alcoholics, older adults, and patients with malignant or intestinal diseases.

Alcohol abuse, which suppresses the metabolic effects of folate, is probably the most common cause of folic acid deficiency anemia. Additional causes include:

- poor diet (common in alcoholics, narcotic addicts, and older people who live alone)
- impaired absorption (due to intestinal dysfunction from such disorders as celiac disease, tropical sprue, regional jejunitis, and bowel resection)
- bacteria competing for available folic acid
- excessive cooking of foods, which destroys the available nutrients
- prolonged drug therapy with such drugs as anticonvulsants, estrogens, and methotrexate

Foods high in folic acid

Folic acid (pteroylglutamic acid, folacin) is found in most body tissues, where it acts as a coenzyme in metabolic processes involving one-carbon transfer. It's essential for formation and maturation of red blood cells and for synthesis of deoxyribonucleic acid. Although its body stores are comparatively small (about 70 mg), this vitamin is plentiful in most well-balanced diets.

However, because folic acid is water soluble and heat labile, it's easily destroyed by cooking. Also, about 20% of folic acid intake is excreted unabsorbed. Insufficient daily folic acid intake (less than 50 mcg per day) usually induces folic acid deficiency within 4 months. Below is a list of foods high in folic acid content; encourage your patient to consume these foods.

Food	mcg/100 g
Asparagus spears	109
Beef liver	294
Broccoli spears	54
Collards (cooked)	102
Orange juice	136
Oatmeal	33
Peanut butter	25
Black beans	128
Wheat germ	99

▶ increased folic acid requirements in patients with neoplastic diseases and some skin diseases such as exfoliative dermatitis.

Signs and symptoms

▶ Severe, progressive fatigue (the hallmark of folic acid deficiency)
▶ Paresthesia or neuropathy in the hands or legs
▶ Dementia (if associated with B_{12} deficiency)
▶ Generalized pallor
▶ Jaundice
▶ Cheilosis and glossitis possible
▶ Shortness of breath
▶ Palpitations
▶ Diarrhea
▶ Nausea
▶ Anorexia
▶ Headaches
▶ Forgetfulness
▶ Irritability
▶ Impaired oxygen-carrying capacity of the blood from lowered hemoglobin levels that may produce complaints of weakness and light-headedness

Diagnostic tests

▶ *Schilling test* and a *therapeutic trial* of vitamin B_{12} injections distinguish between folic acid deficiency anemia and pernicious anemia.
▶ *Blood studies* reveal macrocytosis, decreased reticulocyte count, increased mean corpuscular volume, abnormal platelet count, and serum folate levels below 4 mg/ml.

Treatment

Primary therapies include folic acid supplements replacement (oral or parenteral), elimination of contributing causes, and adherence to a well-balanced diet. (See *Foods high in folic acid.*)

Key nursing diagnoses and outcomes

Imbalanced nutrition: Less than body requirements related to adverse GI effects

Treatment outcome: The patient will no longer show signs and symptoms of folic acid deficiency.

Fatigue related to folic acid deficiency

Treatment outcome: The patient will regain his normal energy level as folic acid deficiency resolves.

Nursing interventions

▶ Plan activities, rest periods, and diagnostic tests to conserve the patient's energy.
▶ Provide good oral hygiene if the patient has glossitis. Recommend a mild or diluted mouthwash and a soft toothbrush.
▶ Provide the patient with nonirritating foods and a well-balanced diet. Offer between-meal snacks.
▶ Monitor the patient's complete blood count, platelet count, and serum folate levels as ordered.
▶ Monitor his electrolyte balance.

PATIENT TEACHING

▶ Emphasize the importance of a well-balanced diet high in folic acid.
▶ Arrange appropriate counseling for alcoholics or other high-risk people with poor dietary habits.
▶ Urge compliance with the prescribed course of therapy. Advise the patient not to stop taking the supplements when he begins to feel better.
▶ Warn the patient to guard against infections, and tell him to report signs and symptoms of infection promptly—especially pulmonary and urinary tract infections—because his weakened condition may increase susceptibility.

FOOT CARE

Daily footbaths and regularly trimmed toenails promote cleanliness, prevent infection, stimulate peripheral circulation, and control odor by removing debris from between toes and under toenails. Foot care is particularly important for bedridden patients and those especially susceptible to foot infection. Increased susceptibility may be caused by peripheral vascular disease, diabetes mellitus, poor nutritional status, arthritis, or any condition that impairs peripheral circulation. In such patients, proper foot care should include meticulous cleanliness and regular observation for signs of skin breakdown.

Toenail trimming is contraindicated in patients with toe infections, diabetes mellitus, neurologic disorders, renal failure, or peripheral vascular disease, unless performed by a physician or podiatrist.

Supplies

▶ Bath blanket
▶ Large basin
▶ Soap
▶ Towel
▶ Linen-saver pad
▶ Pillow
▶ Washcloth
▶ Orangewood stick
▶ Emery board
▶ Cotton-tipped applicator
▶ Cotton
▶ Lotion
▶ Water-absorbent powder
▶ Bath thermometer
▶ Warm water
▶ Gloves
▶ Optional: 2″ × 2″ gauze pads, heel protectors

Implementation

▶ Assemble equipment at the patient's bedside. Wash your hands and put on gloves.
▶ Fill the basin halfway with warm water. Test water temperature with a bath thermometer because patients with diminished peripheral sensation could burn their feet in excessively hot water (over 105° F [40.6° C]) without feeling any warning pain. If a bath thermometer is unavailable, test the water by inserting your elbow. The water temperature should feel comfortably warm.
▶ Cover the patient with a bath blanket. Fanfold the top linen to the foot of the bed.
▶ Place a linen-saver pad and a towel under the patient's feet to keep the bottom linen dry. Then position the basin on the pad.

▶ Insert a pillow beneath the patient's knee to provide support, and cushion the rim of the basin with the edge of the towel to prevent pressure.
▶ Immerse one of the patient's feet in the basin. Wash it with soap; then allow it to soak for about 10 to 20 minutes. Soaking softens the skin and toenails, loosens debris under toenails, and comforts and refreshes the patient.
▶ After soaking the foot, rinse it with a washcloth, remove it from the basin, and place it on the towel.
▶ Dry the foot thoroughly, especially between the toes, to avoid skin breakdown. Blot gently to dry because harsh rubbing may damage the skin.
▶ Empty the basin, refill it with warm water, and clean and soak the other foot.
▶ While the second foot is soaking, give the first one a pedicure. Using the cotton-tipped applicator, carefully clean the toenails. Using an orangewood stick, gently remove any dirt beneath the toenails; avoid injuring subungual skin.
▶ If the patient's toenails should be cut, you may need to consult a podiatrist, according to your facility's policy. File toenails with an emery board to smooth rough edges. Keeping toenails trimmed and filed prevents scratching and injury to the skin on the opposite leg.
▶ If a patient's toenail grows inward at the corners, tuck a wisp of cotton under it to relieve pressure on the toe.
▶ When giving the bedridden patient foot care, unless contraindicated, perform range-of-motion exercises to stimulate circulation and prevent foot contractures or muscle atrophy. Tuck folded 2″ × 2″ gauze pads between overlapping toes to protect the skin from the toenails. Apply heel protectors to prevent skin breakdown. Rinse the foot that has been soaking, dry it thoroughly, and give it a pedicure.
▶ Apply lotion to moisten dry skin, or lightly dust water-absorbent powder between the toes to absorb moisture.
▶ Remove and clean all equipment and dispose of gloves.

Key point While providing foot care, observe the color, shape, and texture of the toenails. If you see redness, drying, cracking, blisters, discoloration, or other signs of traumatic injury, especially in patients with impaired peripheral circulation, notify the physician. Because such patients are vulnerable to infection and gangrene, they need prompt treatment.

Complications

Infection and skin breakdown are potential complications of foot care.

Patient teaching

▶ Inform the patient that you'll wash his feet and provide foot and toenail care.
▶ Instruct the patient to regularly inspect his feet for cuts, cracks, blisters, or red, swollen areas.

Documentation

Record the date and time of bathing and toenail trimming in your notes. Record and report any abnormal findings and any nursing actions you take. Document your patient teaching measures and their effects.

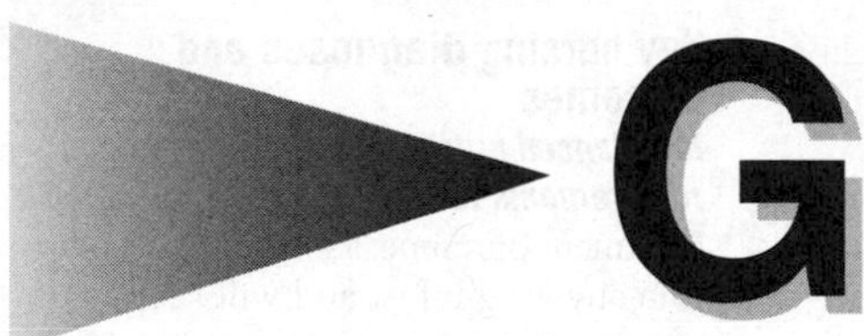

GASTRIC CANCER

Although gastric cancer is common throughout the world in people of all races, its incidence exhibits unexplained geographic, cultural, and gender differences. For example, mortality from this disorder is high in Japan, Iceland, Chile, and Austria. Incidence increases with age and is more prevalent in men.

Gastric cancer occurs more commonly in some parts of the stomach than in others. The pyloric area (50%) and lesser curvature (25%) of the stomach are common sites. Incidence is less common in the cardia (10%), fundus (10%), and greater curvature (5%).

This adenocarcinoma rapidly infiltrates the regional lymph nodes, omentum, liver, and lungs by way of the walls of the stomach, duodenum, and esophagus; the lymphatic system; adjacent organs; the bloodstream; and the peritoneal cavity.

The patient's prognosis depends on the stage of the disease at the time of diagnosis. Early diagnosis and treatment improves prognosis.

Although the cause of gastric cancer is unknown, predisposing factors, such as gastritis with gastric atrophy and gastric ulcers, increase the risk. Genetic factors have also been implicated.

Dietary factors also seem to have an effect. For instance, certain types of food preparation and preservation (especially smoked foods, pickled vegetables, and salted fish and meat) and the physical properties of some foods increase the risk. Furthermore, high alcohol consumption and smoking increase the chances of developing gastric cancer.

Malnutrition occurs when the stomach can't digest protein, and GI obstruction develops as the tumor enlarges. Iron deficiency anemia results as the tumor causes ulceration and bleeding. If the patient has pernicious anemia, the tumor can interfere with the production of intrinsic factor needed for vitamin B_{12} absorption. As the cancer metastasizes to other structures, related complications appear.

Signs and symptoms

- Back pain
- Epigastric pain
- Retrosternal pain areas that's relieved with nonprescription medications
- Vague feeling of fullness, heaviness, and moderate abdominal distention after meals
- Weight loss
- Nausea and vomiting
- Coffee-ground vomitus (if tumor is located in the cardia)
- Weakness and fatigue
- Dysphagia
- Abdominal mass
- Enlarged lymph nodes (supraclavicular and axillary nodes).

Diagnostic tests

- *Barium X-rays* of the GI tract with fluoroscopy show changes that suggest gastric cancer. Changes include a tumor-filling defect in the outline of the stomach, loss of flexibility and distensibility, and abnormal gastric mucosa with or without ulceration.

▶ *Gastroscopy* with fiber-optic endoscope helps rule out other diffuse gastric mucosal abnormalities by allowing direct visualization. Gastroscopic biopsy permits evaluation of gastric mucosal lesions.

▶ A *gastric acid stimulation test* determines whether the stomach secretes acid properly.

▶ *Blood studies* monitor the course of the disease, complications, and the effectiveness of treatment. These include a complete blood count (CBC), chemistry profiles, arterial blood gas analysis, liver function studies, and a carcinoembryonic antigen radioimmunoassay.

▶ Other studies, such as *computed tomography scans, chest X-rays, liver and bone scans,* and *liver biopsy,* evaluate specific organ metastases.

Treatment

Surgery to remove the tumor is the treatment of choice in many cases. Excision of the lesion with appropriate margins is possible in more than one-third of patients. The nature and extent of the lesion determines the type of surgery, which may include gastroduodenostomy, gastrojejunostomy, partial gastric resection, or total gastrectomy. If metastasis has occurred, the omentum and spleen may have to be removed.

Chemotherapy is used, and radiation therapy may be used in combination with chemotherapy if the tumor is nonresectable or partially resectable.

Antiemetics can control nausea, which intensifies as the tumor grows. In more advanced stages, the patient may need sedatives and tranquilizers to control overwhelming anxiety. Pain is controlled with opioid analgesics.

Key nursing diagnoses and outcomes

Imbalanced nutrition: Less than body requirements related to adverse GI effects

Treatment outcomes: The patient will regain any weight lost and will keep his weight within the normal range.

Fatigue related to anemia

Treatment outcomes: The patient will employ measures to prevent and decrease fatigue and will regain his normal energy level when treatment is complete.

Anxiety related to cancer diagnosis

Treatment outcomes: The patient will express his feelings about his diagnosis and prognosis and will use support systems to assist with coping.

Nursing interventions

▶ Provide a high-protein, high-calorie diet and dietary supplements, such as vitamins and iron. Make sure food is cut into small pieces to aid digestion. Offer the patient small, frequent meals.

▶ Encourage his family members to visit during mealtime to create a happy environment. Encourage them to bring some of the patient's favorite foods; wine and brandy may also help stimulate the patient's appetite.

▶ Monitor the patient's nutritional intake. Weigh him regularly and report excessive weight loss to the physician. Watch for signs and symptoms of malnutrition.

▶ Watch for signs of anemia and vitamin B_{12} malabsorption. Monitor CBC and serum vitamin B_{12} levels.

▶ Administer an antacid to relieve heartburn and acid stomach and a histamine-2 receptor antagonist, such as famotidine, to decrease gastric secretions.

▶ Give opioid analgesics, as ordered, to relieve pain.

▶ Administer steroids or antidepressants, as ordered.

▶ Whenever possible, include the patient and his family members or friends in decisions related to the patient's care.

Cultural diversity **In the Japanese culture, the stomach carries great importance, and the people greatly fear diseases that involve the stomach. Observe such a patient for signs of stress, and encourage him to verbalize his fears.**

▶ Prepare the patient for surgery, as indicated.

▶ During radiation therapy, watch for adverse reactions, such as nausea, vomiting, alopecia, malaise, and diarrhea.

▶ During chemotherapy, watch for complications, such as infection, and for expected adverse reactions, such as nausea, vomiting, mouth ulcers, and alopecia.

▶ If all treatments fail, keep the patient comfortable and free from unnecessary pain, and provide psychological support. Encourage him to express his feelings and fears and to ask questions about his illness. Answer such questions honestly; evasive answers will make him retreat and feel isolated.

PATIENT TEACHING

▶ Stress the importance of sound nutrition. Explain that the patient may need vitamins to prevent B_{12} deficiency and iron to prevent or treat anemia.

▶ Provide preoperative teaching for the patient scheduled for surgery.

▶ Explain the ordered treatments to the patient and his family members. Prepare the patient for chemotherapy's adverse effects, such as nausea and vomiting, and suggest measures that may help relieve these problems such as drinking plenty of fluids. Tell him to notify the physician if these effects persist.

▶ Encourage the patient to follow his normal routine as much as possible after recovering from surgery and during radiation therapy and chemotherapy. Leading a near-normal life will help foster feelings of independence and control and will reduce complications of immobility.

▶ Caution the patient to avoid crowds and people with known infections because chemotherapy and radiation therapy diminish the body's natural resistance to infection.

▶ Encourage the patient to learn and practice relaxation and pain management techniques to help control anxiety and discomfort.

▶ If appropriate, direct the patient and his family members to hospital and community support personnel and services. These include social workers, psychologists, cancer support groups, home health care agencies, and hospices.

GASTRIC SURGERY

If chronic ulcer disease doesn't respond to medication, diet therapy, and rest, gastric surgery may be necessary to remove diseased tissue and prevent recurrence of ulcers. This surgery may also be used to excise a malignancy or relieve an obstruction. In an emergency, it may be performed to control severe GI hemorrhage resulting from a perforated ulcer.

Gastric surgery can take various forms, depending on the location and extent of the disorder. For example, a partial gastrectomy may be performed to reduce the amount of acid-secreting mucosa. A bilateral vagotomy may relieve ulcer signs and symptoms and eliminate vagal nerve stimulation of gastric secretions. A pyloroplasty may improve drainage and prevent obstruction. Most commonly, however, two gastric surgeries are combined, such as vagotomy with gastroenterostomy or vagotomy with antrectomy.

Implementation

Surgery begins with an upper abdominal incision such as an upper paramedial incision to expose the stomach and part of the intestine. Total gastrectomy, the removal of the entire stomach, requires a more extensive incision.

The rest of the procedure varies, depending on the type of surgery. (See *Understanding common gastric surgeries*.)

To complete the operation, the surgeon inserts abdominal drains and closes the incision.

Complications

The complications of gastric surgery include hemorrhage, obstruction, dumping syndrome, paralytic ileus, perforation, vitamin B_{12} deficiency, anemia, and atelectasis.

Key nursing diagnoses and outcomes

Imbalanced nutrition: Less than body requirements related to gastric surgery

Treatment outcome: The patient will tolerate oral feedings without experiencing dumping syndrome.

Ineffective breathing pattern related to guarded respirations caused by discomfort from chest or abdominal incision, or both

Treatment outcomes: The patient will maintain adequate ventilation and won't develop respiratory complications, such as pneumonia and atelectasis.

Risk for deficient fluid volume related to nasogastric (NG) drainage and potential for hemorrhage

Treatment outcome: The patient will maintain fluid and electrolyte balance.

Nursing interventions

Before surgery

- Be aware that the extent of preoperative preparation depends on the nature of the surgery. If emergency surgery is necessary, preparation may be limited to immunohematologic studies and measures to control acute hemorrhage, such as cool gastric lavage and administration of vasopressors. Planned surgery allows more extensive preparation.
- Before planned surgery, evaluate and take steps to stabilize the patient's fluid and electrolyte balance and nutritional status — all of which may be severely compromised by chronic ulcer disease or other GI disorders. Monitor intake and output, and draw serum samples for hematologic studies. As ordered, begin I.V. fluid replacement and total parenteral nutrition (TPN). Also, as ordered, prepare the patient for abdominal X-rays. On the night before surgery, administer laxatives and enemas, as necessary. On the morning of surgery, insert an NG tube.
- Make sure the patient or a responsible family member has signed a consent form.

After surgery

- When the patient awakens after surgery, place him in low Fowler's or semi-Fowler's position—whichever he finds more comfortable. Either position will ease breathing and prevent aspiration if he vomits.
- Monitor the patient's vital signs frequently until they're stable; check facility policy for specific guidelines. Watch especially for hypotension, bradycardia, and respiratory changes, which may signal hemorrhage and shock. Periodically check the wound site, NG tube, and abdominal drainage tubes for bleeding.
- Maintain tube feedings or TPN and I.V. fluid and electrolyte replacement therapy, as ordered. Monitor blood studies daily. Watch for signs and symptoms of dehydration, hyponatremia, and metabolic alkalosis, which may result from gastric suctioning. Monitor and record intake and output, including NG tube drainage. Watch for complications associated with TPN or I.V. therapy.
- Auscultate the patient's abdomen daily for the return of bowel sounds. When they return, notify the physician, who will order clamping or removal of the NG tube and gradual resumption of oral feeding. During NG tube clamping, watch for nausea and vomiting; if they

Understanding common gastric surgeries

Besides treating chronic ulcers, gastric surgeries help remove obstructions and neoplasms. Make sure you're familiar with these commonly performed gastric surgeries.

Vagotomy with gastroenterostomy

The surgeon resects the vagus nerves and creates a stoma for gastric drainage. He'll perform selective, truncal, or parietal cell vagotomy, depending on the degree of gastric acid reduction required.

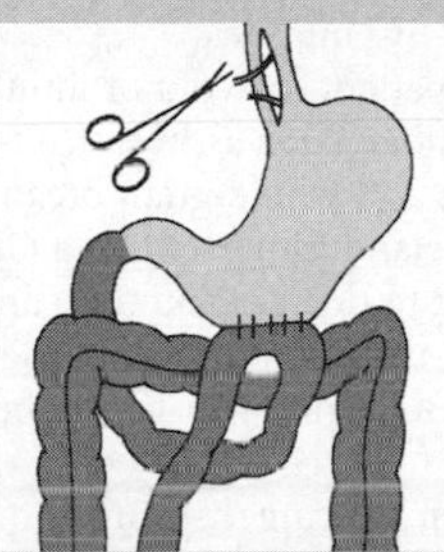

Vagotomy with antrectomy

After resecting the vagus nerves, the surgeon removes the antrum. Then he anastomoses the remaining stomach segment to the jejunum and closes the duodenal stump.

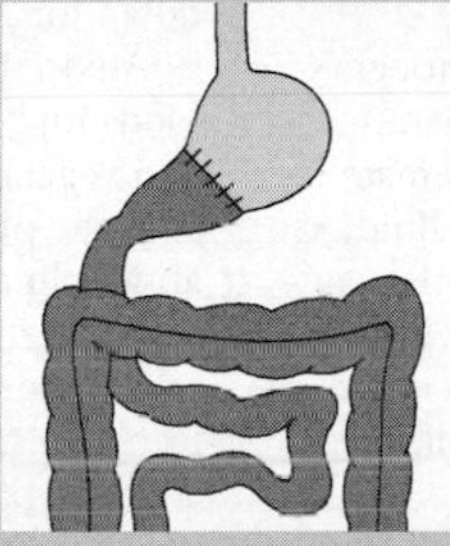

Vagotomy with pyloroplasty

In this procedure, the surgeon resects the vagus nerves and refashions the pylorus to widen the lumen and aid gastric emptying.

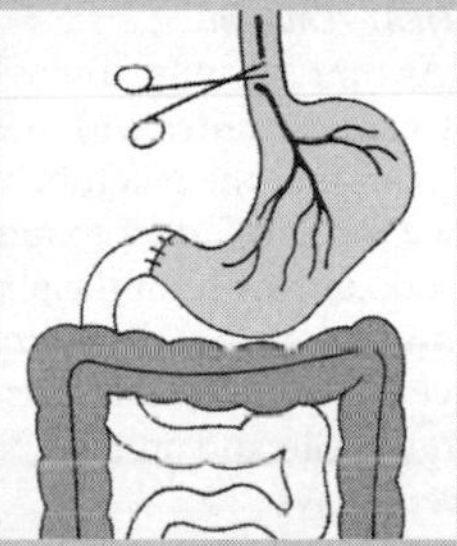

Billroth I

In this partial gastrectomy with a gastroduodenoscopy, the surgeon excises the distal third to half of the stomach and anastomoses the remaining stomach to the duodenum.

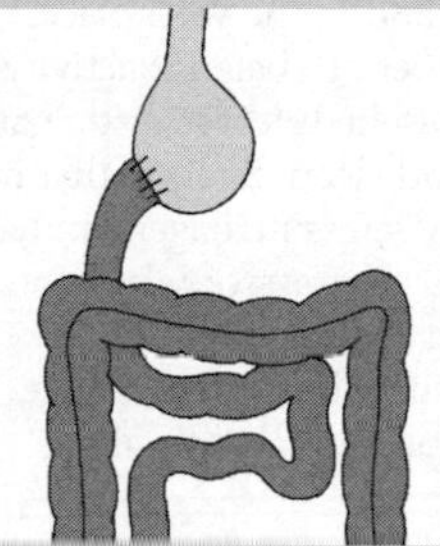

Billroth II

In this partial gastrectomy with a gastrojejunostomy, the surgeon removes the distal segment of the stomach and antrum. Then he anastomoses the remaining stomach and the jejunum and closes the duodenal stump.

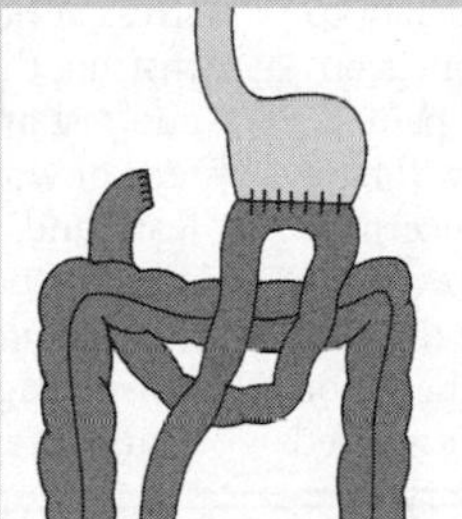

Total gastrectomy

The surgeon removes the entire stomach and attaches the lower end of the esophagus to the jejunum (esophagojejunostomy) at the entrance to the small intestine.

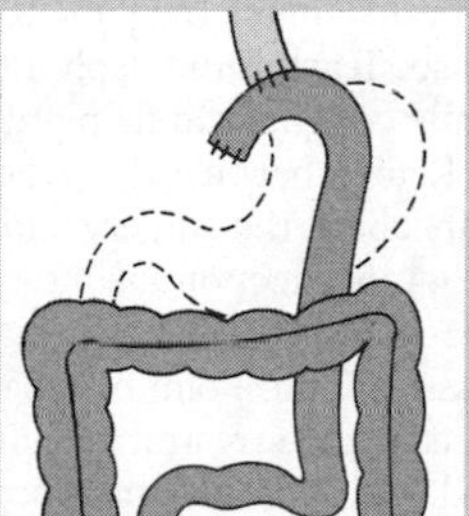

occur, unclamp the tube immediately and reattach it to suction.

▶ Throughout recovery, have the patient cough, deep-breathe, and change position frequently. Provide incentive spirometry, as necessary. Assess his breath sounds frequently to detect atelectasis.

▶ Assess for other complications, including vitamin B_{12} deficiency, anemia (especially common in patients who have undergone total gastrectomy), and dumping syndrome — a potentially serious digestive complication marked by weakness, nausea, flatulence, and palpitations within 30 minutes after a meal.

PATIENT TEACHING

▶ As time permits, discuss postoperative care measures with the patient. Explain that the NG tube will remain in place for 2 to 3 days to remove fluid, blood, and air from the abdominal cavity and to prevent distention; he'll also have abdominal drains inserted at the surgical site and an I.V. line in place for several days.

▶ Discuss how surgery will affect the patient's diet. Explain that he'll gradually resume oral feeding, progressing from clear liquids to solid foods. If gastric surgery is extensive, he may receive TPN for 1 week or longer.

▶ Explain the need for postoperative deep-breathing exercises and coughing to prevent pulmonary complications. Stress the importance of performing these measures even though incisional pain may make the patient reluctant to do so. Teach him to splint his incision while coughing to help reduce pain.

▶ Remember that the patient will have fears about the surgery and concerns about its effect on his lifestyle, even if he doesn't express them. Take the time to reassure him. Point out that other, more conservative treatments haven't worked and that surgery is now necessary to relieve his signs and symptoms and prevent more serious, possibly even life-threatening, complications. Explain that with successful surgery, he should be able to lead a near-normal life with few activity restrictions.

▶ Instruct the patient to notify the physician immediately if he develops any postsurgical signs of life-threatening complications, such as hemorrhage, obstruction, or perforation.

▶ Explain dumping syndrome and ways to avoid it. Advise the patient to eat small, frequent meals evenly spaced throughout the day. He should chew his food thoroughly and drink fluids between meals rather than with them. He should decrease his intake of carbohydrates and salt while increasing fat and protein. After a meal, he should lie down for 20 to 30 minutes.

▶ Advise the patient to avoid or limit foods high in fiber, such as fresh fruits and vegetables and whole-grain breads.

▶ If the physician has prescribed a GI anticholinergic to decrease motility and acid secretion, instruct the patient to take the drug 30 minutes to 1 hour before meals.

▶ If the patient is being discharged on tube feedings, make sure that he and his family member or friend understand how to give the feedings.

▶ Advise the patient to avoid smoking because it alters pancreatic secretions that neutralize gastric acid in the duodenum.

▶ Encourage the patient and his family members to help speed healing and lessen the risk of recurrence by identifying and eliminating sources of emotional stress at home and in the workplace. Instruct the patient to balance activity and rest and to schedule a realistic pattern of work and sleep. Suggest that he learn and apply stress management techniques, such as progressive relaxation and meditation. If the patient finds self-management difficult, encourage him to seek professional counseling.

GASTRITIS

An inflammation of the gastric mucosa, gastritis may be acute or chronic. Acute gastritis, the most common stomach disorder, produces mucosal reddening, edema, hemorrhage, and erosion. Chronic gastritis is common among older patients and patients with pernicious anemia. It's often present as chronic atrophic gastritis, in which all stomach mucosal layers are inflamed, with reduced numbers of chief and parietal cells. However, acute or chronic gastritis can occur at any age.

Acute gastritis has numerous causes, including chronic ingestion of irritating foods, such as hot peppers (or an allergic reaction to them) or alcohol; drugs, such as aspirin and other nonsteroidal anti-inflammatory agents (in large or repeated doses), cytotoxic agents, caffeine, corticosteroids, antimetabolites, phenylbutazone, and indomethacin; ingested poisons, especially ammonia, mercury, carbon tetrachloride, or corrosive substances; and endotoxins released from infecting bacteria, such as staphylococci, *Escherichia coli*, or *Salmonella*.

Acute gastritis may also develop in acute illnesses, especially when the patient has major trauma; burns; severe infection; hepatic, renal, or respiratory failure; or major surgery.

Chronic gastritis usually involves an underlying pathology that results in atrophy of the gastric mucosa. This form of gastritis is commonly seen in association with pernicious anemia, gastric ulcers, and cancer. It's thought to be caused by *Helicobacter pylori*. Chronic gastritis may predispose the patient to gastric ulcers and carcinoma. The incidence of cancer is particularly high in these patients with pernicious anemia.

Although acute gastritis usually resolves when the causative agent is removed, persistent or untreated disease can lead to hemorrhage, shock, obstruction, perforation, peritonitis, and gastric cancer.

Signs and symptoms

Acute gastritis

- Rapid onset of signs and symptoms, such as epigastric discomfort, indigestion, cramping, anorexia, nausea, hematemesis, and vomiting (any lasting from a few hours to a few days)
- Fatigue, grimacing, or restlessness
- With gastric bleeding, paleness, tachycardia, and hypotension
- Abdominal distention, tenderness, and guarding
- Increased bowel sounds

Chronic gastritis

- Signs and symptoms similar to acute gastritis or only mild epigastric discomfort
- Intolerance of spicy or fatty foods
- Mild epigastric pain that's relieved by eating

Diagnostic tests

- *Upper GI endoscopy* (commonly with biopsy) confirms gastritis when done within 24 hours of bleeding. This test is contraindicated after ingestion of a corrosive agent.
- *Laboratory studies* can detect occult blood in vomitus or stools (or both) if the patient has gastric bleeding.
- *Blood studies* show that hemoglobin levels and hematocrit are decreased if the patient has developed anemia from bleeding.
- *H. pylori* and *urea breath tests* note the presence of antibodies to *H. pylori*.

Treatment

An immediate therapeutic priority is to eliminate the cause of gastritis. For example, bacterial gastritis is treated with antibiotics; ingested poisons are neutralized with the appropriate antidote. Once the associated disease is treated or the offending agent is eradicated or neutralized, the gastric mucosa will usually begin to heal.

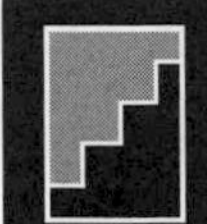

Staying well

Preventing gastritis recurrence

To help your patient prevent the recurrence of gastritis and reduce gastric irritation, give him these tips:

- Take prophylactic medications as ordered.
- Take steroids with milk, food, or antacids.
- Take antacids between meals and at bedtime, and avoid aspirin-containing compounds.

Treatment for acute gastritis is symptomatic and supportive. Healing usually occurs within a few hours to a few days after the cause has been eliminated. Histamine-2 (H_2) receptor antagonists, such as famotidine, may be ordered to block gastric secretion. Antacids may be used as buffering agents.

For critically ill patients, antacids administered hourly with or without H_2-receptor antagonists, may reduce the frequency of acute gastritis episodes. Some patients also require analgesics. Until healing occurs, the patient's oxygen needs, blood volume, and fluid and electrolyte balance must be monitored and maintained.

When gastritis causes massive bleeding, treatment includes blood replacement; iced saline lavage, possibly with norepinephrine; angiography with vasopressin infused in normal saline solution; and, sometimes, surgery.

A last resort, surgery is performed only if more conservative treatments fail. Vagotomy and pyloroplasty have been used with limited success. Rarely, partial or total gastrectomy may be required.

Because patients with chronic gastritis may be asymptomatic or have only vague complaints, no specific treatment may be necessary, except for avoiding aspirin and spicy foods. If signs and symptoms develop or persist, the patient may take antacids. If pernicious anemia is the underlying cause, vitamin B_{12} may be administered parenterally.

If *H. pylori* is implicated as the cause of chronic gastritis, appropriate anti-infective therapy is initiated.

Key nursing diagnoses and outcomes

Imbalanced nutrition: Less than body requirements related to adverse GI effects

Treatment outcomes: The patient will regain any weight lost and will maintain his weight within a normal range.

Risk for deficient fluid volume related to vomiting

Treatment outcome: The patient will maintain normal fluid balance.

Acute pain related to inflammation of gastric mucosa

Treatment outcome: The patient will become pain-free with treatment for gastritis and elimination of potential risk factors.

Nursing interventions

- Provide antiemetics as ordered.
- Administer I.V. fluids, as ordered, to maintain fluid and electrolyte balance.
- When the patient can tolerate oral feedings, provide a bland diet that takes into account his food preferences. Restart feedings slowly.
- Offer smaller, more frequent servings to reduce the amount of irritating gastric secretions.
- Help the patient identify specific foods that cause gastric upset, and eliminate them from his diet.
- Administer antacids and other prescribed medications, as ordered, and note the patient's response.

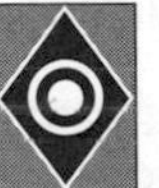

Drug alert About 50% of adults over age 65 have some form of arthritis that requires taking an anti-inflammatory drug that can cause gas-

tritis. Using enteric-coated aspirin or nonacetylated salicylates can decrease GI upset while providing effective pain relief.

- If pain or nausea interferes with the patient's appetite, administer pain medications or antiemetics about 1 hour before meals.
- Monitor the patient's fluid intake and output and electrolyte levels.
- If the patient has received nothing by mouth, assess for the presence of bowel sounds and then watch for returning signs and symptoms as you reintroduce food.

PATIENT TEACHING

- Teach the patient about the disorder and about diagnostic tests and treatments.Explain the relationship between his signs and symptoms and the causative agents so that he'll understand the need to modify his diet or lifestyle. Be attentive to his questions.
- If the patient is scheduled for surgery, reinforce the physician's explanation of the procedure and provide preoperative teaching.
- Give the patient a list of irritating foods to avoid, such as spicy or highly seasoned foods, alcohol, and caffeine. Be sure he understands that these changes are lifelong measures to prevent recurrence of gastritis. If necessary, refer him to the dietitian for further instruction. (See *Preventing gastritis recurrence*.)
- If the patient smokes, encourage him to quit by pointing out that this habit can cause or aggravate signs and symptoms by irritating the gastric mucosa. Refer him to a smoking-cessation program.
- If appropriate, help the patient identify the need for stress reduction. Teach him stress-reduction techniques, such as meditation, deep breathing, progressive relaxation, and guided imagery.
- Urge the patient to seek immediate attention for recurring signs and symptoms, such as hematemesis, nausea, or vomiting.
- Teach family members the importance of supporting the patient as he makes the necessary dietary and lifestyle changes.

GASTROESOPHAGEAL REFLUX DISEASE

Popularly known as heartburn, gastroesophageal reflux is the backflow of gastric or duodenal contents, or both, into the esophagus and past the lower esophageal sphincter (LES), without associated belching or vomiting. Reflux may cause no signs or symptoms or pathologic changes. Persistent reflux may cause reflux esophagitis, an inflammation of the esophageal mucosa. The prognosis varies with the underlying cause.

Normally, gastric contents don't back up into the esophagus because the LES creates enough pressure around the lower end of the esophagus to close it. (The sphincter relaxes after each swallow to allow food into the stomach.) Reflux occurs when LES pressure is deficient or pressure within the stomach exceeds LES pressure. Any of the following predisposing factors may lead to reflux:

- nasogastric intubation for more than 4 days
- any agent that lowers LES pressure: food; alcohol; cigarettes; anticholinergics, such as atropine, belladonna, and propantheline; and other drugs, such as morphine, diazepam, calcium channel blockers, and meperidine.
- hiatal hernia with incompetent sphincter
- any condition or position that increases intra-abdominal pressure.

Reflux esophagitis, the primary complication of gastric reflux, can lead to other sequelae, including esophageal stricture, esophageal ulcer, and replacement of the normal squamous epithelium with columnar epithelium (Barrett's epithelium). A patient with severe reflux esophagitis may also develop anemia from chronic low-grade bleeding of inflamed mucosa.

Pulmonary complications may develop if the patient experiences reflux of gastric contents into his throat and subsequent aspiration. Aspiration pneumonia may result, with its associated high mortality and morbidity among older people. A diminished gag reflex along with a compromised immune system puts them at great risk.

Signs and symptoms

- Heartburn, which worsens with vigorous exercise, bending, or lying down, and is relieved by antacids or by sitting upright
- Regurgitating without associated nausea or belching
- A feeling of fluid accumulation in the throat without a sour or bitter taste (hypersecretion of saliva)
- Odynophagia, possibly followed by a dull substernal ache
- Bright red or dark brown blood in vomitus
- Chronic pain that may mimic angina pectoris, radiating to the neck, jaw, and arm
- Nocturnal hypersalivation, a rare sign that the patient says awakens him with coughing, choking, and a mouthful of saliva

Diagnostic tests

- The *esophageal acidity test* accurately measures the extent of gastroesophageal reflux disease. *Gastroesophageal scintillation testing* may also detect reflux.
- *Esophageal manometry* evaluates the resting pressure of the LES and determines sphincter competence.
- *Acid perfusion test* confirms esophagitis.
- *Esophagoscopy* and *biopsy* help to evaluate the extent of the disease and confirm pathologic changes in the mucosa.
- *Barium swallow* with fluoroscopy reveals normal findings except in patients with advanced disease.

Treatment

Effective management relieves signs and symptoms by reducing reflux through gravity, strengthening the LES with drug therapy, neutralizing gastric contents, and reducing intra-abdominal pressure. Treatment should also include reviewing how the patient's lifestyle or dietary habits may affect his LES pressure and reflux signs and symptoms.

In mild cases, diet therapy may reduce signs and symptoms sufficiently so that no other treatment is required. Positional therapy, which relieves signs and symptoms by reducing intra-abdominal pressure, may be useful in uncomplicated cases.

For intermittent reflux, antacids given 1 hour and 3 hours after meals and at bedtime may be effective. Additional drug therapy may include cholinergic drugs, such as bethanechol, to increase LES pressure and histamine-2 receptor antagonists, such as famotidine or ranitidine, to reduce gastric acidity. A 4-week course of lansoprazole is useful in acute cases. In some cases, sucralfate and metoclopramide have also been beneficial.

Surgery is usually reserved for patients with refractory signs and symptoms or serious complications. Indications include pulmonary aspiration, hemorrhage, esophageal obstruction or perforation, intractable pain, incompetent LES, or associated hiatal hernia. Surgical procedures reduce reflux by creating an artificial closure at the gastroesophageal junction. Several surgical approaches involve wrapping the gastric fundus around the esophagus. Other surgery includes a vagotomy or pyloroplasty (which may be combined with an antireflux regimen) to modify gastric contents.

Key nursing diagnoses and outcomes

Risk for aspiration related to backflow of stomach or duodenal contents, or both

Treatment outcome: The patient will show no signs or symptoms of aspiration.

Acute pain related to irritation of the esophagus

Treatment outcomes: The patient will comply with the prescribed treatment regimen, avoid or minimize contributing factors in his lifestyle, and express feelings of pain relief with antacid therapy.

Deficient knowledge related to gastroesophageal reflux

Treatment outcomes: The patient will express an interest in learning about the disorder, seek information from a knowledgeable source, and communicate an understanding of the disorder and its treatment.

Nursing interventions

- Have the patient sleep with the head of the bed elevated 6″ to 12″ (15 to 30.5 cm).
- After surgery, provide care as you would for any patient who has undergone laparotomy, paying particular attention to the patient's respiratory status because the surgery is performed close to the diaphragm.
- Administer prescribed oxygen.
- Auscultate breath sounds every 4 hours or more frequently as needed.
- Monitor the patient's response to therapy and compliance with treatment.
- Administer prescribed analgesics, and offer the patient emotional and psychological support to help him cope with pain and discomfort.

Cultural diversity **Among Southeast Asians, human suffering is thought to be a natural part of life, and the individual must accept his illness without complaint. Careful assessment skills are especially important with this group because the older patient may not volunteer complaints about his illness.**

PATIENT TEACHING

- Teach the patient about the causes of gastroesophageal reflux, and review his antireflux regimen of medication, diet, and positional therapy.
- Discuss recommended dietary changes. Advise the patient to sit upright after meals and snacks and to eat small, frequent meals. Explain that he should eat at least 2 to 3 hours before lying down. Tell him to avoid highly seasoned food, acidic juices, bedtime snacks, alcoholic beverages, and foods high in fat or carbohydrates because these reduce LES pressure.
- Tell the patient to avoid anything that increases intra-abdominal pressure, such as bending, coughing, vigorous exercise, obesity, constipation, and wearing tight clothing. Tell him to avoid using any substance that reduces sphincter control, including cigarettes, alcoholic beverages, fatty foods, and certain drugs.
- Instruct the patient to avoid lying down immediately after meals and late-night snacks.
- Explain all procedures and medications to the patient and encourage him to ask questions. Supply additional material as needed to support his adherence to the prescribed diet and medication therapy.

GLAUCOMA

A group of disorders, glaucoma is characterized by high intraocular pressure (IOP) that damages the optic nerve. Glaucoma may occur as a primary or congenital disease, or it may be secondary to other diseases or conditions.

Primary glaucoma has two forms: open-angle (also known as chronic, simple, or wide-angle) glaucoma and angle-closure (also known as acute or narrow-angle) glaucoma. Open-angle glaucoma is the most common type of glaucoma affecting older adults.

Secondary glaucoma can develop from such conditions as infections, uveitis, injury, surgery, prolonged drug use (such as with corticosteroids), venous occlusion, and diabetes. Sometimes, new blood vessels may form (neovascularization) and block the drainage of aqueous humor.

One of the leading causes of blindness in the United States, glaucoma accounts for about 12% of newly diagnosed cases of blindness. It most commonly affects people ages 40 to 65; incidence declines with age and is highest among women and blacks. However, early detection and effective treatment contribute to a good prognosis for preserving vision.

Open-angle glaucoma is caused by degenerative changes in the trabecular meshwork. These changes block the flow of aqueous humor from the eye, which causes IOP to rise. The result is optic nerve damage. Open-angle glaucoma accounts for about 90% of all cases of glaucoma and commonly occurs in families.

Angle-closure glaucoma results from reduced outflow of aqueous humor caused by an anatomically narrow angle between the iris and the cornea. This causes IOP to increase suddenly. Attacks of angle-closure glaucoma may be triggered by trauma, pupillary dilation, stress, or any ocular change that pushes the iris forward (a hemorrhage or a swollen lens, for example).

Untreated glaucoma can progress to total blindness.

Signs and symptoms

- Dull headache in the morning
- Mild aching in the eyes
- Loss of peripheral vision (tunnel vision)
- Appearance of colored halos around lights
- Reduced visual acuity (especially at night) that's uncorrected by glasses
- Unilateral eye inflammation
- Cloudy cornea
- Moderately dilated pupil that's nonreactive to light
- Increased IOP, discovered by applying gentle fingertip pressure to the patient's closed eyelids; the eyeball resists such pressure.

Diagnostic tests

- *Tonometry* (with a pneumatic Schiøtz or applanation tonometer) measures IOP and provides a baseline for reference. Normal IOP ranges from 8 to 21 mm Hg. However, patients whose pressure falls within the normal range can develop signs and symptoms of glaucoma, and patients who have abnormally high pressure may have no clinical effects.
- *Slit lamp examination* reveals the effects of glaucoma on the anterior eye structures, including the cornea, iris, and lens.
- *Gonioscopy* determines the angle of the eye's anterior chamber, enabling the examiner to distinguish between open-angle and angle-closure glaucoma. The angle is normal in open-angle glaucoma and abnormal in angle-closure glaucoma. In older patients, however, partial closure of the angle may occur, allowing the two forms of glaucoma to coexist.
- *Ophthalmoscopy* facilitates visualization of the fundus. In open-angle glaucoma, cupping of the optic disk may be seen earlier than in angle-closure glaucoma.
- *Perimetry* or visual field tests determine the extent of peripheral vision loss, which helps evaluate deterioration in open-angle glaucoma.
- *Fundus photography* monitors and records optic disk changes.

Treatment

For open-angle glaucoma, initial drug treatment aims to reduce pressure by decreasing aqueous humor production. The drugs include beta blockers, such as timolol (used cautiously in patients with asthma and those with bradycardia) and betaxolol; epinephrine to dilate the pupil (contraindicated in angle-closure glaucoma); and miotic eyedrops, such as pilocarpine, to promote aqueous humor outflow.

Patients who don't respond to drug therapy may benefit from argon laser trabeculoplasty, in which the ophthalmologist focuses an argon laser beam on the trabecular meshwork of an open angle. This produces a thermal burn that changes the meshwork surface and facilitates the outflow of aqueous humor.

To perform a trabeculectomy, the surgeon dissects a flap of sclera to expose the trabecular meshwork. He removes a small tissue block and performs a peripheral iridectomy, which creates an opening for the outflow of aqueous humor under the conjunctiva and produces a filtering bleb. Postoperatively, subconjunctival injections of fluorouracil may be given to maintain the fistula's patency. The iridectomy relieves pressure by excising part of the iris to reestablish the outflow of aqueous humor. A few days later, the surgeon performs a prophylactic iridectomy on the other (normal) eye to prevent an episode of acute glaucoma in that eye.

Angle-closure (acute angle) glaucoma is an emergency that requires immediate treatment to reduce high IOP. Initial preoperative drug therapy lowers IOP with acetazolamide, pilocarpine (which constricts the pupil, forces the iris away from the trabeculae, and allows fluid to escape), and I.V. mannitol or aoal glycerine (which forces fluid from the eye by making the blood hypertonic). If these medications fail to decrease the pressure, laser iridotomy or surgical peripheral iridectomy must be performed promptly to save the patient's vision.

Narcotic analgesics may be used if the patient has severe pain. After peripheral iridectomy, cycloplegic eyedrops may be given to relax the ciliary muscle and to decrease inflammation, thereby preventing adhesions.

Key nursing diagnoses and outcomes

Disturbed sensory perception (visual) related to increased IOP

Treatment outcomes: The patient will seek medical attention when visual changes occur and will regain and maintain normal vision with treatment.

Risk for injury related to vision disturbances

Treatment outcome: The patient will take precautions to prevent injury because of visual impairment.

Fear related to potential for blindness

Treatment outcomes: The patient will identify sources of fear, seek knowledge about glaucoma from an appropriate source to help reduce his fears, and express an understanding that compliance with the prescribed treatment regimen can prevent further vision loss.

Nursing interventions

- For the patient with angle-closure glaucoma, give drugs as ordered, and prepare him physically and psychologically for laser iridotomy or surgery.
- Remember to administer cycloplegic eyedrops in the affected eye only. In the unaffected eye, these drops may precipitate an attack of angle-closure glaucoma and threaten the patient's residual vision.
- After trabeculectomy, give medications as ordered to dilate the pupil. Also, apply topical corticosteroids as ordered to rest the pupil.
- After surgery, protect the affected eye by applying an eye patch and eye shield, positioning the patient on his back or unaffected side, and following general safety measures.
- Monitor the patient's ability to see clearly. Question him regularly about the occurrence of visual changes.
- Monitor the patient's IOP regularly.
- Monitor the patient's compliance with treatment and lifelong follow-up care.

PATIENT TEACHING

- Stress the importance of meticulous compliance with prescribed drug therapy to maintain low IOP and prevent optic disk changes that cause vision loss.
- Explain all procedures and treatments, especially surgery, to help reduce the patient's anxiety.
- Inform the patient that lost vision can't be restored but that treatment can usually prevent further loss.
- Teach the patient the signs and symptoms that require immediate medical attention, such as sudden vision change or eye pain.
- Tell family members how to modify the patient's environment for safety. For example, suggest keeping pathways clear and reorienting the patient to room layouts, if necessary.
- Discuss the importance of glaucoma screening for early detection and prevention. Point out that all persons over age 35 should have annual tonometric examination.

GLUCOSE MONITORING

Rapid, easy-to-perform reagent strip tests use a drop of capillary blood obtained by fingerstick or earlobe puncture as a sample. These tests can detect or monitor elevated blood glucose levels in patients with diabetes, screen for diabetes mellitus, and help distinguish diabetic coma from nondiabetic coma. In these tests, a reagent patch on the tip of a handheld plastic strip changes color in response to the amount of glucose in the blood sample. Comparing the color change with a standardized color chart provides a semi-quantitative measurement of blood glucose levels; inserting the strip in a portable blood glucose meter provides quantitative measurements that compare in accuracy with other laboratory tests. Some meters store successive test results electronically to help determine glucose patterns.

These tests can be performed in the hospital, physician's office, or patient's home.

Supplies

- Reagent strips
- Gloves
- Portable blood glucose meter, if available
- Gauze pads
- Alcohol pads
- Disposable lancets
- Small adhesive bandage
- Watch or clock with a second hand

Implementation

- Before using reagent strips, check the expiration date on the package and replace outdated strips. Also, check for special instructions related to the specific reagent. Protect the strips from light, heat, and moisture.
- Before using a blood glucose meter, calibrate it and run it with a control sample to ensure accurate test results, if appropriate for that particular device. Make sure you follow the manufacturer's instructions for calibration.
- Select the puncture site, usually the fingertip or earlobe.

Key point To ensure an adequate blood sample, avoid selecting cold, cyanotic, or swollen puncture sites.

- Wash your hands and put on gloves.
- If necessary, dilate the capillaries by applying warm, moist compresses to the area for about 10 minutes.
- Wipe the puncture site with an alcohol pad, and dry it thoroughly with a gauze pad.
- To draw a sample from the patient's fingertip with a disposable lancet (smaller than 2 mm), make the puncture on the side of the fingertip and position the lancet perpendicular to the lines of the patient's fingerprints. Pierce the skin sharply and quickly to minimize the patient's anxiety and pain and to increase blood flow. Alternatively, you may want

to use a mechanical bloodletting device, which uses a spring-loaded lancet.
- After puncturing the finger, make sure you don't squeeze the puncture site, to avoid diluting the sample with tissue fluid.
- Touch a drop of blood to the reagent patch on the strip; make sure you cover the entire patch.
- After collecting the blood sample, briefly apply pressure to the puncture site to prevent painful extravasation of blood into subcutaneous tissues. Ask the patient to hold a gauze pad firmly over the puncture site until bleeding stops.
- Make sure you leave the blood on the strip for exactly 60 seconds.
- Compare the color change on the strip with the standardized color chart on the product container. If you're using a blood glucose meter, follow the manufacturer's instructions. Meter designs vary, but all analyze a drop of blood placed on a reagent strip that comes with the unit, and they provide a digital display of the resulting glucose level.
- After bleeding has stopped, you may apply a small adhesive bandage to the puncture site.

Complications
As a result of glucose monitoring, excessive bleeding at the puncture site or infection may occur.

Patient teaching
- Explain the procedure to the patient and his family members to reduce the patient's fear and promote cooperation.
- Teach the patient proper use of the lancet, the reagent strips and color chart, and the portable blood glucose meter, as necessary. Provide written guidelines.
- Assess whether the patient has the manual dexterity to complete the task. Enlist the assistance of a family member or caregiver, if appropriate.

Documentation
Record the reading from the reagent strip (using a portable blood glucose meter or a color chart) in your notes or on a special flowchart, if available. Also, record the time and date of the test. Document patient teaching and return demonstration.

GRIEF

Grief is a natural, expected reaction to the experience of loss. It most commonly occurs in response to a death or in anticipation of such a loss. Be aware that people grieve in different ways and that every person who experiences a loss has the right to grieve in his own way. Not only is grief experienced differently by each person, but the timing and duration of grief vary as well. Grief may be immediate or delayed, brief or long-lasting.

Signs of grief
Grief can have specific physical and psychological effects. The individual may be restless and unable to sit still. He may also feel a painful inability to initiate and maintain activities of daily living. Social withdrawal may occur in addition to anorexia, GI disturbances, and weight gain or loss. The person may complain of an inability to sleep or hypersomnia and may exhibit lack of strength or physical exhaustion. Crying and tendency to sigh are common. Heart palpitations and other indications of anxiety, nervousness, and tension may occur as well as loss of sexual desire or hypersexuality, lack of energy, and psychomotor retardation. The person may question his existence, mortality, and faith or belief system.

Stages of grief
Initial reactions after the death of a loved one include shock, disbelief, and numbness. The grieving person may be

agitated, cry, engage in aimless activities, be preoccupied with thoughts of the dead person, and feel weak. During this time, support the grieving person through mourning rituals, such as receiving family and friends and planning for the funeral and burial.

Typically, a period of intense distress follows in which the person feels waves of grief. During this time, the person has difficulty concentrating and functioning. This phase may last for weeks or months. As the intensity and frequency of this distress diminish, the individual may come to terms with the loss. This may occur within months or may take a year or longer. Distress may recur, however, with anniversaries and other occasions.

About 20% of people who experience a loss develop major depression or complicated grief that's unresolved. If a family member uses drugs or alcohol to cope, ignores hygiene, develops physical problems, or discusses thoughts of suicide, refer him to his physician or a mental health professional.

Coping with grief

Contact the family within a few weeks of the death to see how they're coping and to answer any questions. Ask how individual family members are coping. Use your knowledge of the grief response to determine whether family members are coping with their loss. Explain the grieving process to the family and explain that what they're feeling is normal. Let the family know of bereavement support groups available in the community.

Tell the person who is having trouble coping to give himself permission to feel the pain and loss and to be patient with the process. Tell him that he should avoid putting pressure and expectations on himself. Encourage the person to accept his emotions and way of healing. Also encourage him to express his feelings, and tell him it's OK to cry. Both are necessary for healing.

In addition, encourage the person to maintain his basic lifestyle and to avoid making major life changes (such as moving, changing jobs, and altering important relationships) within the 1st year of bereavement. This will allow him to maintain a sense of security. The person needs to be reminded to take care of himself, including eating well and exercising. Physical activity is a good way to release tension. Tell him to indulge in small physical pleasures, such as hot baths, naps, and favorite foods, that may reinvigorate him. He should avoid overindulgence in alcohol, however, because alcohol is a depressant that will only make him feel worse in the long run.

To facilitate healing, the person should be encouraged to forgive himself for all the things he said or didn't say and do. Tell him it's also necessary to take breaks from grief. Although it's necessary to work through grief, he doesn't need to constantly focus on it. Encourage him to plan ahead, including preparing for holidays and anniversaries. Tell him to decide if he wants to continue certain traditions or create new ones. Suggest that the person do something symbolic in memory of his loved one. Give information on joining a bereavement support group, which can help him feel less isolated and can give encouragement, information, guidance, comfort, and practical suggestions.

GROUP THERAPY

Group therapy may be more practical and acceptable than individual therapy for those with psychological distress and limited incomes. Feelings of alienation and ineffectiveness are reduced through the sharing of common problems. Group therapy is used to reduce stress-related anxiety, short-term treatment of specific disorders, grief reactions, and conflict resolution. Guided by a group leader (who may be a mental health professional), a group of people experiencing similar emotional problems meet to discuss their concerns with one another.

Implementation

- The group leader should determine the appropriateness of the group for each potential member.
- Ideally, the group should be made up of about 8 to 12 members.
- Meetings should be held anywhere from once weekly to daily for 1 to 1½ hours. The group may meet for several months to years, depending on the needs of the members.
- The leader's role is to provide guidance and clarification of the topics being discussed.
- As the group progresses, the leader steps back and becomes one of the group. Group members may perform some of the leadership functions as they grow and require less support.

Special considerations

Group therapy gives older people a chance to discuss how an illness or the death of a spouse affects their lives and lets them help each other by sharing workable solutions. This form of mental health treatment differs from psychotherapy in that the group consists of peers or family members who have experienced a common problem and the group may or may not have a mental health professional as a facilitator to monitor and focus the discussion. Groups usually meet in churches, senior centers, hospitals, schools, and other public meeting places. Such groups may be free of charge or require a nominal fee.

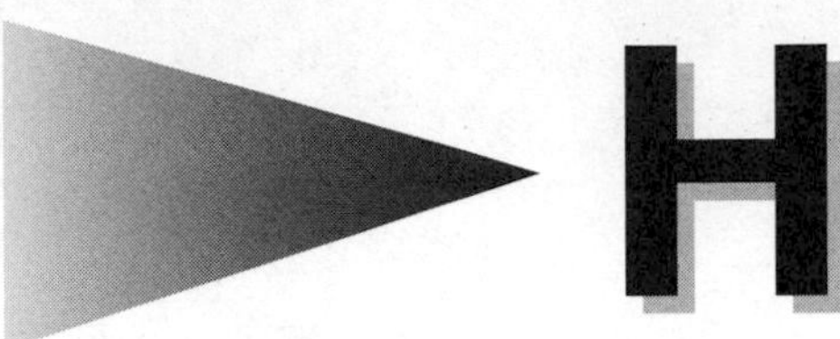

HEARING AIDS

Treatment of sensorineural hearing loss usually involves a hearing aid. A hearing aid is a personal amplifying system that includes a microphone, an amplifier, and a loud speaker. Hearing aids are available in several forms: behind-the-ear aid, in-the-ear aid, and eyeglass hearing aid.

The behind-the-ear hearing aid is suitable for mild to moderate hearing loss. It's durable, easy to conceal, and comfortable to wear. Disadvantages include the close proximity of the microphone to the receiver, which causes feedback and limits the amount of magnification.

The in-the-ear hearing aid fits directly into the ear canal and is supported by the outer ear. It's lightweight and easy to conceal, but it's suitable only for mild hearing loss because it provides less amplification than other aids. The in-the-ear aid also allows some distortion and is less durable. Its small size may make it difficult to operate for someone who has stiff fingers or arms.

The eyeglass hearing aid is used for mild to moderate hearing loss. The hearing unit is built into the arm of an eyeglass frame. The frame can carry a signal from one ear to the other, so amplification is possible in both ears. However, if the person doesn't wear his glasses or if the aid or frame breaks, the wearer may be without both hearing aid and glasses.

Many patients who wear hearing aids complain of speech distortions and amplification of environmental noises. Advances in technology have greatly improved the quality of hearing aids. Some aids contain miniature computer memory chips that help to buffer incoming sounds and filter out background noises.

Hearing loss affects 1 of every 3 persons between ages 65 and 75. Among people age 75 and older, the ratio increases to 1 of every 2 persons. The law requires an examination by a health care provider to rule out disorders of the ear, nose, and throat before audiologic testing is performed.

Financial concerns and lack of Medicare payment are among the reasons older patients aren't fitted with the appropriate devices.

Supplies

- Hearing aid
- Batteries
- Hearing aid case

Implementation

- When you speak to the patient, stand directly in front of him. Speak slowly and distinctly in a low tone; avoid shouting.
- Because the patient may depend on visual clues, make sure he's able to observe activities and people approaching.
- Provide emotional support and encouragement if the patient is learning how to use a hearing aid.

Inserting a hearing aid

▶ Wash your hands.
▶ Make sure the hearing aid is turned off and the volume is turned all the way down.
▶ Examine the earmold to determine whether it's for the right or left ear.
▶ Rotate the earmold slightly forward, and insert the canal portion in the appropriate ear.
▶ Gently push the earmold into the ear while rotating it backward.
▶ Adjust the folds of the ear over the earmold, if necessary. The earmold should fit snugly and comfortably.
▶ After inserting the earmold, adjust the other parts of the hearing aid as needed such as placing a behind-the-ear aid over the ear.
▶ Set the switch to the ON position and slowly turn the volume halfway up. Adjust the volume as necessary.

Removing the hearing aid

▶ Set the switch to the OFF position and lower the volume.
▶ Remove the earmold by rotating forward and pulling outward.
▶ Remove or unclip the hearing aid case.
▶ Store the hearing aid in a safe place.

Complications

Hearing loss can cause embarrassment and may lead to withdrawal from social activities. Profound isolation can have both psychological and physical effects.

Patient teaching

▶ Inform the patient that it may take several weeks or months to feel completely comfortable with his hearing aid, but eventually he'll adjust.
▶ Urge him to be patient with the adjustment period and not be discouraged. Adjustment comes with regular use.
▶ After instruction, have the patient demonstrate insertion and removal of the hearing aid.
▶ Advise the patient of the importance of regular hearing evaluations.

Documentation

Note the type of hearing aid used, your patient-teaching measures and their effect, and the patient's ability to care for and maintain the hearing aid.

HEART FAILURE

In heart failure, the heart fails to pump enough blood to meet the body's metabolic needs. This low cardiac output (CO) triggers a series of compensatory mechanisms, which may lead to pulmonary edema if they fail. (See *Compensatory mechanisms in heart failure*, page 306.) Pump failure usually occurs in a damaged left ventricle (left-sided heart failure). However, it may occur in the right ventricle, either as primary failure or a secondary failure brought on by left ventricular dysfunction. Left- and right-sided heart failure may also develop simultaneously.

Heart failure is usually classified by the site of the failure (left or right ventricle, or both), but it may also be classified by level of CO (high or low), stage (acute or chronic), and direction (forward or backward). These classifications represent different aspects of heart failure, not distinct diseases.

Heart failure in older adults can be precipitated by coronary artery disease (CAD), hypertensive heart disease, cor pulmonale, mitral stenosis, subacute bacterial endocarditis, multisystem complications (renal or hepatic disease, pulmonary disorders), thyrotoxicosis, or adverse drug effects. Among the age-related changes that cause heart failure are reduced elasticity and lumen size of the vessels and rises in blood pressure that interfere with the heart's blood supply.

Most older people with chronic heart failure have CAD. Another cause of chronic heart failure is mechanical dis-

Compensatory mechanisms in heart failure

As the heart's pumping ability becomes increasingly impaired, cardiac output (CO) diminishes. This, in turn, triggers three compensatory mechanisms: ventricular dilation, ventricular hypertrophy, and increased sympathetic activity. Although these mechanisms boost CO, they also force the ventricle to work harder.

Ventricular dilation

An increase in end-diastolic ventricular volume (preload) causes increased stroke work and stroke volume during contraction. As a result, cardiac muscle fibers are stretched beyond optimal limits, leading to pulmonary congestion and pulmonary hypertension, which, in turn, cause right-sided heart failure.

Ventricular hypertrophy

An increase in the muscle mass or diameter of the left ventricle allows the heart to pump against increased resistance to the outflow of blood.

Greater ventricular diastolic pressure now is necessary to fill the enlarged ventricle. This may compromise diastolic coronary blood flow, limiting the oxygen supply to the ventricle and causing ischemia and impaired myocardial contractility.

Increased sympathetic activity

As a response to decreased CO and blood pressure, sympathetic activity increases by enhancing peripheral vascular resistance, contractility, heart rate, and venous return.

Signs of increased sympathetic activity, such as cool extremities and clamminess, may indicate impending heart failure. Increased sympathetic activity also restricts blood flow to the kidneys, which respond by reducing the glomerular filtration rate and increasing tubular reabsorption of sodium and water, in turn expanding circulating blood volume. This renal mechanism, if unchecked, can aggravate congestion and produce overt edema.

turbances in ventricular filling during diastole, with impaired ability of the ventricle to accept blood. Systolic hemodynamic disturbances that increase cardiac workload and limit the heart's ability are also found in older people. Such disturbances include aortic stenosis and systemic hypertension, which increase resistance to ventricular emptying, and mitral or aortic insufficiency, which causes high blood volume. In older people with underlying heart disease, arrhythmias can also cause chronic and acute heart failure. For example, tachyarrhythmias reduce ventricular filling time, bradycardia reduces CO, and other arrhythmias disrupt the synchrony of normal atrial and ventricular filling, leading to heart failure.

Signs and symptoms

- Overwhelming fatigue
- Nocturnal cough
- Dyspnea (initially on exertion)
- Orthopnea
- Weight gain
- Bilateral ankle edema
- Tachycardia
- Restlessness
- Anxiety
- Depression
- Ventricular gallop (heard over the heart's apex)
- Bibasilar crackles
- Ashen, pale, or cyanotic skin that may be cold, warm, or clammy
- Initially, dependent edema, which may progress (right-sided heart failure)
- Distended, rigid neck veins (right-sided heart failure)

▶ Hepatomegaly, which may lead to anorexia, nausea, and vague abdominal pain (right-sided heart failure)

Diagnostic tests

▶ *Electrocardiogram* reflects heart strain or ventricular enlargement, or ischemia. It may also reveal atrial enlargement, tachycardia, and extra systoles.

▶ *Chest X-ray* shows increased pulmonary vascular markings, interstitial edema, or pleural effusion and cardiomegaly.

▶ *Pulmonary artery pressure (PAP) monitoring* demonstrates elevated PAP and pulmonary artery wedge pressure (PAWP), which reflect left-sided end-diastolic pressure in left-sided heart failure and elevated right atrial pressure or central venous pressure in right-sided heart failure.

▶ *Radionuclide angiocardiography* helps assess right-sided heart failure.

▶ *Cardiac catheterization* may show ventricular dilation, coronary artery occlusion, and valvular disorders (such as aortic stenosis) in both left- and right-sided heart failure.

▶ *Echocardiography* may show ventricular hypertrophy, decreased ejection fraction, decreased contractility, and valvular disorders in both left- and right-sided heart failure.

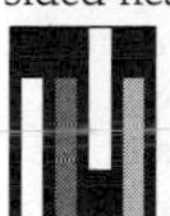

Cultural diversity In the Chinese culture, individuals don't typically display disagreement or discomfort openly. Direct questioning and vigilant assessment skills are necessary to ensure that a patient's quiet nature doesn't mask signs and symptoms that may be life-threatening.

Treatment

People experiencing acute heart failure require immediate care to stabilize their condition, followed by measures to relieve signs and symptoms. Treatment in older adults is the same as for middle-aged people. It seeks to minimize discomfort and prolong life and features medical interventions, such as drug therapy and lifestyle changes, including modifications in diet, fluid intake, exercise, and sleep habits.

Heart failure can usually be controlled quickly by oxygen administration to relieve dyspnea and hypoxia and improve oxygen–carbon dioxide exchange. Angiotensin-converting enzyme (ACE) inhibitors are given to decrease afterload.

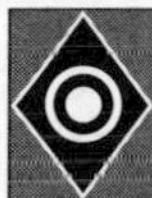

Drug alert Older adult patients may require lower doses of ACE inhibitors because of impaired renal clearance. Monitor for severe hypotension, which signifies a toxic effect.

Diuresis (with diuretics, such as furosemide, hydrochlorothiazide, spironolactone, ethacrynic acid, bumetanide, or triamterene) is used to reduce total blood volume and circulatory congestion.

Drug therapies include inotropic drugs, such as digoxin, to strengthen myocardial contractility; sympathomimetics, such as dopamine and dobutamine, to strengthen contraction and improve CO in acute situations; or amrinone to increase contractility and cause arterial vasodilation. Other choices are vasodilators, such as nitrates to increase CO, and morphine, which is commonly used in acute heart failure to stimulate vasodilation, decrease preload, and reduce anxiety. Beta-adrenergic blockers reduce myocardial workload and oxygen demand by reducing the rate and force of contractions.

Alternating periods of rest and activity are ordered to decrease myocardial demands (chair rest promotes oxygenation and increases diuresis).

Mechanical ventilation may be necessary if, after aggressive treatment, the patient's partial pressure of arterial oxygen (PaO_2) falls below 50 mm Hg, and his partial pressure of arterial carbon dioxide ($Paco_2$) rises above 50 mm Hg.

Key nursing diagnoses and outcomes

Decreased cardiac output related to reduced stroke volume caused by mechanical, structural, or electrophysiologic heart problems

Treatment outcome: The patient will maintain an adequate CO.

Excess fluid volume related to inadequate pumping action of the heart

Treatment outcome: The patient will maintain fluid and electrolyte balance.

Ineffective breathing pattern related to fatigue caused by pulmonary congestion

Treatment outcomes: The patient will regain his baseline respiratory rate, maintain stable respirations and arterial blood gas (ABG) values, and exhibit an ability to conserve energy while performing activities of daily living (ADLs).

Nursing interventions

- Place the patient in Fowler's position and give supplemental oxygen, as ordered, to ease his breathing.
- Auscultate the heart for abnormal sounds and the lungs for crackles or rhonchi.
- Assess the patient's vital signs (for increased respiratory and heart rates and for narrowing pulse pressure) and mental status.
- Provide continuous cardiac monitoring during acute and advanced disease stages to identify and manage arrhythmias promptly.
- Monitor the patient for signs and symptoms of dizziness, syncope, or chest pain.
- Monitor ABG levels. Maintain his Pao_2 above 80 mm Hg and $Paco_2$ at 30 to 40 mm Hg with a normal pH.
- If a PAP monitor is in place, monitor the patient's hemodynamic status. Notify the physician if the cardiac index falls below 2.2 L/minute/m^2 or the PAWP is 18 mm Hg or greater.
- Administer prescribed medications, such as digoxin, diuretics, and ACE inhibitors. Monitor for adverse reactions and toxic effects.
- Restrict fluid intake, as ordered, so that it doesn't exceed fluid output.
- Weigh the patient daily, and observe for peripheral edema and areas of skin breakdown.
- Frequently monitor blood urea nitrogen and serum creatinine, potassium, sodium, chloride, and magnesium levels.
- Organize all activities to provide maximum rest periods.
- Watch for calf pain and tenderness. To prevent deep vein thrombosis due to vascular congestion, help the patient with range-of-motion exercises. Enforce rest, and apply antiembolism stockings.
- Monitor for pulmonary edema, poor response to therapy, increasing acidosis, confusion, and a decreasing level of consciousness. Be prepared to assist with intubation and mechanical ventilation. Resuscitate the patient as needed.
- Provide the patient with a wallet-size card listing medications and emergency phone numbers.

PATIENT TEACHING

- Explain the disorder, its treatment, and any ordered tests to the patient. Many older adults don't understand the concept of chronic illness that can't be cured. As a result, they continually search for a method to "fix" the problem. Explain that heart failure is a chronic disorder and that continued treatment and lifestyle modifications are needed to keep him functional.
- Discuss the need for diet and lifestyle modifications. Stress the importance of regular checkups.
- Stress the need for periodic blood tests to monitor drug levels.
- If the patient is taking digoxin, teach him the signs and symptoms of toxicity,

such as anorexia, vomiting, confusion, slow or irregular pulse rate, and flulike symptoms.

- Stress the importance of taking medications as prescribed. Help the patient simplify his drug regimen and set up a medication schedule. Suggest organizing a week's worth of medication in a pill-box or empty egg carton and using an alarm clock to remind himself when to take medication.
- Tell the patient to notify the physician if his pulse rate is unusually irregular or less than 60 beats/minute; if he experiences dizziness, blurred vision, shortness of breath, persistent dry cough, palpitations, increased fatigue, paroxysmal nocturnal dyspnea, swollen ankles, or decreased urine output; or if he gains 3 to 5 lb (1.4 to 2.3 kg) in 1 week.
- Instruct the patient to report calf pain or tenderness.
- Teach the patient methods to conserve energy while performing ADLs. Suggest that he plan most of his activities for the morning and rest periodically throughout the day. Help the patient delegate tasks.
- Advise the patient to avoid foods high in sodium content, such as canned and commercially prepared foods and dairy products, to curb fluid overload.
- Teach the patient that he must replace the potassium lost through diuretic therapy by taking a prescribed potassium supplement and including potassium-rich foods in his diet, such as bananas, apricots, and orange juice.

Special considerations

Follow-up home care may be needed to assess the patient's compliance with his medication and treatment regimen and lifestyle changes. Home care may also be needed to manage the treatment regimen. Sometimes severe heart failure is managed at home with I.V. infusions of an inotropic drug that affects cardiac contractility, such as dopamine or dobutamine.

HEART VALVE REPLACEMENT

Severe valvular stenosis or insufficiency often requires excision of the affected valve and replacement with a mechanical or biological prosthesis. The mitral and aortic valves are most commonly affected because of the high pressure generated by the left ventricle during contraction.

Indications for valve replacement depend on the patient's signs and symptoms and the affected valve. For example, if the patient has signs and symptoms that can't be managed with drugs and dietary restrictions, a commissurotomy may be performed. If that isn't successful, valve replacement may be done. In aortic insufficiency, valve replacement is usually done once signs and symptoms (palpitations, dizziness, dyspnea on exertion, angina, and murmurs) have developed or if the chest X-ray and electrocardiogram (ECG) reveal left ventricular hypertrophy. In aortic stenosis, which may be asymptomatic, valve replacement may be performed if cardiac catheterization reveals significant stenosis. In mitral stenosis, it's indicated if the patient develops fatigue, dyspnea, hemoptysis, arrhythmias, pulmonary hypertension, or right ventricular hypertrophy. In mitral insufficiency, surgery is usually done when the patient's symptoms (dyspnea, fatigue, and palpitations) interfere with his activities or if insufficiency is acute, as in papillary muscle rupture.

Diseased or damaged mitral or aortic valves may be replaced by either mechanical or biological heart valves. The tilting-disk valve and bileaflet valve are examples of mechanical valves. Both are durable and may exceed the life expectancy of the patient. Because blood flow is turbulent through the valve, many patients require long-term anticoagulant therapy to prevent thrombus formation.

The biological prosthetic heart valve doesn't obstruct blood flow as much as a mechanical valve and is less likely to cause thrombus formation. In addition, it doesn't require prolonged anticoagulant therapy. However, the valve is difficult to insert and less durable (prone to degeneration or calcification, especially in patients with renal disease) than its mechanical counterparts. Biological prosthetic heart valves include human and animal valves.

Implementation

After performing a medial sternotomy and initiating cardiopulmonary bypass, the surgeon cannulates the coronary arteries and perfuses them with a cold cardioplegic solution. For aortic valve replacement, he clamps the aorta above the right coronary artery; for mitral valve replacement, he incises the left atrium to expose the mitral valve.

After excising the diseased valve, the surgeon sutures around the margin of the valve annulus (the ring or encircling structure, which is left intact after valve excision). He then threads the suture material through the sewing ring of the prosthetic valve and, using a valve holder, positions the prosthesis and secures the sutures. Once he's satisfied with prosthetic placement, he removes the patient from the bypass machine. As the heart fills with blood, the surgeon vents the aorta and ventricle for air. Finally, he places epicardial pacemaker leads, inserts a chest tube or tubes, closes the incision, and applies a sterile dressing.

Complications

Although valve replacement surgery carries a low mortality, it can cause serious complications. Hemorrhage may result from unligated vessels, anticoagulant therapy (with mechanical prosthetic valve replacement), or coagulopathy caused by cardiopulmonary bypass during surgery.

Cerebrovascular accident (CVA) may be caused by thrombus formation due to turbulent blood flow through the prosthetic valve or from poor cerebral perfusion during cardiopulmonary bypass. Bacterial endocarditis can develop within days of implantation or months later. Valve dysfunction or failure may occur as the prosthetic device wears out. (This may occur 5 to 10 years after insertion of a biological prosthetic valve and 15 to 20 years after insertion of a mechanical prosthetic valve.)

Key nursing diagnoses and outcomes

Ineffective protection related to decreased blood clotting caused by anticoagulation therapy

Treatment outcomes: The patient will report for regular prothrombin time (PT) and international normalized ratio (INR) measurements and will adjust his anticoagulant dosage, as directed.

Risk for infection related to potential for bacterial endocarditis

Treatment outcome: The patient will express his understanding of what the signs and symptoms of infection are and why he must seek medical attention if these occur.

Nursing interventions

- Reinforce and supplement the physician's explanation of the procedure. Listen to the patient's concerns and encourage him to ask questions.
- Expect to assist with insertion of an arterial line and possibly a pulmonary artery catheter. As ordered, initiate cardiac monitoring.
- Make sure that the patient has signed a consent form and necessary laboratory studies and blood typing and crossmatching have been done.
- Closely monitor the patient's hemodynamic status for signs of compromise.

Watch especially for severe hypotension, decreased cardiac output, and shock. Check and record vital signs every 15 minutes until his condition stabilizes. Frequently assess heart sounds; report distant heart sounds or new murmurs, which may indicate prosthetic valve failure.

▶ Monitor the ECG for disturbances in heart rate and rhythm, such as bradycardia, ventricular tachycardia, and heart block. Such disturbances may signal injury of the conduction system (possible during valve replacement) due to the proximity of the atrial and mitral valves to the atrioventricular node. Arrhythmias may also result from myocardial irritability or ischemia, fluid and electrolyte imbalance, hypoxemia, or hypothermia. If you detect serious abnormalities, notify the physician and be prepared to assist with temporary epicardial pacing.

▶ To ensure adequate myocardial perfusion, maintain the patient's mean arterial pressure within the guidelines set by the physician (for adults, usually between 70 and 100 mm Hg). Also, monitor pulmonary artery and left atrial pressures, as ordered.

▶ Frequently assess the patient's peripheral pulses, capillary refill time, and skin temperature and color, and auscultate for heart sounds. Evaluate tissue oxygenation by assessing breath sounds, chest excursion, and symmetry of chest expansion. Report any abnormalities. Check arterial blood gas values every 2 to 4 hours, and adjust ventilator settings as needed.

▶ Maintain chest tube drainage at the prescribed negative pressure (usually –10 to –40 cm H_2O for adults). Assess chest tubes every hour for signs of hemorrhage, excessive drainage (greater than 200 ml/hour), and sudden decrease or cessation of drainage.

▶ As ordered, administer analgesic, anticoagulant, antibiotic, antiarrhythmic, inotropic, and pressor medications as well as I.V. fluids and blood products. Monitor intake and output and assess for electrolyte imbalances, especially hypokalemia. Once anticoagulant therapy begins, evaluate its effectiveness by monitoring PT and INR daily.

▶ Throughout the patient's recovery period, observe him carefully for complications. Watch especially for signs and symptoms of CVA (altered level of consciousness, pupillary changes, weakness and loss of movement in the extremities, ataxia, aphasia, dysphagia, sensory disturbances), pulmonary embolism (dyspnea, cough, hemoptysis, chest pain, pleural friction rub, cyanosis, hypoxemia), and impaired renal perfusion (decreased urine output and elevated blood urea nitrogen and serum creatinine levels).

▶ After weaning the patient from the ventilator and removing the endotracheal tube, promote chest physiotherapy. Start him on incentive spirometry and encourage him to cough, turn frequently, and deep-breathe. Gradually increase his activities.

PATIENT TEACHING

▶ Tell the patient to immediately report chest pain, fever, or redness, swelling, or drainage at the incision site.

▶ Explain that postpericardiotomy syndrome (fever, muscle and joint pain, weakness, and chest discomfort) can develop after open-heart surgery. Tell the patient to notify the physician if these signs and symptoms occur.

▶ Make sure the patient understands the dose, schedule, and adverse effects of all prescribed drugs.

▶ Teach the patient to carry medical identification with information and instructions on his anticoagulant and antibiotic therapy.

▶ Encourage the patient to follow his prescribed diet, especially the sodium and fat restrictions.

- If the patient smokes, encourage him to stop and recommend smoking cessation groups.
- Teach him how to maintain a balance between activity and rest. Tell the patient to try to sleep at least 8 hours a night, schedule a short rest period each afternoon, and rest frequently during tiring physical activity. As appropriate, tell him he can climb stairs, engage in sexual activity, take baths and showers, and do light housework and other chores. Tell him to avoid lifting objects heavier than 20 lb (9.1 kg), driving a car, doing heavy work, or performing activities that require him to raise his arms over his head, until the physician gives permission. If the physician has prescribed an exercise program, encourage the patient to follow it carefully.
- Instruct the patient to tell his dentist and other health care providers that he has a prosthetic valve before he undergoes dental work or surgery. He'll probably need to take prophylactic antibiotics.

HEAT APPLICATION, DIRECT

Heat applied directly to the patient's body enhances healing by causing vasodilation, which increases blood supply to the affected area. The blood circulation makes more nutrients available for tissue growth and enhances the inflammatory process (leukocytosis, suppuration, and drainage). Heat also reduces pain caused by muscular spasm and decreases congestion in deep visceral organs.

Direct heat may be dry or moist. Dry heat can be delivered at a higher temperature and for a longer time. Devices for applying dry heat include hot-water bottles, electric heating pads, K pads, and chemical hot packs. Moist heat softens crusts and exudates, penetrates deeper than dry heat, doesn't dry the skin, produces less perspiration, and usually is more comfortable for the patient. Devices for applying moist heat include warm compresses for small body areas and warm packs for large areas.

Direct heat treatment is contraindicated for patients at risk for hemorrhage, for those with a sprained limb in the acute stage (because vasodilation would increase pain and swelling), and for those with a condition associated with acute inflammation such as appendicitis.

Key point Use direct heat cautiously on older people because their decreased ability to detect changes in temperature places them at high risk for burns. Heat may also increase vascular permiability and may result in edema. Heat applied to large areas of the body may cause excessive peripheral vasodilation and a subsequent drop in blood pressure.

Use direct heat judiciously, as well, on patients with impaired renal, cardiac, or respiratory function; arteriosclerosis or atherosclerosis; and impaired sensation, all of which are common in older people. Use it with extreme caution on heat-sensitive areas, such as scar tissue or stomas.

Supplies

- Patient thermometer
- Towel
- Adhesive tape or roller gauze
- Gloves (if the patient has an open lesion)

For a hot-water bottle

- Hot tap water
- Pitcher
- Bath (utility) thermometer
- Absorbent, protective cloth covering

Fill the bottle with hot tap water to detect leaks and warm the bottle; then empty it.

Run hot tap water into a pitcher, and measure the water temperature with the bath thermometer. Adjust the temperature as ordered, usually to 105° to 115° F (41° to 46.1° C). Pour the hot water into the bottle, filling it one-half to two-thirds full. Partially filling the bottle keeps it lightweight and flexible enough to mold to the treatment area.

Squeeze the bottle until the water reaches the neck to expel any air that would make the bottle inflexible and reduce heat conduction.

Fasten the top. Cover the bag with an absorbent, protective cloth to provide insulation and absorb perspiration; then secure the cover with tape or roller gauze.

For an electric heating pad

- Absorbent, protective cloth covering

Check the cord for frayed or damaged insulation. Plug in the pad and adjust the control switch to the desired setting. Wrap the pad in a protective cloth covering, and secure the cover with tape or roller gauze. Never place a heating pad under a person; the heat will dissipate and the person may be burned.

For an Aquathermic or a K pad

- Distilled water
- Temperature-adjustment key
- Absorbent, protective cloth covering

Check the cord for safety, as above. Fill the control unit two-thirds full of distilled water. Check for leaks, and then tilt the unit in several directions to clear the pad's tubing of air, which could interfere with even heat conduction. Tighten the cap, and then loosen it a quarter turn to allow heat expansion within the unit.

Make sure the hoses between the control unit and the pad are free from tangles, and place the unit on the bedside table, slightly above the patient so that gravity can assist water flow. Use the key provided to set the temperature. The usual temperature is 105° F.

Place the pad in a protective cloth covering, and secure the cover with tape or roller gauze. Plug in the unit, turn it on, and allow the pad to warm for 2 minutes.

For a disposable chemical hot pack

- Absorbent, protective cloth covering

Select a pack of the correct size. Follow the manufacturer's directions (strike, squeeze, or knead) to activate the heat-producing chemicals. Place the pack in a protective cloth covering, and secure the cover with tape or roller gauze.

For a warm compress or pack

- Basin of hot tap water or container of sterile water, normal saline solution, or another solution
- Hot-water bottle, K pad, or chemical hot pack
- Linen-saver pad
- Compress material (flannel or 4″ × 4″ gauze pads) or pack material (absorbent towels or ABD pads)
- Petroleum jelly
- Sterile cotton-tipped applicators
- Sterile forceps or sterile gloves
- Bowl or basin
- Bath (utility) thermometer
- Waterproof covering, towel, dressing

To prepare a sterile warm compress or pack, warm the container of sterile water or solution by setting it in a sink or basin of hot water.

Measure the solution's temperature with a sterile bath thermometer. If a sterile thermometer is unavailable, pour some heated sterile solution into a clean container, check the temperature with a regular bath thermometer, and then discard the tested solution. Adjust the temperature of the sterile solution by adding hot or cold sterile water to the sink or basin until the solution reaches 105° F. Pour the heated solution into a sterile bowl or basin.

Using sterile technique, soak the compress or pack in the heated solution. If necessary, prepare a hot-water bottle, K pad, or chemical hot pack to keep the compress or pack warm.

To prepare a nonsterile warm compress or pack, fill a bowl or basin with hot tap water or another solution, and measure the temperature of the fluid with a bath thermometer. Adjust the temperature as ordered, usually to 105° F for older patients. Soak the compress or pack in the hot liquid. If necessary, prepare a hot-water bottle, K pad, or chemical hot pack to keep the compress or pack warm.

Implementation

- Check the physician's order and assess the patient's condition.
- Provide privacy, and make sure the room is warm and free from drafts
- Wash your hands thoroughly.
- Record the patient's temperature, pulse, and respiration to serve as a baseline. If heat is being applied to raise the patient's body temperature, monitor his temperature, pulse, and respiration throughout the procedure.
- Expose only the treatment area because vasodilation makes the patient feel chilly.
- If the patient is unconscious, anesthetized, irrational, neurologically impaired, or insensitive to heat for any reason, stay with him throughout the treatment.
- When direct heat is ordered to decrease congestion within internal organs, the application must cover a large enough area to increase blood volume at the skin's surface. For relief of pelvic organ congestion, for example, apply heat over the patient's lower abdomen, hips, and thighs. To achieve local relief, you may concentrate heat only over the specified area.
- Monitor the patient for hypotension when applying heat to a large surface area.

Hot-water bottle, an electric heating pad, a K pad, or a chemical hot pack

- Before applying the heating device, press it against the inner aspect of your forearm to test its temperature and heat distribution. If it heats unevenly, obtain a new device.
- Apply the device to the treatment area and, if necessary, secure it with tape or roller gauze. Make sure that the patient isn't allergic to tape before using it.
- Begin timing the application.
- Assess the patient's skin condition frequently, and remove the device if you observe increased swelling or excessive redness, blistering, maceration, or pronounced pallor or if the patient reports pain or discomfort.
- Refill the hot-water bottle as necessary to maintain the correct temperature.
- Remove the device after 20 to 30 minutes or as ordered.
- Dry the patient's skin with a towel, and re-dress the site if necessary.
- Take the patient's temperature, pulse, and respirations for comparison with baseline values.
- Position the patient comfortably in bed.
- If the treatment is to be repeated, store the equipment in the patient's room out of his reach; otherwise, return the equipment to its proper place.

Warm compress or pack

- Place a linen-saver pad under the treatment area.
- Remove the warm compress or pack from the bowl or basin (using sterile forceps for a sterile procedure).
- Wring excess solution from the compress or pack (using sterile forceps for a sterile procedure). Excess moisture increases the risk of burns.
- Apply the compress gently to the affected site (using forceps, if warranted). After a few seconds, lift the compress (with forceps, if needed) and check the skin for excessive redness, maceration, or blistering. When you're sure the compress isn't causing a burn, mold it firmly to the skin to keep out air, which reduces the temperature and effectiveness of the compress. Work quickly so that the compress retains its heat.
- Apply a waterproof covering (sterile, if warranted) to the compress. Secure the covering with tape or roller gauze to prevent it from slipping.

▶ Place a hot-water bottle, K pad, or chemical hot pack over the compress and waterproof covering to maintain the correct temperature.

▶ Begin timing the application.

▶ Check the patient's skin every 5 minutes for signs of tissue intolerance. Remove the device if the skin shows excessive redness, maceration, or blistering or if the patient feels pain or discomfort. Change the compress as necessary to maintain the correct temperature.

▶ After 15 to 20 minutes or as ordered, remove the compress (using forceps, if warranted). Discard the compress in a waterproof trash bag.

▶ Dry the patient's skin with a towel (sterile, if necessary). Note the condition of the skin and re-dress the area if necessary.

▶ Take the patient's temperature, pulse, and respirations for comparison with baseline values.

▶ Make sure the patient is comfortable.

Complications

Because tissue damage may result from direct heat application, monitor the temperature of the compress carefully. Frequently assess the patient's skin under the heat application device.

Patient teaching

▶ Explain the procedure to the patient, and tell him not to lean or lie directly on the heating device because this reduces air space and increases the risk of burns.

▶ Warn the patient not to adjust the temperature of the heating device or add hot water to a hot-water bottle. If necessary, keep the controls away from a confused or disoriented older patient so that he can't inadvertently touch the temperature setting.

▶ Advise him to report pain or discomfort immediately and to remove the device himself if necessary.

Documentation

Record the time and date of heat application; the type, temperature or heat setting, duration, and site of application; the patient's temperature, pulse, respirations, and skin condition before, during, and after treatment; signs and symptoms of complications; and the patient's tolerance of and reaction to the treatment. Document your patient teaching measures and their effect.

HEMODIALYSIS

Hemodialysis is performed to remove toxic wastes from the blood of patients in renal failure. This potentially life-saving procedure removes blood from the body, circulates it through a purifying dialyzer, and returns the blood to the body. Various access sites can be used for this procedure. (See *Hemodialysis access sites,* page 316.) The most common access device for long-term treatment is an arteriovenous (AV) fistula.

The underlying mechanism in hemodialysis is differential diffusion across a semipermeable membrane, which extracts by-products of protein metabolism, such as urea and uric acid as well as creatinine and excess body water. This process restores or maintains the balance of the body's buffer system and electrolyte level. Hemodialysis thus promotes a rapid return to normal serum values and helps prevent complications associated with uremia.

Hemodialysis provides temporary support for patients with acute reversible renal failure. It's also used for regular long-term treatment of patients with chronic end-stage renal disease. In chronic renal failure, the frequency and duration of treatments depend on the patient's condition. A less common indication for hemodialysis is acute poisoning, such as barbiturate or analgesic overdose.

Specially prepared personnel usually perform this procedure in a hemodialysis unit. However, if the patient is acutely ill and unstable, hemodialysis can be done at bedside in the intensive care

Hemodialysis access sites

Hemodialysis requires vascular access. The site and type of access may vary, depending on the expected duration of dialysis, the surgeon's preference, and the patient's condition.

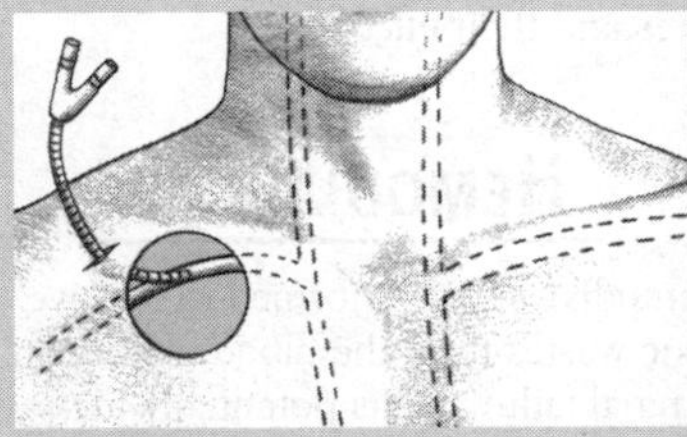

Subclavian vein catheterization

Using the Seldinger technique, the physician or surgeon inserts an introducer needle into the subclavian vein. He then inserts a guide wire through the introducer needle and removes the needle. Using the guide wire, he threads a 5″ to 12″ (12.5- to 30.5-cm) plastic or Teflon catheter (with a Y-hub) into the patient's vein.

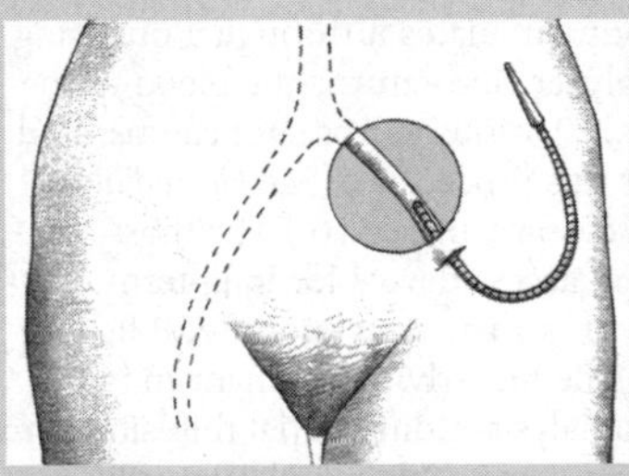

Femoral vein catheterization

Using the Seldinger technique, the physician or surgeon inserts an introducer needle into the left or right femoral vein. He then inserts a guide wire through the introducer needle and removes the needle. Using the guide wire, he threads a 5″ to 12″ plastic or Teflon catheter or two catheters, one for inflow and another placed about ½″ (1.3 cm) distal to the first for outflow.

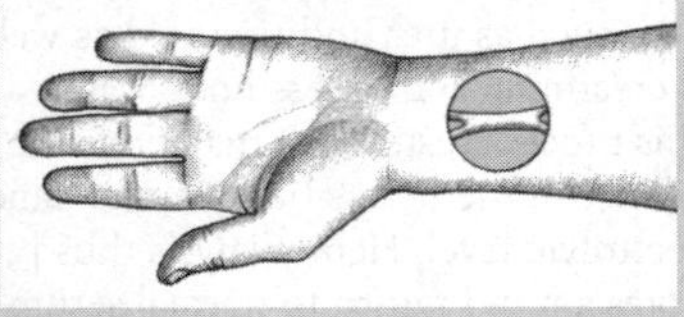

Arteriovenous fistula

To create a fistula, the surgeon first makes an incision into the patient's wrist or lower forearm. Then he makes a small incision in the side of an artery and another in the side of a vein. He sutures the edges of these incisions together to make a common opening ⅛″ to ¼″ (3 to 7 mm) long.

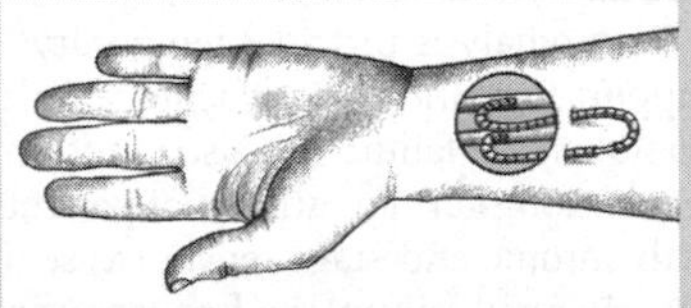

Arteriovenous shunt

To create a shunt, the surgeon makes an incision in the patient's wrist, lower forearm, or (rarely) an ankle. He then inserts a 6″ to 10″ (15- to 25.5-cm) transparent Silastic cannula into an artery and another into a vein. Finally, he tunnels the cannulas out through stab wounds and joins them with a piece of Teflon tubing.

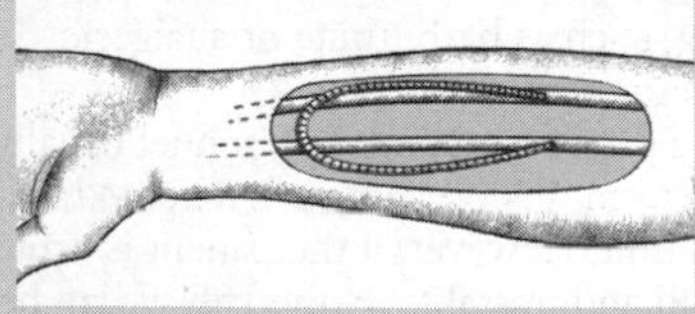

Arteriovenous graft

To create a graft, the surgeon makes an incision in the patient's forearm, upper arm, or thigh. He then tunnels a natural or synthetic graft under the skin and sutures the distal end to an artery and the proximal end to a vein.

unit. Special hemodialysis units are available for use at home but the patient and his family need to complete a home dialysis training program before such use.

Supplies

For preparing the hemodialysis machine

- Hemodialysis machine with appropriate dialyzer
- I.V. solution, administration sets, lines, and related equipment
- Dialysate
- Optional: heparin, 3-ml syringe with needle, medication label, hemostats

For hemodialysis with a double-lumen catheter

- Povidone-iodine pads
- Sterile 4″ × 4″ gauze pads
- Two 5-ml syringes
- Drapes
- Tape
- Heparin bolus syringe
- Clean gloves
- Sterile gloves
- Precut gauze dressings
- Normal saline solution
- Povidone-iodine solution pads
- Heparin flush solution
- Luer-lock injection caps
- Optional: transparent occlusive dressing, skin barrier preparation, tape, materials for culturing drainage

For hemodialysis with an AV fistula

- Two winged fistula needles (each attached to a 10-ml syringe filled with heparin flush solution)
- Linen-saver pad
- Povidone-iodine pads
- Sterile 4″ × 4″ gauze pads
- Tourniquet
- Clean gloves
- Adhesive tape
- Two adhesive bandages
- Povidone-iodine ointment
- Hemostats
- Optional: sterile absorbable gelatin sponges (Gelfoam)

For hemodialysis with an AV shunt

- Sterile drape or barrier shield
- Alcohol pads
- Sterile gloves
- Two sterile shunt adapters
- Sterile Teflon connector
- Two bulldog clamps
- Two 10-ml syringes
- Normal saline solution
- Four short strips of adhesive tape
- Two hemostats
- Povidone-iodine solution and pads
- Elastic gauze bandages
- Gauze pads
- Optional: sterile shunt spreader

Implementation

- Prepare the hemodialysis equipment following the manufacturer's instructions and your facility's protocol. Maintain strict sterile technique to prevent introducing pathogens into the patient's bloodstream during dialysis. Make sure that you test the dialyzer and dialysis machine for residual disinfectant after rinsing. Also, test all the alarms.
- To avoid pyrogenic reactions and bacteremia with septicemia resulting from contamination, use strict sterile technique during preparation of the machine.
- Avoid unnecessary handling of shunt tubing. However, make sure that you inspect the shunt carefully for patency by observing its color. In addition, look for clots and serum and cell separation, and check the temperature of the Silastic tubing. Assess the shunt insertion site for signs and symptoms of infection, such as purulent drainage, inflammation, and tenderness, which may indicate the body's rejection of the shunt. In addition, check to see if the shunt insertion tips are exposed.
- Weigh the patient. To determine ultrafiltration requirements, compare his present weight to his weight after the last dialysis and his target weight. Ideally, no more than 1 to 1.5 kg should be gained between treatments to avoid hypotension associated with removal of

large volumes of fluid. Record his baseline vital signs, taking his blood pressure while he's sitting and standing. Auscultate his heart for rate, rhythm, and abnormalities. Observe respiratory rate, rhythm, and quality. Assess for edema. Check his mental status and the condition and patency of the access site. Also, check for problems since the last dialysis, and evaluate previous laboratory data.

▶ Help the patient into a comfortable position (supine or sitting in a recliner chair with his feet elevated). Make sure that the access site is well supported and resting on a clean drape.

▶ Use standard precautions in all cases to prevent transmission of infection. Wash your hands before beginning.

▶ Obtain blood samples from the patient, as ordered. Samples should be drawn before beginning hemodialysis.

▶ Throughout hemodialysis, carefully monitor the patient's vital signs every 30 to 60 minutes, or more often if indicated. Monitor the patient's weight before and after the procedure to ensure adequate ultrafiltration during treatment.

▶ Continue necessary drug administration during dialysis unless the drug would be removed in the dialysate; if so, administer the drug after dialysis.

Hemodialysis with a double-lumen catheter

▶ Prepare venous access. If extension tubing isn't already clamped, clamp it to prevent air from entering the catheter. Then clean each catheter extension tube, clamp, and luer-lock injection cap with povidone-iodine pads to remove contaminants. Next, place a sterile 4″ × 4″ gauze pad under the extension tubing, and place two 5-ml syringes and two sterile gauze pads on the drape.

▶ Prepare anticoagulant regimen, as ordered.

▶ Identify arterial and venous blood lines, and place them near the drape.

▶ To remove clots and ensure catheter patency, remove catheter caps, attach syringes to each catheter port, open one clamp, and aspirate 1.5 to 3 ml of blood. Close the clamp and repeat the procedure with the other port. Flush each port with 5 ml of heparin flush solution.

▶ Attach blood lines to patient access. First, remove the syringe from the arterial port, and attach the line to the arterial port. Then administer the heparin according to protocol. This prevents clotting in the extracorporeal circuit.

▶ Grasp the venous blood line and attach it to the venous port. Open the clamps on the extension tubing, and secure the tubing to the patient's extremity with tape to reduce tension on the tube and minimize trauma to the insertion site.

▶ Begin hemodialysis according to protocol.

▶ Discontinue after dialysis is complete.

▶ Clamp the extension tubing to prevent air from entering the catheter. Clean all connection points on the catheter and blood lines and all clamps with povidone-iodine pads, to reduce the risk of systemic or local infections.

▶ Place a clean drape under the catheter, and place two sterile 4″ × 4″ gauze pads on the drape beneath the catheter lines. After determining that the patient isn't allergic to iodine, soak the pads with povidone-iodine solution. Then prepare the catheter flush solution with normal saline or heparin flush solution, as ordered.

▶ Put on clean gloves. Then grasp each blood line with a gauze pad and disconnect each line from the catheter.

▶ Flush each port with normal saline solution to clean the extension tubing and catheter of blood. Administer additional heparin flush solution as ordered to ensure catheter patency. Then attach luer-lock injection caps to prevent entry of air or loss of blood.

▶ Clamp the extension tubing.

▶ When hemodialysis is complete, re-dress the catheter insertion site; also re-dress it if it's occluded, soiled, or wet.

Position the patient supine with his face turned away from the insertion site so he doesn't contaminate the site by breathing on it.

▶ Wash your hands and remove the outer occlusive dressing. Then put on sterile gloves, remove the old inner dressing, and discard the gloves and the inner dressing.

▶ Set up a sterile field, and observe the site for drainage. Obtain a drainage specimen for culture if necessary. Notify the physician if the suture appears to be missing.

▶ Put on sterile gloves, and clean the insertion site with an alcohol pad to remove skin oils. Then clean the site with a povidone-iodine pad and allow it to air-dry.

▶ Put a precut gauze dressing over the ointment and under the catheter, and place another gauze dressing over the catheter.

▶ Apply a skin barrier preparation to the skin surrounding the gauze dressing. Then cover the gauze and catheter with a transparent occlusive dressing.

▶ Apply a 4″ to 5″ (10 to 12.5 cm) piece of 2″ tape over the cut edge of the dressing to reinforce the lower edge.

Hemodialysis with an AV fistula

▶ Flush the fistula needles, using attached syringes containing heparin flush solution, and set them aside.

▶ Place a linen saver pad under the patient's arm.

▶ Using sterile technique, clean a 3″ × 10″ (7.5- × 25.5-cm) area of skin over the fistula with povidone-iodine pads. Discard each pad after one wipe. (If the patient is sensitive to iodine, use chlorhexidine gluconate or alcohol instead.)

▶ Apply a tourniquet above the fistula to distend the veins and facilitate venipuncture. Make sure you avoid occluding the fistula.

▶ Put on clean gloves. Perform the venipuncture with a fistula needle. Remove the needle guard and squeeze the wing tips firmly together. Insert the arterial needle at least 1″ (2.5 cm) above the anastomosis, being careful not to puncture the fistula.

▶ Release the tourniquet and flush the needle with heparin flush solution to prevent clotting. Clamp the arterial needle tubing with a hemostat, and secure the wing tips of the needle to the skin with adhesive tape to prevent it from dislodging within the vein.

▶ Perform another venipuncture with the venous needle a few inches above the arterial needle. Flush the needle with heparin flush solution. Clamp the venous needle tubing and secure the wing tips of the venous needle as you did the arterial needle.

▶ Remove the syringe from the end of the arterial tubing, uncap the arterial line from the hemodialysis machine, and connect the two lines. Tape the connection securely to prevent it from separating during the procedure. Repeat these two steps for the venous line.

▶ Release the hemostats and start hemodialysis.

▶ Discontinue after dialysis is complete.

▶ Wash your hands. Turn the blood pump on the hemodialysis machine to 50 to 100 ml/minute.

▶ Put on clean gloves, and remove the tape from the connection site of the arterial lines. Clamp the needle tubing with the hemostat and disconnect the lines. The blood in the machine's arterial line will continue to flow toward the dialyzer, followed by a column of air. Just before the blood reaches the point where the saline solution enters the line, clamp the blood line with another hemostat.

▶ Unclamp the saline solution to allow a small amount to flow through the line. Unclamp the hemostat on the machine line. This allows all blood to flow into the dialyzer where it passes through the filter and back to the patient through the venous line

▶ After blood is retransfused, clamp the venous needle tubing and the machine's venous line with hemostats. Turn off the blood pump.

▶ Remove the tape from the connection site of the venous lines, and disconnect the lines.

▶ Remove the venipuncture needle and apply pressure to the site with a folded 4″ × 4″ gauze pad until all bleeding stops, usually within 10 minutes. Apply an adhesive bandage. Repeat the procedure on the arterial line.

▶ If bleeding continues after you remove an AV fistula needle, apply pressure with a sterile, absorbable gelatin sponge. If bleeding persists, apply a similar sponge soaked in topical thrombin solution.

▶ When hemodialysis is complete, assess the patient's weight, vital signs (including standing blood pressure) and mental status. Then compare your findings with your predialysis assessment data. Document your findings.

▶ Disinfect and rinse the delivery system according to the manufacturer's instructions.

Hemodialysis with an AV shunt

▶ Remove the bulldog clamps and place them within easy reach of the sterile field. Remove the shunt dressing, and clean the shunt, using aseptic technique, as you would for daily care. Clean the bulldog clamps with an alcohol pad.

▶ Assemble the shunt adapters according to the manufacturer's directions.

▶ Clean the arterial and venous shunt connection with povidone-iodine sponges to remove contaminants. Use a separate sponge for each tube, and wipe in one direction only — from the insertion site to the connection sites. Allow the tubing to air-dry.

▶ Put on sterile gloves.

▶ Clamp the arterial side of the shunt with a bulldog clamp to prevent blood from flowing through it. Clamp the venous side to prevent leakage when the shunt is opened.

▶ Open the shunt by separating its sides with your fingers or with a sterile shunt spreader, if available. Both sides of the shunt should be exposed. Always inspect the Teflon connector on one side of the shunt to see if it's damaged or bent. If necessary, replace it before proceeding. Note which side contains the connector so you can use the new one to close the shunt after treatment.

▶ To adapt the shunt to the lines of the machine, attach a shunt adapter and 10-ml syringe filled with about 8 ml of normal saline solution to the side of the shunt containing the Teflon connector. Attach the new Teflon connector to the other side of the shunt with the second adapter. Attach the second 10-ml syringe filled with about 8 ml of saline solution to the same side.

▶ Flush the shunt's arterial tubing by releasing its clamp and gently aspirating it with the saline solution-filled syringe. Then flush the tubing slowly, observing it for signs of fibrin buildup. Repeat the procedure on the venous side of the shunt.

▶ Secure the shunt to the adapter connection with adhesive tape to prevent separation during treatment.

▶ Connect the arterial and venous lines to the adapters, and secure the connections with tape. Tape each line to the patient's arm to prevent unnecessary strain on the shunt during treatment.

▶ Begin hemodialysis according to your unit's protocol.

▶ Discontinue after dialysis is complete.

▶ Wash your hands. Turn the blood pump on the hemodialysis machine to 50 to 100 ml/minute.

▶ Put on the sterile gloves and remove the tape from the connection site of the arterial lines. Clamp the arterial cannula with a bulldog clamp, and then disconnect the lines. The blood in the machine's arterial line will continue to flow toward the dialyzer, followed by a column of air. Just before the blood reaches the point where the normal saline solution enters the line, clamp the blood line with a hemostat.

- Unclamp the saline solution to allow a small amount to flow through the line. Reclamp the saline solution line and unclamp the hemostat on the machine line. This allows all blood to flow into the dialyzer where it's circulated through the filter and back to the patient through the venous line.
- Just before the last volume of blood enters the patient, clamp the venous cannula with a bulldog clamp and the machine's venous line with a hemostat.
- Remove the tape from the connection site of the venous lines. Turn off the blood pump and disconnect the lines.
- Reconnect the shunt cannula. Remove the older of the two Teflon connectors and discard it. Connect the shunt, taking care to position the Teflon connector equally between the two cannulas. Remove the bulldog clamps.
- Secure the shunt connection with plasticized or hypoallergenic tape to prevent accidental disconnection.
- Clean the shunt and its site with the gauze pads soaked with povidone-iodine solution. When the cleaning procedure is finished, remove the povidone-iodine with alcohol pads.
- Make sure blood flows through the shunt adequately.
- Apply a dressing to the shunt site and wrap it securely (but not too tightly) with elastic gauze bandages. Attach the bulldog clamps to the outside dressing.
- After following these procedures, assess the patient's weight, vital signs, and mental status. Then compare your findings with your predialysis assessment data.
- Disinfect and rinse the delivery system according to the manufacturer's instructions.
- Immediately report any machine malfunction or equipment defect.

Complications

Bacterial endotoxins in the dialysate may cause fever. Rapid fluid removal and electrolyte changes during hemodialysis can cause headache, nausea, vomiting, restlessness, hypertension, muscle cramps, backache, and seizures.

Excessive removal of fluid during ultrafiltration can cause hypovolemia and hypotension. Diffusion of the sugar and sodium content of the dialysate solution into the blood can cause hyperglycemia and hypernatremia. These conditions, in turn, can cause hyperosmolarity.

Cardiac arrhythmias can occur during hemodialysis as a result of electrolyte and pH changes in the blood. They can also develop in older patients taking antiarrhythmic drugs because the dialysate removes these drugs during treatment. Angina may develop in patients with anemia or preexisting arteriosclerotic cardiovascular disease because of the physiologic stress on the blood during purification and ultrafiltration.

Reduced oxygen levels resulting from extracorporeal blood flow or membrane sensitivity may require increasing oxygen administration during hemodialysis.

Some complications of hemodialysis can be fatal. For example, an air embolism can result if the dialyzer retains air, if tubing connections become loose, or if the saline solution container empties. Symptoms include chest pain, dyspnea, coughing, and cyanosis.

Hemolysis can result from obstructed flow of the dialysate concentrate or from incorrect setting of the conductivity alarm limits. Signs and symptoms include chest pain, dyspnea, bright red blood, arrhythmias, acute decrease in hematocrit, and hyperkalemia.

Hyperthermia, another potentially fatal complication, can result if the dialysate becomes overheated. Exsanguination can result from separations of the blood lines or from rupture of the blood lines or dialyzer membrane.

Patient teaching

- If the patient is undergoing hemodialysis for the first time, explain the procedure in detail. Encourage the patient to discuss fear, anxiety, and treatment issues he may have related to the disease process and treatment.

▶ Before the patient leaves the hospital, teach him how to care for his vascular access site.

▶ Instruct him to keep the incision clean and dry to prevent infection, and to clean it daily until it heals completely and the sutures are removed (usually 10 to 14 days after surgery).

▶ Teach the patient and his family member or friend that they should notify the physician of pain, swelling, redness, or drainage in the accessed arm. Teach him how to use a stethoscope to auscultate for bruits and how to palpate a thrill.

▶ Explain that once the access site heals, he may use the arm freely.

▶ Remind him not to allow any treatments or procedures on the accessed arm, including blood pressure monitoring or needle punctures. Also, tell him to avoid putting excessive pressure on the arm. He shouldn't sleep on it, wear constricting clothing on it, or lift heavy objects or strain with it. He should also avoid getting wet for several hours after dialysis.

▶ Teach the patient exercises for the affected arm to promote vascular dilation and enhance blood flow. He may start by squeezing a small rubber ball or other soft object for 15 minutes, when advised by the physician.

▶ If the patient will perform hemodialysis at home, thoroughly review all aspects of the procedure with the patient and his family members. Give them the phone number of the dialysis center. Emphasize that training for home hemodialysis is a complex process requiring 2 to 3 months to ensure that the patient or family member performs it safely and competently. Keep in mind that this procedure is stressful.

Documentation

Record the time treatment began and any problems with it. Note the patient's vital signs and weight before and during treatment. Also note the time blood samples were taken for testing, the test results, and treatment for complications. Record the time the treatment was completed and the patient's response to it. Document your patient teaching measures and their effect.

HERPES ZOSTER

Also known as shingles, herpes zoster is a virus that causes acute inflammation of the nerves of the skin, eyes, and ears. Each nerve emanates from the spine, banding and branching around the body to innervate a skin area called a dermatome. The virus produces vesicular skin lesions confined to a dermatome. The herpes zoster rash erupts along the course of the affected nerve fibers, covering the skin in one or several of the dermatomes. The thoracic and lumbar dermatomes are most commonly affected, but others, such as those covering the cervical and sacral areas, can also be affected. Affected dermatomes can vary and overlap.

Herpes zoster is found primarily in adults between ages 50 and 70. It may be more prevalent in people who had chickenpox at a very young age.

The prognosis for people with herpes zoster is good, and most patients recover completely unless the infection spreads to the brain. Researchers are attempting to develop attenuated live-virus vaccines for susceptible populations.

The varicella-zoster virus, a herpesvirus, causes herpes zoster. For unknown reasons and by an unidentified process, the disease erupts when the virus reactivates after dormancy in the cerebral ganglia (extramedullary ganglia of the cranial nerves) or the ganglia of posterior nerve roots. Although the process is unclear, the virus may multiply as it reactivates, and antibodies remaining from the initial infection may fail to neutralize the virus. Without opposition from effective antibodies, the virus continues to multiply in the ganglia, destroys neurons, and spreads along the sensory nerves to the skin.

Herpes zoster ophthalmicus might result in vision loss. Complications of generalized infection might involve acute urine retention and unilateral paralysis of the diaphragm. In postherpetic neuralgia, intractable neuritic pain can persist for years, and scars may be permanent. In rare cases, herpes zoster may be complicated by generalized central nervous system (CNS) infection, muscle atrophy, motor paralysis (usually transient), acute transverse myelitis, and ascending myelitis.

Signs and symptoms

- Fever
- Malaise
- Pain that mimics appendicitis
- Pleurisy
- Musculoskeletal pain

In 2 to 4 days

- Severe, deep pain described as intermittent, continuous, or debilitating, usually lasting from 1 to 4 weeks and occurring in areas bordering the inflamed nerve root ganglia
- Pruritus
- Paresthesia or hyperesthesia (usually affecting the trunk and occasionally the arms and legs)

Within 2 weeks after the initial signs and symptoms

- Small, red, nodular skin lesions that spread unilaterally around the thorax or vertically over the arms or legs. Instead of nodules, you may see vesicles filled with clear fluid or pus. About 10 days after they appear, these vesicles dry, forming scabs. The lesions are most vulnerable to infection after rupture; some may become gangrenous.
- Enlarged regional lymph nodes
- Involvement of the cranial nerves (especially the trigeminal and geniculate ganglia or the oculomotor nerve)
- Vesicle formation in the external auditory canal and ipsilateral facial palsy (with geniculate ganglia involvement), hearing loss, dizziness, and reduced sense of taste
- Eye pain, corneal and scleral damage, and impaired vision (with trigeminal nerve involvement)
- Conjunctivitis, extraocular weakness, ptosis, and paralytic mydriasis (with oculomotor nerve involvement)
- Herpes simplex lesions, commonly found on the tongue, gingivae, cheeks, or genital area. Herpes zoster lesions typically appear in a unilateral distribution around the thorax or vertically over the arms or legs.
- In older patients, recurrent infection or widespread dissemination that calls for an evaluation for underlying lymphoma or other immunodeficiency conditions.

Diagnostic tests

- *Vesicular fluid and infected tissue analyses* typically show eosinophilic intranuclear inclusions and varicella virus. Differentiation of herpes zoster from localized herpes simplex requires staining vesicular fluid and identifying antibodies under fluorescent light.
- With CNS involvement, results of *a lumbar puncture* indicate increased intracranial pressure. *Cerebrospinal fluid analysis* demonstrates increased protein levels and possibly pleocytosis.

Treatment

Oral acyclovir therapy accelerates lesion healing and resolution of zoster-associated pain. Famiciclovir and valacyclovir are also effective. In the immunocompromised patient, herpes zoster should be treated with I.V. acyclovir.

Itching is relieved with antipruritics (such as calamine lotion). The physician may treat neuralgic pain with analgesics (such as aspirin, acetaminophen, or possibly codeine) or use tricyclic antidepressants to help relieve neuritic pain.

Secondary infection may be prevented by applying a demulcent and skin protectant (such as collodion or tincture of benzoin) to unbroken lesions. If bacteria infect ruptured vesicles, treatment consists of an appropriate systemic antibiotic. Herpes zoster that affects trigeminal and corneal structures calls for instilling idoxuridine ointment or another antiviral agent.

Older adults are most likely to experience postherpetic neuralgia. To help patients cope with this intractable pain, a systemic corticosteroid, such as cortisone or corticotropin, may be ordered to reduce inflammation. The physician may also prescribe tranquilizers, sedatives, or tricyclic antidepressants with phenothiazines. Transcutaneous peripheral nerve stimulation, patient-controlled analgesia, or a small dose of radiotherapy may be considered as a last resort for pain control.

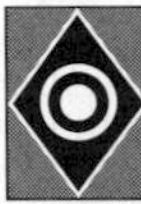

Drug alert **Lower doses of phenothiazines are indicated in older patients, who are more sensitive to the therapeutic and adverse effects, especially cardiac toxicity, tardive dyskinesia, and other extrapyramidal effects. Dosages should be titrated to the patient's response. Monitor these patients closely.**

Key nursing diagnoses and outcomes

Impaired skin integrity related to skin lesions

Treatment outcomes: The patient will demonstrate healing of skin lesions and will regain normal skin integrity.

Acute pain related to inflamed nerve root ganglia

Treatment outcome: The patient will comply with prescribed treatments to eliminate the infection and alleviate pain.

Disturbed sensory perception (tactile) related to paresthesia or hyperesthesia

Treatment outcomes: The patient will take precautions to prevent injury to the affected area and will regain normal sensory function once the infection heals.

Nursing interventions

- Follow standard precautions. Maintain meticulous patient hygiene to prevent spreading the infection to other parts of the body. If the patient has open lesions, follow contact isolation precautions to prevent the spread of infection to immunocompromised patients.
- Be prepared to administer drying therapies, such as oxygen, if the patient has severe disseminated lesions.
- Administer topical treatments as directed. If the physician orders calamine, apply it liberally to your patient's lesions. Avoid blotting contaminated swabs on unaffected skin areas.
- Inspect skin lesions for signs of infection. Use silver sulfadiazine, as ordered, to soften and debride infected lesions.
- Give analgesics exactly as scheduled to minimize severe neuralgic pain. For a patient with postherpetic neuralgia, follow a pain specialist's recommendations to maximize pain relief without risking tolerance to the analgesic.
- Assess the patient for sensory function, noting any areas of paresthesia.
- Keep patient safe from injury to the affected area.

PATIENT TEACHING

- Teach the patient how to apply the prescribed topical medication to the skin.
- Explain that herpes zoster is much less contagious than varicella, but people who haven't had chickenpox may develop it after exposure to a patient with herpes zoster. Stress the need for meticulous hygiene to prevent spreading infection to other parts of the body.
- Inform your patient that treatment consists primarily of drug therapy to relieve pain and promote healing of the

skin lesions. Reassure him that herpetic pain eventually subsides.

- Teach him how to apply cool compresses for additional relief from pain and itching.
- Suggest diversionary or relaxation activities to take the patient's mind off the pain and pruritus.
- To decrease discomfort from oral lesions, tell the patient to use a soft toothbrush, eat soft foods, and use a saline- or bicarbonate-based mouthwash and oral anesthetics.
- Stress the need for rest during the acute phase.
- Teach the patient to be aware of the areas of paresthesia so as not to cause injury. For example, watch application of heat to areas so as not to cause a burn.

HIATAL HERNIA

Commonly producing no signs or symptoms, hiatal hernia (hiatus hernia) is a defect in the diaphragm that permits a portion of the stomach to pass through the diaphragmatic opening into the chest. Three types of hiatal hernia can occur: sliding hernia, paraesophageal (rolling) hernia, or mixed hernia.

In a sliding hernia, both the stomach and the gastroesophageal junction slip up into the chest, so the gastroesophageal junction is above the diaphragmatic hiatus. This type of hernia causes signs and symptoms if the lower esophageal sphincter (LES) is incompetent, which permits gastric reflux and heartburn.

In a paraesophageal, or rolling, hernia, a part of the greater curvature of the stomach rolls through the diaphragmatic defect. This type of hernia usually doesn't cause gastric reflux and heartburn because the closing mechanism of the LES is unaffected. In a mixed hernia, features of both the sliding and rolling hernias occur.

The incidence of this disorder increases with age. By age 60, about 60% of people have hiatal hernias. However, most have no signs or symptoms; the hernia is an incidental finding during a barium swallow. Or, it may be detected by tests that follow the discovery of occult blood. The prevalence (especially of the paraesophageal type) is higher in women than in men.

In a sliding hernia, the muscular collar around the esophageal and diaphragmatic junction loosens, permitting the lower portion of the esophagus and the upper portion of the stomach to rise into the chest when intra-abdominal pressure increases. This muscle weakening may be associated with normal aging, or it may be secondary to esophageal carcinoma, kyphoscoliosis, trauma, or surgery. A sliding hernia may also result from certain diaphragmatic malformations that may cause congenital weakness.

The exact cause of a paraesophageal hiatal hernia isn't fully understood. One assumption holds that the stomach isn't properly anchored below the diaphragm, permitting the upper portion of the stomach to slide through the esophageal hiatus when intra-abdominal pressure increases.

Increased intra-abdominal pressure can be caused by such conditions as ascites, pregnancy, obesity, constrictive clothing, bending, straining, coughing, Valsalva's maneuver, and extreme physical exertion.

If the hiatal hernia is associated with gastroesophageal reflux, the esophageal mucosa may become irritated, leading to esophagitis, esophageal ulceration, hemorrhage, peritonitis, and mediastinitis. Aspiration of refluxed fluids may lead to respiratory distress, aspiration pneumonia, or cardiac dysfunction from pressure on the heart and lungs.

Other complications include esophageal stricture and incarceration, in which a large portion of the stomach is caught above the diaphragm. Incarceration may lead to perforation, gastric ulcer, and strangulation and gangrene of the herniated stomach portion.

Signs and symptoms

- Heartburn, beginning 1 to 4 hours after eating and aggravated by reclining, belching, or conditions that increase inter-abdominal pressure
- Regurgitation or vomiting
- Retrosternal or substernal chest pain resembling angina pectoris (typically after meals or at bedtime)
- Feeling of fullness after eating
- A feeling of breathlessness or suffocation

Diagnostic tests

- *Chest X-ray* occasionally shows an air shadow behind the heart in a large hernia and infiltrates in the lower lung lobes if the patient has aspirated the refluxed fluids.
- *Barium swallow* with fluoroscopy reveals an outpouching containing barium at the lower end of the esophagus.
- *Blood studies* may show decreased serum hemoglobin levels and hematocrit.
- *Esophageal motility studies* reveal esophageal motor or lower esophageal pressure abnormalities before surgical repair of the hernia.
- *Endoscopy* and *biopsy* are used to differentiate between hiatal hernia, varices, and other small gastroesophageal lesions. These tests are also used to identify the mucosal junction and the edge of the diaphragm indenting the esophagus and can be used to rule out cancer that might otherwise remain undetected.
- *pH studies* are used to assess for reflux of gastric contents.
- An *acid perfusion test* is used to distinguish heartburn, for example, by distinguishing the pain caused by esophagitis from those caused by cardiac disorders.

Treatment

The goals of treatment are to relieve symptoms by minimizing or correcting the incompetent LES (if present) and to manage and prevent complications. Medical therapy to reduce gastroesophageal reflux consists of medications, activity modifications, and dietary measures.

Antacids, which help neutralize refluxed fluids, are probably the best treatment for intermittent reflux. Intensive antacid therapy may call for hourly administration; however, the choice of antacids should take into account the patient's bowel function.

Histamine-2 receptor antagonists modify the acidity of the fluid refluxed into the esophagus. Bethanechol is given to strengthen LES tone. Metoclopramide has also been used to stimulate smooth-muscle contraction, increase LES tone, and decrease reflux after eating.

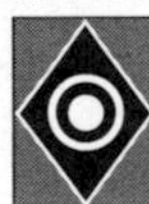

Drug alert Bethanechol should be given with caution to older adults with cardiac or pulmonary disease because of the increased risk of adverse effects, such as heart failure, bradycardia, chest pain, edema, dyspnea, bronchospasm, and pharyngitis.

The patient is urged to make lifestyle changes, such as to restrict any activity that increases intra-abdominal pressure and to stop smoking because it stimulates gastric acid production. A modified diet that includes smaller, more frequent meals and no spicy or irritating foods helps reduce reflux.

Rarely, surgery is required when signs and symptoms persist despite medical treatment or if complications develop. Indications for surgery include esophageal stricture, significant bleeding, pulmonary aspiration, or incarceration or strangulation of the herniated stomach portion. Techniques vary greatly, but most forms of surgery create an artificial closing mechanism at the gastroesophageal junction to strengthen the barrier function of the LES. The surgeon may use an abdominal or a thoracic approach. Many older patients are poor candidates for surgical intervention, so conservative measures may be their only treatment option.

Generally, a sliding hernia without an incompetent sphincter produces no reflux or signs or symptoms and therefore requires no treatment. A large rolling hernia, however, should be surgically repaired (even if it produces no signs or symptoms) because of the high risk of complications, especially strangulation.

Key nursing diagnoses and outcomes

Risk for aspiration of refluxed stomach fluids

Treatment outcome: The patient will comply with the prescribed drug regimen to reduce gastroesophageal reflux.

Impaired swallowing related to esophagitis, esophageal ulceration, or stricture

Treatment outcome: The patient will regain ability to swallow normally through medical or surgical therapy.

Acute pain related to esophageal irritation caused by refluxed stomach fluids

Treatment outcomes: The patient will express pain relief after taking medications as prescribed and will take precautions to minimize reflux of stomach contents.

Nursing interventions

- Administer prescribed antacids and other medications.
- Reduce intra-abdominal pressure and prevent aspiration by having the patient sleep in a reverse Trendelenburg position (with the head of the bed elevated 6″ to 12″ [15 to 30.5 cm]).
- Assess the patient's response to nonsurgical treatment.
- Observe for pulmonary aspiration by monitoring for cough and the color of sputum.
- If necessary, prepare the patient for surgery and provide appropriate preoperative and postoperative care.
- Observe for postsurgical complications, especially significant bleeding, pulmonary aspiration, or incarceration or strangulation of the herniated stomach portion.
- After endoscopy, watch for signs and symptoms of perforation (falling blood pressure, rapid pulse, shock, and sudden pain) caused by the endoscope.
- Monitor daily weights.

PATIENT TEACHING

- To enhance compliance, teach the patient about his disorder. Explain significant signs and symptoms, diagnostic tests, and prescribed treatments.
- Discourage the use of constrictive clothing. Many older women wear constrictive garments, such as a girdle, which may aggravate their condition.
- Review prescribed medications, explaining their desired actions and possible adverse effects. Tell the patient that he'll need medications for hiatal hernia treatment indefinitely, even after surgical repair.
- Teach the patient dietary changes to reduce reflux. For example, tell him to eat small, frequent, bland meals to reduce stomach bulk and acid secretion. Advise him to avoid beverages and foods that intensify his signs and symptoms, such as alcohol and spicy foods.
- Explain how gravity can help to prevent reflux. Encourage the patient to delay lying down for 2 hours after eating. Suggest that he elevate the head of his bed on 6″ (15-cm) blocks at home.
- Instruct the patient to avoid activities that increase intra-abdominal pressure, such as coughing and straining.

HIP FRACTURE

Hip fractures — the most common fall-related injuries resulting in hospitalization — are a leading cause of disability among older adults. They are one of many events that may permanently change your patient's level of functioning and independence. Many who survive a hip fracture never return to their prefracture ambulatory status.

Fractures in the older person are related to falls and preexisting conditions, such as cancer metastasis, osteoporosis, and other skeletal diseases. The most common site of fracture is the head of the femur, with women having a higher incidence than men. Older adults' bones fracture more easily because they are more brittle. They also heal more slowly, increasing the risk of immobility complications.

Poor footing, uneven surfaces, improper use of assistive devices, inappropriate footwear, or slippery conditions can cause falls. People who are confused and restrained with side rails or body vests can sometimes experience hip fractures while simply attempting to get out of bed. The aging adult with bony metastasis or severe osteoporosis can fracture his hip by twisting in bed.

Complications of a hip fracture can be devastating and include pneumonia, venous thrombosis, pressure ulcers, and voiding dysfunction. These complications can delay or prevent rehabilitation and may require that the patient be admitted to a nursing home.

Signs and symptoms

- History of a fall or other trauma to the bones
- Pain in the affected hip and leg, exacerbated by any movement
- Fractured leg, usually rotated outward, apparently shorter than the other leg, and with limited or abnormal range of motion
- Possible edema and discoloration of surrounding tissue
- In an open fracture, bone protruding through the skin

Diagnostic tests

- *X-rays* are used to diagnose most fractures. Pictures are usually taken from two angles.
- *Computed tomography scans* may be ordered for complicated fractures to pinpoint the abnormalities.

Treatment

Treatment of the patient with a hip fracture focuses on restoring function and motion to the injured leg. Activity and weight bearing are limited to allow the fracture to mend properly and, depending on the location, the fracture is treated with immobilization or joint replacement.

Skin traction may be ordered preoperatively to decrease muscle spasms. If the patient won't be treated surgically, bed rest with immobility is ordered initially. Narcotic or nonnarcotic analgesics are ordered to treat pain.

Physical therapy is used to teach the patient non-weight-bearing transfers, and a therapist works with the patient as his weight-bearing status changes.

Key nursing diagnoses and outcomes

Acute pain related to injury to hip

Treatment outcome: The patient will be pain-free.

Fear related to helplessness and outcome of treatment of hip injury

Treatment outcomes: The patient will express his anxiety and demonstrate coping skills.

Risk for impaired skin integrity related to surgery and immobility caused by injury

Treatment outcomes: The patient will protect skin and receive care for any incisions or lesions.

Nursing interventions

- In an emergency, if the bone is protruding from the skin, immediately apply a sterile dressing to cover the bone and open wound, stabilize the leg, and notify the physician.
- Maintain the patient's proper body alignment and use an abductor splint or trochanter roll between his legs to pre-

vent loss of alignment. A footboard and sandbags also help maintain proper positioning. Use logrolling techniques to turn your patient in bed.

▶ Administer pain medications as ordered.

▶ Offer your patient opportunities to express fears and concerns. Answer all questions honestly.

▶ Encourage his participation in his own care; stress the importance of improving mobility and regaining independence.

▶ If the patient has skin traction, remove it daily to check the skin for redness or other signs or symptoms of breakdown. Maintain alignment of the traction, and check the setup to ensure that the weights are hanging freely, not touching the bottom of the bed or the floor.

▶ Keep the patient's skin clean and dry.

▶ Turn your patient often, and consider using a sheepskin or alternating pressure mattress to prevent skin breakdown.

▶ Inspect skin thoroughly for breaks in integrity and treat them immediately.

▶ If an incision is present, perform daily wound care, inspect for signs and symptoms of infection, and treat accordingly.

▶ Good nutrition promotes healing and increases resistance. Encourage the older person to eat as much of his meals as possible. Offer high-protein, high-calorie snacks.

▶ As soon as the physician permits, help the patient move about. Reassure him that the healed limb is safe to use. Plan progress in small steps. Start by helping him stand at the bedside. At the next session, have him walk to a nearby chair, as prescribed. Your patient's early involvement in physical therapy is vital to his successful recovery.

PATIENT TEACHING

▶ Teach the patient and his family member or friend to reposition the limb frequently. Teach them how to maintain proper body alignment.

▶ Teach them to inspect skin daily and report any break in skin integrity.

▶ Instruct the family members on proper wound care and inspection of an incision site for infection.

▶ Review all pain medications, actions, and potential adverse effects. Make sure that you evaluate the effectiveness of the medication. If ineffective, change medications until adequate pain relief is obtained.

▶ If the patient is taking a narcotic analgesic such as codeine, advise him to avoid activities that require alertness. Also, tell him to report a rash, itching, or GI upset. Because older people are more prone to constipation, a direct adverse effect of narcotic use, have him talk to his physician about using a stool softener.

▶ Tell the patient who is taking a nonsteroidal anti-inflammatory drug that the drug may cause GI upset and bleeding. Instruct him to report loss of appetite, nausea, vomiting, diarrhea, or other signs and symptoms of GI distress. Tell him to call his physician immediately if he has black, tarry stools, or bloody vomitus.

▶ Explain the physiology of healing bones to help the patient understand the importance of activity restrictions and lifestyle changes.

▶ Inform the patient and family members about available services to lend support and offer counseling about the patient's anxieties.

HIP REPLACEMENT

Total or partial replacement of the hip joint with a synthetic prosthesis restores mobility and stability and relieves pain. The benefits of hip replacement include not only improved, pain-free mobility but also an increased sense of independence and self-worth.

The most common indication for hip replacement is primary degenerative arthritis. The procedure is also used for

Looking at total hip replacement

To form a totally artificial hip, the surgeon cements a prosthetic head in place in the femoral shaft to articulate with a studded cup, which he then cements into the deepened acetabulum. He may avoid using cement by implanting a prosthesis with a porous coating that promotes bony ingrowth.

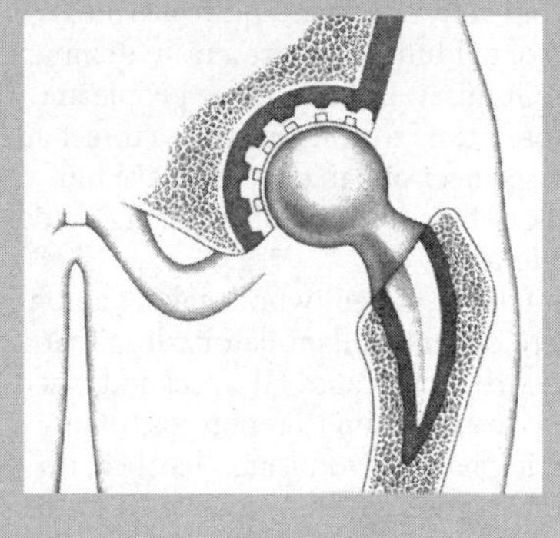

patients with other forms of severe chronic arthritis, extensive joint trauma, and hip fractures. A protruding acetabulum associated with rheumatoid arthritis, osteomalacia, or Paget's disease are less common indications. (See *Looking at total hip replacement.*)

Implementation

During the procedure, the surgeon must remove the head of the femur, exposing the marrow cavity of the femur's shaft. The femoral component of the prosthesis is inserted into the cavity, at an angle that allows its head to articulate with the acetabular cup. The acetabular cup is attached to the pelvic bones.

Hip replacement is performed using either a cemented or noncemented technique. With a cemented prosthesis, the surgeon cements the head of the prosthesis into a position that allows articulation with a studded cup, which he then cements into the deepened acetabulum. Because of the many complications associated with methyl methacrylate cement, porous-coated prostheses were developed.

In a porous-coated prosthesis, the smooth metal surface is studded with metal beads and sprayed with a bone-stimulating material. The coated beads are designed to stimulate bone growth between the beads to hold the prosthesis in place. The incidence of loosening with this technique is no higher than that found with the cemented technique.

Complications

After hip replacement, fractures can occur if the prosthesis is too large for the marrow cavity or if an incorrect angle is used. The patient may suffer a dislocation from excess forward or backward motion of the hip or a loosening prosthesis.

As a result of surgery, cerebrovascular accident and myocardial infarction are possible, and fat embolism may develop within 72 hours. Infection is a concern. Hypovolemic shock from blood loss during surgery is a rare complication.

Complications are linked to the methyl methacrylate cement used, such as pulmonary edema, arterial thrombosis, pseudoaneurysms, hematomas, cardiac arrest, hypertension, and fracture of the cement in the joint, displacing the head of the prosthesis.

Key nursing diagnoses and outcomes

Anxiety related to lack of knowledge about hip replacement surgery

Treatment outcomes: The patient will state his understanding of hip replacement surgery and will have all of his questions addressed before the procedure.

Risk for infection related to foreign object introduced into sterile joint cavity
Treatment outcome: The patient will exhibit no signs or symptoms of infection, such as fever (may not occur in the older patient), increased pain, or redness and swelling at injection site.

Acute pain related to hip replacement surgery
Treatment outcome: The patient will become pain-free after healing has occurred.

Nursing interventions

- After surgery, assess the patient's vital signs frequently and report any abnormal findings.
- Maintain bed rest for the prescribed period.
- Maintain the hip in proper alignment, using a triangular abduction pillow.
- Assess the patient's level of pain and provide analgesics.
- Monitor for signs and symptoms of fat embolism, including apprehension, diaphoresis, fever, dyspnea, pulmonary effusion, tachycardia, cyanosis, seizures, and petechial rash on the chest and shoulders.
- Inspect the incision site frequently for signs and symptoms of infection.
- Assess neurovascular and motor status distal to the site.
- Check for signs and symptoms of dislocation, such as sudden severe pain, shortening of the involved leg, or external rotation of the leg.
- Reposition the patient often (keeping the hip in proper alignment) to enhance his comfort and prevent pressure ulcers. Encourage frequent coughing and deep breathing to prevent pulmonary complications.
- Assist the patient in exercising the affected leg.
- Assess the patient's home for safety and functionality. Available seating, bathroom setup, location of bedrooms and bathrooms, and number of steps should be evaluated.

PATIENT TEACHING

- Before surgery, advise the patient that physical therapy may begin as early as the day of surgery. Teach the patient about weight-bearing limitations.
- After surgery, demonstrate the use of the abductor pillow, splints, and assistive devices.
- Instruct the patient on transfer and pivoting techniques.
- Reinforce the need to follow an exercise program.
- Review prescribed limitations of activity.
- Advise the patient to report any signs or symptoms of infection or a sudden increase in pain.
- Provide the patient with written instructions for incision care.
- Provide referrals for home physical therapy and needed equipment.

HOME SAFETY

For older people living in the community, local visiting nurse associations, hospitals, or health or fire departments can arrange home safety checks. They can also teach family members or other caregivers how to check for and eliminate hazards in the home.

Home safety measures
If you're doing a home safety check, look for the following:

- Are frequently used objects placed within functional reach of the older adult? (Objects used infrequently should be put away and retrieved by someone other than the patient when they're needed.)
- Are pots and pans and other kitchen equipment light enough so that an older person can handle them easily, even when they contain food?

- Are assistive devices for housekeeping, personal hygiene, and dressing readily available? Has the patient been taught to use them properly?
- Is lighting adequate? Are night-lights present for safe ambulation at night?
- Have throw rugs been removed and loose tiles or floor boards repaired?
- Do stairways have good indirect or diffused lighting and secure handrails? If stairs are uneven, in poor repair, or very steep, see that they're repaired or ensure that the older person doesn't use them. (You'll have to make other arrangements for getting the person to different levels of the house.)
- Is the floor free from cords and wires and small objects that the older person could trip over? (Pets and small children should also be kept out of the way when older people are moving about.)
- Are electric cords in good condition?
- Is furniture arranged so that the older person can see it clearly, and is it then left in place? If a piece of furniture is hard to distinguish from its surroundings, place an item of contrasting color on it — for example, a colorful throw over the back of a chair that otherwise blends into the wallpaper.
- Are smoke detectors in place on every floor and are they in working order?

Crime prevention measures

The older person and his family members must take measures to keep themselves safe from crime. To help the older person avoid being a crime victim, look for the following when assessing their home environment:

- Does the older person keep doors and windows locked at all times?
- If he moved into a previously occupied house or apartment, were the locks changed? If there's a chance that the previous occupant may have a key, have the locks changed.
- Does the older person have a door peephole to view someone at the door without opening it?
- Does he keep a large amount of money in the house? If he does, encourage him to put it in the bank or a safe-deposit box.

Special considerations

If preventive measures fall short, your patient must be able to report a crime or activate the emergency medical service. To activate an emergency response in a timely manner, help him post emergency numbers by the phone. Alternatively, if the phone is programmable, program the numbers into the phone so that the patient doesn't have to dial so many numbers. If he has a visual impairment, recommend a large-dial telephone.

Make sure that at least one telephone is placed in a low position so that the patient can reach it even if he can't stand. If he lives alone, suggest that he obtain a telephone alert system. These systems usually require the patient to wear a device around his neck. If he needs help and can't reach a phone, he can push a button on the device. System operators then call the patient to assess his condition. If he doesn't answer the phone, the system activates emergency aid. Urge the patient to ask his insurance company if any part of this service is reimbursable.

HYPEROSMOLAR HYPERGLYCEMIC NONKETOTIC SYNDROME

Also known as hyperosmolar coma or hyperosmolar nonketotic coma, this acute metabolic complication of diabetes is a medical emergency and the most common acute complication affecting older diabetes patients. Hyperosmolar hyperglycemic nonketotic syndrome (HHNS) is characterized by severe hyperglycemia (blood glucose levels above

800 mg/dl), hyperosmolarity (serum osmolarity over 280 mOsm/L), and severe dehydration from osmotic diuresis. It commonly causes impaired consciousness — typically coma or near coma.

When it isn't diagnosed early enough for effective treatment, HHNS causes high mortality.

HHNS begins with insulin deficiency, which hinders glucose uptake by fat and muscle cells and causes glucose to accumulate in the blood. At the same time, the liver responds to the demands of the energy-starved cells by converting glycogen to glucose and releasing glucose into the blood, further increasing the blood glucose level. When this level exceeds the renal threshold, excess glucose is excreted in the urine.

The insulin-deprived cells respond by rapidly metabolizing protein, which depletes intracellular potassium and phosphorous and liberates too many amino acids. The liver converts these amino acids into urea and glucose. The result of these grossly elevated blood glucose levels is increased serum osmolarity and glycosuria, which lead to osmotic diuresis. The massive fluid loss from diuresis causes electrolyte imbalances and dehydration, which further increase osmolarity and diuresis. The glomerular filtration rate decreases and the amount of glucose excreted diminishes, further raising the serum glucose level. The cycle continues, causing additional hyperosmolarity and dehydration.

Various acute and chronic illnesses and other conditions — such as acute pancreatitis, severe burns, uremia, hypothermia, and thyrotoxicosis — can precipitate HHNS by causing stress, which increases the body's insulin needs. Previously undiagnosed or untreated diabetes (possibly because the older patient doesn't buy medications or take them regularly) is a common cause of HHNS.

Drug alert The use of alcohol or certain drugs — including phenytoin, thiazide diuretics, steroids, mannitol, propranolol, immunosuppressants, diazoxide, glucagon, furosemide, ethacrynic acid, and cimetidine — may precipitate HHNS.

Certain medical procedures, such as peritoneal dialysis, total parenteral nutrition, prolonged mannitol-induced diuresis, and nasogastric tube feedings with high-protein mixtures, also increase the risk of HHNS.

Signs and symptoms

- Urinary incontinence
- Abdominal discomfort
- Nausea or vomiting
- Change in level of consciousness (LOC); in some cases, stupor and lethargy first
- Rapid respiratory rate
- Tacky mucous membranes
- Hypotension
- Decreased bowel sounds
- Extreme thirst
- Seizures

Diagnostic tests

- *Random blood glucose testing* reveals extreme hyperglycemia.
- *Arterial blood gas analysis* reveals mild metabolic acidosis.

Treatment

Fluid and electrolyte replacement and insulin therapy are used. Fluid replacement is even more important than insulin therapy. Expect to give abundant I.V. fluids — hypotonic saline solution or, if the patient has hypovolemic shock, isotonic saline solution. Insulin therapy immediately follows, and low insulin dosage, usually given by continuous infusion, gradually decreases hyperglycemia and hyperosmolarity.

Electrolyte replacement aims to replace ions lost through osmotic diuresis. Normal saline solution replaces sodium and chloride. Once fluid replacement begins to shift potassium back to the cells and lower the serum potassium level, parenteral potassium replacement is ordered.

Key nursing diagnoses and outcomes

Risk for injury related to complications

Treatment outcome: The patient will experience no injury from HHNS.

Deficient knowledge related to diabetes mellitus and the complex treatment regimen

Treatment outcomes: The patient will express an understanding of his prescribed treatment regimen and will demonstrate skill in managing it.

Nursing interventions

- Check for a patent airway and adequate circulation.
- Administer I.V. fluids as ordered.

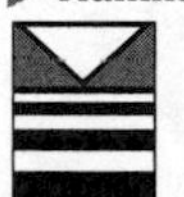

Key point Because the older adult is at higher risk for fluid overload, make sure that you assess his fluid tolerance while you administer fluids. Also assess his lungs for crackles. Notify the physician immediately if you find them, and be prepared to slow the infusion rate. In addition, monitor for cerebral edema as water moves back into the brain cells.

- Begin the insulin infusion as ordered.

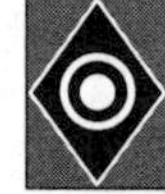

Drug alert Patients with HHNS are more sensitive to insulin than patients with diabetic ketoacidosis, so expect to give them smaller doses.

- Monitor blood glucose levels closely to help avoid hypoglycemia, and document the infusion rate and blood glucose levels regularly. When the blood glucose level approaches 250 mg/dl, you'll probably give I.V. glucose and discontinue the insulin infusion. Give further insulin subcutaneously, as ordered.
- Monitor electrolyte levels every 4 hours, and administer replacement therapy as ordered. Be alert for signs and symptoms of hypokalemia (cardiovascular irregularities, arrhythmias, decreased peristalsis, and weakness).
- Record your patient's vital signs every 15 minutes until he's stable. Report any drop in blood pressure or increase in heart rate or respiratory rate to the physician. Monitor LOC and intake and output.

PATIENT TEACHING

- Review with the patient the importance of taking prescribed medications on time. If the physician has ordered home glucose monitoring, make sure the patient is comfortable using the device and have him do a return demonstration. Arrange for a visiting nurse to check on his technique and disease knowledge.
- For a newly diagnosed diabetic patient, your teaching should include information about diet, medications, exercise, monitoring techniques, hygiene, and how to recognize and prevent hypoglycemia and hyperglycemia.
- Stress the importance of keeping follow-up appointments with the physician. To encourage compliance with lifestyle changes, emphasize the importance of blood glucose control in maintaining long-term health.

HYPERTENSION

Hypertension is marked by an intermittent or sustained elevation of diastolic or systolic blood pressure. Serial blood pressure measurements of 150/95 mm Hg or greater in a person over age 50 confirm hypertension. The incidence of hypertension rises with age. In older adults, hypertension generally results from vasoconstriction associated with aging, which produces peripheral resistance. Other causes include hyperthyroidism, parkinsonism, Paget's disease, anemia, and thiamine deficiency. Hypertension affects more than 60 million adults in the United States. Blacks are twice as likely as whites to be affected, and they're four times as likely to die of the disorder.

Aside from characteristic high blood pressure, hypertension is classified according to its type, cause, and severity. The two major types are called essential (also called primary or idiopathic) hypertension, which accounts for 90% to 95% of cases, and secondary hypertension, which results from renal disease or another identifiable cause. Malignant hypertension is a severe, fulminant form that commonly arises from both essential and secondary hypertension.

Along with the normal physiologic changes of aging, other risk factors for hypertension include diabetes, race, family history, and gender. Lifestyle factors, such as obesity, high salt intake, excess alcohol intake, and oral contraceptive use, also put the patient at increased risk.

The exact cause of essential hypertension is unknown. Family history, race, stress, obesity, a diet high in sodium or saturated fat, use of tobacco or oral contraceptives, sedentary lifestyle, and aging have all been studied to determine their role in the development of hypertension. Secondary hypertension may result from renovascular disease, renal parenchymatous disease, pheochromocytoma, primary hyperaldosteronism, Cushing's syndrome, diabetes mellitus, coarctation of the aorta, neurologic disorders, and dysfunction of the thyroid, pituitary, or parathyroid glands.

Signs and symptoms

- No history of signs or symptoms until disorder is revealed during evaluation for other problems
- Awakening with a headache in the occipital region, which subsides spontaneously after a few hours — a symptom usually associated with severe hypertension
- Dizziness
- Memory loss
- Palpitations
- Fatigue
- Impotence

With vascular involvement

- Nosebleeds
- Bloody urine
- Weakness
- Blurred vision
- Chest pain and dyspnea, which may indicate cardiac involvement
- Slow tremors
- Nausea
- Vomiting
- A rise in the diastolic blood pressure when the person changes from a sitting to a standing position (suggesting essential hypertension)
- A fall in blood pressure with a change from the sitting to the standing position (indicating secondary hypertension)
- Peripheral edema, in late stages when heart failure is present
- Hemorrhages, exudates, and papilledema revealed in ophthalmoscopic evaluation in late stages (if hypertensive retinopathy is present)
- Stenosis or occlusion, detected upon auscultation of the carotid artery for bruits
- Abdominal bruit, heard just to the right or left of the umbilicus midline, or in the flanks if renal artery stenosis is present; bruits also heard over the abdominal aorta and femoral arteries
- Palpable pulsating mass in the abdomen, suggesting an abdominal aneurysm
- Enlarged kidneys, pointing to polycystic disease, a cause of secondary hypertension

Diagnostic tests

- *Urinalysis* may show protein, red blood cells, or white blood cells, sug-

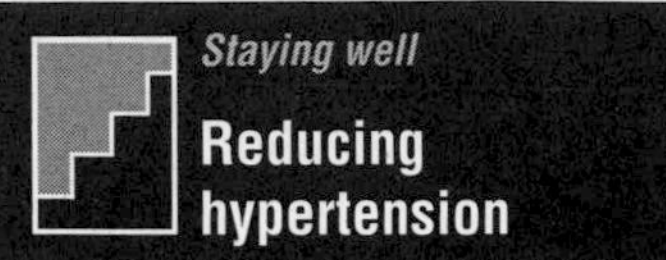

Staying well

Reducing hypertension

Lifestyle factors may play a large part in the development and control of hypertension. Recommend these lifestyle modifications to your patient to help him reduce hypertension:

- Suggest stress-reduction groups and an exercise program (such as aerobic walking) to improve cardiac status and reduce obesity and serum cholesterol levels.
- Encourage changes in dietary habits. Help the obese patient plan a weight-loss diet.
- Tell the patient to avoid high-sodium foods, such as pickles, potato chips, canned soups, and cold cuts; table salt; and foods high in cholesterol and saturated fat.

gesting renal disease, or glucose, suggesting diabetes mellitus.

▶ *Excretory urography* may reveal renal atrophy, indicating chronic renal disease. One kidney that is more than ⅝″ (1.5 cm) shorter than the other suggests unilateral renal disease.

▶ *Blood studies* that show serum potassium levels lower than 3.5 mEq/L may indicate adrenal dysfunction (primary hyperaldosteronism). Blood urea nitrogen levels that are normal or elevated to more than 20 mg/dl and serum creatinine levels that are normal or elevated to more than 1.5 mg/dl suggest renal disease.

▶ *Electrocardiography* may show left ventricular hypertrophy or ischemia.

▶ *Chest X-rays* may demonstrate cardiomegaly.

▶ *Opthalmoscopy* reveals arteriovenous nicking and, in hypertensive encephalopathy, edema.

▶ An *oral captopril challenge* may be done to test for renovascular hypertension. This functional dignostic test depends on the abrupt inhibition of circulatory angiotensin II by angiotensin-converting enzyme inhibitors, removing the major support for perfusion through a stenotic kidney. The acutely ischemic kidney immediately releases renin and undergoes a marked decrease in glomerular filtration rate and renal blood flow.

▶ *Renal arteriography* may show renal artery stenosis.

Treatment

Although essential hypertension has no cure, drugs and modifications in diet and lifestyle can control it. Generally, nondrug treatment, such as lifestyle modification, is tried first, especially in early, mild cases. If this is ineffective, treatment progresses in steps to include various types of antihypertensives. Many older adults with hypertension can be treated with diuretics alone.

Most blacks respond poorly to beta-adrenergic blocking agents; however, for unclear reasons, they respond well to a combination of a diuretic and an angiotensin-converting enzyme inhibitor.

Treatment of secondary hypertension includes correcting the underlying cause and controlling hypertensive effects.

Key nursing diagnoses and outcomes

Risk for injury related to complications of hypertension

Treatment outcome: The patient will avoid dysfunction of any organ system, especially the cardiovascular and renal systems.

Deficient knowledge related to hypertension and its treatment

Treatment outcome: The patient will express an understanding of hypertension and the methods used to control it.

Noncompliance related to the lifelong need for antihypertensive therapy and the misconception that such therapy is needed only during symptomatic periods
Treatment outcome: The patient will comply with the prescribed treatments, as shown by normal blood pressure and absence of organ dysfunction.

Nursing interventions

▶ If the patient is hospitalized with hypertension, find out if he was taking his prescribed antihypertensive medication.
▶ Administer diuretics and antihypertensive drugs as ordered.

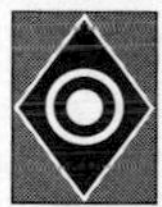

Drug alert Older patients are at an increased risk for the adverse effects of antihypertensives, especially orthostatic hypotension. They may need lower doses.

▶ When routine blood pressure screening reveals elevated pressure, make sure the sphygmomanometer cuff size is appropriate for the patient's upper arm circumference. Take the pressure in both arms in lying, sitting, and standing positions. Ask the patient if he smoked, drank a beverage containing caffeine, or was emotionally upset before the test.

PATIENT TEACHING

▶ Focus your teaching on helping the person learn to live with and control his hypertension. Emphasize that lifelong therapy is needed, even when overt signs and symptoms of ill health are absent. (See *Reducing hypertension*.)
▶ Teach the person to use a self-monitoring blood pressure cuff and to record the reading at least twice weekly in a journal for review by the physician at every office appointment. Tell him to take his blood pressure at the same hour each time with relatively the same type of activity preceding the measurement.
▶ To encourage compliance with antihypertensive therapy, suggest establishing a daily routine for taking medication. Warn the person that uncontrolled hypertension may cause stroke and heart attack. Tell him to keep a record of the drugs he takes and the effectiveness of each, and to discuss this information with the physician during follow-up visits.
▶ Explain that suddenly stopping drug therapy is dangerous. Instruct him to report any adverse effects to the physician immediately.
▶ Advise the person to avoid high-sodium antacids and over-the-counter cold and sinus medications containing harmful vasoconstrictors.
▶ For people who smoke tobacco, describe the effects of smoking and the importance of quitting, or refer the person to a smoking-cessation program. Explain the proper use of nicotine-containing patches, chewing gum, or nasal spray.
▶ Advise the person to limit daily consumption of alcohol to 1 oz.
▶ Continue to monitor the patient's blood pressure and compliance with treatment. Provide positive reinforcement and psychosocial support, as needed.

Special considerations

Expense of treatment is typically an important variable affecting whether the older adult is compliant with his medication regimen. Fixed-dose combination products may help simplify the regimen, at a lower cost.

HYPOTENSION, ORTHOSTATIC

Orthostatic hypotension is a major cause of confusion and falls in older people and a major cause of death. The disorder is characterized by a decline of 20 mm Hg or more in systolic blood pressure or a 10 mm Hg drop in diastolic pressure, when assuming an upright position. Although the baroreceptor reflex is present in older patients, it's usually slowed. Therefore, even a small cardiovascular abnormality may produce orthostatic hypotension in the older patient on bed rest with a subacute or chronic illness. Many conditions can cause older adults to experience orthostatic hypotension, such as:

- cerebrovascular disease
- Parkinson's disease
- Shy-Drager syndrome
- chronic alcohol abuse
- Wernicke's encephalopathy
- diabetes mellitus
- heart block
- blood loss
- fluid depletion caused by salt and water loss
- medications, such as tricyclic antidepressants, methyldopa, diuretics, phenothiazines, prazosin, hydralazine, clonidine, antihypertensives sympatholytic agents, and ganglionic blocking agents.

Signs and symptoms

- Dizziness when arising from a lying or sitting position
- Sudden drop in blood pressure with a change in position (arising from a lying or sitting position)

Diagnostic tests

- *Blood pressure measurements* with the patient in lying, sitting, and standing positions will show a drop in pressure as the patient rises.

Treatment

Evaluation of the patient's present drug regimen is important. If a particular drug is responsible for the orthostatic hypotension, he may need a new drug therapy.

Elastic support stockings applied before arising and isometric exercises may prevent orthostatic hypotension. Fluid replacement helps, if volume depletion is the problem.

Key nursing diagnoses and outcomes

Risk for injury related to dizziness and light-headedness associated with orthostatic hypotension

Treatment outcome: The patient will be free from injury from orthostatic hypotension.

Deficient knowledge related to orthostatic hypotension

Treatment outcomes: The patient will express an understanding of his prescribed treatment regimen and will demonstrate skill in managing it.

Nursing interventions

- Monitor the patient's blood pressure in various positions (lying, sitting, and standing).
- Review the patient's current drug therapy.
- Help the patient get out of bed slowly, after he sits on the edge of the bed for a few minutes before standing.

PATIENT TEACHING

- Teach the patient and his family member or friend about his disease process.
- Tell the patient to change positions slowly when going from a lying or sitting position to a standing position.

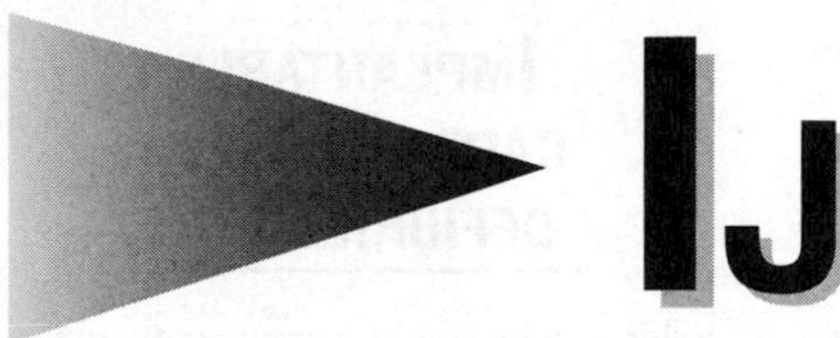

Imagery

Imagery is a mind-body technique in which patients use their imaginations to promote relaxation, relieve symptoms (or better cope with them), and heal disease. It's successfully used to control pain and enhance immune function. It's also used as an adjunctive therapy for several diseases. Imagery is widely used in cancer patients to help mobilize the immune system, to alleviate the nausea and vomiting associated with chemotherapy, to relieve pain and stress, and to promote weight gain. It's used in many cardiac rehabilitation programs and centers specializing in chronic pain. imagery can also be effective in helping patients tolerate medical procedures.

According to imagery advocates, people with strong imaginations, those who can literally "worry themselves sick," are excellent candidates for using imagery to positively affect their health.

Two of the more popular imagery techniques are palming and guided imagery. In palming, the patient places his palms over his closed eyes and tries to fill his entire field of vision with only the color black. He tries to picture the black changing to a color he associates with stress, such as red, and then mentally replaces that color with one he finds soothing, such as pale blue. In guided imagery, the patient is asked to visualize a goal he wants to achieve and to then picture himself taking action to achieve it. This type of therapy is intended to complement traditional cancer treatments rather than replace them.

As an active means of relaxation, imagery is a central part of almost all stress-reduction techniques. Additionally, it's a useful self-care tool. With proper instruction, patients can use imagery to relieve stress, enhance immune function to fight a cold virus, and improve their sense of well-being.

Implementation

- Provide the patient with a private, quiet environment that's free from distractions. Also provide a comfortable place in which to lie down.
- If you're using a taped imagery sequence, make sure the tape player is working and that the room has an electrical outlet.
- Help the patient into a comfortable position and explain the exercise. Answer any questions the patient may have.
- When the patient is comfortable, instruct him to close his eyes. Lower the lights if possible.
- Use a steady, soothing, low voice throughout the exercise.
- Instruct the patient to take a few deep breaths and to imagine that with each breath he's taking in calmness and peacefulness and releasing tension, discomfort, and worry. Tell him to let his breath find its own rate and rhythm and to continue to breathe in calmness and peacefulness and breathe out tension and worry.
- Help the patient relax his body. Instruct him to imagine that he's breath-

ing calmness into his feet and legs and releasing tension with each exhalation. Continue this sequence moving from feet to head, having him breathe in calmness to each successive body part.

▶ As you complete this portion of the exercise, remind the patient to let his whole body sink into a peaceful, relaxed state.

▶ Tell the patient to imagine himself in a place that's peaceful and beautiful, perhaps somewhere he has visited or a special place where he would like to be. Encourage him to notice details of this place, such as colors, shapes, and living things found there. Have him think about the sounds and smells of the place and pay attention to any feelings of peacefulness and relaxation.

▶ While remaining quiet, allow the patient to spend as long as he wants in this place; tell him that when he's ready, he should allow the images to fade and slowly bring himself back to the outer world.

▶ If the patient is willing, discuss the experience with him, concentrating on the positive feelings of relaxation and peace.

▶ Document the length of the session, the imagery path used, and the patient's response.

Special considerations

▶ To enhance the effects of imagery, consider adding a smell to trigger the image that the patient is trying to experience.

▶ Occasionally, an imagery session may lead a person to remember an unpleasant period or event in his life. If this occurs, stop the session and encourage the patient to tell you what he was seeing and feeling. If the patient becomes upset, stay with him. When possible, notify the doctor.

▶ Imagery is contraindicated in psychotic patients.

▶ Be aware that patients with respiratory problems may have difficulty controlling their breathing.

IMPLANTABLE CARDIOVERTER-DEFIBRILLATOR

Older adults with recurrent ventricular tachycardia or fibrillation who can't be managed adequately with antiarrhythmic drugs may benefit from an implantable cardioverter-defibrillator (ICD). An ICD is an electronic device that's implanted in the body to continually monitor the heart for bradycardia, ventricular tachycardia (VT), and ventricular fibrillation (VF). The device administers either shocks or paced beats to treat these dangerous arrhythmias. In general, ICDs are indicated for patients in whom drug therapy, surgery, or catheter ablation has failed to prevent arrhythmias.

The ICD system consists of a programmable pulse generator and one or more leadwires. The leads are insulated wires that carry the heart signal to the pulse generator and deliver electrical energy from the pulse generator to the heart. The pulse generator is a small computer powered by a battery. The generator is responsible for monitoring the heart's electrical signals and delivering electrical therapy when it identifies an abnormal rhythm. It also stores information on the heart's activity before, during, and after an arrhythmia and tracks which treatment was delivered and the outcome of that treatment. Many devices also store electrograms, electrical tracings that are similar to electrocardiograms (ECGs). With an interrogation device, a doctor can retrieve this information to evaluate ICD function and battery status and to adjust ICD system settings.

Today's advanced devices can detect a wide range of arrhythmias and automatically respond with the appropriate therapy, such as bradycardia pacing (both single- and dual-chamber), antitachycardia pacing, cardioversion, and defibrilla-

Types of ICD therapies

Implantable cardioverter-defibrillators (ICDs) can deliver a range of therapies, depending on the arrhythmias detected and how the device is programmed. Therapies include antitachycardia pacing, cardioversion, defibrillation, and bradycardia pacing.

Therapy	Description
Antitachycardia pacing	A series of small, rapid electrical pacing pulses used to interrupt ventricular tachycardia and return the heart to its normal rhythm; not appropriate for all patients and initiated by the doctor after appropriate evaluation of electrophysiology studies
Cardioversion	A low- or high-energy shock (up to 34 joules) that's timed to the R wave to terminate ventricular tachycardia and return the heart to its normal rhythm
Defibrillation	A high-energy shock (up to 34 joules) to the heart to terminate ventricular fibrillation and return the heart to its normal rhythm
Bradycardia pacing	Electrical pacing pulses used when the natural electrical signals are too slow (most ICD systems can pace one chamber [VVI pacing] of the heart at a preset rate; some systems will sense and pace both chambers [DDD pacing])

tion. ICDs that provide therapy for atrial arrhythmias, such as atrial fibrillation, are under evaluation. (See *Types of ICD therapies*.)

Implementation

ICD implantation is most commonly performed in the cardiac catheterization laboratory by a specially trained cardiologist. Occasionally, a patient who requires other surgery, such as coronary artery bypass, may have the device implanted in the operating room. (See *Location of an ICD*, page 342.)

Complications

Early complications include serous or bloody drainage from the insertion site, swelling, ecchymosis, incisional pain, and impaired mobility. Other complications include venous thrombosis, embolism, infection, pneumothorax, pectoral or diaphragmatic muscle stimulation from the ICD, arrhythmias, cardiac tamponade, heart failure, and abnormal ICD operation with lead dislodgment. Late complications include failure to function, resulting in untreated ventricular fibrillation and cardiac arrest.

Key nursing diagnoses and patient outcomes

Anxiety related to lack of understanding of ICD unit function

Treatment outcomes: The patient will express fears and concerns related to the ICD and will cope with anxiety by obtaining information about ICD function from appropriate sources.

Decreased cardiac output related to decreased left ventricular filling time caused by arrhythmia resulting from failure of ICD

Treatment outcomes: The patient won't exhibit signs of decreased cardiac output, such as hypotension and altered tissue perfusion. The patient will recover a

Location of an ICD

To insert an implantable cardioverter-defibrillator (ICD), the cardiologist makes a small incision near the collarbone and accesses the subclavian vein. The leadwires are inserted through the subclavian vein, threaded into the heart, and placed in contact with the endocardium.

The leads are connected to the pulse generator, which is placed under the skin in a specially prepared pocket in the right or left upper chest. (Placement is similar to that used for a pacemaker.) The cardiologist then closes the incision and programs the device.

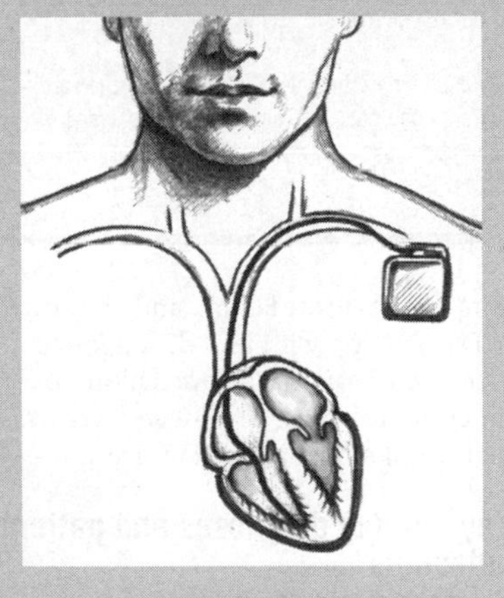

normal cardiac rhythm that will remain normal.

Risk for injury related to potential for ICD malfunction

Treatment outcomes: The patient will identify reportable signs and symptoms of ICD malfunction, have ICD function checked regularly, and report impaired physical mobility.

Nursing interventions

Care of a patient with an ICD includes monitoring device function, providing emergency care if indicated, observing precautions, and recognizing complications.

Before the procedure

- If the patient is scheduled for ICD implantation, ensure that he and his family understand the doctor's explanation of the need for the device, the potential complications, and the alternatives. Make sure they also understand ICD terminology and functioning.
- Before implantation, obtain baseline vital signs and record a 12-lead ECG or rhythm strip. Evaluate radial and pedal pulses and assess the patient's mental status.
- Restrict food and fluids for 12 hours before the procedure.
- Explain to the patient that he may receive a sedative before the procedure and will probably have his upper chest shaved and scrubbed with an antiseptic solution. Inform him that when he arrives in the cardiac catheterization laboratory, his hands may be restrained so that they don't inadvertently touch the sterile area and his chest or abdomen will be draped with sterile towels.
- Check that the patient or a responsible family member has signed a consent form.
- Document any arrhythmias in a monitored patient.
- Notify the doctor if a change in pulse pattern or rate occurs in an unmonitored patient or if a monitored patient exhibits an arrhythmia.
- Be prepared to initiate cardiopulmonary resuscitation (CPR), if indicated, when a life-threatening arrhythmia occurs.
- Administer medications, as ordered, and prepare to assist with medical procedures (such as defibrillation) if indicated.

After the procedure

- When caring for a patient with an ICD, it's important to know how the device is programmed. This information is available through a status report that can

Analyzing the function of an ICD

To evaluate the function of an implantable cardioverter-defibrillator (ICD), compare the electrocardiogram monitor strips with the device status report. The example demonstrates proper device function for ventricular tachycardia (VT) according to the programmed parameters. When VT occurs, the device is programmed to first deliver antitachycardia pacing consisting of eight pacing stimuli, six separate times. If the VT doesn't terminate in response to the antitachycardia pacing or deteriorates to ventricular fibrillation, the device is programmed to deliver a shock. The episode of VT converts to normal sinus rhythm with the first cardioversion.

Status report

VT therapy	1	2	3	4
Therapy status:	On	On	On	On
Therapy type:	ATP	CV	CV	CV
Initial # pulses:	8			
# Sequences	6			
Energy (joules)		10	34	34
Waveform		Biphasic	Biphasic	Biphasic

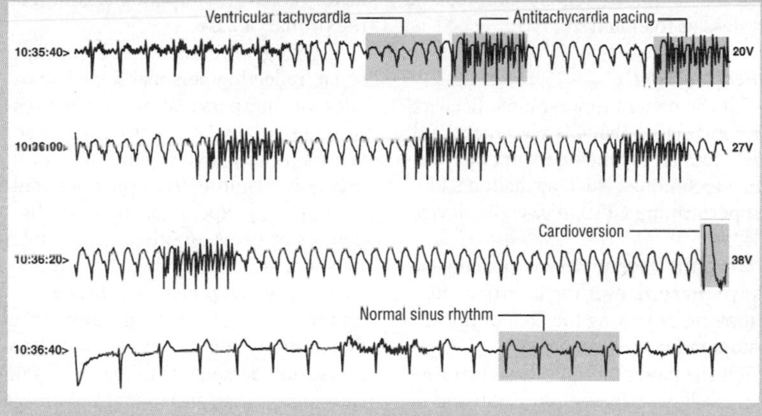

be obtained and printed when the doctor or specially trained technician interrogates the device. Program information includes:
- type and model of ICD
- status of the device (on or off)
- detection rates
- therapies that will be delivered: pacing, antitachycardia pacing, cardioversion, and defibrillation.

▶ If the patient experiences an arrhythmia or the device delivers a therapy, this information helps the nurse evaluate the functioning of the device. (See *Analyzing the function of an ICD.*)

▶ If the patient experiences a cardiac arrest, initiate CPR and advanced cardiac life support.

▶ If the ICD delivers a shock while you're performing chest compressions, you may feel a slight shock. Wearing latex gloves can eliminate this.

▶ It's also safe to externally defibrillate the patient as long as the paddles aren't placed directly over the pulse generator. The anteroposterior paddle position is preferred.

▶ Be on guard for signs of a perforated ventricle, with resultant cardiac tamponade. Ominous signs include persistent hiccups, distant heart sounds, pulsus paradoxus, hypotension accompanied by narrow pulse pressure, increased venous pressure, bulging neck veins, cyanosis, decreased urine output, restlessness, and complaints of fullness in the chest. Report any of these signs immediately and prepare the patient for emergency surgery.

- Assess the area around the incision for swelling, tenderness, and hematoma, but don't remove the occlusive dressing for the first 24 hours without a doctor's order. When you do remove the dressing, check the wound for drainage, redness, and unusual warmth or tenderness.
- After the first 24 hours, begin passive range-of-motion exercises if ordered and progress as tolerated.

Patient teaching

- Tell the patient to wear a medic alert band indicating the ICD placement and to educate family members in emergency techniques (such as dialing 911 and performing CPR) in case the device fails.
- Warn the patient to avoid placing excessive pressure over the insertion site or moving or jerking the area until the postoperative visit.
- Tell the patient to follow normal routines as allowed by the physician and to increase exercise as tolerated.
- Remind the patient to carry information regarding his ICD at all times and to inform airline clerks when he travels as well as individuals performing diagnostic functions (such as computed tomography scans and magnetic resonance imaging).
- Explain that electrical or electronic devices may cause disruption of the device.
- Stress the importance of follow-up care and checkups with the patient's physician.

IMPOTENCE

Impotence is also known as erectile dysfunction. A man with this disorder can't attain or maintain penile erection sufficient to complete intercourse. The patient with primary impotence has never achieved a sufficient erection; secondary impotence, more common and less serious, implies that he has succeeded in completing intercourse in the past. Erectile dysfunction affects all age-groups but frequency increases with age.

Psychogenic factors cause approximately 50% to 60% of erectile dysfunction; organic factors underlie the rest. In some patients, psychogenic and organic factors coexist, hampering isolation of the primary cause.

Psychogenic causes may be intrapersonal, reflecting personal sexual anxieties, or interpersonal, reflecting a disturbed sexual relationship. Intrapersonal factors usually involve guilt, fear, or depression, resulting from previous traumatic sexual experience, rejection by parents or peers, or other factors. Interpersonal factors may stem from differences in sexual preferences between partners, lack of communication, insufficient knowledge of sexual function, or nonsexual personal conflicts. Stress may cause temporary situational impotence.

Organic causes may include chronic disorders, such as cardiopulmonary disease, diabetes mellitus, multiple sclerosis, or renal failure; spinal cord trauma; complications of surgery; drug- or alcohol-induced dysfunction; and rarely, genital anomalies or central nervous system defects. (See *Characterizing the male climacteric.*)

Signs and symptoms

- Sudden or gradual loss of erectile function
- Complaints of severe depression
- Anxiety, with sweating and palpitations

Diagnostic tests

▶ Diagnosis must rule out chronic disease, such as diabetes mellitus and other vascular, neurologic, or urogenital problems. Personal sexual history is the key to differentiating between primary and secondary impotence.

Treatment

Sex therapy, largely directed at reducing performance anxiety, may cure psychogenic impotence. Such therapy should include both partners.

The course and content of sex therapy depend on the specific cause of the disorder and the nature of the relationship. In other cases of organic impotence, treatment focuses on reversing the cause, if possible. Some people benefit from the recently approved drug Sildenafil Citrate, which causes smooth-muscle relaxation and increased blood flow to the penis. This drug may have limited use among older adults because it can't be combined with nitrates. Certain patients suffering from organic impotence may benefit from surgically inserted inflatable or noninflatable penile implants. Others with low testosterone levels benefit from testosterone injections.

Key nursing diagnoses and outcomes

Sexual dysfunction related to stress or underlying cause

Treatment outcome: The patient will voice feelings about his sexual dysfunction.

Ineffective sexuality patterns related to illness or medical treatment

Treatment outcome: The patient will express feelings associated with his sexuality and self-concept.

Nursing interventions

▶ Help the patient feel comfortable about discussing his sexuality.

▶ Assess the patient's sexual health during your initial nursing interview.

▶ Monitor the patient's current drug regimen. Erectile dysfunction may be an adverse effect of his current therapy.

PATIENT TEACHING

▶ Teach the patient about sexual dysfunction and its possible causes.

▶ After penile implant surgery, instruct the patient to avoid intercourse until the incision heals, which usually takes 6 weeks.

> **Characterizing the male climacteric**
>
> This list reviews the physiologic changes that characterize the climacteric in the older male.
>
> - Testosterone production declines.
> - Pleasure sensations become less genitally localized and more generalized.
> - Erections require more time and stimulation to achieve.
> - Erections aren't as full or as hard.
> - The prostate gland enlarges and its secretions diminish.
> - Seminal fluid decreases.
> - Ejaculatory force diminishes.
> - Contractions in the prostate gland and penile urethra during orgasm vary in length and quality.
> - The refractory period following ejaculation may lengthen from minutes to days.

INCONTINENCE MANAGEMENT

In older adults, incontinence commonly follows any loss or impairment of urinary or anal sphincter control. The incontinence may be transient or perma-

Correcting urinary incontinence with bladder retraining

The incontinent patient typically feels frustrated, embarrassed, and sometimes hopeless. Fortunately, though, his problem can usually be corrected by bladder retraining—a program that aims to establish a regular voiding pattern. To implement such a program, follow these guidelines.

Assess elimination patterns

First assess the patient's intake pattern, voiding pattern, and reason for each accidental voiding (for example, a coughing spell).

Establish a voiding schedule

Encourage the patient to void regularly—every 2 hours, for example. Once he can stay dry for 2 hours, increase the time between voidings by 30 minutes each day until he achieves a 3- to 4-hour voiding schedule.

Teach the patient to practice relaxation techniques, such as deep breathing, which helps decrease the sense of urgency.

Record results and remain positive

Keep a record of continence and incontinence for about 5 days. This may reinforce your patient's efforts to remain continent.

Remember, your positive attitude as well as your patient's are crucial to his successful bladder retraining.

Take steps for success

Here are some additional tips to help boost the patient's success.

- Be sure to locate the patient's bed near a bathroom or portable toilet. Leave a light on at night. If the patient needs assistance getting out of a bed or a chair, promptly answer the call for help.
- Encourage the patient to wear his usual clothing. This confirms your confidence in his ability to stay dry. If necessary, use high-quality incontinence products to decrease the risk of skin breakdown.
- Encourage the patient to drink 1½ to 2 qt (1.5 to 2 L) of fluid, preferably water, each day. Lowering fluid intake won't reduce or prevent incontinence; it will promote infection. Limiting fluid intake after 6 p.m., however, will help the patient remain continent during the night.
- Reassure your patient that periodic incontinent episodes don't signal failure of the program. Encourage persistence, tolerance, and a positive attitude.

nent. In all, about 10 million adults experience some form of urinary incontinence; this includes about 50% of the 1.5 million people in extended care facilities. Fecal incontinence affects up to 10% of the patients in such facilities.

Contrary to popular opinion, urinary incontinence isn't a disease and isn't part of normal aging. It may be caused by confusion, dehydration, fecal impaction, or restricted mobility. It's also a sign of various disorders, such as prostatic hyperplasia, bladder calculus, bladder cancer, urinary tract infection (UTI), cerebrovascular accident (CVA), diabetic neuropathy, Guillain-Barré syndrome, multiple sclerosis, prostatic cancer, prostatitis, spinal cord injury, and urethral stricture. It may also result from urethral sphincter damage after prostatectomy. What's more, certain drugs, including diuretics, hypnotics, sedatives, anticholinergics, antihypertensives, and alpha-adrenergic blockers, may trigger urinary incontinence.

Urinary incontinence is classified as acute or chronic. Acute urinary incontinence results from disorders that are potentially reversible, such as delirium, dehydration, urine retention, restricted mobility, fecal impaction, infection or inflammation, drug reactions, and polyuria. Chronic urinary incontinence occurs as four distinct types: stress, overflow, urge, or functional incontinence. With stress incontinence, leakage results from sudden physical strain, such as a sneeze, cough, or quick movement. In overflow incontinence, urine retention causes dribbling because the distended bladder can't contract strongly enough to force a urine stream. In urge incontinence, the patient can't control the impulse to urinate. Finally, functional (total) incontinence results when urine leaks, even though the bladder and urethra function normally. This condition is usually related to cognitive or environmental factors, such as mental impairment or lack of appropriate or timely care.

Fecal incontinence, the involuntary passage of feces, may occur gradually (as it does in dementia) or suddenly (as it does in spinal cord injury). It most commonly results from fecal stasis and impaction secondary to reduced activity, inappropriate diet, or untreated painful anal conditions. It can also result from chronic laxative use, reduced fluid intake, and neurologic deficit. Pelvic, prostatic, or rectal surgery can also cause fecal incontinence as can medications, including antihistamines, psychotropics, and iron preparations. Not usually a sign of serious illness, fecal incontinence can seriously impair an older patient's physical and psychological well-being.

Patients with urinary or fecal incontinence should be carefully assessed for underlying disorders. Most can be treated — some can be cured. Treatment aims to control the condition through bladder or bowel retraining or other behavior management techniques, diet modification, kegels or pelvic muscle exercise, drug therapy and, possibly, surgery. Corrective surgery for urinary incontinence includes transurethral resection of the prostate in men, repair of the anterior vaginal wall or retropelvic suspension of the bladder in women, urethral sling, and bladder augmentation.

Supplies

- Bladder retraining record sheet
- Gloves
- Stethoscope (to assess bowel sounds)
- Lubricant
- Moisture barrier cream
- Incontinence pads
- Bedpan
- Specimen container
- Label
- Laboratory request form
- Optional: stool collection kit, urinary catheter

Implementation

- Whether the patient reports urinary or fecal incontinence, or both, you'll need to perform initial and continuing assessments to plan effective interventions. (See *Correcting urinary incontinence with bladder retraining*.)

For urinary incontinence

- Ask the patient when he first noticed urine leakage and whether it began suddenly or gradually. Have him describe his typical urinary pattern: Does incontinence usually occur during the day or at night? Ask him to rate his urinary control: Does he have moderate control, or is he completely incontinent? If he sometimes urinates with control, ask him to identify when and how much he usually urinates.
- Evaluate related problems, such as urinary hesitancy, frequency, and urgency; nocturia; and decreased force or interrupted urine stream. Ask the patient to describe any previous treatment he had for incontinence or measures he performed by himself. Also ask about medications, including nonprescription drugs.
- Assess the patient's environment. Is a toilet or commode readily available, and how long does the patient take to reach

Strengthening pelvic floor muscles

Stress incontinence is the most common kind of urinary incontinence in women and usually results from weakening of the urethral sphincter. In men, it may sometimes occur after a radical prostatectomy.

You can help a patient prevent or minimize stress incontinence by teaching about pelvic floor (Kegel) exercises to strengthen the pubococcygeal muscles. Here's how.

Learning the exercises

First, teach the patient how to locate the muscles of the pelvic floor. Instruct her to tense the muscles around the anus, as if to retain stool or intestinal gas, without using the abdominal muscles.

Next, teach the patient to tighten the muscles of the pelvic floor to stop the flow of urine while urinating and then to release the muscles to restart the flow. Biofeedback-assisted pelvic muscle exercises are effective in providing the patient with information about correct muscle use.

Once learned, these exercises can be done anywhere at any time.

Establishing a regimen

Suggest starting out by contracting the muscles and holding the contraction for 10 seconds. Then direct the patient to relax for 10 seconds before slowly tightening the muscles and then releasing them. Stress that contraction and relaxation exercises are essential to muscle retraining.

Typically, the patient starts with 15 contractions in the morning and afternoon and 20 contractions at night. Or the patient may exercise for 10 minutes, three times a day, working up to 25 contractions at a time as strength improves.

Advise the patient not to use stomach, leg, or buttock muscles. Also discourage leg crossing or breath holding during these exercises.

it? Once the patient is in the bathroom, assess manual dexterity — for example, how easily does he manipulate his clothes?

- Evaluate the patient's mental status and cognitive function.
- Quantify the patient's normal daily fluid intake.
- Review the patient's medication and diet history for drugs and foods that affect digestion and elimination.
- Review or obtain the patient's medical history, noting especially any incidence of UTI, prostate disorders, spinal injury or tumor, CVA, or bladder, prostate, or pelvic surgery and, in the female, number and route of births. Also, assess for disorders, such as delirium, dehydration, urine retention, restricted mobility, fecal impaction, infection, inflammation, or polyuria.
- Inspect the urethral meatus for obvious inflammation or anatomic defects. Have the female patient bear down while you note any urine leakage. Gently palpate the abdomen for bladder distention, signaling urine retention. If possible, have the patient examined by a urologist.
- Obtain specimens for appropriate laboratory tests, as ordered. Label each specimen container and send it to the laboratory with a request form.
- Begin incontinence management by implementing an appropriate bladder retraining program.
- To manage stress incontinence, implement an exercise program to help strengthen the pelvic floor muscles. (See *Strengthening pelvic floor muscles*.)
- To manage functional incontinence, frequently assess the patient's mental

and functional status. Regularly remind the patient to void. Respond to his calls promptly, and help him get to the bathroom as quickly as possible. Provide positive reinforcement.

- To ensure healthful hydration and to prevent UTI, make sure that the patient maintains adequate daily fluid intake (six to eight 8-oz glasses of fluid). Restrict fluid intake after 6 p.m.

For fecal incontinence

- Ask the patient with fecal incontinence to identify its onset, duration, and severity. Also, have him identify any discernible incontinence patterns — for instance, whether it occurs at night or with diarrhea. Focus the history on GI, neurologic, and psychological disorders.
- Note the frequency, consistency, and volume of stool passed within the past 24 hours and obtain a stool specimen, if ordered. Protect the patient's bed with an incontinence pad.
- Assess the patient for chronic constipation and GI and neurologic disorders as well as laxative abuse. Also, inspect the abdomen for distention, and auscultate for bowel sounds. If not contraindicated, put on gloves and check for fecal impaction (which may be a factor in overflow incontinence).
- Assess the patient's medication regimen. Check for medications that affect bowel activity, such as aspirin, some anticholinergic antiparkinson agents, aluminum hydroxide, calcium carbonate antacids, diuretics, iron preparations, opiates, tranquilizers, tricyclic antidepressants, and phenothiazines.
- For the neurologically capable patient with chronic incontinence, provide bowel retraining.
- Maintain effective hygienic care to increase the patient's comfort and prevent skin breakdown and infection. Clean the perineal area frequently, and apply a moisture barrier cream. Control foul odors as well.

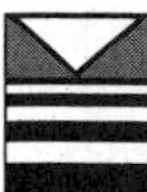

Key point Schedule extra time to provide encouragement and support for the patient. He may feel shame, embarrassment, and powerlessness because he has lost control.

Complications

Skin breakdown and infection may result from incontinence. Psychological problems caused by incontinence include social isolation, loss of independence, lowered self-esteem, and depression.

Patient teaching

- Advise the patient to consume a fiber-rich diet, with raw, leafy vegetables (such as carrots and lettuce), unpeeled fruits (such as apples), and whole grains (such as wheat or rye breads and cereals). If the patient has a lactase deficiency, suggest calcium supplements to replace calcium lost by eliminating dairy products from the diet.
- Encourage adequate fluid intake.
- Teach the older patient to gradually eliminate laxative use, if necessary. Point out, as needed, that using laxative agents to promote regular bowel movement may have the opposite effect — producing either constipation or incontinence over time. Suggest using natural laxatives, such as prunes or prune juice, instead.
- Promote regular exercise by explaining how it helps to regulate bowel motility. Even a nonambulatory patient can perform some exercises while sitting or lying in bed.
- To rid the bladder of residual urine, teach the patient to perform Valsalva's maneuver or Credé's method, or institute clean intermittent catheterization. Use an indwelling urinary catheter only as a last resort, because of the risk of UTI.

Documentation

Record all bladder and bowel retraining efforts, noting scheduled bathroom times, food and fluid intake, and elimination amounts, as appropriate. Record the duration of the patient's continent periods. Note any complications, including emotional problems, and signs and symptoms of skin breakdown and infection. Document treatment given for complications. Note your patient teaching measures and their effects.

INDWELLING URINARY CATHETER INSERTION

Also known as a Foley or retention catheter, an indwelling urinary catheter remains in the bladder to provide continuous urine drainage. A balloon inflated at the catheter's distal end prevents it from slipping out of the bladder after insertion. Indwelling catheters are usually used to relieve bladder distention caused by urine retention and to allow continuous urine drainage when the urinary meatus is swollen from surgery or local trauma. Other indications for an indwelling catheter include urinary tract obstruction (by a tumor or enlarged prostate), urine retention or infection from neurogenic bladder paralysis caused by spinal cord injury or disease, and any illness in which the patient's urine output must be monitored closely.

An indwelling catheter is inserted using sterile technique and only when absolutely necessary—it shouldn't be used to manage incontinence. Insertion should be performed with extreme care to prevent injury and infection.

Supplies

- Sterile indwelling catheter (latex or silicone #10 to #22 French; average adult sizes are #16 to #18 French)
- Syringe filled with 5 to 8 ml of normal saline solution
- Washcloth
- Towel
- Soap and water
- Two linen-saver pads
- Sterile gloves
- Sterile drape
- Sterile fenestrated drape
- Sterile cotton balls and plastic forceps
- Povidone-iodine or other antiseptic cleaning agent
- Urine receptacle
- Sterile water-soluble lubricant
- Sterile drainage collection bag
- Intake and output sheet
- Adhesive tape
- Prepackaged sterile disposable indwelling kits
- Optional: urine-specimen container and laboratory request form, leg band with Velcro closure, gooseneck lamp

Implementation

- Check the order on the patient's chart to determine if a catheter size or type has been specified. Then wash your hands, select the appropriate equipment, and assemble it at the patient's bedside.
- Provide privacy. Check his chart and ask when he voided last. Percuss and palpate the bladder to establish baseline data. Ask the patient if he feels the urge to void.
- So that you can see the urinary meatus clearly in poor lighting, place a gooseneck lamp next to the patient's bed.
- Place the female patient in the supine position, with her knees flexed and separated and her feet flat on the bed, about 2′ (61 cm) apart. If she finds this position uncomfortable, have her flex one knee and keep the other leg flat on the bed. You may need an assistant to help the patient stay in position or to direct the light. If necessary, ask the patient to lie on her side with her knees drawn up to her chest during the catheterization procedure. This position may be especially helpful for older or disabled patients such as those with severe contractures.

- Place the male patient in the supine position with his legs extended and flat on the bed. Ask the patient to hold the position to give you a clear view of the urinary meatus and to prevent contamination of the sterile field.
- Make sure the patient isn't allergic to povidone-iodine solutions.
- Put on gloves and use the washcloth to clean the patient's genital area and perineum thoroughly with soap and water. Dry the area with the towel.
- Place the linen-saver pads on the bed between the patient's legs and under the hips. Take off the gloves and wash your hands. To create the sterile field, open the prepackaged kit or equipment tray and place it between the female patient's legs or next to the male patient's hip. If the sterile gloves are the first item on the top of the tray, put them on. Place the sterile drape under the patient's hips. Then drape the patient's lower abdomen with the sterile fenestrated drape so that only the genital area remains exposed. Take care not to contaminate your gloves.
- Open the rest of the kit or tray. Put on the sterile gloves if you haven't already done so.
- Tear open the packet of povidone-iodine or other antiseptic cleaning agent, and use it to saturate the sterile cotton balls. Be careful not to spill the solution on the equipment.
- Open the packet of water-soluble lubricant and apply it to the catheter tip; attach the drainage bag to the other end of the catheter. (If you're using a commercial kit, the drainage bag may be attached.) Make sure that all tubing ends remain sterile and that the clamp at the emptying port of the drainage bag is closed to prevent urine leakage from the bag. Some drainage systems have an air-lock chamber to prevent bacteria from traveling to the bladder from urine in the drainage bag.
- Before inserting the catheter, inflate the balloon with normal saline solution to inspect it for leaks. To do this, attach the saline-filled syringe to the luer-lock port; then push the plunger and check for seepage as the balloon expands. Aspirate the saline to deflate the balloon. Also, inspect the catheter for resiliency. Rough, cracked catheters can injure the urethral mucosa during insertion, which can predispose the patient to infection.

Catheterizing the female patient

- Separate the labia majora and labia minora as widely as possible with the thumb, middle, and index fingers of your nondominant hand so that you have a full view of the urinary meatus. Keep the labia well separated throughout the procedure so that they don't obscure the urinary meatus or contaminate the area once it's cleaned.
- With your dominant hand, pick up a sterile cotton ball with the plastic forceps and wipe one side of the urinary meatus with a single downward motion. Wipe the other side with another cotton ball, in the same way. Then wipe directly over the meatus with still another cotton ball. Take care not to contaminate your sterile glove.
- Advance the catheter about 2″ to 3″ (5 to 7.5 cm). Continue to hold the labia apart until urine begins to flow.
- Pick up the catheter with your dominant hand, and prepare to insert the lubricated tip into the urinary meatus. To facilitate insertion by relaxing the sphincter, ask the patient to cough as you insert the catheter. Tell her to breathe deeply and slowly to further relax the sphincter and prevent spasms. Hold the catheter close to its tip to ease insertion and control its direction.

Catheterizing the male patient

- Hold the penis with your nondominant hand. If the patient is uncircumcised, retract the foreskin. Then gently lift and stretch the penis to a 60- to 90-degree angle. Hold the penis in this way throughout the procedure to straighten the urethra and maintain a sterile field.

▶ Use your dominant hand to clean the glans with a sterile cotton ball held in the forceps. Clean in a circular motion, starting at the urinary meatus and working outward.

▶ Repeat the procedure using another sterile cotton ball and taking care not to contaminate your sterile glove.

▶ Pick up the catheter with your dominant hand, and prepare to insert the lubricated tip into the urinary meatus. To facilitate insertion by relaxing the sphincter, ask the patient to cough as you insert the catheter. Tell him to breathe deeply and slowly to further relax the sphincter and prevent spasms. Hold the catheter close to its tip to ease insertion and control its direction.

▶ Advance the catheter about 6″ to 8″ (15 to 20.5 cm) until urine begins to flow. If the foreskin was retracted, make sure that you replace it to prevent compromised circulation and painful swelling.

Key point Never force a catheter during insertion. Maneuver it gently as the patient bears down or coughs. If you still meet resistance, stop the procedure and notify the physician. Strictures, sphincter spasms, misplacement in the vagina, or an enlarged prostate may cause resistance.

▶ If the physician orders a urine specimen for laboratory analysis, obtain it from the urine receptacle with a specimen collection container and send it to the laboratory with the appropriate laboratory request form.

▶ When urine stops flowing, attach the saline-filled syringe to the luer-lock port.

▶ Observe the patient carefully for adverse reactions such as hypovolemic shock caused by removing excessive volumes of residual urine. Check facility policy beforehand to determine the maximum amount of urine that may be drained at one time (some hospitals limit the amount to between 700 and 1,000 ml). Whether or not to limit the amount of urine drained is currently controversial. Clamp the catheter at the first sign of an adverse reaction, and notify the physician.

▶ Push the plunger and inflate the balloon to keep the catheter in place in the bladder.

▶ Never inflate a balloon without first establishing urine flow, which assures you that the catheter is in the bladder, not in the urethral channel.

▶ Hang the collection bag below bladder level to prevent urine reflux into the bladder, which can cause infection, and to facilitate gravity drainage of the bladder. Make sure the tubing doesn't get tangled in the bed's side rails.

▶ Tape the catheter to the female patient's thigh to prevent possible tension on the urogenital trigone. Tape the catheter to the male patient's thigh or lower abdomen to prevent pressure on the urethra at the penoscrotal junction, which can lead to formation of urethrocutaneous fistulas. Taping the catheter also prevents traction on the bladder and alteration in the normal direction of urine flow in males.

▶ As an alternative to taping, secure the catheter to the patient's thigh using a leg band with a Velcro closure. This decreases skin irritation, especially in patients with long-term indwelling catheters.

▶ Dispose of all used supplies properly.

▶ Inspect the catheter and tubing periodically while they're in place to detect compression or kinking that could obstruct urine flow.

▶ Empty the urine receptacle or bag as often as necessary. Excessive fluid volume may require more frequent emptying to prevent traction on the catheter, which would cause the patient discomfort, and to prevent injury to the urethra and bladder wall.

▶ Change catheters as often as facility policy requires. Some facilities encourage changing catheters at regular intervals, such as every 30 days, if the patient will have long-term continuous drainage.

Complications

Urinary tract infection (UTI) can result from the introduction of bacteria into the bladder. Improper insertion can cause traumatic injury to the urethral and bladder mucosa. Bladder atony or spasms can result from rapid decompression of a severely distended bladder.

Patient teaching

▶ Explain the procedure to the patient to reduce fear and promote cooperation.
▶ Explain the basic principles of gravity drainage so that the patient realizes the importance of keeping the drainage tubing and collection bag lower than his bladder at all times.
▶ If the patient is to be discharged with a long-term indwelling catheter, teach him and a family member or friend all aspects of daily catheter maintenance, including care of the skin and urinary meatus, signs and symptoms of UTI or obstruction, how to irrigate the catheter (if appropriate), and the importance of adequate fluid intake to maintain patency.
▶ Explain that a home care nurse should visit every 4 to 6 weeks, or more often if needed, to change the catheter.

Documentation

Record the date and time of insertion and the size and type of indwelling catheter used. Also, describe the amount, color, and other characteristics of urine emptied from the bladder. Your facility may require only the intake and output sheet for fluid-balance data. If large volumes of urine have been emptied, describe the patient's tolerance for the procedure. Note whether a urine specimen was sent for laboratory analysis. Document your patient teaching measures.

INFLUENZA

Also called the grippe or the flu, influenza is an acute, highly contagious infection of the respiratory tract. Although it affects all age-groups, influenza is more serious in older people and people with chronic diseases. In these groups, it can sometimes lead to death.

Influenza is caused by three types of viruses. Type A, the most prevalent form, strikes every year, with new serotypes causing epidemics every 3 years. Type B also strikes annually but causes epidemics only every 4 to 6 years. Type C is endemic and causes only sporadic cases.

The infection is transmitted by inhaling a respiratory droplet from an infected person or by indirect contact, such as drinking from a contaminated glass. The virus then invades the epithelium of the respiratory tract, causing inflammation and desquamation.

A remarkable feature of the influenza virus is its ability to mutate into different strains so that those at high risk have no immunologic resistance.

The most common complication of influenza is pneumonia, which can be primary viral pneumonia or secondary to bacterial infection. Influenza may also cause myositis, exacerbation of chronic obstructive pulmonary disease, Reye's syndrome and, rarely, myocarditis, pericarditis, transverse myelitis, and encephalitis.

Signs and symptoms

After incubation of 24 to 48 hours

▶ Sudden onset of chills, fever (may not appear in an older person)
▶ Headache
▶ Malaise
▶ Myalgia
▶ Nonproductive cough
▶ Laryngitis, hoarseness

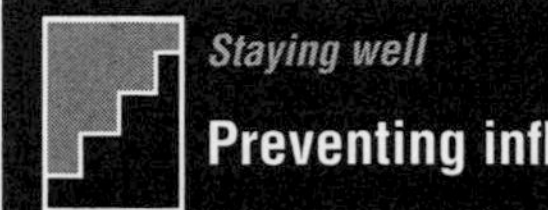

Staying well

Preventing influenza

To help your patient avoid getting influenza, be sure to cover these points:

- Discuss influenza immunization. Suggest that older patients get an annual inoculation at the start of flu season (late autumn). Explain that each year's vaccine is based on the previous year's virus and usually is about 75% effective.
- Tell a patient receiving the vaccine about possible adverse reactions (discomfort at the vaccination site, fever, malaise and, rarely, Guillain-Barré syndrome). The vaccine also shouldn't be given to anyone who's allergic to eggs, feathers, or chickens because it's made from chicken embryos. (Amantadine is an effective alternative for these people.)

▶ Red, watery eyes
▶ Clear nasal discharge
▶ Erythema of the nose and throat without exudate

As infection progresses

▶ Fatigue
▶ Frequent cough
▶ Tachypnea, cyanosis, and shortness of breath (with pulmonary complications)
▶ Purulent or bloody sputum (with bacterial infection)
▶ Cervical adenopathy and tenderness
▶ Transient gurgles or crackles
▶ Breath sounds possibly diminished in areas of consolidation

Diagnostic tests

▶ *Laboratory tests* of nose and throat cultures and a *blood analysis* showing increased serum antibody titers can help confirm the diagnosis.
▶ *Blood tests* in uncomplicated cases show a decreased white blood cell count and an increased lymphocyte count.
▶ Once an epidemic has been confirmed, diagnosis requires only observation of clinical signs and symptoms.

Treatment

The patient with uncomplicated influenza needs bed rest, adequate fluids, acetaminophen or aspirin to relieve fever and muscle pain, and an antitussive to relieve nonproductive coughing. He may be given the antiviral drug amantadine, which has effectively reduced the duration of type A infection.

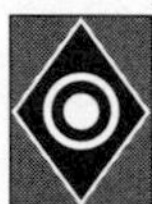

Drug alert Older patients receiving amantadine are more susceptible than others to the drug's neurologic adverse effects, such as depression, fatigue, confusion, dizziness, hallucinations, anxiety, irritability, ataxia, insomnia, headache, and light-headedness. Dividing the daily dose into two doses may decrease this risk.

In influenza complicated by pneumonia, the patient needs supportive care, including fluid and electrolyte replacement, oxygen, assisted ventilation, and appropriate antibiotics for bacterial superinfection.

Key nursing diagnoses and outcomes

Fatigue related to infectious process

Treatment outcome: The patient will employ measures to minimize fatigue and regain his normal energy level after the influenza has resolved.

Risk for deficient fluid volume related to fever and potential for pneumonia

Treatment outcome: The patient will maintain adequate hydration.

Hyperthermia related to infectious process

Treatment outcome: The patient will regain and maintain a normal temperature after the influenza has resolved.

Nursing interventions

▶ Administer analgesics, antipyretics, and decongestants, as ordered.

- Provide cool, humidified air, but change the water daily to prevent *Pseudomonas* superinfection.
- Monitor vital signs and note any increase in temperature.
- Provide tepid sponge bath to help reduce fever.
- Watch for signs and symptoms of developing pneumonia, such as crackles, increased fever, chest pain, dyspnea, and coughing accompanied by purulent or bloody sputum.
- Administer I.V. fluids, as ordered, and encourage the patient to drink plenty of fluids. Monitor the patient's fluid intake and output for signs and symptoms of dehydration.
- Help the patient gradually return to his normal level of activity.

PATIENT TEACHING

- Influenza usually doesn't require hospitalization. Teach the home patient about supportive care measures and signs and symptoms of serious complications. (See *Preventing influenza.*)
- Suggest a warm bath or a heating pad to relieve myalgia.
- Advise your patient to make rest his priority to shorten the course of influenza and reduce the risk of complications such as pneumonia. Encourage him to rest in bed as much as possible and to take frequent rest periods until he's fully recovered.
- Teach the patient the importance of increased fluids to prevent dehydration, especially if he has a fever.
- Inform family members of the need to encourage fluids if the patient isn't capable of administering fluids to himself.
- Advise the patient to use a vaporizer to provide cool, moist air, but tell him to clean the reservoir and change the water every 8 hours.
- Teach the patient how to dispose of tissues properly, and demonstrate proper hand-washing technique to prevent the virus from spreading.

INFORMED CONSENT

Generally, the health care provider's right to treat a patient—except in emergencies and other unanticipated situations—is based on a contract that arises through the mutual consent of the parties in the relationship. Consent is the voluntary authorization by a patient or the patient's legal representative to do something to the patient. The key to valid consent is the patient's comprehension.

Consent concerns the health care provider's right to treat an individual, not the manner in which treatment is delivered. Thus, one can deliver safe, competent care and still be sued for lack of consent. For example, a patient may sue for battery (or unconsented touching) if he hasn't given consent for a procedure and a health care provider performs it anyway. The patient may bring a lawsuit and be awarded damages even if the therapy is performed correctly and the patient's health improves because of the procedure or treatment. The trend, though, in negligence or malpractice cases is to raise the issue of consent by arguing that the patient didn't fully comprehend the information presented or that all pertinent information wasn't given.

A health care provider has a duty to obtain consent before treating a patient. Consent isn't implied by a patient's request for information or clarification; it must be actively sought by the health care practitioner. The rights to consent and to refuse consent are based on a long-recognized, common-law right of people to be free from harmful or offensive touching of their bodies. In a landmark 1914 case, *Schloendorff v. Society of New York Hospitals,* the court declared the reason for consent, which is still quoted today: "Every human being of adult years has a right to determine what shall be done with his own body, and a surgeon who performs an operation without his patient's consent commits an assault for which he is liable in damages."

Special considerations

Consent versus informed consent

Consent, technically, is an easy yes or no: "Yes, I'll allow the surgery" or "No, I want to try medications first, and then maybe I'll allow the surgery." Yet the patient may not fully understand what he's allowing. The law concerning consent in health care situations is therefore based on informed consent. The doctrine of informed consent was developed from negligence law when courts realized that in some cases, though consent was given, not enough information was provided for the patient to make an informed decision.

Informed consent mandates that the health care practitioner disclose needed facts in terms that the patient can reasonably understand so that he can make an informed choice. The information should include descriptions of available alternatives to the proposed treatment and the risks and dangers of each.

Failure to disclose the needed facts in understandable terms doesn't negate consent that's been given, but it does make the practitioner potentially liable for negligence. In 1957, the California courts found a physician negligent for failing to explain the potential risks of a vascular procedure to a patient who was paralyzed by the procedure (*Salgo v. Leland Stanford, Jr. University Board of Trustees*).

If a practitioner fails to obtain any consent, he may be sued for battery; if he fails to obtain informed consent, he may be sued for negligence.

Some courts have extended the right to informed consent to what might be called "informed refusal." A practitioner may be liable for failure to inform a patient of the risks of not consenting to a therapy or diagnostic test. *Truman v. Thomas* (1980) was one of the first cases to recognize this important corollary to informed consent. In that case, the court awarded damages against a physician for failure to tell the patient about the potential risks of not consenting to a recommended Papanicolaou (Pap) test.

Inclusions in informed consent

To be informed, a patient must receive—in terms that he can understand—the following information:

- brief but complete explanation of the treatment or procedure to be performed
- name and qualifications of the person (and any assistants) who is to perform the procedure
- description of any serious harm, pain, or discomforting adverse reactions that can occur during and after the procedure (including death if that's a realistic outcome)
- explanation of alternative therapies to the procedure or treatment, including the risk associated with doing nothing
- explanation that the patient can refuse the therapy or procedure without having alternative care or support discontinued
- fact that the patient can still refuse even after a procedure or therapy has begun; for example, scheduled radiation treatments may be cancelled if a patient decides against completing a planned series.

Forms of informed consent

Consent may be given in several forms: expressed or implied, written or oral, complete or partial.

Expressed consent is authority given by direct words, written or oral—for example, after the nurse informs a patient that an I.V. infusion is going to be given, the patient says, "Okay, but could you put the needle in my left arm because I'm right-handed?" Expressed consent is the type health care providers usually seek and receive.

Implied consent is consent that's inferred by the patient's conduct or that's legally presumed in emergency situations. This principle has its foundation in the classic case of *O'Brien v. Cunard*

Steamship Company (1899), in which a ship's female passenger joined a line of people receiving vaccinations. She neither questioned nor refused the injection; in fact, she willingly held out her arm for the vaccination. Later, she unsuccessfully brought suit for battery. A reasonable practitioner would infer that by extending her arm and saying nothing, the patient both understood the therapy and consented by action. Health care practitioners often use implied consent for minor procedures and routine care.

Implied consent is presumed in emergency situations—when a delay in providing care would result in the loss of life or limb, and the patient can't make his wishes known. An important element in allowing emergency consent is that the health care provider has no reason to think that consent wouldn't be given were the patient able to give or deny consent. For example, the health care provider isn't permitted to wait until the patient loses consciousness to order treatment that the patient had previously refused, such as a blood transfusion for a known Jehovah's Witness patient.

Consent may also be implied by law, as when the patient is a minor and the parent or the state—standing in the place of a parent—consents to treatment. The law implies the minor's consent for the treatment.

Consent may be given orally or in writing. Unless state law mandates written consent, the law views oral and written consent as equally valid. As a precaution, health care providers should recognize that oral consent is much more difficult to prove in court. As a convenience and to prevent such court cases, most health care facilities require written consent.

Consent may be partial or complete; a patient may authorize the entire treatment or procedure or only part of it. For instance, if the patient authorizes a breast biopsy but refuses to sign the consent form for a mastectomy based on the biopsy results, only a biopsy may be performed. The health care practitioner would then need to have a separate consent form signed before performing a mastectomy.

Standards of informed consent

Various jurisdictions apply standards of disclosure for informed consent in one of three manners. These have evolved to ensure that patients are informed in their decisions and to allow a means for determining the adequacy of the disclosure.

MEDICAL COMMUNITY STANDARD

Most states use a medical community standard, sometimes referred to as the reasonable medical practitioner standard. This standard evolved from the landmark *Karp v. Cooley* case (1974) and is based on a model of medical paternalism. It requires that a practitioner "disclose facts which a reasonable medical practitioner in a similar community and of the same school of medical thought would have disclosed regarding the proposed treatment." This standard is fluid and changing, based on the prevailing medical thought and community, and is established in court through expert medical witness testimony. Generally, the patient must be told of inherent risks, but not necessarily unexpected risks, that could occur after the treatment or procedure is initiated. Disclosure must include serious injuries that could occur. In general, courts favor more rather than fewer facts for full disclosure.

OBJECTIVE PATIENT STANDARD

The other two tests are based on a reasonable patient standard. One is the objective patient standard (also known as the prudent patient standard or material risk standard) and is based on disclosure of the risks and benefits that a prudent person in the given patient's position would deem material. Material facts are those that can make a significant difference to the reasonable and prudent patient. In *Joswick v. Lenox Hill Hospital* (1986) and *Arato v. Avedon* (1993), the courts decided that a person must have enough information on which to base a decision, including material risks. In *Korman v. Mallin* (1993), the court stated that determining materiality is a two-step process: first, defining the existence and nature of the risk and the likelihood of occurrence; and second, determining whether the probability of harm is a risk that a reasonable patient would consider.

SUBJECTIVE PATIENT STANDARD

The second reasonable patient standard is the subjective patient standard (or the individual patient standard). This requires full disclosure of the facts that a particular patient—rather than a reasonable person—would want to know. A judge and jury must determine what risks were or weren't material to a particular patient's decision with respect to treatment that's accepted or refused. No expert testimony is required on the scope of disclosure, although such expert testimony may be required to establish risks and alternatives to therapy. Only a handful of states has adopted this standard.

OTHER PRACTICES

Some states have attempted to bypass the three tests of disclosure by statutorily defining what must be disclosed to a patient before therapy or surgery. These medical disclosure laws mandate that certain risks and consequences be printed on the face of the consent form in language that the patient can be reasonably expected to understand.

Some states haven't adopted one standard for disclosure, instead relying on a case-by-case analysis. Others restrict informed consent to certain types of procedures, such as operative or surgical procedures (*Jones v. Philadelphia College of Osteopathic Medicine,* 1993).

PROPOSED STANDARD

A newer collaborative model for informed consent has been proposed (*Piper,* 1994) in which the patient and physician would define jointly what informed consent means to them. Such a standard would assign at least four responsibilities to patients:

- to communicate their values and expectations of treatment to the physician
- to ask questions and seek clarification in patient-physician discussions
- to evaluate signs and symptoms and report subjective impressions of how well treatment is satisfying their individual goals and values
- to make reasonable efforts to participate appropriately in treatment.

This model would ensure that patients' values and concerns about death and dying are communicated to the primary health care provider while the patient is competent or that they're communicated to the primary health care provider by the patient's surrogate.

Arguments for standards of full disclosure center on four key points:

- The patient assumes all potential risks because it's his body and life that are affected.
- Informed consent mandates increased communication between the patient and the health care provider. With increased communication, the caregiver is less apt to violate the informed consent standards and more likely to fully answer the patient's questions.
- Informed consent improves the consumer's health awareness and ultimately encourages better health care practices.
- Informed consent improves the quality of medical care because the health care provider explains all risks and benefits of the proposed procedure and outlines alternatives, thus aiding selection of the best type and quality of care.

To bring a successful malpractice suit based on informed consent, the plaintiff must be able to prove all of the following:

- the physician's duty to know of a risk or alternative treatment
- the physician's duty to disclose the risk or alternative treatment
- a breach of the duty to disclose
- if the case is in a reasonable patient standard jurisdiction, that a reasonable person in the plaintiff's position wouldn't have consented to the treatment if the risk had been known
- that the undisclosed risk caused harm or that the harm wouldn't have occurred if an alternative treatment plan was selected
- that the plaintiff suffered damages.

Exceptions to informed consent

The courts recognize four exceptions to the need for informed consent when consent is still required: emergency situations, therapeutic privilege, patient waiver, and prior patient knowledge. The practitioner still needs consent to prevent charges of battery, but the informed consent requirements are relaxed.

Therapeutic privilege, which has its origins in the common-law defense of necessity, allows primary health care providers to withhold information and any disclosures that they feel would be detrimental to the patient's health. The detriment must be more than a suspicion that the information would lead to the patient's refusal; it must be a recognized and documented increase of anxiety in the patient. In using this exception, physicians must be able to show that full disclosure of material facts would be likely to hinder or complicate necessary treatment, cause severe psychological harm, or be so upsetting as to render a rational decision by the patient impossible.

Therapeutic privilege typically comes into play only when the patient is severely and emotionally disturbed and his current medical status presents an imminent danger to his life. Some courts hold that a relative must concur with the patient's decision to consent and that the relative must be given full disclosure, whereas other courts hold that no relative need give concurrent consent. Once the risk to the patient has abated, the physician or independent practitioner must fully disclose the previously withheld information to the patient.

The courts may be more tolerant of therapeutic privilege when it applies to an older patient who has periods of confusion alternating with competence or who is slower to realize the full intent of a proposed medical therapy. Courts insist that the patient's next of kin or another family member be consulted when using this exception to informed consent.

The patient may also waive the right to full disclosure and still consent to a procedure. The caveat is that the health care provider may not suggest such a waiver. To be valid, the waiver must be initiated by the patient.

Prior patient knowledge means that the risks and benefits were fully explained the first time the patient consented to a procedure. Liability doesn't exist for nondisclosure of risks that are public or common knowledge or that the patient had previously experienced.

Accountability for obtaining informed consent

The physician or independent practitioner is responsible for obtaining informed consent. Health care facilities have no responsibility for obtaining informed consent unless the physician or independent practitioner is an employee or agent of the facility or the facility knew or should have known about the lack of informed consent and took no action. Court cases and state statutes have repeatedly upheld this principle. In one case, the court concluded that the patient should discuss risks of procedures with the physician, who "is the best person to inform the patient about the procedure and where to obtain proper services and facilities."

Attorneys argue both sides of the accountability issue as it relates to hospitals and other health care settings, but most medical professionals feel that to allow liability—and thus allow the hospital to monitor consulting procedures and the disclosure of material facts—would destroy the professional relationship with the patient.

THE NURSE'S ROLE

Nurses who aren't independent practitioners may be involved in obtaining informed consent. Because consent must be obtained for all procedures and treatments, not just medical procedures, the impact of this doctrine is vast. This does not mean that nurses must obtain written consent each time they give an injection or turn a patient. Most nursing interventions rely on oral expressed consent or implied consent that may be readily inferred through the patient's actions.

The doctrine of informed consent means that nurses must continually assess a patient's competence and communicate with him, explaining procedures and obtaining his permission. It also means that they must respect a patient's refusal to allow a certain procedure. However, state laws vary on allowing patients to refuse life-sustaining treatment. In some cases, even if a patient refuses life-sustaining treatment, a nurse could face charges for honoring or failing to honor this request. If a patient is unable to communicate, permission may be derived from his admission to the hospital or obtained from his legal representative.

A major concern for nurses involves obtaining consent for nursing procedures when the primary procedure is performed by another practitioner. For example, who is responsible for teaching postoperative care—the primary practitioner or the nursing staff? Postoperative teaching is considered a nursing procedure, but a physician performs the surgery (primary procedure). The answers from a legal perspective are far from clear.

The best way to handle this dilemma is probably for the nurse to give postoperative care information after the patient has consented to the surgical procedure. This approach prevents interference with the physician-patient relationship and conflicting explanations. Another approach is to provide postoperative teaching materials and films that orient the patient to the entire procedure after consent has been given and before the procedure. This approach may be augmented by having a nurse answer questions or provide clarification as needed. Many facilities have implemented this approach for major procedures and operations, such as heart catheterization, vascular arteriography, and open-heart surgery.

Another concern for health care professionals is obtaining informed consent for medical procedures that are provided entirely by another practitioner. In the past, nurses obtained consent for surgical or medical therapies performed by physicians. Some facilities still permit nurses to obtain the patient's signature on a consent form, but most avoid potential liability by prohibiting nurses from doing this.

DELEGATING RESPONSIBILITY

Still, physicians may legally delegate to a nurse the responsibility for obtaining a patient's informed consent. However, the physician does so at some peril because most medical practice acts hold the physician responsible for obtaining informed consent. Thus, any deficiencies in the informed consent obtained by the nurse may be imputed back to the physician.

The general rule is that the responsibility for obtaining a patient's informed consent rests with the person who will carry out the procedure. This is usually the attending physician. Any additional information that the patient requests should be supplied by the physician, and the nurse should contact the physician immediately rather than attempt to talk a reluctant patient into a proposed procedure.

Many facilities prohibit physicians from delegating responsibility for obtaining informed consent to a nurse because once the nurse becomes an integral part of the informed consent process, the facility also assumes liability under the doctrine of respondeat superior.

The nurse also has an important role if the patient wishes to revoke consent that was previously given or if it becomes obvious that the patient's signed consent form doesn't meet the standards of informed consent. Most nurses have been faced with the problem of what to do when a patient doesn't understand a procedure or believes it poses no major risks or adverse consequences.

LEGAL CONSEQUENCES

The health care professional and the facility may incur liability if the standards of informed consent haven't been met. If a patient changes his mind about consenting to a procedure or fails to understand the procedure and any risks it poses, the nurse should contact her immediate supervisor and the responsible physician. Both need to be informed of a patient's change of mind or lack of com prehension.

If the physician performs a procedure without the patient's informed consent and the patient sues for battery, the courts might hold the nurse responsible if:

- the nurse took part in the battery by assisting with the procedure
- the nurse knew the procedure was taking place and didn't try to stop it.

If the physician fails to provide adequate information for consent and the patient sues the physician for negligent nondisclosure, the courts might hold the nurse responsible if, knowing the physician hadn't provided enough information to the patient, the nurse fails to try to stop the procedure by informing a superior.

Consent forms

Two types of consent forms are commonly used. A blanket consent form that a patient is required to sign before admission is sufficient for routine and customary care. Consent to perform routine and customary care may also be implied by the patient's voluntary admission into the hospital, so the initial blanket consent form is needed only for insurance coverage and assignment of benefits.

A specific consent form provides specific information, such as the name and description of the procedure to be performed. It usually also states that the person who signed the form was told about the medical procedure, its risks and benefits, and any alternatives and that all questions have been answered. With this type of form, the physician and facility can show that no battery occurred because consent was given. However, the plaintiff may still be able to convince a court that informed consent wasn't given.

A second type of specific consent form might prevent the latter possibility. This is a detailed consent form that lists the procedure, consequences, risks, and alternatives. Many states now mandate this type of form. Most of these forms include the following elements:

- name and full description of the proposed procedure
- description of probable consequences of the proposed procedure
- description of risks and alternatives to the proposed procedure, including nontreatment
- signature of the competent patient or a legal representative
- signatures of one or two witnesses, depending on state law.

When using such detailed forms, the nurse should remember three things. First, witnesses aren't required for consent to be valid. Witnesses merely attest to the competence of the patient signing the form and to the genuineness of the signature, not to the fact that the patient had all the information needed to make an informed choice. Although the nurse need not be a witness to make the consent form valid, observing the signing of the consent form would make the nurse an excellent witness if a medical malpractice case arose.

Second, consent may be withdrawn at any time. Nothing in the written form precludes a patient's right to withdraw consent at will. Third, consent forms aren't conclusive evidence of informed consent. Several challenges to this notion have surfaced — for example, that technical language prevented the patient from understanding what was signed; that the signature wasn't voluntarily given, but was coerced or forced; and that the competence of the signer was impaired by medications.

A consent form is considered valid until it's withdrawn by the patient or until the patient's condition or authorized treatments change significantly. Some facilities use a 30-day guideline, but most prefer to have no set guidelines, particularly with patients who may require prolonged hospitalization or rehabilitation at a skilled nursing facility.

Who must consent?

Informed consent becomes a moot point if the wrong person consents to a procedure or therapy.

COMPETENT ADULT

The basic rule is that if a patient is an adult according to state law, only that person can give or refuse consent. In most states, 18 is the age at which one is considered an adult, although some actions — for example, marriage — may qualify a younger person to act as an adult. The adult giving or refusing consent must be competent to sign or refuse to sign the necessary consent forms.

Competence legally means that the court hasn't declared a person to be incompetent and the person is generally able to understand the consequences of his actions. A person's legal competence is usually based on an assessment by a physician or other health care professional, in many cases at the time informed consent is requested. Other health care professionals should be consulted if the patient is mentally retarded or has an obvious mental disorder or a disease that affects mental functions. In the case of an older patient, especially one who has alternating periods of confusion and competence, it's advisable to document how the health care provider assessed the patient for competence at the time of consent or refusal of consent. A simple entry clarifying the patient's competence may well prevent a lawsuit.

Courts generally hold that there is a strong presumption of continued competence. Exceptions may involve a person who is disoriented at times or confined to a mental institution. In these cases, the court is likely to seek evidence to show whether the person is capable of understanding the alternatives to a procedure as well as the consequences of refusing consent to it.

There are two exceptions to the legal adult's right to give or to refuse informed consent. The facility must seek and abide by the decision of a court-appointed guardian or a person with a valid, written power of attorney. Such persons present themselves to the facility administration if they have previously been appointed and if the adult patient is incapable of giving or refusing consent.

LEGAL GUARDIAN

A legal guardian or representative is a person who is legally responsible for giving or refusing consent for an incompetent adult. A guardian or representative has a narrower range of permissible choices than he would if deciding for himself. Some states insist that the known choices of a patient be considered first. Any expressed wishes concerning therapy or refusal of therapy made while the patient was still fully competent should be evaluated and followed if at all possible. A values history form completed by the patient while still competent may prevent treatment delays and needless questions about patient preferences.

To appoint a legal guardian or representative, the court must first declare an adult incompetent. The court then appoints either a temporary or permanent guardian. If the court has reason to believe the adult is only temporarily incapacitated, it appoints a guardian to act until the adult is able to resume managing personal affairs.

Three types of guardians may be appointed. A person may assume guardianship of property, which allows him to take care of financial matters but gives him no authority to make medical decisions for the incompetent patient. Guardianship of person permits medical decisions to be made, but the guardian has no financial responsibilities. A plenary guardianship allows the guardian to make all types of decisions about the incompetent person's medical and financial needs.

Because the language and requirements for guardianships vary from state to state, health care providers should ensure that their state requirements are met before relying on the guardianship papers as presented. A guardian is usually selected from a patient's family in the belief that such a person has the patient's best interests at heart and is in a position to best know the patient's desires. If the spouse of an incompetent adult is also old and ill, an adult child may be the appointed guardian.

In cases where a person hasn't been adjudicated as incompetent by a court of law, some states will ask family members to make decisions for the incompetent patient. The order of selection in cases involving older patients is usually: (1) spouse; (2) adult children or grandchildren; (3) adult brothers and sisters; and (4) adult nieces and nephews. Other states require durable power of attorney for valid, informed consent to health care or other formal procedures.

The practitioner should validate state laws and judicial decisions because family consent may not be valid in a handful of states. Lack of valid consent may lead to a court battle, especially if the practitioner acts on family consent and family members disagree about which course of action to take.

INTESTINAL OBSTRUCTION

Commonly a medical emergency, intestinal obstruction is the partial or complete blockage of the small- or large-bowel lumen. Complete obstruction in any part of the bowel, if untreated, can cause death within hours from shock and vascular collapse. Intestinal obstruction is most likely after abdominal surgery or in persons with congenital bowel deformities. Approximately 10% of older adults admitted with an acute abdomen are diagnosed with either a partial or complete intestinal obstruction.

Intestinal obstruction is caused by either mechanical or nonmechanical (neurogenic) blockage of the lumen. Causes of mechanical obstruction include adhesions; external, internal, or strangulated hernias (usually associated with small-bowel obstruction); carcinomas (usually associated with large-bowel obstruction); fecal impaction, foreign bodies, such as fruit pits, gallstones, or worms; compression of the bowel wall from stenosis; intussusception; volvulus of the sigmoid or cecum; tumors; and atresia.

Nonmechanical obstruction is usually caused by paralytic ileus (the most common intestinal obstruction). Paralytic ileus (also referred to as *adynamc ileus*) is a physiologic form of intestinal obstruction that usually develops in the small bowel after abdominal surgery. Other nonmechanical causes of obstruction include electrolyte imbalances; toxicity, such as that associated with uremia or generalized infection; neurogenic abnormalities such as spinal cord lesions; and thrombosis or embolism of mesenteric vessels.

Although intestinal obstruction may occur in several forms, the underlying pathophysiology for all forms is similar. Intestinal obstruction can lead to perforation, peritonitis, septicemia, secondary infection, metabolic alkalosis or acidosis, hypovolemic or septic shock and, if untreated, death.

Signs and symptoms

Mechanical obstruction

- History of abdominal surgery, radiation therapy, or gallstones
- Medical history of Crohn's disease, diverticular disease, or ulcerative colitis
- Family history of colorectal cancer
- Hiccups
- Colicky pain
- Nausea
- Vomiting of fecal contents or orange-brown foul-smelling material
- Constipation
- Distended abdomen
- Borborygmi and rushes
- Abdominal tenderness (rebound tenderness with strangulation) or peritoneal irritation
- History of constipation
- Peritonitis

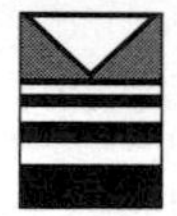

Key point If an older patient with an intestinal obstruction tells you that he has had a recent change in his bowel or bladder habits or that he has noticed blood in his stools, inform the physician immediately. Such signs and symptoms suggest that colon cancer may be causing the obstruction.

Nonmechanical obstruction

- History of recent abdominal surgery or severe illness
- Mild, continuous abdominal discomfort
- Vomiting consisting of gastric and bile contents
- Generalized abdominal distention
- Minimal or absent bowel sounds
- Constipation and hiccups

Diagnostic tests

- *Abdominal X-rays* reveal a distended, air-filled colon.
- *Blood tests* show that serum sodium, chloride, and potassium levels are decreased; white blood cell (WBC) counts are normal or slightly elevated; serum amylase level is increased; and hemoglobin levels and hematocrit are increased.
- *Sigmoidoscopy, colonoscopy*, or *barium enema* may help determine the cause, but all are contraindicated if a perforation is suspected.

Treatment

Surgery is usually the treatment of choice in cases of complete mechanical obstruction. The type of surgery depends on the cause of blockage. For example, if a tumor is obstructing the intestine, a colon resection with anastomosis is performed; if adhesions are obstructing the lumen, these are lysed.

When surgery is chosen, preparation includes correction of fluid and electrolyte imbalances, treatment of shock and peritonitis with fluid resuscitation, and administration of broad-spectrum antibiotics. Decompression is begun preoperatively with the insertion of a nasogastric (NG) tube attached to low-pressure intermittent or continuous suction. This tube relieves vomiting, reduces abdominal distention, and prevents aspiration.

Postoperative care involves careful patient monitoring and interventions geared to the type of surgery. Total parenteral nutrition (TPN) may be ordered if the patient has a protein deficit from chronic obstruction, postoperative or paralytic ileus, or infection.

Nonsurgical treatment may be attempted in some patients with partial obstruction, particularly those who suffer recurrent partial obstruction or who developed it after surgery or a recent episode of diffuse peritonitis. Nonsurgical treatment usually includes decompression with an NG tube attached to low-pressure intermittent or continuous suction, correction of fluid and electrolyte deficits, and administration of broad-spectrum antibiotics. Occasionally, a patient will require TPN.

Throughout nonsurgical treatment, the patient's condition must be closely monitored. If he fails to improve or his condition deteriorates, surgery is required.

Another indication for nonsurgical treatment is nonmechanical obstruction from paralytic ileus. Most of these cases occur postoperatively and disappear spontaneously in 2 to 3 days. However, if the disorder doesn't resolve within 48 hours, treatment consists of decompression with an NG tube attached to low-pressure intermittent or continuous suction. (Decompression occasionally can be achieved by colonoscopy or rectal tube insertion.) Oral intake is restricted until bowel function resumes; then the diet is gradually advanced from liquids to solids.

When paralytic ileus develops secondary to another illness, such as severe infection or electrolyte imbalance, the primary problem must also be treated. Again, if conservative treatment fails, surgery is required.

In both surgical and nonsurgical treatment, drug therapy includes antibiotics and analgesics or sedatives, such as meperidine or phenobarbital (but not opiates because they inhibit GI motility).

Key nursing diagnoses and outcomes

Imbalanced nutrition: Less than body requirements related to inability to eat

Treatment outcomes: The patient will maintain his weight within a normal range and will resume his oral intake after the obstruction is alleviated.

Risk for deficient fluid volume related to inability to ingest oral fluids

Treatment outcome: The patient won't demonstrate any signs or symptoms of dehydration.

Acute pain related to the pressure and irritation resulting from an intestinal obstruction

Treatment outcome: The patient will express relief of pain following analgesic administration and become pain-free after the obstruction is alleviated.

Nursing interventions

- Assess the patient's level of pain, administer analgesics as needed, and assess the effectiveness of treatment.
- Administer broad-spectrum antibiotics as ordered.
- Change the patient's position at least every 2 hours. Maintain the patient in semi-Fowler's or Fowler's position.
- Watch for signs of dehydration (thick, swollen tongue; dry, cracked lips; dry oral mucous membranes; hypotension; decreased urine output).
- Monitor vital signs and intake and output.
- Monitor electrolyte, blood urea nitrogen, and creatinine levels.
- Watch for signs and symptoms of secondary infection, such as fever and chills or increased WBCs.
- Measure and record the patient's abdominal girth every 8 hours.
- Monitor and record the presence or absence of bowel sounds.
- Allow the patient to have nothing by mouth until the obstruction is alleviated. Some patients may be allowed a small amount of ice chips to moisten the mouth.
- Insert an NG tube as ordered and attach the tube to low-pressure, intermittent suction. Monitor the NG tube drainage for color, consistency, and quantity.
- Maintain I.V. therapy, as ordered.
- Provide blood replacement therapy as necessary.

▶ Observe closely for signs of shock (pallor, tachycardia, change in level of consciousness, hypotension).
▶ Watch for metabolic alkalosis (changes in sensorium; slow, shallow respirations; hypertonic muscles; tetany) or acidosis (shortness of breath on exertion; disorientation; and, later, deep, rapid breathing, weakness, and malaise).

PATIENT TEACHING

▶ Teach the patient about his disorder, focusing on his type of intestinal obstruction, its cause, and its signs and symptoms. Listen to his questions and take time to answer them.
▶ Explain necessary diagnostic tests and treatments. Make sure the patient understands that these procedures are necessary to relieve the obstruction and reduce pain. Instruct him in pretest guidelines; for example, advise him to lie on his left side for about a half hour before X-rays are taken.
▶ Explain to the patient why he's on nothing-by-mouth status.
▶ Prepare the patient and his family members for the possibility of surgery. Provide preoperative teaching, and reinforce the physician's explanation of the surgery. Demonstrate techniques for coughing and deep breathing, and teach the patient how to use incentive spirometry.
▶ Tell the patient what to expect postoperatively.
▶ Review the proper use of prescribed medications, focusing on their correct administration, desired effects, and possible adverse effects.
▶ Emphasize the importance of following a structured bowel regimen, particularly if the patient had a mechanical obstruction from fecal impaction. Encourage him to eat a high-fiber diet and to exercise daily.
▶ Reassure the patient who had an obstruction from paralytic ileus that recurrence is unlikely. However, remind him to report any recurrence of abdominal pain, abdominal distention, nausea, or vomiting.
▶ If the patient has a GI tube or an NG tube in place and is at risk for pulling the tube out, instruct a family member to sit with the patient to remind him to leave the tube in place. Suggest using distraction techniques to keep the patient from thinking about the tube, and advise covering the tube with the patient's sheet to keep the tube out of his sight.

INTRAMUSCULAR INJECTION

Intramuscular (I.M.) injections deposit medication deep into muscle tissue, which is well vascularized and can absorb it quickly. This route of administration provides rapid systemic action and absorption of relatively large doses (up to 5 ml in appropriate sites). I.M. injections are recommended for patients who are uncooperative or can't take medication orally and for drugs that are altered by digestive juices. Because muscle tissue has few sensory nerves, I.M. injection allows less painful administration of irritating drugs.

The site for an I.M. injection must be chosen carefully, taking into account the patient's general physical status and the purpose of the injection. I.M. injections shouldn't be administered at inflamed, edematous, or irritated sites or at those containing moles, birthmarks, scar tissue, or other lesions. I.M. injections may also be contraindicated in patients with impaired coagulation mechanisms, and in patients with occlusive peripheral vascular disease, edema, and shock, because these conditions impair peripheral absorption. I.M. injections require sterile technique to maintain the integrity of muscle tissue.

The prescribed medication must be sterile. The needle may be packaged separately or already attached to the syringe. Needles used for I.M. injections are longer than subcutaneous needles because they must reach deep into the muscle. Needle length also depends on the injection site, the patient's size, and the amount of subcutaneous fat covering the muscle. In addition, the needle gauge for I.M. injections should be larger to accommodate viscous solutions and suspensions.

Oral or I.V. routes are preferred for administration of drugs that are poorly absorbed by muscle tissue, such as phenytoin, digoxin, chlordiazepoxide, diazepam, and haloperidol.

Supplies

- Patient's medication record and chart
- Prescribed medication
- Diluent or filter needle, if needed
- 3- to 5-ml syringe
- 20G to 25G 1″ to 3″ needle
- Gloves
- Alcohol pads

Implementation

- Verify the order on the patient's medication record by checking it against the physician's order. Also, note if the patient has any allergies, especially before the first dose.
- Check the prescribed medication for color and clarity. Also, note the expiration date. Never use medication that's cloudy or discolored or that contains a precipitate, unless the manufacturer's instructions allow it. Remember also that for some drugs (such as suspensions) the presence of drug particles is normal. Observe for any abnormalities. If in doubt, check with the pharmacist.
- Choose equipment appropriate to the prescribed medication and injection site, and make sure it works properly. The needle should be straight, smooth, and free from burrs.
- Wipe the stopper of the medication vial with an alcohol pad, and then draw up the prescribed amount of medication using the three-label check system: Read the label as you select the medication, as you draw up the medication, and after you have completed drawing up the medication to verify the correct dosage.
- Next, draw about 0.2 cc of air into the syringe according to your facility's policy. When the syringe is inverted during the injection, the air bubble rises to the plunger end of the syringe and follows the medication into the injection site. The air clears the needle of medication and helps prevent leakage into the subcutaneous tissue following injection by creating an air block that reduces reflux (tracking) along the needle path.
- Confirm the patient's identity by asking his name and checking his wrist band for name, room number, and bed number.
- Provide privacy for the patient.
- Wash your hands.

Giving the injection

- Select an appropriate injection site. The gluteal muscles (gluteus medius and minimus and the upper outer corner of the gluteus maximus) are used most commonly for healthy adults, although the deltoid muscle may be used for a small-volume injection (2 ml or less). Remember to always rotate injection sites for patients who require repeated injections.
- Position and drape the patient appropriately, making sure the site is well-exposed and that lighting is adequate.
- Loosen the protective needle sheath, but don't remove it.
- Gently tap the chosen injection site to stimulate nerve endings and minimize pain when the needle is inserted.
- Clean the skin at the site with an alcohol pad. Move the pad outward in a circular motion to a circumference of about 2″ (5 cm) from the injection site. Then allow the skin to dry to avoid introducing alcohol into the needle puncture, which causes pain. Keep the alcohol pad for later use.
- Put on gloves. With the thumb and index finger of your nondominant hand,

gently stretch the skin of the injection site taut.

▶ Holding the syringe in your dominant hand, remove the needle sheath by slipping it between the free fingers of your nondominant hand and then drawing back the syringe.

▶ Position the syringe at a 90-degree angle to the skin surface, with the needle a couple of inches from the skin. Because the older person may have a decrease in muscle mass, the site of injection and the length of the needle should be appropriate for his size. Even for older adults, the ventrogluteal site provides a well-developed muscle free from nerves and blood vessels. If the needle length can't be chosen, such as in the case of commercially prefilled unit dose syringes, alter the angle of injection when entering the muscle mass. Patients who use wheelchairs have atrophied lower-extremity muscles, so the deltoid muscle may be a better choice to them if the volume of the injection is 1 ml or less. (See *Modifying I.M. injections*.)

▶ Tell the patient that he will feel a prick as you insert the needle. Then quickly and firmly thrust the needle through the skin and subcutaneous tissue, deep into the muscle.

▶ Support the syringe with your nondominant hand, if desired. Pull back slightly on the plunger with your dominant hand to aspirate for blood. If no blood appears, place your thumb on the plunger rod and slowly inject the medication into the muscle. A slow, steady injection rate allows the muscle to distend gradually and accept the medication under minimal pressure. You should feel little or no resistance against the force of the injection. The air bubble in the syringe should follow the medication into the injection site.

▶ If blood appears in the syringe on aspiration, the needle is in a blood vessel. If this happens, stop the injection, withdraw the needle, prepare another injection with new equipment, and inject another site. Don't inject the bloody solution.

▶ After the injection, gently but quickly remove the needle at a 90-degree angle.

▶ Using a gloved hand, cover the injection site immediately with the used alcohol pad, apply gentle pressure, and unless contraindicated, massage the relaxed muscle to help distribute the drug and promote absorption.

▶ Remove the alcohol pad, and inspect the injection site for signs of active bleeding or bruising. If bleeding continues, apply pressure to the site; if bruising occurs, you may apply ice.

▶ Watch for adverse reactions at the site for 30 minutes after the injection.

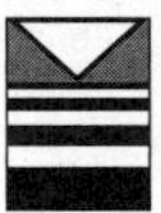

Key point The older patient will probably bleed or ooze after the injection because of decreased tissue elasticity. A small pressure bandage may be helpful.

▶ Discard all equipment according to standard precautions and your facility's policy. Don't attempt to recap needles; dispose of them in an appropriate sharps container to avoid needle-stick injuries.

Complications

Accidental injection of concentrated or irritating medications into subcutaneous tissue, or into other areas where it can't be fully absorbed, can cause sterile abscesses to develop. Such abscesses result from a natural immune response in which phagocytes attempt to remove the foreign matter.

Failure to rotate sites in patients who require repeated injections can lead to deposits of unabsorbed medications. Such deposits can reduce the desired pharmacologic effect and may lead to abscess formation or tissue fibrosis.

I.M. injections can damage local muscle cells, causing elevated serum creatine kinase (CK) levels, that can be confused with the elevated enzymes resulting from damage to cardiac muscle, as in myocardial infarction (MI). To distinguish between skeletal and cardiac mus-

Modifying I.M. injections

Before you give an I.M. injection to an older person, consider the physical changes that accompany aging and choose your equipment, site, and technique accordingly.

Choosing a needle

An older person usually has less subcutaneous tissue and less muscle mass than a younger adult — especially in the buttocks and deltoids. Therefore, you might need to use a shorter needle than you would for a younger adult.

Selecting a site

An older patient typically has more fat around the hips, abdomen, and thigh areas. This makes the vastus lateralis muscle and ventrogluteal area (gluteus medius and minimus, but not gluteus maximus muscles) primary injection sites. The illustration below shows an injection being given in the vastus lateralis muscle.

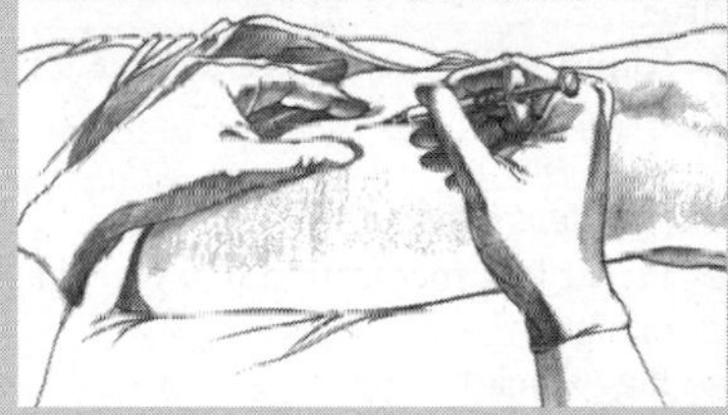

The ventrogluteal site is preferred because it is easily accessed without repositioning the patient excessively and is free from major nerves and blood vessels. The muscle remains large enough for injection even in very slender patients and is located well away from areas of contamination if the patient is incontinent. The deltoid site is usually a poor site for all but infrequent administration of very small amounts.

You should be able to palpate the muscle in these areas easily. However, if the patient is extremely thin, gently pinch the muscle to elevate it and to avoid putting the needle completely through it (which will alter the absorption and distribution of the drug).

Caution: Never give an I.M. injection in an immobile limb because of poor drug absorption and the risk that a sterile abscess will form at the injection site.

Checking technique

To avoid inserting the needle into a blood vessel, pull back on the plunger and look for blood before injecting the drug. Because of age-related vascular changes, older patients are also at greater risk for hematomas. To check bleeding after an I.M. injection, you may need to apply direct pressure over the puncture site for a longer time than usual. Gently massage the injection site to aid drug absorption and distribution. However, avoid site massage with certain drugs given by the Z-track injection technique, such as iron dextran or hydroxyzine hydrochloride.

cle damage, diagnostic tests for suspected MI must identify the isoenzyme of CK specific to cardiac muscle and include tests for lactate dehydrogenase and aspartate aminotransferase. If it's important to measure these enzyme levels, suggest that the physician switch to I.V. administration, with dosages adjusted accordingly.

In the geriatric patient, reduced or absent subcutaneous sensation may prevent the patient from being aware of a complication at the injection site.

Drug alert Because older patients have decreased muscle mass, I.M. medications can be absorbed more quickly than expected. Monitor the patient closely for more immediate effects than expected.

Patient teaching

- Explain the procedure to the patient to reduce his fear and promote cooperation.
- Always encourage the patient to relax the muscle you'll be injecting because injections into tense muscles are more painful and may bleed more readily.

Documentation

Chart the drug administered and the dose, date, time, route, and injection site. Also, note the patient's tolerance of the injection and its effects, including any adverse effects. Keep a rotation record that lists all available injection sites, divided into various body areas, for patients who require repeated injections. Document your patient-teaching measures.

I.V. MEDICATION ADMINISTRATION

I.V. medications are given through a peripheral I.V. site using one of three methods: direct or bolus, intermittent or piggyback, and continuous. The bolus method delivers a one-time dose of a drug, whereas the intermittent and continuous methods deliver the necessary dose over a given period.

Follow the same procedure for reconstituting, mixing, and adding medications to an I.V. solution for an older person as you would for any adult.

A bolus injection is given directly through a primary I.V. tubing or through an intermittent infusion device such as a saline lock. Because it allows the patient more freedom to move around, a saline lock is generally used more than a keep-vein-open line.

The most common way to administer I.V. drugs, intermittent infusion allows you to maintain therapeutic blood levels using small volumes (25 to 250 ml) over several minutes to a few hours. You can deliver an intermittent infusion through a piggyback line or a saline lock or through a primary line.

A continuous, or primary, I.V. infusion helps maintain a constant therapeutic drug level. This method may be the least irritating to the patient. There is also less handling of the equipment, which means a lower infection risk. However, fluid overload can occur if the rate and volume aren't carefully monitored. Also, vein selection and maintenance of the I.V. site might be difficult because of the condition of the older person's veins.

Supplies

- Patient's medication record and chart
- Gloves
- Alcohol pads
- Tape

Bolus injection

- Needle (20G or smaller) or needleless connector with a syringe containing normal saline solution
- Syringe containing the prescribed drug
- Saline- or heparin-filled syringe for flushing

Intermittent infusion

- Prescribed medication in a piggyback minibag
- Piggyback tubing
- 20G needle (or smaller) or a recessed needle device
- Syringe filled with 1 ml of heparin or saline flush solution (according to facility procedure)
- Two needles with syringes filled with 2 ml of normal saline solution
- I.V. pole.

Continuous infusion

- Prescribed medication in a container of I.V. solution
- Administration set
- Infusion pump or controller, if appropriate.

Implementation

- Needleless systems are available to prevent accidental needle sticks. The procedure for using them is the same as for using syringes with needles. Check with your facility for availability and recommendations.
- Check the condition of the patient's veins. In many cases they're fragile and easily injured, making routine site rotation difficult.
- Put on gloves.

To give a bolus injection through a primary I.V. line

- Keep in mind that drugs given by bolus injection produce an immediate effect. Be alert for signs and symptoms of adverse reactions.
- Close the flow clamp on the I.V. tubing and clean the port closest to the insertion site with an alcohol pad.
- When you're giving a bolus injection of a drug that's incompatible with dextrose 5% in water, flush the device with normal saline solution.
- Puncture the center of the port with the needle attached to the medication syringe. Aspirate slightly to check for a blood return. Be especially careful not to manipulate the venipuncture site because the older patient's veins are very fragile.
- Inject the medication slowly over the recommended time interval. Observe the site as you are injecting for any puffiness or swelling, which might indicate possible infiltration. If this occurs, stop the injection and evaluate the I.V. site; if necessary, remove the I.V. line and restart in another area.
- Remove the syringe and the needle or needleless system, and discard it immediately to prevent needle sticks.

To give a bolus injection through a heparin lock

- Wipe the injection port of the heparin lock with an alcohol pad, and insert the needle attached to the saline-filled syringe.
- Whenever you insert or remove a needle from a heparin lock, make sure that you stabilize the device to prevent trauma to the vein and dislodgment.
- Check for a blood return. If none appears, apply a tourniquet tightly above the injection site, keeping it in place for about 1 minute, and then aspirate again. If blood still doesn't appear, remove the tourniquet and inject the saline solution. Monitor the patient's skin under the tourniquet to minimize the risk of bruising and possible injury.
- If you feel resistance or see swelling, stop the injection immediately. Resistance indicates occlusion; swelling indicates infiltration. If these occur, insert a new heparin lock.
- If you feel no resistance, watch for signs and symptoms of infiltration, such as stiffness or pain at the site, as you slowly inject the saline solution. If these occur, insert a new heparin lock.
- If you aspirate blood, slowly inject the saline solution and continue observing for signs of infiltration. The saline solution flushes out any heparin solution that's incompatible with the medication.
- Withdraw the needle and the syringe.
- Insert the needle attached to the medication syringe.
- Inject the medication at the required rate. Then remove the needle from the injection port. Watch the patient closely for his response to the medication and for any adverse reactions.
- Insert the needle of the remaining saline-filled syringe into the injection port and slowly inject the saline solution. This flushes all the medication through the device.
- Remove the needle and insert and inject the heparin or saline flush solution to prevent clotting in the device (according to facility procedure).
- Discard all needles immediately to prevent needle sticks.

To give a piggyback infusion through a heparin lock

▶ Remove the I.V. administration tubing from the box.

▶ Straighten the tubing and close the roller clamp. Remove the protective cap from the end, and attach the 20G needle. You may also use a needleless system or a click-lock I.V. system.

▶ Remove the protective cap from the diaphragm of the minibag and remove the cap from the I.V. tubing spike. Insert the spike into the diaphragm of the minibag. Hang the bag on the I.V. pole.

▶ Squeeze the drip chamber of the I.V. tubing, and allow the chamber to fill halfway.

▶ Remove the cap from the needle and open the roller clamp when the solution reaches the tip of the needle. Cover the needle with its protective cap.

▶ Clean the port on the heparin lock with an alcohol pad. Flush the lock with 1 to 2 ml of normal saline solution. Remove the needle cap and insert it into the heparin lock. Securely tape this connection to reduce the risk of dislodging the needle. Check the I.V. site for infiltration.

▶ Adjust the roller clamp to infuse the medication over the recommended time interval. Keep in mind the patient's fluid status when determining the length of time for the infusion.

▶ When the infusion is complete, remove the needle from the heparin lock. Clean the heparin lock port with an alcohol pad, and inject the saline solution. Follow with the heparin flush solution, if used.

▶ Discard any uncapped needles immediately to avoid needle sticks.

To give a piggyback infusion through a primary line

▶ Follow the first four steps for administering a piggyback infusion through a heparin lock.

▶ When you're giving a dose through the primary I.V. line, both medications or solutions must be compatible.

▶ Clean the Y-port above the roller clamp of the primary I.V. tubing with an alcohol pad. Insert the needle of the piggyback tubing into the port, and tape the connection securely.

▶ Hang the primary I.V. bag or bottle lower than the minibag, using the extension hook included in the piggyback tubing box.

▶ Open the roller clamp on the piggyback tubing. Adjust the roller clamp of the primary bag to set the infusion rate of the minibag. To avoid fluid overload and adverse reactions, don't allow the infusion to run too fast.

▶ While the minibag is infusing, the primary I.V. solution won't run.

▶ When the minibag is finished, the primary I.V. solution resumes; make sure you readjust the rate of the primary solution.

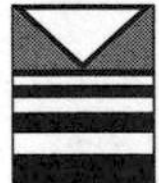

Key point Make sure you use the appropriate amount of fluid for the piggyback medication. Keep in mind the older patient's size, body mass, and fluid status. Using the smallest amount of fluid possible may be more appropriate for the older patient to prevent fluid overload.

To give a continuous infusion

▶ Attach the administration set to the solution container, and prime the tubing.

▶ Attach the tubing to the pump or controller, if appropriate.

▶ Put on gloves and remove the protective cap at the end of the administration set. Then attach the set to the venipuncture device.

▶ Begin the infusion and regulate the flow for the ordered rate.

▶ Frequently monitor the flow rate and the patient.

Complications

Infiltration and a reaction to the administered drug are the most common complications. In addition, repeated needle sticks into the ports increase the risk of contaminating the tubing or heparin lock cap. Giving a large volume of fluid can change a patient's electrolyte levels and result in fluid overload.

Patient teaching

- Explain the procedure to the patient and his family member or friend to reduce the patient's fear and promote cooperation.
- Explain the therapeutic use of the drug and any potential adverse effects.

Documentation

Record the amount and type of drug on the medication records. Note the amount of I.V. solution, if any, on the intake and output records. Note the date and duration of administration, and rate of infusion, if appropriate. Note the patient's response, where applicable. Document your patient-teaching measures and their effects.

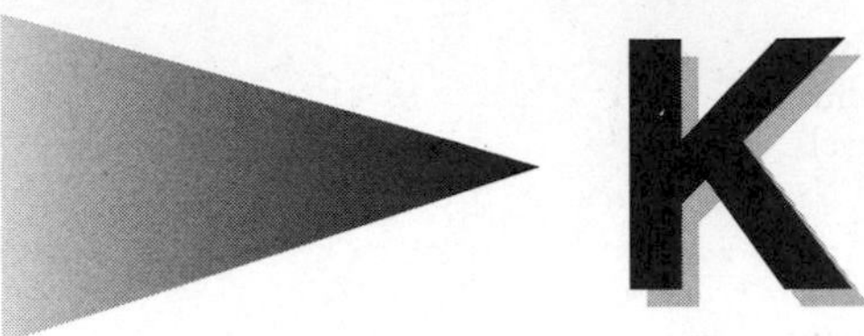

Keratoses

Tumors of the epidermis that affect older people, keratoses are classified as either actinic, a precancerous type (caused by excessive exposure to sunlight), or seborrheic, a benign type (caused by the proliferation of immature epithelial cells). Actinic keratoses require monitoring because they turn malignant in 1 in 1,000 cases.

Signs and symptoms

Actinic keratoses

- Small, light-colored lesions, usually gray or brown on exposed areas of the skin
- Cutaneous horns with a slightly reddened and swollen base (if keratin accumulates in them)

Seborrheic keratoses

- Dark, oily-looking lesions when located in the sebaceous regions of the face, neck, and trunk
- Light-colored, dry-looking lesions when located in less sebaceous regions
- May be as small as a pinhead or as large as a quarter and have a "stuck" appearance
- Increase in size and number as the patient ages

Diagnostic tests

- *Skin biopsy* is performed to make sure that the lesion isn't cancerous.

Treatment

Actinic keratoses

Freezing agents or acids are applied to remove the lesions. Electrodesiccation or surgical incision ensures thorough removal.

Seborrheic keratoses

Lesions can be frozen with liquid nitrogen or curetted, if needed, but generally don't require specific treatment.

Key nursing diagnoses and outcomes

Impaired skin integrity related to skin lesions

Treatment outcome: The patient will regain skin integrity when the keratoses have been eradicated.

Deficient knowledge related to cause and treatment of keratoses

Treatment outcome: The patient will communicate an understanding of the treatment of keratoses.

Disturbed body image related to skin lesions

Treatment outcome: The patient will express positive feelings about himself.

Nursing interventions

- Listen to the patient's fears and concerns, and offer reassurance when appropriate. Remain with the patient during periods of severe stress and anxiety.
- Provide wound care as ordered after treatment.

PATIENT TEACHING

- Explain all procedures and treatments to the patient and his family. Encourage the patient to ask questions, and then answer them honestly.
- Teach the patient to periodically examine his skin and to have lesions removed promptly.
- Instruct the patient to avoid exposure to sunlight or ultraviolet rays.
- Reinforce the importance of wearing sunscreen with a skin protection factor of at least 15.

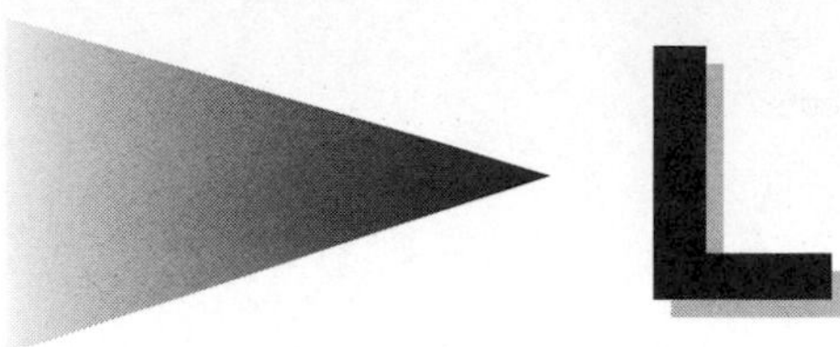

Leukemia

Beginning as a malignant proliferation of white blood cell (WBC) precursors, or blasts, in bone marrow or lymph tissue, leukemia results in an accumulation of these cells in peripheral blood, bone marrow, and body tissues. This accumulation is marked by the uncontrollable spread of abnormal, small lymphocytes in lymph tissue, blood, and bone marrow.

Leukemia can be classified as acute or chronic with four main types: acute myelogenous leukemia (AML), chronic myelogenous leukemia, acute lymphocytic leukemia, and chronic lymphocytic leukemia (CLL). The most common forms among older adults are AML, which causes rapid accumulation of myeloid precursors (myeloblasts), and CLL.

Acute myelogenous leukemia

In the United States, AML affects about 9,400 people annually, with an increased incidence after age 40. AML is slightly more common in men than women. Untreated, AML is invariably fatal, usually because of complications resulting from leukemic cell infiltration of bone marrow or vital organs. With treatment, the prognosis varies.

The exact cause of AML is unknown. However, radiation (especially prolonged exposure), certain chemicals and drugs, viruses, genetic abnormalities, and chronic exposure to benzene are likely contributing factors.

Although the pathogenesis isn't clearly understood, immature, nonfunctioning WBCs appear to accumulate first in the tissue where they originate (lymphocytes in lymph tissue, granulocytes in bone marrow). These immature WBCs then spill into the bloodstream, from which they infiltrate other tissues.

AML increases the risk of infection and, eventually, organ malfunction through encroachment or hemorrhage.

Chronic lymphocytic leukemia

A generalized, progressive disease, CLL is marked by the uncontrollable spread of abnormal small lymphocytes in lymphoid tissue, blood, and bone marrow. Once these cells infiltrate bone marrow, lymphoid tissue, and organ systems, clinical signs begin to appear.

CLL occurs most commonly in adults ages 60 to 65, with a slightly greater prevalence in men (2.5 to 1). It accounts for almost one-third of new leukemia cases annually. It's the most benign and the most slowly progressive form of leukemia. However, the prognosis is poor if anemia, thrombocytopenia, neutropenia, bulky lymphadenopathy, and severe lymphocytosis develop. Gross bone marrow replacement by abnormal lymphocytes is the most common cause of death, usually within 4 to 5 years of diagnosis.

Although the cause of CLL is unknown, researchers suspect hereditary factors because a higher incidence has been recorded within families. Undefined chromosomal abnormalities and certain immunologic defects, such as ataxia-telangiectasia or acquired agammaglobulinemia, are also suspected. A history of radiation exposure may also be a factor.

The most common complication of CLL is infection, which can be fatal. In the end stage of the disease, possible complications include anemia, progressive splenomegaly, leukemic cell replacement of the bone marrow, and profound hypogammaglobulinemia, which usually terminates with fatal septicemia.

Signs and symptoms

Acute myelogenous leukemia

- Sudden onset of high fever and abnormal bleeding (such as bruising after minor trauma, nosebleeds, gingival bleeding, purpura, ecchymoses, and petechiae)
- Fatigue and night sweats
- Weakness and lassitude
- Recurrent infections and chills
- Abdominal or bone pain
- Pallor on inspection
- Tachycardia, decreased ventilation, palpitations, and systolic ejection murmur on auscultation
- Lymph node, liver, or spleen enlargement on palpation

Chronic lymphocytic leukemia

- In the early stages: fatigue, malaise, fever, weight loss, frequent infections; macular or nodular eruptions (evidence of skin infiltration) on inspection; enlargement of lymph nodes, liver, and spleen, along with bone tenderness and edema from lymph node obstruction on palpation
- As the disease progresses: anemia, pallor, weakness, dyspnea, tachycardia, palpitations, bleeding, and infection from bone marrow involvement
- Poor appetite and abdominal fullness due to spleen or liver enlargement
- In the late stages: signs of opportunistic fungal, viral, or bacterial infections

Diagnostic tests

Acute myelogenous leukemia

- *Bone marrow aspiration* showing a proliferation of immature WBCs confirms acute leukemia. If the aspirate is dry or free from leukemic cells but the patient has other typical signs of leukemia, a bone marrow biopsy—usually of the posterior superior iliac spine—must be performed.
- *Blood studies* reveal thrombocytopenia and neutropenia; WBC differential determines the cell type.
- *Lumbar puncture* detects meningeal involvement.
- *Computed tomography* (CT) *scan* shows the affected organs.
- *Cerebrospinal fluid analysis* detects abnormal WBC invasion of the central nervous system.

Chronic lymphocytic leukemia

- *Blood tests* reveal numerous abnormal lymphocytes. In the early stages, the patient has a mildly but persistently elevated WBC count. Granulocytopenia is the rule, although the WBC count climbs as the disease progresses. Other results include a hemoglobin count under 11 g/dl, decreased serum globulin levels, neutropenia (less than 1,500/µl), lymphocytosis (more than 10,000/µl) and thrombocytopenia (less than 150,000/µl).
- *Bone marrow aspiration* and *biopsy* show lymphocytic invasion.
- *CT scan* identifies affected organs.

Treatment

Systemic chemotherapy, aimed at eradicating leukemic cells and inducing remission, is used when fewer than 5% of blast cells in the marrow and peripheral blood are normal. The specific chemotherapeutic and radiation treatment varies with the diagnosis.

Acute myelogenous leukemia

For AML, treatment consists of a combination of I.V. daunorubicin and cytarabine. If these drugs fail to induce remission, treatment involves some or all of the following: a combination of cyclophosphamide, vincristine, prednisone, or methotrexate; high-dose cytarabine alone or with other drugs; amsacrine; etoposide; and azacitidine and mitoxantrone.

For meningeal infiltration in AML, the patient receives an intrathecal instillation of methotrexate or cytarabine and cranial irradiation.

Chronic lymphocytic leukemia

Systemic chemotherapy includes alkylating agents, usually chlorambucil or cyclophosphamide, and sometimes corticosteroids (prednisone) when autoimmune hemolytic anemia or thrombocytopenia occurs.

When CLL causes obstruction or organ impairment or enlargement, local radiation therapy can reduce organ size and splenectomy can help relieve the symptoms. Allopurinol can prevent hyperuricemia, a relatively rare finding.

Both forms

For both of these leukemias, antibiotic, antifungal, and antiviral drugs and granulocyte injections may be given to control infection. Transfusions of platelets are given to prevent bleeding; transfusions of red blood cells are given to prevent anemia. Bone marrow transplantation is performed in some patients.

Key nursing diagnoses and outcomes

Fatigue related to hematologic abnormalities

Treatment outcome: The patient will incorporate measures to modify his level of fatigue into his daily routine.

Risk for infection related to abnormal WBC count

Treatment outcome: The patient will remain free from infection.

Risk for injury related to thrombocytopenia

Treatment outcome: The patient will incorporate bleeding precautions into his daily routine until he regains a normal platelet count.

Nursing interventions

- Develop a care plan that emphasizes comfort, minimizes the adverse effects of chemotherapy, promotes preservation of veins, manages complications, and provides teaching and psychological support.

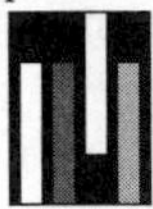

Cultural diversity In the Asian population, it's customary *not* to tell the patient if he has an incurable disease. Instead, the head of the family is given this information.

- Before treatment begins, help establish an appropriate rehabilitation program for the patient during remission.
- Minimize stress by providing a calm, quiet atmosphere that's conducive to rest and relaxation.
- Administer prescribed pain medications as needed. Provide comfort measures, such as position changes and distractions, to alleviate the patient's discomfort.
- Watch for bleeding. If bleeding occurs, apply ice compresses and pressure, and elevate the affected extremity. Also, avoid giving the patient aspirin or aspirin-containing drugs or rectal suppositories, taking a rectal temperature, or performing a digital rectal examination.
- Prepare the patient for a bone marrow transplant, as indicated.
- Control mouth ulceration by providing frequent mouth care and saline rinses.
- Administer blood products as needed.

Infection control

- Place the patient in a private room, and impose isolation precautions if necessary (although the benefits of these precautions are controversial).

Coordinate care so that the patient doesn't come into contact with staff members who care for other patients who have infections or infectious diseases.

▶ Don't use an indwelling urinary catheter or give I.M. injections; they provide an avenue for infection.

▶ Keep the patient's skin and perianal area clean, apply mild lotions or creams to keep the skin from drying and cracking, and thoroughly clean the skin before all invasive skin procedures.

▶ Change I.V. tubing according to your facility's policy.

▶ Use strict sterile technique when starting an I.V. line. If the patient is receiving total parenteral nutrition, provide scrupulous central venous catheter care.

▶ Watch for signs of meningeal infiltration (confusion, lethargy, and headache). If this complication develops, the patient will need intrathecal chemotherapy.

▶ Monitor the patient's temperature every 4 hours. If his temperature rises above 101° F (38.3° C) and his WBC count decreases, he'll need prompt antibiotic therapy.

▶ Screen staff members and visitors for contagious diseases, and watch for and report signs of infection in the patient.

▶ After intrathecal drug instillation, check the lumbar puncture site often for bleeding.

▶ Watch for signs of thrombocytopenia (easy bruising and nosebleeds; bleeding gums; and black, tarry stools) and anemia (pale skin, weakness, fatigue, dizziness, and palpitations).

PATIENT TEACHING

▶ Explain the course of the disease to the patient.

▶ Tell him that if chemotherapy causes weight loss and anorexia, he'll need to eat and drink high-calorie, high-protein foods and beverages. If he loses his appetite, advise him to eat small, frequent meals. If chemotherapy and adjunctive prednisone instead cause weight gain, he'll need dietary counseling.

▶ Advise the patient to limit his activities and to plan rest periods during the day.

▶ Teach the patient and his family members how to recognize signs and symptoms of infection (fever, chills, cough, and sore throat) and that they must report an infection to the physician at once. Stress the importance of keeping sick visitors away from the patient.

▶ Explain to the patient that his blood may not have enough platelets for proper clotting, and teach him the signs of abnormal bleeding (bruising, petechiae, and rectal bleeding). Explain that he can apply pressure and ice to the area to stop such bleeding. Also, teach him steps he can take to prevent bleeding. Urge him to report excessive bleeding or bruising to the physician.

▶ Instruct the patient to use a soft toothbrush and to avoid hot, spicy foods and commercial mouthwashes, which can irritate the mouth ulcers that result from chemotherapy.

▶ If the patient needs a bone marrow transplant, reinforce the physician's explanation of the treatment, its possible benefits, and its potential adverse effects. Teach him about total body irradiation and the chemotherapy that he'll undergo before transplantation. Tell him what to expect after the transplantation.

▶ Refer the patient to the social services department, home health care agencies, and support groups such as the American Cancer Society.

LIFE-REVIEW THERAPY

Life review involves the review of remote memories, the expression of related feelings, the recognition of conflicts, and the relinquishment of viewpoints that are self-inhibiting. During periods of crisis and transition, life review occurs naturally for many persons.

Life-review therapy facilitates the exploration of feelings and meanings of situations. It's most commonly used to achieve resolution and identify the potential for new directions. Much can be learned about a patient's history, communication style, relationships, coping mechanisms, strengths, fears, affect, and adaptive capacity by thoughtful listening. This therapy shouldn't be confrontational or involve interpretation for the older adult.

An effective life review resolves, at least partially, some past conflicts that hold significance for the present and the future. In very elderly people, this therapy will most likely alter views of what has been rather than what will be.

This therapy is beneficial not only to older people, but also to young adults. Children can join the older person and hear about history from those who were there and experienced the event.

Implementation

- Provide opportunities for the patient to recapitulate events in his life.
- Support the search for meaning, problem solving, and emotional gratification.
- Facilitate expression by sharing some of your own life experiences.
- Facilitate connections between past hopes, present events, and future expectations.

Special considerations

The psychologically disturbed older adult may be reluctant or unable to reminisce fluently. He may need assistance in expressing his life experiences.

LUNG CANCER

The most common forms of lung cancer are classified as small-cell or non–small-cell cancers. The most common site is the wall or epithelium of the bronchial tree.

Although lung cancer is largely preventable, it's the most common cause of cancer death in men. In women, lung cancer surpasses breast cancer as a leading cause of death. Only about 13% of patients with lung cancer survive 5 years after diagnosis.

Lung cancer's exact cause remains unclear. Risk factors include tobacco smoking, exposure to carcinogenic and industrial air pollutants (asbestos, arsenic, chromium, coal dust, iron oxides, nickel, radioactive dust, and uranium), and genetic predisposition.

Disease progression and metastasis cause various complications. When the primary tumor spreads to intrathoracic structures, complications may include tracheal obstruction; esophageal compression with dysphagia; phrenic nerve paralysis with hemidiaphragm elevation and dyspnea; sympathetic nerve paralysis with Horner's syndrome; eighth cervical and first thoracic nerve compression that causes arm and shoulder pain on the affected side, along with atrophy of the arm and hand muscles (Pancoast's syndrome); lymphatic obstruction with pleural effusion; and hypoxemia.

Other complications include anorexia and weight loss (sometimes leading to cachexia), digital clubbing, and hypertrophic osteoarthropathy. Endocrine syndromes may result when the tumor secretes hormones or hormone precursors.

Signs and symptoms

- Coughing (induced by tumor stimulation of nerve endings) or partial airway obstruction
- Hemoptysis
- Dyspnea (from tumor obstructing air flow)
- Hoarseness (from tumor or tumor-bearing lymph nodes pressing on the laryngeal nerve)
- Shortness of breath when walking or exerting effort
- Finger clubbing

▶ Edema of the face, neck, and upper torso
▶ Dilated chest and abdominal veins (superior vena cava syndrome)
▶ Weight loss
▶ Fatigue
▶ Enlarged lymph nodes and liver on palpation
▶ Dullness over the lung fields (with pleural effusion) on auscultation
▶ Decreased breath sounds, wheezing, and pleural friction rub (with pleural effusion) on auscultation

The patient may have a history of exposure to carcinogens. If he's a smoker, determine pack years.

Diagnostic tests

▶ *Chest X-rays* usually show an advanced lesion and can detect a lesion up to 2 years before signs and symptoms appear.
▶ *Cytologic sputum analysis*, which is 75% reliable, requires a sputum specimen expectorated from the lungs and tracheobronchial tree, *not* from postnasal secretions or saliva.
▶ *Bronchoscopy* can locate the tumor site. Bronchoscopic washings provide material for cytologic and histologic studies. The flexible fiber-optic bronchoscope increases test effectiveness.
▶ *Needle biopsy* of the lungs relies on biplanar fluoroscopic visual control to locate peripheral tumors before withdrawing a tissue specimen for analysis. The biopsy allows a firm diagnosis in 80% of patients.
▶ *Tissue biopsy* of metastatic sites (including supraclavicular and mediastinal nodes and pleura) helps to assess disease extent. Based on histologic findings, staging determines the disease's extent and prognosis and helps direct treatment.
▶ *Thoracentesis* allows chemical and cytologic examination of pleural fluid.

Additional studies include chest tomography, magnetic resonance imaging (MRI), bronchography, esophagography, angiocardiography (contrast studies of bronchial tree, esophagus, and cardiovascular tissues), mediastinoscopy, or thoracoscopy. Tests that can detect metastasis include a bone scan (abnormal findings may lead to a bone marrow biopsy, which is typically recommended in patients with small-cell carcinoma), a computed tomography scan or MRI of the brain, liver function studies, and gallium scans of the liver and spleen.

Treatment

Various combinations of surgery, radiation therapy, and chemotherapy improve the prognosis and prolong patient survival. Because lung cancer is usually advanced at diagnosis, treatment may be only palliative in nature.

Surgery is the primary treatment for stage I, stage II, or selected stage III non–small-cell cancers, unless the tumor is inoperable or other conditions (such as cardiac disease) rule out surgery. Most small-cell lung cancers can't be cured by surgery alone. Surgery may involve partial lung removal (wedge resection, segmental resection, lobectomy, radical lobectomy) or total removal (pneumonectomy, radical pneumonectomy).

Preoperative radiation therapy may reduce tumor bulk to allow for surgical resection and may also improve response rates. Radiation therapy (possibly combined with surgery and chemotherapy) is ordinarily recommended for stage I and stage II lesions if surgery is contraindicated and for stage III disease that's confined to the involved hemithorax. Postoperative radiation therapy usually begins about 1 month after surgery (to allow the wound to heal). It's directed to the chest area most likely to develop metastasis. Brachytherapy is another form of radiation therapy that may be used. It involves implantation of radioactive material into the tumor or adjacent airway.

Chemotherapy drug combinations using cisplatin (most common), carboplatin (related to cisplatin), gemcitabine, paclitaxel, docetaxel, etoposide, or vinorelbine can be employed in the treatment of non–small-cell lung cancer cases. For small-cell lung cancer cases, gemcitabine, paclitaxel, vinorelbine, topotecan, and teniposide are being studied.

Immunotherapy and gene therapy are investigational. Nonspecific regimens using bacille Calmette-Guérin vaccine or, possibly, *Corynebacterium parvum* offer the most promise.

In laser therapy, also largely investigational, a laser beam is directed through a bronchoscope to destroy local tumors.

Key nursing diagnoses and outcomes

Anticipatory grieving related to poor prognosis

Treatment outcomes: The patient will express his feelings about his diagnosis and the potential for death and will use appropriate behaviors to cope with the threat of death.

Fatigue related to hypoxia caused by impaired gas exchange

Treatment outcome: The patient will demonstrate energy-conservation measures.

Impaired gas exchange related to pulmonary dysfunction

Treatment outcome: The patient will obtain optimum oxygenation.

Nursing interventions

- Provide comprehensive supportive care and patient teaching to minimize complications and speed the patient's recovery from surgery, radiation therapy, and chemotherapy.
- Be sure to explain all procedures before performing them. This will help reduce the patient's anxiety.
- Urge the patient to voice his concerns, and schedule time to answer his questions.
- Ask the dietary department to provide soft, nonirritating, protein-rich foods. Encourage the patient to eat high-calorie between-meal snacks.
- Give antiemetics and antidiarrheals as needed during chemotherapy, and evaluate their effectiveness.
- Schedule patient care to help the patient conserve his energy.
- Arrange for home care assistance to decrease stress and promote energy.
- Impose reverse isolation if bone marrow suppression develops during chemotherapy.
- Monitor the patient's respiratory status, and administer oxygen as needed. Obtain arterial blood gas analyses regularly, as ordered.
- Administer analgesics as ordered to decrease pain and promote increased lung expansion.

PATIENT TEACHING

- Explain all treatments and their outcomes. Review all medications, including their actions and potential adverse effects.
- Allow a family member or friend to be with the patient for as many procedures as possible.
- Advise the patient to schedule activities throughout the day to avoid fatigue. Encourage the patient to follow a diet that increases his energy.
- Tell the patient to report signs of difficulty breathing.
- Encourage smokers to quit; refer them to local branches of the American Cancer Society or Smokenders.
- Teach the patient's family members to include rest periods with his daily activities.
- Recommend support groups or counseling for the patient and his family members to help them cope with the stress of illness.

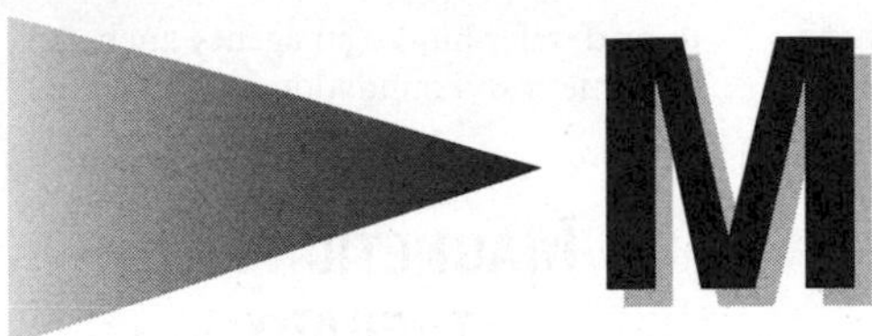

Macular degeneration

Commonly affecting both eyes, macular degeneration is a leading cause of blindness among all age-groups in the United States. At least 10% of older Americans have irreversible central vision loss caused by age-related macular degeneration. Two primary forms are the atrophic (also called involutional or dry) form, which accounts for about 70% of cases, and the exudative (also called hemorrhagic or wet) form.

Age-related macular degeneration is caused by hardening and obstruction of the retinal arteries, usually associated with age-related degenerative changes. Thus, formation of new blood vessels (neovascularization) in the macular area obscures central vision. The disorder can also be genetic or the result of an injury, inflammation, or infection.

Age-related macular degeneration may result in blindness. Bilateral macular lesions may lead to nystagmus.

Signs and symptoms

- Appearance of a blank spot (scotoma) in the center of a page while reading
- Intermittent blurring of central vision that gradually worsens
- Distorted appearance of straight lines

Diagnostic tests

- *Indirect ophthalmoscopy* through a dilated pupil discloses changes in the macular region of the fundus.
- *Fluorescein angiography* may identify (in sequential photographs) leaking vessels in the subretinal neovascular net.
- *Amsler grid tests* can detect visual distortion (metamorphopsia) on a daily basis, if appropriate.

Treatment

No cure currently exists for the atrophic form of macular degeneration. In 5% to 10% of patients with the exudative form, argon laser photocoagulation may slow the progression of severe vision loss.

Key nursing diagnoses and outcomes

Fear related to loss of vision

Treatment outcomes: The patient will identify and verbalize his fears.

Disturbed sensory perception (visual) related to decreased central vision

Treatment outcomes: The patient will resume a functional lifestyle and adjust to decreased vision.

Risk for injury related to decrease in vision

Treatment outcome: The patient will take precautions to protect himself from injury.

Nursing interventions

- Adjust the patient's activity according to his visual ability, and help with care if necessary.
- Adjust the patient's environment as needed to improve independent living and maintain safety. For example, keep utensils in an easily accessible spot and

provide bright lighting. If you're caring for the patient in his home, arrange the household for his comfort and visual ability; try to keep all activities on one level of the house.

- Identify yourself and others when you're with the patient.
- Assess improvement in the patient's sight with treatment, and adjust care accordingly.
- Help the patient obtain optical aids for low vision, such as magnifiers and special lamps.
- Allow the patient to express his fear, anxiety, and frustration about his vision loss, and offer reassurance.
- Stress the importance of regular ophthalmologic examinations to monitor the degree of visual impairment and to determine which aids may be prescribed to improve visual acuity.

PATIENT TEACHING

- Explain all procedures and tests, and encourage the patient to ask questions.
- Teach the patient's family about his vision loss and how to decrease his anxiety.
- Teach the patient and his family how to adjust his environment and lifestyle to compensate for decreased vision.
- Review safety precautions with the patient and his family. Instruct them to keep the environment free from clutter and to inform the patient of any change in household setup.
- Remind his family members that they may need to explain activities to the patient so that he can participate appropriately.
- Teach the patient how to adjust activities to promote independence. Include his family members in his care.
- Remind his family members that stimuli can help or confuse the patient and that they need to observe him and adjust their actions accordingly.
- Explain that macular degeneration usually doesn't affect peripheral vision, which should be adequate for performing routine activities. If the patient likes to read, refer him to an agency such as the American Foundation for the Blind.

MAGNETIC FIELD THERAPY

Magnetic field therapy (also called biomagnetic therapy, magnet therapy, or magnetotherapy) involves the use of magnetic fields to prevent and treat disease and to treat injuries. Its goal is to restore a person's internal bioelectromagnetic balance. With successful therapy, the patient should learn to maintain this internal balance without the need for continued external intervention.

One theory of magnetic therapy suggests that diseased cells have lost their magnetic equilibrium and that topically applied magnets work on a molecular level to restore this equilibrium within the cells. This, in turn, benefits surrounding cells and the entire organism.

Another theory, based on the magnetic nature of red blood cells, supposes a magnetically induced increase in blood and oxygen supply to diseased tissues. This improved circulation helps adjust pH, increase nutrient availability, and relieve congestion and pain.

Practitioners claim that therapeutic magnets benefit a wide range of conditions from acute and chronic pain, strains, and swelling to systemic illness. It has been recognized in sports medicine particularly for its effectiveness in relieving sprains and strains. Magnetic field therapy has also been used in conjunction with other therapies, such as nutrition, herbs, and acupuncture. Practitioners agree that biomagnetic therapy effectively relieves pain, swelling, and discomfort, but they disagree on whether therapeutic effects are best obtained using the bionorth (–) pole, the biosouth (+) pole, or both. They also disagree about which gauss strengths are most appropriate.

Implementation

▶ Magnets used for magnetic field therapy should be high-quality medical magnets. True bionorth and biosouth poles can be determined using a simple compass. The bionorth pole is attracted to the biosouth, or positive, pole; the biosouth pole, to the bionorth, or negative, pole. Gauss meters are also available for measuring the magnet's external field strength.

▶ Magnetic field therapy handbooks describe the best placement and magnet strength for self-treatment of various illnesses.

▶ The simplest home remedy for pain involves applying a low- to medium-gauss (800 gauss or less) magnet to the area of discomfort and leaving it in place until well after the discomfort disappears. The longer the treatment, the quicker the healing and the greater the symptom relief. If the pain decreases with treatment, the magnet is correctly oriented; if the pain increases, even if the magnet's bionorth side is facing the patient, the magnet needs to be turned over.

▶ Magnetic therapy may be of short duration (1 to 2 hours) or it may be used overnight or for 24 hours or more for maximum effect.

Special considerations

▶ Biosouth magnetic energy should only be used under medical supervision because some investigators believe that the brain can become overstimulated, producing seizures, hallucinations, insomnia, hyperactivity, and magnetic addiction. It has also been claimed that positive magnetic energy may stimulate the growth of tumors and microorganisms.

▶ Recognize that magnets may alter magnetic instruments, such as pacemakers, battery-powered wristwatches, hearing aids, and other equipment in use around a patient. Keep magnets away from magnetic resonance imaging machines and away from patients who have metallic parts in their body. Post signs above a patient's bed to warn other staff and visitors.

▶ Because of the complex range of symptoms commonly experienced by geriatric patients, you should encourage these patients to continue to seek conventional treatment and to report any alternative therapies they're using.

▶ Patients with pacemakers or defibrillators shouldn't use magnetic beds, and no magnets should be placed closer than 6″ (15.2 cm) to such devices to avoid interfering with their function.

▶ Because magnet polarity is important in treatment, caution the patient to use a magnetometer or a compass to check the poles on the magnets he plans to use.

▶ Inform patients to avoid using magnets on the abdomen for 60 to 90 minutes after meals to allow peristalsis to take place.

▶ Monitor a patient who is undergoing magnetic field therapy for potential adverse effects and the subsequent need to decrease or discontinue use.

▶ Inform patients that more and stronger magnets aren't necessarily better for magnetic field therapy.

▶ Warn patients to remove all magnets before undergoing surgery because the magnets may cause life-threatening instrument malfunction.

▶ If your patient is treating himself with magnets, teach him about safe magnet use. Inform him that magnets may alter magnetic instruments (such as pacemakers and hearing aids), that magnets shouldn't be banged or dropped, that they shouldn't be heated above 500° F (260° C) because doing so can decrease their strength, and that different-sized magnets shouldn't be kept together because doing so can alter their strength.

▶ Magnets should be kept away from computer hard drives and magnetic media — such as diskettes, recording tapes, credit or bank cards, videos, and compact disks — to prevent damage to or erasure of contents.

MAMMOGRAPHY

Mammography is a radiographic technique used to detect breast cysts or tumors, including those not palpable on physical examination. Film mammography, the most commonly used screening modality, uses X-ray film. Digital mammography is also available. A biopsy of suspicious areas may be required to confirm a malignant tumor. Other methods of breast imaging (ultrasound, magnetic resonance imaging, positron-emission tomography scanning, electrical impedance studies) are utilized in cases in which an abnormality is noted on screening or during cancer investigation.

Breast cancer prevention guidelines recommend that women over age 50 have a mammogram once every 1 to 2 years. Although 90% to 95% of malignant breast tumors can be detected by mammography, this test produces many false-positive results. If a lesion is found, the mammogram may be repeated or a breast biopsy may be necessary.

Supplies

- Mammograph
- X-ray film
- Plastic compressor

Implementation

- The patient is asked to rest one of her breasts on a table above an X-ray cassette.
- The compressor is placed on the breast, and the patient is instructed to hold her breath.
- A radiograph of the craniocaudal view is taken.
- The machine is rotated, the breast is compressed again, and a radiograph of the lateral view is taken.
- The procedure is repeated on the other breast.
- After the films are developed, they're checked to make sure they're readable.

Complications

Mammography can produce many false-positive results, creating anxiety for the patient as well as the need for further testing.

Patient teaching

- Inform the patient that she should tell the staff if she has breast implants, so the proper technologist will be available.
- Tell the patient that the test usually takes 15 to 30 minutes to complete.
- Instruct her to not wear any body powder, creams, or deodorant the day of the procedure.
- Tell her she may experience some discomfort during the procedure, because the breast must be compressed to get the best image.

Documentation

- Document patient teaching as well as the patient's tolerance of the procedure.

MASTECTOMY

A mastectomy is performed primarily to remove malignant breast tissue and any regional lymphatic metastasis. It may be combined with radiation therapy and chemotherapy. Until recently, radical mastectomy was the treatment of choice for breast cancer. Now, several different types of mastectomy can be performed, depending on the size of the tumor and the presence of metastasis. (See *Types of mastectomy*.)

Implementation

In a total mastectomy, the surgeon removes the entire breast without dissecting the lymph nodes. He may apply a skin graft if necessary. In a modified radical mastectomy, the surgeon may use one of several techniques to remove the entire breast. He also resects all axillary lymph nodes, while leaving the pectoralis major muscle intact. He may remove the pectoralis minor muscle. If the

Types of mastectomy

If a tumor is confined to breast tissue and no lymph node involvement is detected, a lumpectomy or a *total (simple) mastectomy* may be performed. A total mastectomy may also be used palliatively for advanced, ulcerative cancer and as a treatment for extensive benign disease.

A *modified radical mastectomy,* the standard surgery for stage I and II lesions, removes small, localized tumors. It has replaced radical mastectomy as the most widely used surgical procedure for treating breast cancer. Besides causing less disfigurement than a radical mastectomy, it reduces postoperative arm edema and shoulder problems.

A *radical mastectomy* controls the spread of larger metastatic lesions. Later, breast reconstruction may be performed using a portion of the latissimus dorsi. Rarely, an *extended radical mastectomy* may be used to treat cancer in the medial quadrant of the breast or in subareolar tissue. This procedure is done to prevent metastasis to the internal mammary lymph nodes.

Skin-sparing mastectomy, which preserves breast skin and replaces cancerous tissue with other body tissue, is an option for women who have noninvasive cancer that's localized in the breast. Recurrence with this type of surgery is extremely low and it allows the patient to leave the hospital with a totally reconstructed breast, which provides many psychological benefits.

Sentinel lymph node biopsy is a new procedure that can potentially minimize the risk of future lymphodema in the arm on the affected side. The surgeon injects blue dye or radioisotope into the lymphatic system and then examines the lymph nodes either visually (for blue dye) or with a Geiger counter (for the radioisotope). The lymph node closest to the operative breast is biopsied. If it has evidence of metastasis, it's removed. Other nodes are examined and removed as needed. If no evidence of metastasis exists, further lymph node removal isn't warranted.

patient has small lesions and no metastasis, the surgeon may perform breast reconstruction immediately or a few days later.

In a radical mastectomy, the surgeon removes the entire breast, axillary lymph nodes, underlying pectoral muscles, and adjacent tissues. He covers the skin flaps and exposed tissue with moist packs for protection and, before closure, irrigates the chest wall and axilla.

In an extended radical mastectomy, the surgeon removes the breast, underlying pectoral muscles, axillary contents, and upper internal mammary (mediastinal) lymph node chain.

After closing the mastectomy site, the surgeon may make a stab wound and insert a drain or catheter. The drain or catheter removes blood that may collect under the skin flaps, where it could prevent healing and lead to infection. Less commonly, he may use large pressure dressings instead. If a graft was needed to close the wound, he'll probably place a pressure dressing over the donor site.

In a skin-sparing mastectomy, surgery involves an oncologic surgeon and a plastic surgeon. Before surgery, the plastic surgeon marks the spot on the breast where the incision should be made for the best cosmetic outcome. If necessary, the oncologic surgeon modifies the incision site to ensure successful cancer surgery.

An incision is made around the nipple area, starting with an entry about the size of a half-dollar. During the procedure, the skin around the nipple area stretches and allows the surgeon enough room to remove the breast tissue. After successful removal of the breast tissue, the plastic surgeon reconstructs the breast using abdominal or back tissue and muscle to fill the space where the tumor was located. Then he closes the incision in a cosmetically pleasing manner.

Complications

After any type of mastectomy, infection and delayed healing are possible. However, the major complication of radical mastectomy and axillary dissection is lymphedema, which may occur soon after surgery and persist for years. Dissection of the lymph nodes draining the axilla may interfere with lymphatic drainage of the arm on the affected side, resulting in chronic edema.

Key nursing diagnoses and outcomes

Risk for infection related to lymph fluid stasis caused by lymphedema secondary to mastectomy with axillary lymph node dissection

Treatment outcomes: The patient will take precautions to prevent lymphedema and will maintain a normal temperature and white blood cell count.

Disturbed body image related to loss of a breast

Treatment outcomes: The patient will demonstrate control over her situation by participating in care decisions after the mastectomy and will express positive feelings about herself.

Nursing interventions

▶ Review the surgeon's explanation of the procedure, and prepare the patient for postoperative care. Explain that a drain or catheter and suction may be used to drain the incision and that the arm on her affected side will be elevated. She'll have to sit up and turn in bed by pushing up (but not pulling) with her unaffected arm. Tell her that she'll begin arm and shoulder exercises shortly after surgery. Demonstrate the exercises and have her repeat them.

▶ Take arm measurements on both sides to obtain baseline data. If the patient will have a radical mastectomy, explain that the skin on the anterior surface of one thigh may be shaved and prepared in case she needs a graft.

▶ Verify that the patient has signed a consent form.

▶ When the patient returns to the unit, elevate her arm on a pillow to enhance circulation and prevent edema. Periodically check the suction tubing to ensure proper function, and observe the drainage site for erythema, induration, and drainage. Using sterile technique, measure and record drainage every 8 hours. Keep in mind that drainage should change from sanguineous to serosanguineous fluid. After 2 to 3 days, you may need to milk the drain periodically to prevent clots from occluding the tubing.

▶ As ordered, teach the patient arm exercises to prevent muscle shortening and contracture of the shoulder joint and to promote lymph drainage. The surgeon will determine the optimal time for initiating these exercises, based on the degree of healing, presence of a drainage tube, and tension placed on skin flaps and sutures with movement. You can usually initiate arm flexion and extension on the first postoperative day and then add exercises each day, depending on the patient's needs and the procedure performed.

▶ Plan an exercise program with the patient. Such exercises may include climbing the wall with her hands, arm swinging, and rope pulling.

▶ To prevent lymphedema, make sure no blood pressure readings, injections, or venipunctures are performed on the affected arm. Place a sign bearing this message at the head of the patient's bed.

▶ Because mastectomy causes emotional distress, teach the patient to conserve her energy and to recognize early signs of fatigue. Gently encourage her to look at the operative site by describing its appearance and allowing her to express her feelings. Be sure to be present when she looks at the wound for the first time.

▶ Arrange for a volunteer who has had a mastectomy to talk with the patient. Contact the American Cancer Society's rehabilitation program, Reach to Recovery.

▶ After 2 to 3 days, initiate a fitting for a temporary breast pad. Soft and lightweight, the pad may be inserted into a bra without stays or underwires.

▶ If appropriate, explain breast reconstruction.

PATIENT TEACHING

▶ Tell the patient to use the affected arm as much as possible and to avoid keeping it in a dependent position for a prolonged period.

▶ Reinforce the importance of performing range-of-motion exercises daily. Instruct the patient to do them with both arms to maintain symmetry and prevent additional deformities.

▶ Emphasize the importance of not allowing blood pressure readings, injections, or venipunctures on the affected arm.

Key point Inform the patient that preventing lymphedema is critical. Explain that swelling may follow even minor trauma to the arm on her affected side. Tell her to promptly wash cuts and scrapes on the affected side and to contact the physician immediately if erythema, edema, or induration occurs.

▶ Remind the patient that her energy level will wax and wane. Instruct her to be alert for signs of fatigue and to rest frequently during the day for the first few weeks after discharge.

▶ Teach the importance of monthly selfexamination of the unaffected breast and the mastectomy site. Demonstrate the correct examination technique, and have the patient repeat it.

▶ Explain the importance of keeping scheduled postoperative appointments.

▶ If necessary, provide information regarding a permanent prosthesis, which can be fitted 3 to 4 weeks after surgery. Prostheses are available in a wide range of styles, skin tones, and weights from lingerie shops, medical supply stores, and department stores.

▶ Reassure the patient that she can wear the same type of clothing she wore before her surgery.

▶ Refer the patient to a local chapter of the American Cancer Society for information about support groups in her area.

MECHANICAL VENTILATION

A mechanical ventilator moves air in and out of a patient's lungs. However, although the equipment serves to ventilate a patient, it doesn't ensure adequate gas exchange. Mechanical ventilators may use either positive or negative pressure to ventilate patients.

Positive-pressure ventilators exert positive pressure on the airway, which causes inspiration while increasing tidal volume (VT). The inspiratory cycles of these ventilators may vary in volume, pressure, or time. For example, a volume-cycled ventilator — the type used most commonly — delivers a preset volume of air each time, regardless of the amount of lung resistance. A pressure-cycled ventilator generates flow until the machine reaches a preset pressure, regardless of the volume delivered or the time required to achieve the pressure. A time-cycled ventilator generates flow for a preset amount of time. A high-frequency ventilator uses high respiratory rates and low VT to maintain alveolar ventilation.

Negative-pressure ventilators act by creating negative pressure, which pulls the thorax outward and allows air to flow into the lungs. Examples of such ventilators are the iron lung, the cuirass (chest shell), and the body wrap. Negative-pressure ventilators are used mainly to treat neuromuscular disorders, such as Guillain-Barré syndrome, myasthenia gravis, and poliomyelitis.

Other indications for ventilator use include central nervous system disorders, such as cerebral hemorrhage and spinal cord transsection, adult respiratory distress syndrome, pulmonary edema, chronic obstructive pulmonary disease, flail chest, and acute hypoventilation.

Supplies

- Oxygen source
- Air source that can supply 50 psi
- Mechanical ventilator
- Humidifier
- Ventilator circuit tubing, connectors, and adapters
- Condensation collection trap
- Spirometer, respirometer, or electronic device to measure flow and volume
- In-line thermometer
- Probe for gas sampling and measuring airway pressure
- Bacterial filter
- Gloves
- Hand-held resuscitation bag with reservoir
- Suction equipment
- Sterile distilled water
- Equipment for arterial blood gas (ABG) analysis
- Soft restraints, if indicated
- Optional: oximeter

Implementation

- Specialized training is necessary to safely operate a ventilator. In most facilities, respiratory therapists assume responsibility for setting up the ventilator. If your facility doesn't have a respiratory therapist to set up the ventilator, check the manufacturer's instructions.
- In most cases, you'll need to add sterile distilled water to the humidifier and connect the ventilator to the appropriate gas source.
- Verify the physician's order for ventilator support. If the patient isn't already intubated, prepare him for intubation.
- Perform a complete physical assessment, and draw blood for ABG analysis to establish a baseline.
- Suction the patient if necessary.
- Plug the ventilator into the electrical outlet and turn it on. Adjust the settings on the ventilator as ordered. Make sure that the ventilator's alarms are set as ordered and that the humidifier is filled with sterile distilled water.
- Put on gloves if you haven't already. Connect the endotracheal tube to the ventilator. Observe for chest expansion, and auscultate for bilateral breath sounds to verify that the patient is being ventilated.
- If necessary, apply soft wrist restraints to the patient to avoid accidental self-extubation.
- Monitor the patient's ABG values after the initial ventilator setup (usually 20 to 30 minutes), after any changes in ventilator settings, and as the patient's clinical condition indicates to determine whether the patient is being adequately ventilated and to avoid oxygen toxicity. Be prepared to adjust ventilator settings depending on ABG analysis.
- Check the ventilator tubing frequently for condensation, which can cause resistance to airflow and which may also be aspirated by the patient. As needed, drain the condensate into a collection trap, or briefly disconnect the patient from the ventilator (ventilating him with a handheld resuscitation bag if necessary) and empty the water into a receptacle. Don't drain the condensate into the humidifier because the condensate may be contaminated with the patient's secretions.
- Check the in-line thermometer to make sure that the temperature of the air delivered to the patient is close to body temperature.
- When monitoring the patient's vital signs, count spontaneous breaths as well as ventilator-delivered breaths.

▶ Change, clean, or dispose of the ventilator tubing and equipment according to facility policy to reduce the risk of bacterial contamination. Typically, ventilator tubing should be changed every 48 to 72 hours and sometimes more often.

▶ When ordered, begin to wean the patient from the ventilator.

▶ Make sure that the ventilator alarms are on at all times. These alarms alert the nursing staff to potentially hazardous conditions and changes in patient status. If an alarm sounds and the problem can't be identified easily, disconnect the patient from the ventilator and use a handheld resuscitation bag to ventilate him. (See *Responding to ventilator alarms,* page 392.)

▶ Provide emotional support to the patient during all phases of mechanical ventilation to reduce anxiety and promote successful treatment. Even if the patient is unresponsive, continue to explain all procedures and treatments to him.

▶ Unless contraindicated, turn the patient from side to side every 1 to 2 hours to facilitate lung expansion and removal of secretions. Perform active or passive range-of-motion exercises on all extremities to reduce the hazards of immobility. If the patient's condition permits, position him upright at regular intervals to increase lung expansion. When moving the patient or the ventilator tubing, be careful to prevent condensation in the tubing from flowing into the lungs because aspiration of this contaminated moisture can cause infection. Provide care for the patient's artificial airway as needed.

▶ Assess the patient's peripheral circulation, and monitor his urine output for signs of decreased cardiac output. Watch for signs and symptoms of fluid volume excess or dehydration.

▶ Place the call button within the patient's reach, and establish a method of communication, such as a communication board, because intubation and mechanical ventilation impair the patient's ability to speak. An artificial airway may help the patient speak by allowing air to pass through his vocal cords.

▶ Administer a sedative, as ordered, to relax the patient.

▶ Administer a neuromuscular blocking agent, as ordered, to eliminate spontaneous breathing efforts that can interfere with the ventilator's action. Remember that the patient receiving a neuromuscular blocking agent requires close observation because of his inability to breathe or communicate.

▶ If the patient is receiving a neuromuscular blocking agent, make sure that he also receives a sedative. Neuromuscular blocking agents cause paralysis without altering the patient's level of consciousness (LOC). Reassure the patient and his family that the paralysis is temporary. Also make sure that emergency equipment is readily available in case the ventilator malfunctions or the patient is extubated accidentally. Continue to explain all procedures to the patient, and take extra steps to ensure his safety, such as raising the side rails when turning the patient and covering and lubricating his eyes.

▶ Ensure that the patient gets adequate rest and sleep because fatigue can delay weaning from the ventilator. Provide subdued lighting, safely muffle equipment noises, and restrict staff access to the area to promote quiet during rest periods.

▶ When weaning the patient, continue to observe for signs of hypoxia. Schedule weaning to fit comfortably and realistically with the patient's daily regimen. Avoid scheduling sessions after meals, baths, or lengthy therapeutic or diagnostic procedures. Have the patient help you set up the schedule to give him some sense of control over a frightening procedure. As the patient's tolerance for weaning increases, help him sit up out of bed to improve his breathing and sense of well-being. Suggest diversionary activities to take his mind off breathing.

Responding to ventilator alarms

Signal	Possible causes	Interventions
Low pressure alarm	■ Tube disconnected from ventilator	■ Reconnect the tube to the ventilator.
	■ Endotracheal (ET) tube displaced above vocal cords or tracheostomy tube extubated	■ Check tube placement and reposition if needed. If extubation or displacement has occurred, ventilate the patient manually and call the physician immediately.
	■ Leaking tidal volume from low cuff pressure (from an underinflated or ruptured cuff or a leak in the cuff or one-way valve)	■ Listen for a whooshing sound around the tube, indicating an air leak. If you hear one, check cuff pressure. If you can't maintain pressure, call the physician; he may need to insert a new tube.
	■ Ventilator malfunction	■ Disconnect the patient from the ventilator, and ventilate him manually if necessary. Obtain another ventilator.
	■ Leak in ventilator circuitry (from loose connection or hole in tubing, loss of temperature-sensitive device, or cracked humidification jar)	■ Make sure all connections are intact. Check for holes or leaks in the tubing and replace if necessary. Check the humidification jar and replace if cracked.
High pressure alarm	■ Increased airway pressure or decreased lung compliance due to worsening disease	■ Auscultate the lungs for evidence of increasing lung consolidation, barotrauma, or wheezing. Call the physician if indicated.
	■ Patient biting on oral ET tube	■ Insert a bite block if needed.
	■ Secretions in airway	■ Look for secretions in the airway. To remove them, suction the patient or have him cough.
	■ Condensate in large-bore tubing	■ Check tubing for condensate and remove any fluid.
	■ Intubation of right mainstem bronchus	■ Check tube position. If it has slipped, call the physician; he may need to reposition it.
	■ Patient coughing, gagging, or attempting to talk	■ If the patient fights the ventilator, the physician may order a sedative or neuromuscular blocking agent.
	■ Chest wall resistance	■ Reposition the patient to see if it improves chest expansion. If repositioning doesn't help, administer the prescribed analgesic.
	■ Failure of high-pressure relief valve	■ Have the faulty equipment replaced.
	■ Bronchospasm	■ Assess the patient for the cause. Report to the physician and treat as ordered.

Complications

Mechanical ventilation can cause tension pneumothorax from barotrauma, decreased cardiac output, oxygen toxicity, infection, fluid volume excess caused by humidification, and GI complications, such as distention or bleeding from stress ulcers.

Patient teaching

▶ Explain the procedure to the patient and his family to help reduce anxiety and fear. Assure them that staff members are nearby to provide care.

▶ If the patient will be discharged on a ventilator, evaluate the caregiver's ability and motivation to provide such care. Well before discharge, develop a teaching plan that will address the patient's needs. For example, include information about ventilator care and settings, artificial airway care, suctioning, respiratory therapy, communication, nutrition, therapeutic exercise, signs and symptoms of infection, and ways to troubleshoot minor equipment malfunctions. In most cases, 24-hour in-home professional nursing care is needed to ensure patient safety.

▶ Evaluate the patient's need for adaptive equipment, such as a hospital bed, a wheelchair or walker with a ventilator tray, a patient lift, and a bedside commode.

▶ Determine whether the patient needs to travel; if so, select appropriate portable and backup equipment.

▶ Before discharge, have the patient's caregiver demonstrate his ability to use the equipment. At discharge, contact a durable medical equipment vendor and a home health nurse to follow up with the patient. Also refer the patient to community resources, if available.

Documentation

Document the date and time that mechanical ventilation was initiated. Name the type of ventilator used and note its settings. Describe the patient's subjective and objective responses to mechanical ventilation (including vital signs, breath sounds, use of accessory muscles, intake and output, and weight). List any complications that occurred and any nursing actions taken. Record all pertinent laboratory data, including ABG analysis results and oxygen saturation levels. Also document your patient-teaching measures and their effect.

During weaning, record the date and time of each session, the weaning method, and baseline and subsequent vital signs, oxygen saturation levels, and ABG values. Again describe the patient's subjective and objective responses (including LOC, respiratory effort, arrhythmias, skin color, and need for suctioning).

List all weaning complications and nursing actions taken. If the patient was receiving pressure support ventilation or using a T-piece or tracheostomy collar, note the duration of spontaneous breathing and the patient's ability to maintain the weaning schedule. If the patient was receiving intermittent mandatory ventilation, with or without pressure support ventilation, record the control breath rate, the time of each breath reduction, and the rate of spontaneous respirations.

MEDITATION

The ancient art of meditation—focusing one's attention on a single sound or image or on the rhythm of one's own breathing—has been found to have positive effects on health. By directing attention away from worries about the future or preoccupation with the past, meditation reduces stress, a major contributing factor in many health problems. Stress reduction in turn results in a wide range of physiologic and mental health benefits, from decreased oxygen consumption, heart rate, and respiratory rate to improved mood, spiritual calm, and heightened awareness.

Most meditation approaches fall into one of two techniques: concentrative meditation or mindful meditation. Concentrative meditation involves focusing on an image, a sound (called a mantra), or one's own breathing in order to achieve a state of calm and heightened awareness. Transcendental meditation is a form of concentrative meditation in which the individual repeats a mantra over and over again while sitting in a comfortable position. When other thoughts enter his mind, he's instructed to notice them and return to the mantra. Concentrating on the mantra prevents distracting thoughts.

Mindful meditation takes the opposite approach. Instead of focusing on a single sensation or sound, the individual is aware of all sensations, feelings, images, thoughts, sounds, and smells that pass through his mind without actually thinking about them. The goal is a calmer, clearer, nonreactive state of mind.

Meditation has a wide variety of indications. It's used to enhance immune function in patients with cancer, acquired immunodeficiency syndrome, and autoimmune disorders and has been successful in treating drug and alcohol addiction as well as posttraumatic stress disorder. Anxiety disorders, pain, and stress are also commonly treated with meditation. Meditation can also be used with dietary and lifestyle changes for patients with hypertension or heart disease.

Implementation

▶ To assist your patient with meditation, you'll need a private, quiet environment that's free from distractions and offers a comfortable place for your patient to sit or recline.

▶ If you'll be helping the patient with meditation, begin by explaining the procedure and answering any questions. Tell the patient that he can stop the exercise if he becomes uncomfortable. Help him into a comfortable position. If he's in a sitting position, ask him to keep his back straight and let his shoulders droop.

▶ Using a calm, soothing, low voice, instruct the patient to close his eyes, if doing so feels comfortable. Tell him to focus on his abdomen, feeling it rise each time he inhales and fall each time he exhales. Tell him to concentrate on his breathing. Explain that if his mind wanders off his breathing, he should simply bring it back, regardless of what the thought was.

▶ Have the patient practice the exercise for 15 minutes every day for 1 week; then evaluate its benefits with him.

▶ Document the session, the instructions you gave the patient, and his response.

Special considerations

▶ Be aware that meditation may elicit negative emotions, disorientation, or memories of early childhood abuse or other traumas. If this occurs, try to find out what the feeling or memory concerns and direct the patient to a safer, more pleasant thought or memory. If this isn't possible, stop the session, notify the physician, and stay with the patient until he's calm and controlled.

▶ Use meditation cautiously in schizophrenic patients and in those with attention deficit hyperactivity disorder.

▶ Remind the patient that meditation isn't a substitute for medical treatment. If he's taking a prescribed medication, such as an antihypertensive, tell him to continue taking it.

▶ Be aware that patients with respiratory problems may have difficulty with meditation techniques that focus on breathing.

MELANOMA, MALIGNANT

A neoplasm that arises from melanocytes, malignant melanoma is potentially the most lethal of the skin cancers. It accounts for 3% of all cancers and its incidence is rapidly increasing. Melanoma is slightly more common in women than in men and is unusual in children. Peak incidence occurs between ages 50 and 70, although the incidence in younger age-groups is increasing.

This cancer has a strong tendency to metastasize. Melanoma spreads through the lymphatic and vascular systems and metastasizes to the regional lymph nodes, skin, liver, lungs, and central nervous system. Its course is unpredictable, however, and recurrence and metastasis may not appear for more than 5 years after resection of the primary lesion. The prognosis varies with the tumor thickness. In most patients, superficial lesions are curable, whereas deeper lesions tend to metastasize.

Common sites for melanoma are the head and neck in men, the legs in women, and the backs of people exposed to excessive sunlight. Up to 70% of malignant melanomas arise from a preexisting nevus. Complications result from disease progression to the lungs, liver, or brain.

There are four types of melanomas:

▶ *Superficial spreading melanoma*, the most common type (accounting for 50% to 70% of cases), usually develops between ages 40 and 50. These tumors may grow horizontally for years, but the prognosis worsens when vertical growth occurs.

▶ *Nodular melanoma* usually develops between ages 40 and 50 and accounts for 12% to 30% of cases. It grows vertically, invades the dermis, and metastasizes early.

▶ *Acral-lentiginous melanoma* is the most common melanoma among Hispanics, Asians, and Blacks. It occurs on the palms and soles and in sublingual locations.

▶ *Lentigo maligna melanoma* is relatively rare, accounting for 4% to 10% of cases. This is the most benign, slowest growing, and least aggressive of the four types. It usually occurs in areas heavily exposed to the sun and affects people between ages 60 and 70. This melanoma arises from a lentigo maligna on an exposed skin surface.

Several factors may influence the development of melanoma:

▶ excessive exposure to sunlight—Melanoma occurs most commonly in sunny, warm areas and typically develops on body parts that are exposed to the sun.

▶ skin type—Most people who develop melanoma have blond or red hair, fair skin, and blue eyes; are prone to sunburn; and are of Celtic or Scandinavian ancestry. Melanoma is rare among Blacks; when it does develop, it usually arises in lightly pigmented areas (the palms, plantar surface of the feet, or mucous membranes).

▶ genetic factors—Atypical moles in a patient with two family members with melanoma carries an extremely high lifetime risk of melanoma.

▶ family history—Melanoma occurs slightly more commonly within families.

▶ past history—A person who has had one melanoma is at greater risk for developing a second.

Signs and symptoms

▶ Sore that doesn't heal

▶ Persistent lump or swelling

▶ Changes in preexisting skin markings, such as moles, birthmarks, scars, freckles, or warts

▶ In superficial spreading melanoma, lesions on the ankles or the inside surfaces of the knees that may appear red, white, or blue over a brown or black background; may have an irregular, notched margin; and may ulcerate and bleed

▶ In nodular melanoma, a uniformly discolored nodule that may resemble a grayish blackberry (occasionally, flesh-colored with flecks of pigment around its base, which may be inflamed)

▶ In acral-lentiginous melanoma, rich brown, tan, and black lesions on the palms and soles and possibly an irregular tan or brown stain on the nail that diffuses from the nail bed

▶ In lentigo maligna melanoma, a long-standing, large (3 to 6 cm) lesion on the face, on the back of the hand, or under the fingernails that has ulcerated; may look like a freckle of tan, brown, black, whitish, or slate color with possibly irregular scattered black nodules on the surface

Diagnostic tests

▶ *Excisional biopsy* and full-depth *punch biopsy* with *histologic examination* can distinguish malignant melanoma from a benign nevus, seborrheic keratosis, or pigmented basal cell epithelioma and can also determine the tumor's thickness and stage.

▶ *Baseline laboratory studies* may include complete blood count with differential, erythrocyte sedimentation rate, platelet count, and liver function studies, in addition to urinalysis.

Depending on the depth of tumor invasion and any metastatic spread, baseline diagnostic studies may also include such tests as chest X-rays, computed tomography (CT) scans of the chest and abdomen, and a gallium scan. Signs of bone metastasis may require a bone scan; central nervous system metastasis, a CT scan of the brain. Magnetic resonance imaging may be used to assess metastasis.

Treatment

A patient with malignant melanoma always requires surgical resection to remove the tumor. A 1-cm margin is recommended for thin melanomas (less than 1 mm thick) and a 2- to 3-cm margin for intermediate and thick melanomas (more than 1 mm thick). The extent of resection depends on the size and location of the primary lesion. Closure of a wide resection may require a skin graft. Plastic surgery techniques can provide excellent cosmetic repair. Surgical treatment may also include regional lymphadenectomy.

Deep primary lesions may merit adjuvant chemotherapy. The most consistently used drugs are dacarbazine and carmustine. After surgical removal of a mass, intra-arterial isolation perfusions are performed to prevent recurrence and metastatic spread.

Although experimental, biotherapy, consisting of treatment with bacille Calmette-Guérin vaccine, offers hope to patients with advanced melanoma. Immunotherapy combats cancer by boosting the body's disease-fighting systems.

Chemotherapy is useful only in metastatic disease. Dacarbazine and the nitrosoureas have generated some response. Similarly, radiation therapy is usually reserved for metastatic disease. It doesn't prolong survival but may reduce tumor size and relieve pain.

Regardless of treatment, melanomas require close long-term follow-up care to detect metastasis and recurrence. Statistics show that about 13% of recurrences develop more than 5 years after primary surgery.

Key nursing diagnoses and outcomes

Impaired skin integrity related to skin cancer

Treatment outcome: The patient will maintain a skin care routine to prevent or minimize the risk of melanoma recurrence that includes inspecting his skin daily for changes and seeking medical attention if changes occur.

Anxiety related to potential for metastasis

Treatment outcomes: The patient will express his feelings of anxiety and will cope with his diagnosis and the requirements of follow-up care without exhibiting severe signs of anxiety.

Nursing interventions

▶ Listen to the patient's fears and concerns, and stay with him during periods of stress and anxiety. Include the patient and his family members in care decisions.

▶ Provide positive reinforcement as the patient attempts to adapt to his disease.

▶ Provide a diet that's high in protein and calories. If the patient is anorectic, provide small, frequent meals. Consult with the dietitian to incorporate foods that the patient enjoys into his diet.

▶ After surgery, take precautions to prevent infection. If surgery included lymphadenectomy, apply a compression stocking and instruct the patient to keep the extremity elevated to minimize lymphedema.

▶ Watch for complications associated with interferon, such as fever, chills, malaise, and fatigue.
▶ In advanced metastatic disease, control and prevent pain with regularly scheduled administration of analgesics.
▶ When appropriate, refer the patient and his family to community support services, such as a local chapter of the American Cancer Society or a hospice.

PATIENT TEACHING
▶ Make sure the patient understands the procedures and treatments associated with his diagnosis. Review the physician's explanation of treatment alternatives. Honestly answer any questions the patient or his family members may have about surgery, interferon, chemotherapy, and radiation therapy.
▶ Tell the patient what to expect before and after surgery, what the wound will look like, and what type of dressing he'll have. Warn him that the donor site for a skin graft may be as painful as the tumor excision site, if not more so.
▶ Teach the patient and his family members relaxation techniques to help relieve anxiety, and encourage them to continue these after discharge.
▶ Emphasize the need for close follow-up care for years to detect recurrence early. Teach the patient how to recognize the signs of recurrence.
▶ To help prevent recurrence of melanoma, stress the detrimental effects of exposure to sunlight. Instruct the patient to wear protective clothing and sunscreen with a minimum skin protection factor of 15. Urge him to avoid becoming sunburned or using tanning salons.

METABOLIC ACIDOSIS

Metabolic acidosis is a physiologic state of excess acid accumulation and deficient base bicarbonate that's caused by an underlying disorder. Symptoms result from the body's attempts to correct the acidotic condition through compensatory mechanisms in the lungs, kidneys, and cells. Severe or untreated metabolic acidosis can lead to coma, arrhythmias, cardiac arrest, and death.

Metabolic acidosis usually results from excessive burning of fats in the absence of usable carbohydrates. This can be caused by diabetic ketoacidosis (DKA), chronic alcoholism, malnutrition, or a low-carbohydrate, high-fat diet — all of which produce more ketoacids than the metabolic process can handle.

Other causes of acid accumulation include:
▶ anaerobic carbohydrate metabolism — A decrease in tissue oxygenation or perfusion (as occurs with pump failure after myocardial infarction or with pulmonary or hepatic disease, shock, or anemia) forces a shift from aerobic to anaerobic metabolism, causing a corresponding rise in lactic acid level.
▶ renal insufficiency and failure (renal acidosis) — Underexcretion of metabolized acids or inability to conserve base bicarbonate results in excess acid accumulation or deficient base bicarbonate.
▶ diarrhea and intestinal malabsorption — Loss of sodium bicarbonate from the intestines causes the bicarbonate buffer system to shift to the acidic side.
▶ massive rhabdomyolysis — High quantities of organic acids added to the body with the breakdown of cells causes high anion gap acidosis.
▶ poisoning and drug toxicity — Common causative agents, such as salicylates, ethylene glycol, and methyl alcohol, may produce acid-base imbalance.
▶ hypoaldosteronism or use of potassium-sparing diuretics — These conditions inhibit distal tubular secretion of acid and potassium.

Signs and symptoms
▶ Changes in level of consciousness (LOC) — from lethargy, drowsiness, and confusion to stupor and coma

Test values in metabolic acidosis

If your patient has metabolic acidosis, expect the following abnormal arterial blood gas values:

- pH below 7.35
- decreased partial pressure of carbon dioxide, representing compensation for acidosis
- bicarbonate level below 24 mEq/L in acute metabolic acidosis
- anion gap above 14 mEq/L from increased acid production or renal insufficiency.

▶ Kussmaul's respirations (as the lungs attempt to compensate by blowing off carbon dioxide)

▶ In underlying diabetes mellitus, fruity breath odor from catabolism of fats and excretion of accumulated acetone through the lungs

▶ Diminished muscle tone and deep tendon reflexes on neuromuscular assessment

Diagnostic tests

For key laboratory test values, see *Test values in metabolic acidosis*. Other characteristic findings include the following:

▶ *Urinalysis* indicates a pH of 4.5 or below in the absence of renal disease.

▶ *Blood tests* show elevated serum potassium levels as hydrogen ions move into the cells and potassium moves out of the cells to maintain electroneutrality; increased blood glucose and serum ketone levels in diabetes mellitus; and elevated plasma lactic acid levels in lactic acidosis.

Treatment

For acute metabolic acidosis, treatment may include I.V. administration of sodium bicarbonate (when arterial pH is less than 7.2) to neutralize blood acidity. For chronic metabolic acidosis, oral bicarbonate may be given.

Other measures include careful evaluation and correction of electrolyte imbalances and correction of the underlying cause. For example, DKA requires insulin administration and fluid replacement. Mechanical ventilation may be required to ensure adequate respiratory compensation.

Key nursing diagnoses and outcomes

Disturbed thought processes related to neurologic dysfunction

Treatment outcomes: The patient will remain safe and free from injury and will exhibit orientation to time, place, and person.

Ineffective breathing pattern related to pulmonary dysfunction

Treatment outcomes: The patient will maintain adequate ventilation and oxygenation and will avoid hypoxia.

Nursing interventions

▶ Provide care to eliminate the underlying cause of metabolic acidosis. For example, administer insulin and I.V. fluids, as ordered, to reverse DKA.

▶ Administer sodium bicarbonate, as prescribed, and keep sodium bicarbonate ampules handy for emergency administration.

▶ Orient the patient frequently, as needed. Reduce unnecessary environmental stimulation. Ensure a safe environment if he's confused. Keep the bed in the lowest position, with the side rails raised.

▶ Provide good oral hygiene. Use sodium bicarbonate washes to neutralize mouth acids, and lubricate the patient's lips with petroleum jelly.

▶ Frequently assess the patient's vital signs, laboratory test results, and LOC because changes can occur rapidly.

▶ Monitor the patient's respiratory function. Check his arterial blood gas values frequently.

- If the patient has DKA, watch for secondary changes caused by hypovolemia such as decreasing blood pressure.
- Record the patient's intake and output accurately to monitor renal function. Watch for signs of excessive serum potassium levels, such as weakness, flaccid paralysis, and arrhythmias (which may lead to cardiac arrest). After treatment, check for overcorrection of hypokalemia.

PATIENT TEACHING

- To prevent DKA, teach the patient with diabetes how to routinely test blood glucose levels or how to test his urine for glucose and acetone. Encourage strict adherence to insulin or oral antidiabetic therapy, and reinforce the need to follow the prescribed dietary therapy.
- As needed, teach the patient and his family members about prescribed medications, including their mechanism of action, dosage, and possible adverse effects. Provide verbal and written instructions.

METABOLIC ALKALOSIS

Metabolic alkalosis is a clinical state marked by decreased amounts of acid or increased amounts of base bicarbonate. It always occurs secondary to an underlying cause and is commonly associated with hypocalcemia and hypokalemia, which may account for the signs and symptoms. With early diagnosis and prompt treatment, the prognosis is good. However, untreated metabolic alkalosis may result in coma, atrioventricular arrhythmias, and death.

Underlying causes of acid loss include vomiting, nasogastric (NG) tube drainage or lavage without adequate electrolyte replacement, fistulas, and the use of steroids and certain diuretics (furosemide, thiazides, and ethacrynic acid). Hyperadrenocorticism is another cause of severe acid loss. Cushing's disease, primary hyperaldosteronism, and Bartter's syndrome, for example, all lead to retention of sodium and chloride and urinary loss of potassium and hydrogen.

Excessive retention of base can be caused by excessive intake of bicarbonate of soda or other antacids (usually for treatment of gastritis or peptic ulcer), excessive intake of absorbable alkali (as in milk-alkali syndrome, typically seen in patients with peptic ulcers), administration of excessive amounts of I.V. fluids with high concentrations of bicarbonate or lactate, massive blood transfusions, or respiratory insufficiency.

Signs and symptoms

- Irritability, belligerence, and paresthesia
- Apathy, confusion, seizures, stupor, or coma if alkalosis is severe
- Tetany if serum calcium levels are borderline or low
- Decreased respiratory rate and depth (as a compensatory mechanism)
- Hyperactive reflexes and muscle weakness if serum potassium levels are markedly low
- Arrhythmias in hypokalemia

The patient history may reveal excessive ingestion of alkali antacids and extracellular fluid (ECF) volume depletion, which is frequently associated with conditions leading to metabolic alkalosis (for example, vomiting or NG tube suctioning).

Diagnostic tests

- *Arterial blood gas analysis* reveals a blood pH over 7.45 and a bicarbonate level over 29 mEq/L. Partial pressure of carbon dioxide over 45 mm Hg indicates attempts at respiratory compensation.
- *Serum electrolyte studies* usually show low potassium, calcium, and chloride levels.
- *Electrocardiography (ECG)* discloses a low T wave merging with a P wave and atrial or sinus tachycardia.

Treatment

Correcting the underlying cause of metabolic alkalosis is the goal of treatment. Mild metabolic alkalosis generally requires no treatment. Potassium chloride and normal saline solution (except with heart failure) are usually sufficient to replace losses from gastric drainage. Rarely, therapy for severe alkalosis includes cautious I.V. administration of ammonium chloride to release hydrogen chloride and restore the concentration of ECF and chloride levels.

Electrolyte replacement with potassium chloride and discontinuation of diuretics correct metabolic alkalosis resulting from potent diuretic therapy.

Oral or I.V. acetazolamide, which enhances renal bicarbonate excretion, may be prescribed to correct metabolic alkalosis without rapid volume expansion. Because acetazolamide also enhances potassium excretion, the patient may be given potassium before he takes this drug.

Key nursing diagnoses and outcomes

Disturbed thought processes related to neurologic dysfunction

Treatment outcomes: The patient will remain safe and free from injury and will become oriented to time, place, and person.

Decreased cardiac output related to atrioventricular arrhythmias

Treatment outcomes: The patient will maintain hemodynamic stability and will avoid manifestations of profoundly decreased cardiac output, such as shock and tissue ischemia.

Nursing interventions

- When administering I.V. solutions containing potassium salts, dilute potassium with the prescribed I.V. solution and use an I.V. infusion pump. Infuse 0.9% ammonium chloride I.V. no faster than 1 L over 4 hours; faster administration may cause hemolysis of red blood cells (RBCs). Avoid administering excessive amounts of these solutions because this could cause overcorrection leading to metabolic acidosis. Don't give ammonium chloride to a patient who has signs of hepatic or renal disease.
- Observe seizure precautions, and provide a safe environment for the patient with altered thought processes. Orient the patient as needed.
- Irrigate the patient's NG tube with normal saline solution instead of plain water to prevent loss of gastric electrolytes.
- Monitor I.V. fluid concentrations of bicarbonate or lactate. Observe the infusion rate of I.V. solutions containing potassium salts to prevent damage to blood vessels. Monitor I.V. solutions containing ammonium chloride to prevent RBC hemolysis. Watch for signs of phlebitis.
- Assess the patient's laboratory values, including pH and serum bicarbonate, potassium, and calcium levels. Notify the physician if you detect significant changes or if the patient responds poorly to treatment.
- Observe the ECG for arrhythmias.
- Watch closely for signs of muscle weakness, tetany, or decreased activity.
- Check the patient's vital signs frequently, and record intake and output to evaluate respiratory, fluid, and electrolyte status. Keep in mind that the respiratory rate usually slows in an effort to compensate for alkalosis. Tachycardia may indicate electrolyte imbalance, especially hypokalemia.
- Assess the patient's level of consciousness frequently.

PATIENT TEACHING

- To prevent metabolic alkalosis, warn the patient not to overuse alkaline agents.
- If the patient has an ulcer, teach him how to recognize signs of milk-alkali syndrome, including a distaste for milk, anorexia, weakness, and lethargy.

▶ If potassium-wasting diuretics or potassium chloride supplements are prescribed, make sure the patient understands the drug regimen, including the purpose, dosage, and possible adverse effects.

MUSIC THERAPY

Music therapy uses the universal appeal of rhythmic sound to communicate, explore, and heal. It can take the form of creating music, singing, moving to music, or just listening.

Music therapy benefits patients with developmental disabilities, mental health disorders, dementia, substance addictions, and chronic pain. Studies have demonstrated the positive effects of music in reducing pain and procedural anxiety and in dental anesthesia.

Patients who listen to classical music prior to surgery, and then again in the recovery room, reported minimal postoperative disorientation. Music has also been successfully used to communicate with Alzheimer's patients and head trauma victims when other approaches failed. In a study on the effects of music on Alzheimer's patients, those who listened to big band music during the day were more alert and happier and had better long-term recollection than the control group. Throughout the illness, music can reorient confused patients. In the final stages of the disease, it provides psychological comfort.

Implementation

▶ Arrange a comfortable environment.
▶ Choose music that's appropriate to the patients and the session objectives. The music should be meaningful to the participants.
▶ If your session will involve making music, collect instruments appropriate for the group.
▶ For sessions involving singing, choose music that's known to the group members. Provide words for the songs, either in writing or by repeating them to the group.
▶ Introduce the participants to each other. Explain the purpose of the session, and encourage everyone to participate as they feel able.
▶ When the group is ready, start the music and position yourself so you're facing the group.
▶ If the group will be listening to music, watch the reactions of the participants. If they're making the music, circulate among the group members and offer individual support.
▶ Encourage the participants to discuss the feelings they experienced while listening to the music. Praise their efforts.
▶ After the session, document the type of activity and the group's response.

Special considerations

Music is especially effective as a means of reminiscence therapy for older people. For many of them, the music they enjoyed in their youth hasn't been part of their lives for decades.

MYOCARDIAL INFARCTION

Myocardial infarction (MI) results from reduced blood flow through a coronary artery, which causes myocardial ischemia and necrosis. The infarction site depends on the vessels involved. For instance, occlusion of the circumflex coronary artery causes a lateral wall infarction; occlusion of the left anterior coronary artery causes an anterior wall infarction. True posterior and inferior wall infarctions are caused by occlusion of the right coronary artery or one of its branches. Right ventricular infarctions also can result from right coronary artery occlusion, can accompany inferior infarctions, and may cause right-sided heart failure. In transmural (Q-wave) MI, tissue damage extends through all myocardial layers; in subendocardial (non-Q-wave) MI, usually only the innermost layer is damaged.

Although MI is more common in men than premenopausal women, the incidence equalizes after women go through menopause. In North America and Western Europe, MI is one of the most common causes of death, which usually results from cardiac damage or complications. The mortality rate for people over age 70 is twice that for younger adults. Sudden death may be the first and only indication of MI.

Age-related changes in the cardiovascular system, along with other risk factors, predispose the older person to MI. Additional risk factors for this age-group include eating a large meal and physical exertion. Older people are also at greater risk for silent MI, which commonly triggers sudden death from arrhythmias. Because of the high incidence and mortality of MI, teaching about prevention is a critical aspect of your nursing care.

Occlusion of the coronary arteries may result from atherosclerosis, thrombosis, platelet aggregation, or coronary artery stenosis or spasm. Predisposing factors include aging; diabetes mellitus; elevated serum, triglyceride, low-density lipoprotein, and cholesterol levels; decreased serum high-density lipoprotein levels; excessive intake of saturated fats, carbohydrates, or salt; hypertension; obesity; family history of coronary artery disease (CAD); sedentary lifestyle; smoking; stress; and type A personality (aggressive, competitive attitude, addiction to work, chronic impatience).

Elderly people are more prone to complications and death from an MI. Possible cardiac complications include arrhythmias, cardiogenic shock, heart failure (leading to pulmonary edema), pericarditis, ventricular aneurysm, and rupture of the atrial or ventricular septum, ventricular wall, or valves.

Signs and symptoms

- Mild pain that's confused with indigestion (or no pain at all)
- Dyspnea (common presenting symptom in people over age 85), possibly accompanied by anxiety or confusion
- With CAD, reports of increasing anginal frequency, severity, or duration (especially when not precipitated by exertion, a heavy meal, or exposure to cold and wind)
- Feeling of impending doom
- Nausea and vomiting
- Jugular vein distention with right-sided heart failure
- Palpitations or worsening heart failure
- Cerebrovascular accident (CVA)
- Syncope or dizziness
- Acute renal failure
- Subtle changes, such as excessive fatigue, altered mental status, unusual behavior, and changes in eating patterns
- Within the first hour after an anterior MI, sympathetic nervous system hyperactivity, such as tachycardia and hypertension (in about 25% of patients)
- With an inferior MI, parasympathetic nervous system hyperactivity, such as bradycardia and hypotension (in up to 50% of patients)
- On auscultation, S_4, S_3, paradoxical splitting of S_2, and decreased heart sounds (in patients with ventricular dysfunction); systolic murmur of mitral insufficiency (in papillary muscle dysfunction secondary to infarction); or pericardial friction rub (especially in transmural MI or pericarditis)
- Low-grade fever a few days after the MI

Diagnostic tests

- *Serial 12-lead electrocardiography* (ECG) may be normal or inconclusive in the first few hours after an MI and difficult to interpret in an older patient with preexisting heart disease. Characteristic abnormalities include serial ST-segment depression in subendocardial MI and ST-segment elevation and Q waves, representing scarring and necrosis, in transmural MI.
- *Blood studies* usually show an elevated serum creatine kinase (CK) level, espe-

cially the CK-MB isoenzyme, the cardiac muscle fraction of CK. In older people, the CK level and other laboratory test results can be confusing because of their typically lean body mass. In malnourished older people, cardiac enzyme levels may not be elevated high enough to confirm a diagnosis of MI. Myoglobin (the hemoprotein found in cardiac and skeletal muscle) is released with muscle damage and may be detected as early as 2 hours after MI. Troponin I, a structural protein found in cardiac muscle, is elevated only in cardiac muscle damage. It's more specific than the CK-MB level. Troponin levels increase within 4 to 6 hours of myocardial injury and may remain elevated for 5 to 11 days.

- *Echocardiography* shows ventricular wall dyskinesia in a transmural MI and helps evaluate the ejection fraction.
- *Technetium-99m pertechnetate scan* can identify acutely damaged muscle by picking up accumulations of radioactive nucleotide, which appear as a hot spot on the film
- *Myocardial perfusion imaging with thallium 201* reveals a cold spot in most patients during the first few hours after a transmural MI.
- *Thyroid studies, arterial blood gas analysis,* and *complete blood count* may reveal underlying conditions that trigger ischemic episodes.

Treatment

The goals of treatment are to relieve chest pain, stabilize heart rhythm, and reduce cardiac workload. Drug therapy includes I.V. morphine for pain and sedation, inotropic drugs (such as dobutamine and amrinone) to treat reduced myocardial contractility, and beta-adrenergic blockers (such as propranolol and timolol) to help prevent reinfarction. Anticoagulation therapy may be indicated if atrial fibrillation is present.

Nitroglycerin (sublingual, topical, transdermal, or I.V.); calcium channel blockers, such as nifedipine, verapamil, or diltiazem (sublingual, oral, or I.V.); or isosorbide dinitrate (sublingual, oral, or I.V.) may also be administered to relieve pain by redistributing blood to ischemic areas of the myocardium, increasing cardiac output, and reducing myocardial workload. Atropine I.V. or a temporary pacemaker is used for heart block or bradycardia. Amiodarone or lidocaine may be used for ventricular arrhythmias. If ineffective, procainamide or magnesium may be indicated.

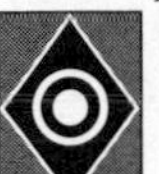

Drug alert Because of age-related changes, older adults are more susceptible to the toxic effects of lidocaine, such as confusion, seizures, respiratory depression, and hypotension. Older patients should be given lower doses and monitored closely for these effects.

Oxygen is usually administered (by face mask or nasal cannula) at a modest flow rate for 24 to 48 hours; a lower concentration is necessary if the patient has chronic obstructive pulmonary disease. Bed rest with the head of the bed elevated 20 to 30 degrees and a bedside commode is enforced to decrease the cardiac workload.

Pulmonary artery catheterization may be performed to detect left- or right-sided heart failure and to monitor response to treatment, but it isn't routinely done. An intra-aortic balloon pump may be inserted for cardiogenic shock.

Revascularization therapy is used more commonly for patients under age 70 who don't have a history of CVA, bleeding, GI ulcers, marked hypertension, recent surgery, or chest pain lasting longer than 6 hours. Thrombolytic therapy must begin within 3 hours of the onset of symptoms, using intracoronary or systemic (I.V.) streptokinase or tissue plasminogen activator (tPA). The best response occurs when treatment begins within the first hour after onset of symptoms. Cardiac catheterization, percutaneous transluminal coronary angioplasty (PTCA), and coronary artery bypass grafting may also be performed.

Key nursing diagnoses and outcomes

Ineffective (cardiac) tissue perfusion related to narrowing or closure of one or more coronary arteries

Treatment outcome: The patient will regain adequate cardiac tissue perfusion.

Risk for injury related to complications of MI

Treatment outcome: The patient will avoid permanent deficits caused by complications of MI.

Chronic pain related to myocardial tissue ischemia

Treatment outcome: The patient won't have chest pain after treatment.

Nursing interventions

- When the patient is admitted to the intensive care unit, monitor and record his ECG readings, vital signs, temperature, and heart and breath sounds.
- Assess pain and give analgesics, as ordered. Record the severity, location, type, and duration of pain. Don't give I.M. injections because absorption from the muscle is unpredictable and I.V. administration provides more rapid relief.
- Check the patient's blood pressure after giving nitroglycerin, especially after the first dose.
- Continuously monitor ECG readings to detect rate changes and arrhythmias. Analyze rhythm strips and place a representative strip in the patient's chart if any new arrhythmias are documented, if chest pain occurs, or at least every shift or according to your facility's protocol.
- During episodes of chest pain, obtain ECG readings and vital signs and pulmonary artery catheter measurements (if applicable) to determine changes.
- Be alert for crackles, cough, tachypnea, and edema, which may indicate impending left-sided heart failure. Carefully monitor daily weight, intake and output, respiratory rate, serum enzyme levels, ECG readings, and blood pressure.
- Auscultate for adventitious breath sounds periodically (patients on bed rest frequently have atelectatic crackles, which may disappear after coughing) and for S_3 or S_4 gallops.
- Organize patient care and activities to maximize uninterrupted rest periods.
- Ask the dietitian to provide a clear liquid diet until nausea subsides. A low-cholesterol, low-sodium diet, without caffeinated beverages may be ordered.
- Provide a stool softener to prevent straining during defecation, which causes vagal stimulation and may slow the heart rate. Allow the patient to use a bedside commode, and provide privacy.
- Assist with range-of-motion exercises. If the patient is immobilized by a severe MI, turn him often. Antiembolism stockings help prevent venostasis and thrombophlebitis.
- Provide emotional support, and help reduce stress and anxiety; administer tranquilizers as needed.
- If the patient has undergone PTCA, keep the sheath line open with a heparin drip. In addition, platelet inhibitors (Aggrastat, Intergrilin, ReoPro) may be infused through a peripheral line for 12 hours. Observe for generalized and site bleeding. Keep the leg with the sheath insertion site immobile, and maintain strict bed rest. Check peripheral pulses in the affected leg frequently. Provide analgesics for back pain if needed.
- After thrombolytic therapy, administer continuous heparin, if ordered and according to facility guidelines. This may include measuring partial thromboplastin time and monitoring the patient for evidence of bleeding. Check ECG rhythm strips for reperfusion arrhythmias, and treat them according to your facility's protocol. If the artery reoccludes, the patient will experience the same symptoms as before. If this occurs, prepare the patient for return to the cardiac catheterization laboratory.

PATIENT TEACHING

- Explain all procedures to the patient and his family, and answer their questions. Describe the intensive care unit environment and routine. Remember that you may need to repeat explanations once the emergency has resolved.

▶ To promote compliance with the prescribed drug regimen and other treatment measures, thoroughly explain drug dosages and the reason for drug therapy. Inform the patient of the drug's adverse effects, and advise him to watch for and report signs of toxicity (anorexia, nausea, vomiting, mental depression, vertigo, blurred vision, and yellow vision if he's receiving a cardiac glycoside).

▶ Review dietary restrictions with the patient. If he must follow a low-sodium or low-fat and low-cholesterol diet, provide a list of foods to avoid. Ask the dietitian to speak to the patient and family.

▶ Urge the patient to participate in a cardiac rehabilitation program. The physician and the exercise physiologist should determine the level of exercise, discuss it with the patient, and secure his agreement to a stepped-care program.

▶ Counsel the patient to resume sexual activity progressively. Don't overlook this aspect of care with older adults. Most older adults are sexually active but may not feel comfortable asking about this topic. The patient may need to take nitroglycerin before sexual intercourse to prevent chest pain.

▶ Tell him to report typical or atypical chest pain. Post-MI syndrome may develop, producing chest pain that must be differentiated from recurrent MI, pulmonary infarction, and heart failure.

▶ If appropriate, stress the need to stop smoking. If necessary, refer the patient to a smoking cessation program. (See *Lifestyle changes for a healthy heart.*)

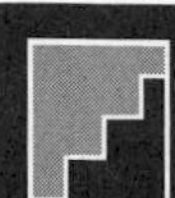

Staying well

Lifestyle changes for a healthy heart

Dietary and lifestyle changes can reduce a patient's risk of high blood pressure, heart attack, and other forms of heart disease. If the patient already has high blood pressure or heart disease, suggest these changes to improve his health, strengthen his heart and, possibly, even help him live longer.

- If applicable, stop smoking and avoid second-hand smoke. Speak with a physician about nicotine patches or gum. Contact the American Cancer Society, American Heart Association, or American Lung Association for support groups and information.
- Eat a diet low in saturated fat and cholesterol. The risk of heart disease increases as blood cholesterol levels rise.
- Eat a diet rich in potassium, calcium, magnesium, and protein. Limit sodium intake. Eat plenty of fresh fruits and vegetables and high-fiber foods.
- Lose weight if necessary.
- Exercise regularly and be active. Strive for at least 30 minutes of continuous aerobic exercise daily. If that isn't possible, exercise three times per day for 10 minutes. Consult with your physician before starting an exercise program.
- Limit alcohol intake to one drink per day for women and two drinks per day for men.
- Reduce stress.
- Speak with your physician about hormone replacement therapy (for postmenopausal women).
- Control your blood glucose levels if you have diabetes.

Special considerations

▶ The incidence of asymptomatic MI increases with age. Although pain is still considered to be the classic symptom of MI in older adults, the pain may be vaguely described and poorly localized (such as in patients with diabetes, elderly patients, and women). It may be isolated in such areas as the throat, shoulder, and abdomen. Shortness of breath commonly occurs with or without fatigue in elderly patients.

▶ In older adults, 10% of CVAs are associated with an MI.

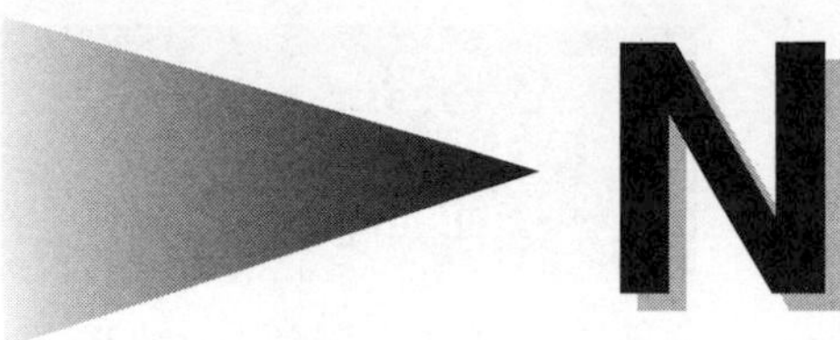

NUTRITIONAL NEEDS

Eating is a complex biological, social, cultural, and behavioral phenomenon. A person's dietary preferences and eating habits profoundly affect his nutritional status and health. Of course, good nutrition is essential to your patient, no matter his age. However, because of various interrelated factors — inactivity, low income, lack of transportation, social isolation, need for special diets, and the disappearance of corner grocery stores — older people are especially vulnerable to malnutrition. Normal age-related changes (diminished sense of thirst or need to drink, diminished sense of smell and taste) place even elderly patients with stable incomes, transportation, and available grocery stores at risk for malnutrition.

In many ambulatory care settings, nutritional assessment consists primarily of obtaining a 24-hour dietary recall and comparing it to the Food Guide Pyramid. However, this is at best a cursory assessment of food intake over a limited period. Nutrition assessments in the acute care setting are usually a part of the nurse's admission assessment and are rather superficial — usually limited to learning food preferences and allergies. Daily food intake is documented on flow sheets and the dietitian is consulted as needed.

Few assessment instruments are specific to older people. The Minimum Data Set for Nursing Home Resident Assessment and Care Screening has a nutritional component. The Nutrition Screening Initiative, a joint venture of the American Academy of Family Physicians, the American Dietetic Association, and the National Council on Aging, includes screening methods and interventions to prevent and remedy nutritional deficiencies specifically in older adults. The Nutrition Screening Initiative is widely used in outpatient settings. This program begins with a self-administered questionnaire that highlights areas of known risk for nutritional deficiencies. After the questionnaire is scored, at-risk patients are referred for more extensive screening. This includes another questionnaire (Screen 1) administered by a health professional. It further explores the known risk areas using the mnemonic device DETERMINE:

- Disease or depression
- Eating poorly
- Tooth loss or mouth pain
- Economic hardship
- Reduced social contact and interaction
- Multiple medications
- Involuntary weight loss or gain
- Need for assistance with self-care
- Elder at an advanced age.

A second screening test (Screen 2) elicits in-depth information about nutritional status as well as specific biochemical, clinical, and diagnostic test data using the mnemonic device ABCDEF:

- Anthropometric (height and weight) — Some studies have found an association between weight loss over time and mortality (the greater the weight loss, the higher the mortality risk), particularly in cognitively impaired older patients with self-care deficits. The question of what's the most appropriate scale for height-, weight-, and age-related measurements in older persons is still unsettled.

- Biochemical — A serum albumin level less than 3.5 mg/dl is a good nonspecific indicator of poor nutritional status, as are low hemoglobin, hematocrit, and serum cholesterol levels. Prealbumin is the most accurate indicator, however, because it reveals the most recent nutritional status (past 7 to 14 days). Serum vitamin B_{12} level can rule out B_{12} deficiency.
- Clinical, physical, and medical history — Assessments are needed to complete the medical history, including medications, herbal products, and over-the-counter products. These factors may influence nutritional intake. A complete physical, including laboratory studies, and clinical nursing assessments should also be completed. Report signs and symptoms of malnutrition or other abnormalities to the patient's physician.
- Dietary history — A food diary includes a list of all food and drink consumed in a 24-hour period, the use of supplements, sources for obtaining food, food storage, and cooking facilities.
- Empathy — This involves active listening, probing about diet, and allowing the patient ample time to divulge problems.
- Functional assessment — This assessment determines if the patient is dependent on others for help with activities of daily living (ADLs) or instrumental ADLs, including shopping and meal preparation, or is at risk for nutritional problems because of cognitive impairment.

Once you've assessed your patient's nutritional status, you can begin to formulate interventions.

Dietary guidelines

Most national educational programs on the subject of nutrition, including Healthy People 2010, Dietary Guidelines for Americans, and the Food Guide Pyramid, are aimed at the general population, not specifically at older adults.

The Food Guide Pyramid, introduced by the U.S. Department of Agriculture (USDA) in 1992, offers graphic as well as written information on recommended daily allowances of six food groups; it supersedes the older Basic Four Food Groups recommendations, which didn't address the issues of fat, cholesterol, sodium, or essential minerals in the diet. Although the pyramid includes information on portion sizes as well as the suggested number of servings for older adults, this data is commonly omitted or presented on a separate page. As a result, many consumers disregard portion size under the impression that they're following a healthy diet as long as they follow the basic guidelines shown in the pyramid.

Researchers at Tufts University have developed a new Food Guide Pyramid that they believe more accurately reflects the nutritional needs of healthy adults ages 70 and older. They recommend adding a base to the pyramid of eight or more 8-oz (236.6 ml) glasses of water each day to counteract the decreased thirst sensation that occurs with aging. Their pyramid is topped by the dietary supplements calcium and vitamin D, which are recommended to enhance bone health, and vitamin B_{12}, which promotes nerve function. The rest of their Food Guide Pyramid is the same as the 1992 Food Guide Pyramid, except that there are no maximum limits.

A more pertinent USDA source, Food Facts For Older Adults, applies established dietary guidelines to community-dwelling older adults and includes healthy recipes, shopping and food preparation tips, and further nutrition resources. Even the system of Recommended Dietary Allowances (RDAs) formulated by the National Research Council, which offers specific caloric guidelines for older people, groups this information under a single "age 51-plus" category. However, scientists believe that elderly patients have greater needs for some nutrients than those recommended in the RDAs. Specifically, greater intakes of folic acid and vitamins B_6 and B_{12} are necessary to reduce the decline in cognitive function related to the aging process. Moreover, by maintaining normal homocysteine levels, higher levels of folic acid and vitamins B_6 and B_{12} reduce the risk for coronary heart disease. A lack of vitamin B_{12} and folate may be associated with age-related hearing loss. Research has also shown that older adults have higher protein needs than the RDAs (1 to 1.3 g/kg body weight versus 0.8 g/kg).

Previous RDAs are being replaced by Dietary Reference Intakes (DRIs), which divide adults older than age 50 into two groups: ages 51 to 70 and ages 71 and older. The DRIs for several vitamins and nutrients are greater than the RDAs. For nutrients for which DRIs aren't available, the RDA values should be used. Thus, health care providers who work with older adults should consult a nutritionist if they suspect a problem in this area.

Special considerations

Your care will be based on nutritional assessment findings and the setting in which the older person lives. In general, you'll need to focus on the following areas: preventing dehydration, ensuring adequate calcium and fiber intake, preventing drug interactions with foods, dealing with feeding problems (such as food preparation, use of utensils, oral and dental hygiene, and swallowing difficulties), and educating the patient and caregivers about nutritional requirements.

Preventing dehydration

First and foremost, advise your patient to drink plenty of fluids—at least 30 oz (1,000 ml) per day, unless contraindicated. If he's taking prescription diuretics, warn him not to decrease fluid intake, even if he feels that frequent elimination restricts his mobility or ability to socialize. Also advise him that drinking alcoholic or caffeinated beverages increases diuresis, thereby increasing the need for fluids.

If your patient has urinary incontinence, make sure he doesn't purposely limit fluid intake in an attempt to reduce incontinence episodes. Advise the mobile patient to drink extra fluids during activity in hot weather to replace losses caused by perspiration and evaporation.

Older patients are at particularly high risk for dehydration because of their diminished thirst perception and any combination of physical, cognitive, speech, mobility, and visual impairments. You can take a number of steps to avoid dehydration in such patients. (See *Preventing dehydration.*)

Ensuring adequate calcium and fiber intake

Calcium, found in dairy products, tofu, leafy green vegetables, oysters, salmon, and sardines, is essential for maintaining bone density and preventing osteoporosis. Encourage your patient to obtain adequate calcium by consuming several servings of the foods listed above every day. In addition, you can easily boost your patient's dietary calcium by adding 1 or 2 tsp of nonfat dry milk to regular milk, cereals, and yogurt.

Adequate fiber is important in promoting regular bowel movements and may help prevent colon cancer. Some dietary fiber sources (such as oat bran) also lower cholesterol. Significant sources of dietary fiber are whole grain cereals and breads, raw fruits, leafy vegetables, and legumes. Over-the-counter products that add fiber to the diet, such

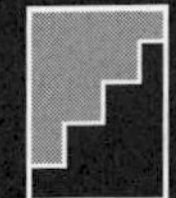

Staying well

Preventing dehydration

To maintain adequate hydration, elderly patients need between 1,000 and 3,000 ml of fluid per day. Less than 1,000 ml daily may lead to constipation, which can contribute to urinary incontinence, and more concentrated urine, which predisposes the patient to urinary tract infections. Follow these guidelines to make sure your patient is adequately hydrated.

Monitoring and assessment

- Monitor intake and output. Ensure an intake of at least 1,500 ml of oral fluids and urine output of 1,000 to 1,500 ml per 24 hours.
- Assess skin turgor and mucous membranes.
- Monitor vital signs, especially pulse rate, respiratory rate, and blood pressure. An increase in pulse and respiratory rates with decreased blood pressure may indicate dehydration.
- Monitor laboratory test results, such as serum electrolyte, blood urea nitrogen, and creatinine levels; hematocrit; and urine and serum osmolarity. Also check for signs of acidosis.
- Weigh the patient at the same time daily, using the same scale, and with the patient wearing the same type of clothes.
- Auscultate bowel sounds for any increase in activity. Also monitor stools for character: Hard stools may indicate dehydration; loose, watery stools indicate loss of water.
- Be aware of diagnostic studies that affect intake and output (for example, those requiring laxative or enema use can cause fluid loss), and replace any lost fluids.

Providing fluids

- Provide fluids frequently throughout the day, for example, every hour and with a bedtime snack.
- Provide modified cups that the patient can handle; help patients who have difficulty.
- Offer the patient fluids other than water; find out the types of beverages he likes and the preferred temperatures (for example, ice cold or room-temperature drinks).
- Monitor coffee intake; coffee acts as a diuretic and may cause excessive fluid loss.
- If the patient can't take oral fluids, request an order for I.V. hydration.

as FiberCon crackers and Metamucil, are also available. When using these products, adequate fluid intake is necessary to prevent intestinal obstruction.

Preventing drug interactions with foods

Because your patient may be taking many different drugs to treat various conditions, the risk of drug-nutrient interactions is high. Drugs can affect the patient's nutritional status by altering nutrient absorption, metabolism, utilization, or excretion. Likewise, various foods, beverages, and mineral or vitamin supplements can affect the absorption and effectiveness of drugs. These interactions must be considered when evaluating your patient's drug regimen.

Dealing with feeding problems

Patients with nutritional problems will respond to interventions that match the type of facility they're in.

ACUTE CARE SETTINGS

You'll need to monitor nutritional status, hydration status, and the effects of medical treatments daily. Some older patients initially have food or fluid restrictions and require parenteral supplementation.

If a patient is anorectic, ask his family members and other visitors to bring special foods from home that may improve his appetite. In addition, encourage his family members to collaborate in feeding a dependent patient. The family involvement can help promote the patient's recovery, enhance his feeling of well-being, and stimulate him to eat more.

Before discharge, teach the patient and his family about desirable nutritional practices and any prescribed therapeutic diets. Note the patient's dietary needs and preferences as well as special feeding techniques or assistive devices on the transfer form or postdischarge referral form to ensure continuity of care.

LONG-TERM CARE SETTINGS

Frail older people in group residential and long-term care settings pose a different set of nutritional challenges. Research shows that these older adults are interested in food preparation, service, and quality. They usually look forward to mealtimes and are easily disappointed if food doesn't meet their expectations.

People of different ethnic and cultural backgrounds have specific dietary preferences. In many cases, appropriate dietary adjustments can determine whether the patient will eat at all. If you can't arrange for a special diet, encourage family members or friends to bring in suitable foods that can be heated and served at mealtimes.

Oral health concerns, such as poor oral hygiene, loose or missing teeth, or absent or ill-fitting dentures, can also contribute to feeding problems. Make every effort to secure needed dental care for your patient and to replace lost or ill-fitting dentures. If this isn't possible because of profound disability or economic constraints, the patient will need a pureed diet.

Dysphagia (difficulty swallowing) can seriously compromise an older person's nutritional status.

Key point Be alert for signs of dysphagia, such as coughing while eating or while drinking a thin liquid such as water. Other signs are eating slowly, weight loss, recurrent pneumonia, or a gurgling voice during or after eating. The patient with dysphagia may try to compensate by turning away or refusing further food, which can easily be misinterpreted as lack of appetite.

To help the patient with dysphagia, teach him the "chin-tuck and swallow" technique, add thickeners to liquids (or provide thicker liquids such as tomato juice), or give pureed foods. If indicated, have the patient evaluated for swallowing problems by a speech therapist.

Many patients in long-term care settings need help to feed themselves. Typically, they're fed by nursing assistants supervised by the nurse. It may be sufficient to set up a feeding table, provide modified utensils and cups, help the patient open containers, and cut up food. Try not to do more than the patient needs. Too much help can encourage dependence and promote functional loss, especially in cognitively impaired patients.

One study of functional feeding of patients with dementia found the following measures were sufficient to promote self-feeding without prolonging mealtimes: reducing interruptions and distractions, placing residents at a dining table, using placemats and namecards, providing finger foods, placing food directly in front of the patient, maintaining consistency in mealtime activities, and prompting and cueing the patient to eat.

Patient teaching

As a health care provider, you'll need to educate your patients about the crucial role of nutrition in maintaining their physical health. As you select written materials, consider the ethnic background, educational level, visual capabilities, and primary language of the intended reader.

If the patient has recently been discharged from an acute-care or rehabilitation facility, contact the dietitian there to find out if the patient has special dietary needs. If you work in a community setting, find out about available nutrition support resources, such as congregate meals (provided at a church or senior center, for example, under auspices of the Older Americans Act), home-delivered meals (such as Meals On Wheels), and in-home services for meal preparation.

For the older person who lives alone but is mobile, encourage meal sharing or swapping with similar people in the vicinity to improve nutrition for all involved and to increase socialization. Use other appropriate community programs, such as case management by the area Agency on Aging, social services to help poor people obtain food stamps, surplus food distribution programs, food pantries, church-related groups, and nutrition services provided by local or state health departments.

In addition, anorexia and weight loss are symptoms that need to be evaluated medically to rule out underlying causes, such as carcinoma or somatic manifestations of depression.

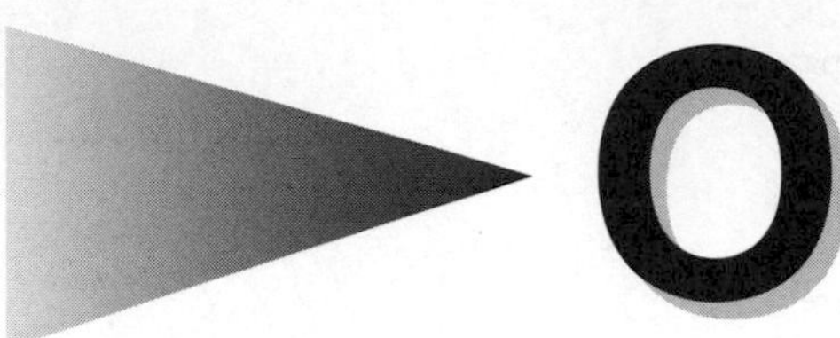

Obsessive-compulsive disorder

Marked by repetitive performance of acts or rituals, such as hand washing, house cleaning, checking doorknobs, and making lists, obsessive-compulsive disorder (OCD) can begin at any stage in adulthood. A person with OCD may have a very rigid personality and insist on performing everyday tasks in an unvarying order. This rigid behavior, which usually develops over a lifetime, can be exacerbated if the person experiences a serious stressful event.

The person with OCD performs the rituals out of a need for control and order and as a means of coping with anxiety. If he's prevented from carrying out his pattern of ritual activity, he may become anxious or agitated. Any environmental alteration (such as transfer to a nursing home or a visit from a stranger in the patient's home care setting) may trigger a need for treatment.

OCD is typically a chronic condition with remissions and flare-ups. Mild forms of the disorder are relatively common in the general population.

Signs and symptoms

- Repetitive acts or rituals (in older adults, commonly manifested as morbid fears and obsessions with bodily functions)
- Self-doubt, indecision, and ambivalence

Diagnostic tests

Diagnosis of OCD is made when the patient's signs and symptoms meet the criteria set forth in the American Psychiatric Association's *Diagnostic and Statistical Manual of Mental Disorders,* 4th edition.

Treatment

Counseling helps the patient cope with anxiety related to this disorder. Clomipramine is a tricyclic antidepressant used to treat OCD. Fluvoxamine, a selective serotonin reuptake inhibitor (SSRI), is also approved for treating OCD, although most SSRIs should be effective. Fluoxetine, sertraline, and paroxetine are other commonly prescribed SSRIs. It may take 5 to 10 weeks for SSRI effects to become apparent.

Other treatments include relaxation techniques, such as imagery and meditation.

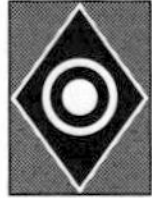

Drug alert If the physician prescribes clomipramine for your patient, be especially alert for cardiac problems and hallucinations.

Key nursing diagnoses and outcomes

Disturbed thought processes related to repetitious thoughts and actions

Treatment outcome: The patient will have more controlled thought processes.

Anxiety related to loss of control of actions

Treatment outcome: The patient will express relief of tension and control over feelings of helplessness.

Nursing interventions

- Identify actions that are compulsively repetitive.
- Investigate coping skills used for other situations of anxiety.
- Administer drugs as ordered and monitor their effectiveness.
- Follow the treatment regimen prescribed by the patient's mental health care provider.
- Involve the patient's family members in the treatment plan so they can help the patient control his actions.

PATIENT TEACHING

- Teach the patient and his family members about his illness and the importance of following the prescribed treatment plan.
- Teach the patient about the importance of identifying alternative coping mechanisms to replace the compulsive behavior in times of anxiety.

ORAL MEDICATION ADMINISTRATION

Most drugs are administered orally because oral administration is usually the safest, most convenient, and least expensive method. Medications for oral administration are available in many forms: tablets, enteric-coated tablets, capsules, syrups, elixirs, oils, liquids, suspensions, powders, and granules. Some require special preparation before administration such as mixing with juice to make them more palatable; oils, powders, and granules usually require such preparation.

Oral drugs are sometimes prescribed in higher dosages than their parenteral equivalents because, after absorption through the GI system, they're immediately broken down by the liver before they reach the systemic circulation. However, oral dosages normally prescribed for adults may be dangerous for older adults.

Drug alert Drug dosages for the geriatric patient may need to be reduced because of age-related changes affecting the drug's pharmacokinetics.

Oral administration is contraindicated for unconscious patients; it may also be contraindicated for patients with nausea and vomiting and in those unable to swallow.

Supplies

- Patient's medication record and chart
- Prescribed drug
- Medication cup
- Optional: appropriate vehicle, such as jelly or applesauce, for crushed pills; juice, water, or milk and drinking straw for liquid medications; mortar and pestle for crushing pills

Implementation

- Verify the order on the patient's medication record by checking it against the physician's order.
- Wash your hands.
- Check the label on the drug three times before you administer it: first, when you take the container from the shelf or drawer; again, before you pour the drug into the medication cup; and again before returning the container to the shelf or drawer. If you're administering a unit-dose drug, check the label for the final time at the patient's bedside, immediately after pouring the drug and before discarding the wrapper.
- Use care in measuring the prescribed dose of liquid oral drugs.
- Don't give drugs from a poorly labeled or unlabeled container. Don't attempt to label or reinforce drug labels yourself.
- Never give a drug poured by someone else.
- Confirm the patient's identity by asking his name and checking the name,

Altering tablets and capsules

When caring for an older person, you may crush tablets or capsules to help him swallow them more easily. But first find out whether a liquid preparation of the same drug is available. If not, determine whether crushing affects the drug's action, and follow these guidelines.

Which forms shouldn't be altered

Avoid crushing sustained-release (also known as *extended-release* or *controlled-release*) drugs. However, some of these drugs can be scored and broken. Also avoid crushing capsules that contain tiny beads of a drug. However, you may empty the beads into a beverage, pudding, or applesauce.

Don't crush or score enteric-coated tablets, which usually are shiny or candy-coated, because they're designed to prevent GI upset. Finally, avoid altering buccal and sublingual tablets.

Crushing tablets

If you need to crush a tablet, try to use a chewable form, which is easier to crush. Then use a mortar and pestle or a pill crusher, press the tablet between two spoons, or place it in a small plastic bag and crush it with a rolling pin. Unless contraindicated, mix the drug with 1 tsp or 1 tbs of pureed fruit or pudding.

Breaking tablets

If you need to break a tablet, use one that's scored. Use an instrument that can't cause injury, such as a spatula, rather than a knife.

If a tablet isn't scored, it should be crushed, weighed, and dispensed by the pharmacist. Also follow this procedure when breaking a tablet into smaller pieces than the score allows or when giving the patient part of a capsule.

room number, and bed number on his wristband.

- Assess the patient's condition, including level of consciousness and vital signs, as needed. Changes in condition may warrant withholding drugs.
- If the patient questions you about the drug or dosage, check his drug record again. If the drug is correct, reassure him. Make sure you tell him about any changes in his drug or dosage. Teach him about possible adverse effects, and ask him to report anything he feels may be an adverse effect.
- To avoid damaging or staining the patient's teeth, give acid or iron preparations through a straw. An unpleasant-tasting liquid can usually be made more palatable if taken through a straw because the liquid contacts fewer taste buds.
- Give the patient his drug and, as needed, an appropriate food or liquid to aid swallowing, minimize adverse effects, or promote absorption. Suggest that he take a few sips of fluid first, if not contraindicated, to moisten the mucous membranes and aid in swallowing. Keep in mind that older adults have decreased saliva production, which might cause a dry mouth.
- Help the patient place the drug in his mouth if needed. If he has difficulty swallowing (common because of a diminished gag reflex and decreased saliva production), have him place the drug on the back of his tongue and drink some fluid. If necessary, gently massage the upper neck area just below the chin or have him use the chin-tuck method to aid swallowing.
- If appropriate, crush the drug to facilitate swallowing. (See *Altering tablets and capsules*.)
- If the patient has dentures, encourage him to wear them as much as possible to

maintain the gum line and the fit of the dentures. You need not remove them for medication administration unless they fit poorly and collect debris in loose-fitting areas.

▶ Always give the most important drug first, and allow time for the patient to take it. Should he tire or refuse to take any more drugs, he'll already have taken the most important one.

▶ Stay with the patient until he has swallowed the drug. If he seems confused or disoriented, check his mouth to make sure he has swallowed it. Return and reassess the patient's response within 1 hour after giving the drug.

▶ Never return unwrapped or prepared drugs to stock containers. Instead, dispose of them and notify the pharmacy. Keep in mind that the disposal of any narcotic drug must be cosigned by another nurse, as mandated by law.

Complications

Aspiration is a potential complication of oral drug administration. To help prevent aspiration, ensure that the patient has completely swallowed the medication, elevate the head of the bed, and mix the drug in applesauce rather than a thin liquid.

Patient teaching

Teach the patient about the drugs he's receiving, including uses, dosages, and possible adverse effects.

Documentation

Note the drug administered, dose, date and time, and the patient's reaction, if any. If the patient refuses a drug, document the refusal and notify the patient's physician, as needed. Also note if a drug was omitted or withheld for other reasons, such as radiology or laboratory tests, or if, in your judgment, the drug was contraindicated at the ordered time. Sign out all narcotics given on the appropriate narcotics control record. Document your patient-teaching measures.

Osteoarthritis

The most common form of arthritis, osteoarthritis causes deterioration of joint (articular) cartilage and formation of new bone at the margins and subchondral areas of the joints. The chronic degeneration, which is caused by a breakdown of chondrocytes, occurs most commonly in weight-bearing joints, especially in the hips and knees.

Osteoarthritis occurs equally in both sexes and affects 83% to 87% of people between ages 55 and 64. More than one-half of all people over age 30 have some features of primary osteoarthritis. And nearly all people over age 60, when examined radiographically, exhibit evidence of the disorder, although fewer than one-half experience symptoms.

In osteoarthritis, the breakdown of cartilage begins long before symptoms appear. As the disease progresses, whole sections of cartilage may disintegrate, osteophytes (bony spurs) form, and fragments of cartilage and bone float freely in the joint. Progression rates vary; joints may remain stable for years in the early stage of deterioration.

Depending on the site and severity of joint involvement, the patient's disability can range from minor limitation of the fingers to near immobility in some people with hip or knee disease. Some joints, such as hips and knees, can be replaced to improve mobility and function.

Primary osteoarthritis may be related to aging. Although researchers don't understand exactly why, wear and tear on the joints as a person ages is thought to play a major role in its development. Other factors that may lead to primary osteoarthritis are obesity and repetitive overuse of a joint. For example, a baseball player may develop osteoarthritis of the shoulder. In some older adults, however, the disease may be hereditary.

Secondary osteoarthritis usually follows a specific event or circumstance,

Signs of osteoarthritis

Heberden's nodes appear on the dorsolateral aspect of the distal interphalangeal joints. Usually hard and painless, these bony and cartilaginous enlargements typically occur in middle-aged and older osteoarthritis patients. Bouchard's nodes, similar to Heberden's nodes but less common, appear on the proximal interphalangeal joints.

HEBERDEN'S NODES

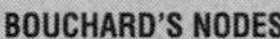

BOUCHARD'S NODES

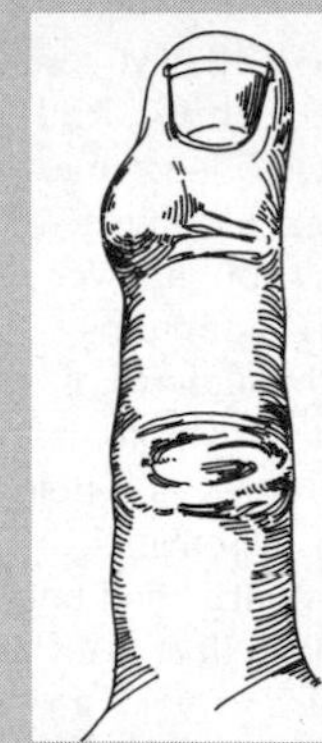

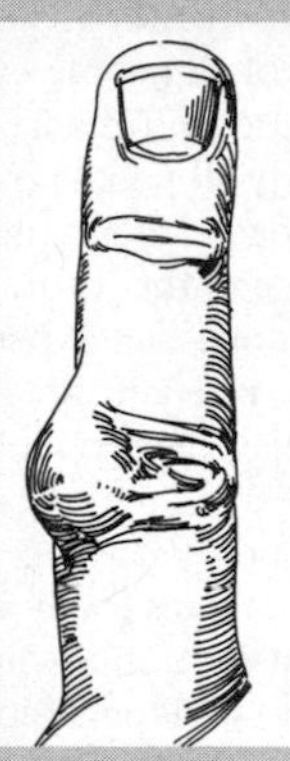

most commonly a traumatic injury or a congenital abnormality such as hip dysplasia. Endocrine disorders (such as diabetes mellitus), metabolic disorders (such as chondrocalcinosis), and other types of arthritis also can lead to secondary osteoarthritis.

Possible complications of osteoarthritis include flexion contractures, subluxation and deformity, ankylosis, bony cysts, gross bony overgrowth, central cord syndrome (with cervical spine osteoarthritis), nerve root compression, and cauda equina syndrome.

Signs and symptoms

Early osteoarthritis

- No symptoms or a mild, dull ache when the joint is used
- Relief of discomfort with rest

Advanced disease

- Pain that becomes more frequent, even during rest, and typically worsens as the day progresses
- Deep, aching joint pain after exercising or bearing weight on the affected joint
- Relief of pain with rest

General signs and symptoms

- Stiffness in the morning and after exercise
- Aching during changes in weather
- Contractures
- Limited movement
- A "grating" feeling when the joint moves
- Joint swelling, muscle atrophy, and deformity of the involved areas on inspection
- Joint tenderness or instability and limited movement on palpation
- Gait abnormalities (when arthritis affects hips or knees)
- In osteoarthritis of the interphalangeal joints, hard nodes on the distal and proximal joints that are painless at first, but eventually become red, swollen, and tender. The most common of these nodes, Heberden's nodes, occur on the dorsolateral aspect of the distal interphalangeal joint. Bouchard's nodes, which occur less commonly, appear on the proximal interphalangeal joint. The fingers may become numb and lose dexterity. (See *Signs of osteoarthritis*.)

Diagnostic tests

- *X-rays* may be normal in the early stages. Later films may show a narrowing of the joint space or margin, cystlike bony deposits in the joint space and margins, sclerosis of the subchondral space, joint deformity caused by degeneration or articular damage, bony growths at weight-bearing areas, and joint fusion in people with erosive, inflammatory osteoarthritis.
- *Synovial fluid analysis* can rule out inflammatory arthritis.

▶ *Radionuclide bone scans* also can rule out inflammatory arthritis by showing normal uptake of the radionuclide.

▶ *Arthroscopy* identifies soft-tissue swelling by showing internal joint structures.

▶ *Magnetic resonance imaging* produces clear, cross-sectional images of the affected joint and adjacent bones and can illustrate disease progression.

▶ *Neuromuscular tests* may disclose reduced muscle strength (such as reduced grip strength).

Treatment

Treatment, which commonly includes drug therapy, is aimed at controlling pain, restoring joint alignment, and strengthening muscles that support affected joints. Aspirin, nonsteroidal anti-inflammatory drugs, and salicylates are the most commonly used medications to treat osteoarthritis. In some older adults, intra-articular injections of corticosteroids may be necessary. Such injections, given every 4 to 6 months, may delay nodal development in the hands.

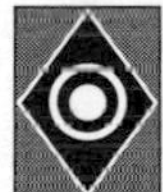

Drug alert The effects of salicylates on renal prostaglandins may cause fluid retention and edema, a significant disadvantage in older patients, especially those with heart failure.

Injections into the knee joint of such drugs as synvisc Hylan G-F20 and Hyalgan (sodium hyaluranate) are being used to artifically replace hyaluronic acid, a naturally occurring lubricant and shock absorber.

Adequate rest balanced with activity is an important component of treatment. Physical therapy methods include massage, moist heat, paraffin dips for the hands, supervised exercise to maintain muscle tone and posture and to decrease muscle spasms and atrophy, and protective techniques for preventing undue joint stress. Weight reduction may help an obese patient. Crutches, braces, a cane, a walker, a cervical collar, or traction may reduce stress and increase mobility.

Patients with a severe disability or uncontrollable pain may undergo surgery. Possible procedures include partial or total arthroplasty, replacement of a deteriorated part of the joint with a prosthetic appliance (common in severe hip and knee disease); arthrodesis, surgical fusion of the bones (used primarily in the spine); osteoplasty, scraping and lavaging deteriorated bone from the joint; and osteotomy, removing a wedge of bone (usually in the lower leg) to change alignment and relieve stress.

Key nursing diagnoses and outcomes

Impaired physical mobility related to joint deterioration

Treatment outcomes: The patient will avoid complications, such as contractures, venous stasis, and skin breakdown, and will achieve the highest mobility level possible.

Chronic pain related to joint deterioration

Treatment outcome: The patient will express relief of pain after analgesic administration.

Anxiety related to the potential crippling effects of osteoarthritis

Treatment outcomes: The patient will express his feelings of anxiety and develop effective coping behaviors.

Nursing interventions

▶ Provide emotional support and reassurance to help the patient cope with limited mobility. Give him opportunities to voice his feelings about the disease and its effect on his functioning.

▶ Include the patient and his family in all phases of his care. Answer their questions as honestly as you can.

▶ Encourage the patient to perform as much self-care as his immobility and pain allow. Provide him with adequate time to perform activities at his own pace.

▶ Assess the patient's pain pattern. Administer anti-inflammatory drugs and other drugs, as ordered, and monitor his response.
▶ To help promote sleep, adjust pain medications to allow for maximum rest. Provide the patient with sleep aids, as needed, such as a pillow, bath, or back rub.
▶ Help the patient identify techniques and activities that promote rest and relaxation. Encourage him to perform them.
▶ For joints in the hand, provide hot soaks and paraffin dips to relieve pain, as ordered.
▶ For cervical spinal joints, adjust the patient's cervical collar to avoid constriction.
▶ For lumbosacral spinal joints, provide a firm mattress (or bed board) to decrease morning pain.
▶ For the hip, use moist heat pads to relieve pain and administer antispasmodic drugs, as ordered.
▶ For the knee, assist with prescribed range-of-motion (ROM) exercises twice daily to maintain muscle tone. Also help perform progressive resistance exercises to increase the patient's muscle strength.
▶ Provide elastic supports or braces if needed.
▶ Check crutches, cane, braces, or walker for proper fit. A patient with unilateral joint involvement should use an orthopedic appliance (such as a cane or walker) on the unaffected side.
▶ Positively reinforce the patient's efforts to adapt. Point out improving or stabilizing physical functioning.

PATIENT TEACHING

▶ Instruct the patient to take drugs exactly as prescribed. Tell him which adverse reactions to report immediately.
▶ As necessary, refer the patient to an occupational therapist or a home health nurse to help him cope with activities of daily living. Although not covered by most insurance policies (except in conjunction with a skilled home care provider), homemaker services may spare him strenuous activities and relieve some anxiety about coping with his illness.
▶ Instruct the patient to plan for adequate rest during the day, after exertion, and at night.
▶ Encourage him to learn and use energy conservation methods, such as well-paced activities, simplified work procedures, and protected joints.
▶ Advise against overexertion. Although benefits of isometric and mild exercise for osteoarthritis are well known, excessive exercise can cause more pain and degeneration.
▶ Tell the patient that he should take care to stand and walk correctly, to minimize weight-bearing activities, and to be especially careful when stooping or picking up objects.
▶ Instruct the patient to wear well-fitting support shoes and to repair worn heels.
▶ Advise him to have safety devices installed at home such as grab bars in the bathroom.
▶ Teach him to do ROM exercises, performing them as gently as possible.
▶ Advise maintaining proper body weight to minimize strain on joints.
▶ Teach the patient how to use crutches or other orthopedic devices properly. Stress the importance of proper fitting and regular professional readjustment of such devices. Warn him that because of impaired sensation, he could develop tissue damage from these aids without feeling any discomfort.
▶ Suggest that the patient sit on cushions and use an elevated toilet seat. Both reduce the stress of rising from a seated position.
▶ Teach the patient and his family diversional activities to decrease the perception of pain.
▶ Recommend support groups or counseling to improve coping techniques.

OSTEOPOROSIS

In osteoporosis, a metabolic bone disorder, the rate of bone resorption accelerates and the rate of bone formation decelerates, resulting in decreased bone mass. The bones lose calcium and phosphate, becoming porous, brittle, and abnormally vulnerable to fracture. The immobility that follows a fracture can exacerbate osteoporosis. It occurs in one of nine people over age 65 in the United States.

Osteoporosis may be primary or secondary to an underlying disease. Primary osteoporosis may be classified as idiopathic, type I, or type II. Idiopathic osteoporosis affects children and adults. Type I (postmenopausal) osteoporosis usually affects women ages 51 to 75. Related to the loss of estrogen's protective effect on bone, type I osteoporosis results in trabecular bone loss and some cortical bone loss. Vertebral and wrist fractures are common. Type II (senile) osteoporosis usually occurs between ages 70 and 85 and is characterized by trabecular and cortical bone loss and consequent fractures of the proximal humerus, proximal tibia, femoral neck, and pelvis.

The cause of primary osteoporosis is unknown. However, several contributing factors are suspected: mild but prolonged negative calcium balance, which can occur from inadequate dietary calcium intake; declining gonadal adrenal gland function and estrogen deficiency, which causes faulty protein metabolism; and a sedentary lifestyle.

Secondary osteoporosis may result from prolonged therapy with steroids or heparin, bone immobilization or disuse (as occurs with hemiplegia), alcoholism, malnutrition, rheumatoid arthritis, liver disease, malabsorption, scurvy, lactose intolerance, hyperthyroidism, osteogenesis imperfecta, and Cushing's disease. Patients with hyperparathyroidism have loss of cortical bone as well.

Bone fractures are the major complication of osteoporosis. They occur most commonly in the vertebrae, femoral neck, and distal radius.

Signs and symptoms

- Pain in the back that developed slowly over several years or that occurred suddenly (for example, after bending down)
- With vertebral collapse, backache and pain radiating around the trunk that's aggravated by any movement
- Dowager's hump (clinical hallmark of osteoporosis), caused by increased spinal curvature from repeated vertebral fractures
- Loss of height
- Muscle spasm, especially in the lumbar region
- Decreased spinal movement (flexion more limited than extension)

Diagnostic tests

Differential diagnosis must exclude other causes of rarefying bone disease, especially those that affect the spine, such as metastatic cancer and advanced multiple myeloma.

- *Bone mineral density testing* can help screen for osteoporosis, especially in postmenopausal women ages 65 and older.
- *X-rays* show characteristic degeneration in the lower thoracolumbar vertebrae. The vertebral bodies may appear flatter and denser than usual. Loss of bone mineral appears in later disease.
- *Dual or single photon absorptiometry* allows measurement of bone mass, which helps to assess the extremities, hips, and spine.
- *Blood studies* show normal serum calcium, phosphorus, and alkaline phosphatase levels and possibly elevated parathyroid hormone levels.
- *Bone biopsy* may be performed to directly examine osteoporotic changes in bone cells.
- *Computed tomography scan* allows accurate assessment of spinal bone loss.

▶ *Bone scans* that use a radionuclide agent display injured or diseased areas as darker portions.

Treatment

To control bone loss, relieve pain, and prevent further fractures, treatment focuses on a physical therapy program of gentle exercise and activity, and drug therapy to slow disease progression. Supportive devices, such as a back brace, aid mobility.

Estrogen may be prescribed within 3 years after menopause to decrease the rate of bone resorption. Sodium fluoride may be given to stimulate bone formation. Calcium and vitamin D supplements may help support normal bone metabolism. Calcitonin may be used to reduce bone resorption and slow the decline of bone mass.

Bisphosphonates, such as alendronate and etidronate are approved to restore lost bone. Studies show that etidronate used for 2 weeks every 4 months increases bone mass. Selective estrogen receptor modulators, such as raloxifene, are also indicated for prevention and treatment.

Surgery (open reduction and internal fixation) can correct pathologic fractures of the femur. Colles' fracture requires reduction and immobilization with a cast for 4 to 10 weeks.

Key nursing diagnoses and outcomes

Risk for injury related to potential for fractures

Treatment outcomes: The patient will incorporate safety precautions into her daily life and will avoid fractures.

Impaired physical mobility related to decreased spinal flexion

Treatment outcomes: The patient will seek assistance with activities of daily living and will achieve the highest level of physical mobility possible.

Chronic pain related to stress on a bone with decreased bone mass

Treatment outcome: The patient will express relief of pain.

Nursing interventions

▶ When designing your care plan, consider the patient's fragility. Focus on careful positioning, ambulation, and prescribed exercises.
▶ Make ancillary personnel in the facility aware of how easily the patient's bones can fracture.
▶ Impose safety precautions such as keeping side rails up on the patient's bed.
▶ Check the patient's skin daily for redness, warmth, and new pain sites, which may indicate new fractures.
▶ Provide emotional support and reassurance to help the patient cope with limited mobility. Give her opportunities to voice her feelings. If possible, arrange for her to interact with others who have similar problems.
▶ Encourage the patient to perform as much self-care as her immobility and pain allow. Allow her adequate time to perform these activities at her own pace.
▶ Encourage the patient to engage in activities that involve mild exercise; help her to walk several times daily. As appropriate, perform passive range-of-motion exercises or encourage her to perform active exercises.
▶ Make sure the patient attends scheduled physical therapy sessions.
▶ Provide a balanced diet rich in nutrients that support skeletal metabolism, such as vitamin D, calcium, and protein.
▶ Administer analgesics and heat to relieve pain, as ordered.
▶ Monitor the patient's pain level, and assess her response to analgesics, heat therapy, and diversional activities.

PATIENT TEACHING

▶ Thoroughly explain osteoporosis to the patient and her family. If they don't understand the disease process, they may feel needless guilt, thinking that they could have acted to prevent bone fractures.

- Demonstrate proper body mechanics. Show the patient how to stoop before lifting anything and how to avoid twisting movements and prolonged bending.
- Tell the patient to report any new pain sites immediately, especially after a traumatic injury.
- Teach the patient how to use a back brace properly, if appropriate.
- Encourage the patient to install safety devices, such as grab bars and railings, at home.
- Urge the patient to eat a diet rich in calcium, and give her a list of calcium-rich foods. Explain that type II osteoporosis may be prevented by adequate dietary calcium intake and regular exercise. Hormonal and fluoride treatments may also help prevent osteoporosis.
- If the patient takes a calcium supplement, encourage liberal fluid intake to help maintain adequate urine output and thereby avoid renal calculi, hypercalcemia, and hypercalciuria.
- Advise the patient to sleep on a firm mattress and to avoid excessive bed rest.
- Explain that secondary osteoporosis may be prevented by effective treatment of underlying disease, early mobilization after surgery or trauma, decreased alcohol consumption, careful observation for signs of malabsorption, and prompt treatment of hyperthyroidism.
- Reinforce the patient's efforts to adapt, and show her how her condition is improving or stabilizing. As necessary, refer her to an occupational therapist or a home health nurse to help her cope with activities of daily living.
- Make sure the patient and her family clearly understand the prescribed drug regimen. Tell them how to recognize significant adverse reactions, and instruct them to report them immediately.
- Teach the patient and her family members diversional activities to change the patient's perception of pain.
- Instruct the patient to avoid activities that aggravate pain and create more stress on joints.

OSTOMY CARE

A patient with an ascending or transverse colostomy or an ileostomy must wear an external pouch to collect emerging fecal matter, which will be watery or pasty. Besides collecting waste matter, the pouch helps to control odor and to protect the stoma and peristomal skin. Most disposable pouching systems can be used from 2 to 7 days. Some models last even longer.

The pouch should be changed immediately if a leak develops. Every pouch should be emptied when it's one-third to one-half full. The patient with an ileostomy may empty his pouch four or five times daily. The best time to change the pouching system is when the bowel is least active, usually between 2 and 4 hours after meals. After a few months, most patients can predict the best changing time.

In selecting a pouching system, consider which system provides the best adhesive seal and skin protection for the individual patient. Select a pouch type to suit the stoma's location and structure, the availability of supplies, wear time, consistency of effluent, and the patient's personal preference, girth, size, contours, visual acuity, manual dexterity, activity, and finances.

Pouching systems may be drainable or closed-bottomed, disposable or reusable, adhesive-backed, and one-piece or two-piece, convex or nonconvex, and cut-to-fit or presized.

Supplies

- Pouching system
- Stoma measuring guide
- Stoma paste (if drainage is watery to pasty or stoma secretes excess mucus)
- Plastic bag
- Water

- Washcloth and towel
- Closure clamp
- Toilet or bedpan
- Water or pouch-cleaning solution
- Gloves
- Facial tissues
- Optional: ostomy belt, paper tape, mild nonmoisturizing soap, skin shaving equipment, liquid skin sealant, pouch deodorant

Implementation

For all the procedures discussed below, provide privacy and emotional support.

To fit the pouch and skin barrier

- For a pouch with an attached skin barrier, measure the stoma with the stoma measuring guide. Select the opening size that matches the stoma.
- For an adhesive-backed pouch with a separate skin barrier, measure the stoma with the measuring guide and select the opening that matches the stoma. Trace the selected size opening onto the paper back of the skin barrier's adhesive side. Cut out the opening. (If the pouch has precut openings, which can be handy for a round stoma, select an opening that's ⅛″ [0.3 cm] larger than the stoma. If the pouch comes without an opening, cut the hole ⅛″ wider than the measured tracing.) The cut-to-fit system works best for an irregularly shaped stoma.
- For a two-piece pouching system with flanges, see *Applying a skin barrier and pouch.*
- Avoid fitting the pouch too tightly because the stoma has no pain receptors. A constrictive opening could injure the stoma or skin tissue without the patient feeling discomfort. Also avoid cutting the opening too big because this could expose the skin to fecal matter and moisture.
- The patient with a descending or sigmoid colostomy who has formed stools and whose ostomy doesn't secrete much mucus may choose to wear only a pouch. In this case, make sure the pouch opening closely matches the stoma size.
- Between 6 weeks and 1 year after surgery, the stoma will shrink to its permanent size. At that time, pattern-making preparations will be unnecessary unless the patient gains weight, has additional surgery, or injures the stoma.

To apply or change the pouch

- Collect all the equipment.
- Wash your hands and put on gloves.
- Remove and discard the old pouch. Gently wipe the stoma and peristomal skin with a facial tissue.
- Carefully wash and dry the peristomal skin. Inspect the peristomal skin and stoma. If necessary, shave surrounding hair (in a direction away from the stoma) to promote a better seal and avoid skin irritation from hair pulling against the adhesive.
- For a pouching system with flanges, align the lip of the pouch flange with the bottom edge of the skin barrier flange. Gently press around the circumference of the pouch flange, beginning at the bottom, until the pouch securely adheres to the barrier flange. (The pouch will click into its secured position.) Holding the barrier against the skin, gently pull on the pouch to confirm the seal between flanges.
- Consider using a liquid skin sealant, if available, to give skin tissue additional protection from drainage and adhesive irritants.
- Encourage the patient to stay quietly in position for about 5 minutes to improve adherence. Body warmth also helps to improve adherence and soften a rigid skin barrier.
- Attach an ostomy belt to further secure the pouch, if desired. (Some pouches have belt loops, and others have plastic adapters for belts.)
- Leave some air in the pouch to allow drainage to fall to the bottom.
- Apply the closure clamp, if necessary.

Applying a skin barrier and pouch

A skin barrier and ostomy pouch can be fitted properly in a few steps. The illustrations below show a commonly used two-piece pouching system with flanges.

Measure the stoma using a measuring guide.

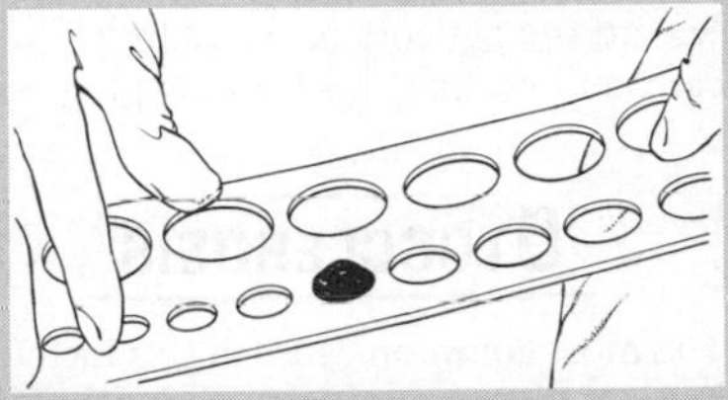

Trace the appropriate circle carefully on the back of the skin barrier.

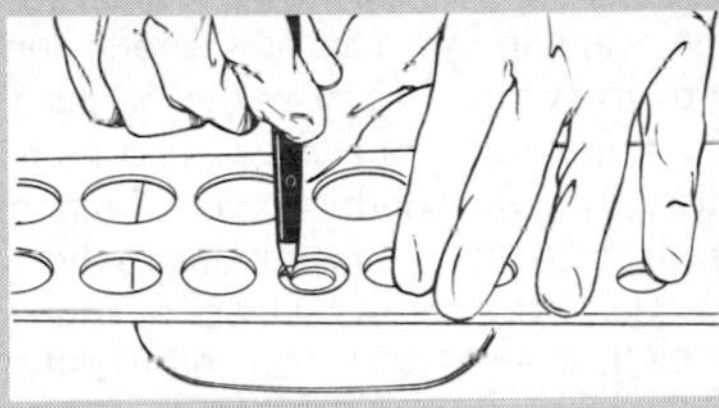

Cut the circular opening in the skin barrier. Bevel the edges to keep them from irritating the patient.

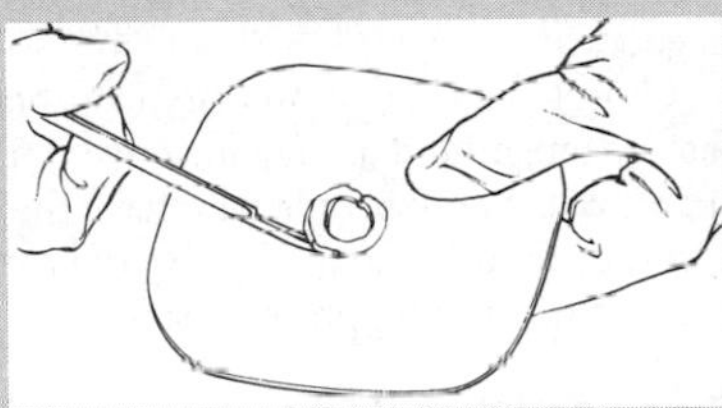

Remove the backing from the skin barrier and moisten it or apply barrier paste, as needed, along the edge of the circular opening.

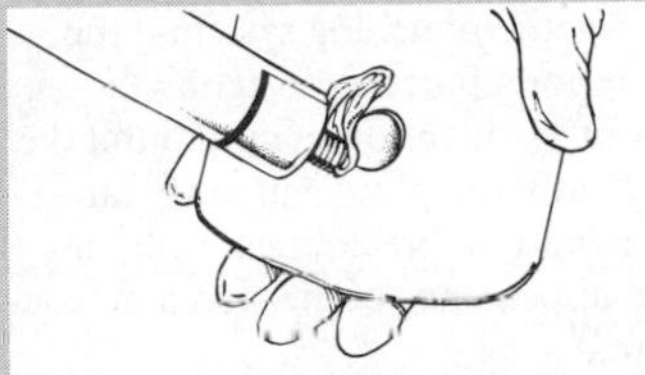

Center the skin barrier over the stoma, adhesive side down, and gently press it to the skin.

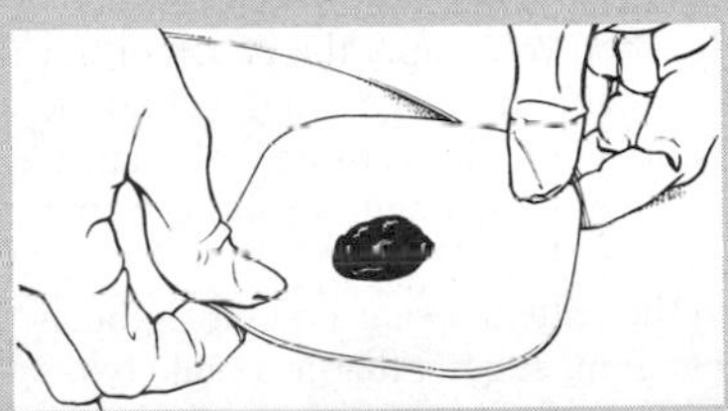

Gently press the pouch opening onto the ring until it snaps into place.

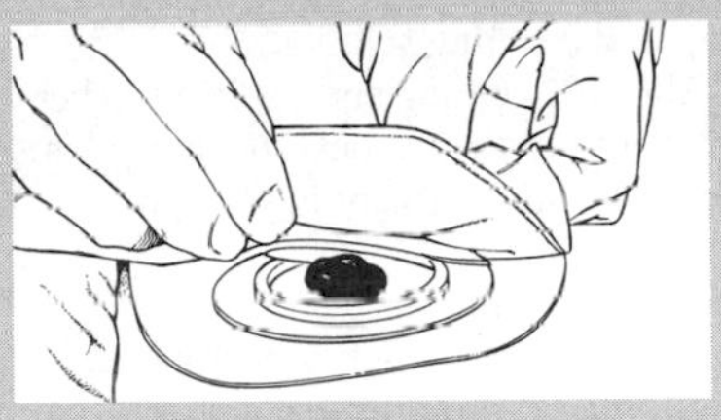

- If desired, apply paper tape in a picture-frame fashion to the pouch edges for additional security.

To empty the pouch

- Tilt the bottom of the pouch upward and remove the closure clamp.
- Turn up a cuff on the lower end of the pouch, and allow it to drain into the toilet or bedpan.
- Wipe the bottom of the pouch and reapply the closure clamp.
- If desired, you can rinse the bottom portion of the pouch with cool tap water. Don't aim the water up near the top of the pouch because this could loosen the seal on the skin.
- A two-piece flanged system can also be emptied by unsnapping the pouch. Let the drainage flow into the toilet.

▶ Release flatus through the gas release valve if the pouch has one. Otherwise, release flatus by tilting the pouch bottom upward, releasing the clamp, and expelling the flatus. To release flatus from a flanged system, loosen the seal between the flanges.
▶ Never make a pinhole in a pouch to release gas. This destroys the odor-proof seal.
▶ Remove the pouching system if the patient reports burning or itching beneath it or purulent drainage around the stoma. Notify the physician or therapist of skin irritation, breakdown, rash, or unusual appearance of the stoma or peristomal area.
▶ Use commercial pouch deodorants, if desired. However, most pouches are odorfree, and odor should be evident only when you empty the pouch or if it leaks. Before discharge, suggest that the patient avoid odor-causing foods, such as fish, eggs, asparagus, cabbage, beans, onions, and garlic.
▶ If the patient wears a reusable pouching system, suggest that he obtain two or more systems so that he can wear one while the other dries after being cleaned with soap and water or a commercially prepared cleaning solution.
▶ After performing and explaining the procedure to the patient, encourage his increasing involvement in self-care.

Complications

Failing to fit the pouch properly over the stoma or improper use of a belt can injure the stoma. Be alert for a possible allergic reaction to adhesives and other ostomy products.

Patient teaching

▶ Explain the procedure to the patient. As you perform each step, explain what you're doing and why because the patient will eventually perform the procedure himself.
▶ Refer the patient to resource groups that assist patients with ostomies.

Documentation

Record the date and time of the pouching system change; note the character of drainage, including color, amount, type, and consistency. Also describe the appearance of the stoma and the peristomal skin. Document your patient teaching and describe the teaching content. Record the patient's response to self-care, and evaluate his learning progress.

OTOSCLEROSIS

The most common cause of conductive hearing loss among older adults, otosclerosis is the slow formation of spongy bone in the otic capsule, particularly at the oval window. This otosclerotic bone growth eventually causes the footplate of the stapes to become fixed in position, disrupting the conduction of vibrations from the tympanic membrane to the cochlea. Otosclerosis is twice as common in women as in men and usually begins between ages 15 and 50. Occurring unilaterally at first, the disorder may progress to bilateral conductive hearing loss. With surgery, the prognosis is good.

Otosclerosis may result from a genetic factor transmitted as an autosomal dominant trait. Many people who have this disorder report a family history of hearing loss (excluding presbycusis).

Signs and symptoms

▶ Gradual hearing loss in one ear, which may have progressed to both ears, without middle ear infection
▶ Tinnitus
▶ Ability to hear a conversation better in a noisy environment than in a quiet one (paracusis of Willis)

Diagnostic tests

▶ *Otoscopic examination* reveals a normal-appearing tympanic membrane. Occasionally, however, a faint pink blush may be seen through the membrane from the vascularity of the active otosclerotic bone.

▶ *Rinne test* demonstrates that a bone-conducted tone is heard longer than an air-conducted tone. (Normally, the reverse is true.) As otosclerosis progresses, bone conduction also deteriorates.

▶ *Weber's test* shows sound lateralizing to the more damaged ear. (See *Reviewing Weber's and Rinne tests,* page 426.)

▶ *Audiometric testing* reveals hearing loss ranging from 60 dB in early stages to total loss as the disease progresses.

Treatment

In most cases, treatment consists of stapedectomy (removal of the stapes) and insertion of a prosthesis to restore partial or total hearing. This procedure is performed on one ear at a time, beginning with the ear that has sustained greater damage. Antibiotics are given postoperatively to prevent infection. Other surgical procedures include fenestration and stapes mobilization, all require normal cochlear function.

Sometimes further hearing loss can be prevented by giving the patient sodium fluoride and calcium supplements to promote recalcification and arrest spongy bone formation. Hearing aids may be an acceptable alternative and enable the patient to hear conversation in normal surroundings.

Key nursing diagnoses and outcomes

Disturbed sensory perception (auditory) related to otosclerotic bone growth

Treatment outcome: The patient will have improved hearing.

Anxiety related to diminished hearing

Treatment outcomes: The patient will express feelings of anxiety related to hearing loss and will develop coping mechanisms to deal with them.

Nursing interventions

▶ Answer your patient's questions, encourage him to discuss his concerns about hearing loss, and offer reassurance when appropriate.

▶ Be aware that hearing loss may cause frustration and anger. Allow the patient to express his emotions, and make sure his family members are aware of the patient's emotional needs.

▶ If the patient has difficulty understanding procedures and treatments because of hearing loss, provide clear, concise explanations. Also provide written materials if possible. Face the patient when speaking; enunciate clearly, slowly, and in a normal tone; and give the patient time to grasp what you've said. Supply a pencil and paper to aid communication, and alert staff members to the communication problem.

▶ After stapedectomy, follow the physician's orders regarding specific postoperative positioning of the patient. He may be placed on the unaffected side to prevent graft displacement or on the affected side to facilitate drainage. Some physicians allow any position that doesn't cause vertigo.

▶ After surgery, keep the bed's side rails raised and help the patient walk. Administer prescribed drugs for pain, and assess the patient's response.

PATIENT TEACHING

▶ Teach the patient and his family members about the causes of hearing loss.

▶ Stress the importance of taking prescribed medications, and explain how they may improve hearing.

▶ Teach the patient's family members ways to improve communication with him.

▶ For a patient undergoing surgery, provide preoperative and postoperative teaching.

▶ After surgery, advise the patient to move slowly to prevent vertigo; to avoid any activities that provoke dizziness,

Reviewing Weber's and Rinne tests

The two most common tests used to detect hearing loss and provide preliminary information about its type are Weber's test and the Rinne test. Both tests use a tuning fork.

Weber's test

Weber's test determines whether your patient hears the tone of the tuning fork in only one ear. In this test, you'll place the base of a vibrating tuning fork at the vertex of his head or midline on his forehead (as shown below). Alternative sites include the bridge of the nose, the central incisors, or the mandibular symphysis.

TUNING FORK POSITION FOR WEBER'S TEST

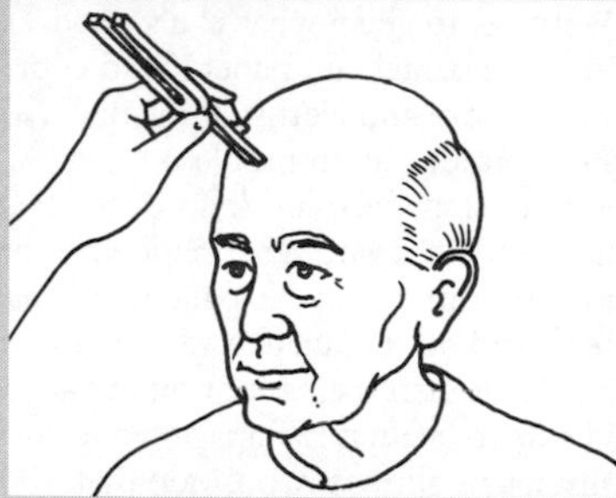

Does the patient hear the tone equally well in both ears? If he does, he has normal hearing. However, if the tone is louder in one ear, he may have conductive hearing loss in that ear. That's because the tone lateralizes to the affected ear through bone conduction, while background noise prevents similar detection by the unaffected ear.

Although this test is inconclusive for sensorineural hearing loss, if your patient has one normal ear and he hears the tone equally or more loudly in that ear, he may have sensorineural hearing loss in the other ear.

The Rinne test

The Rinne test evaluates your patient's ability to hear sounds through bone conduction and air conduction. For this test, you'll place the vibrating tuning fork against his mastoid process and hold it there until he no longer hears the tone (as shown below). This tests bone conduction.

FIRST TUNING FORK POSITION FOR THE RINNE TEST

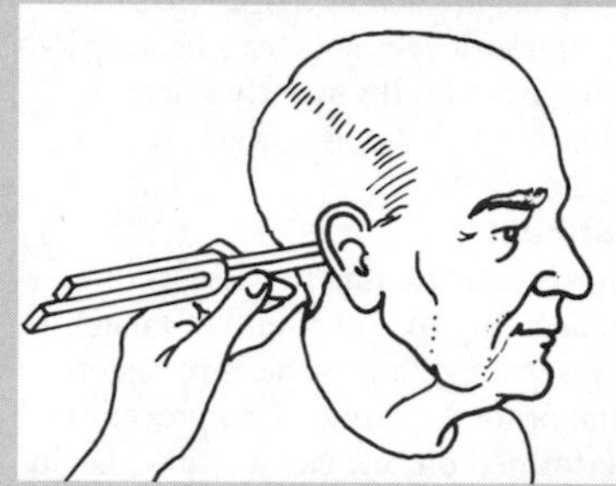

Next, you'll quickly move the vibrating tuning fork to a position in front of his ear canal, but not touching his auricle (as shown below), until he no longer hears the tone. This tests air conduction. Then you'll repeat the test on his other ear.

SECOND TUNING FORK POSITION FOR THE RINNE TEST

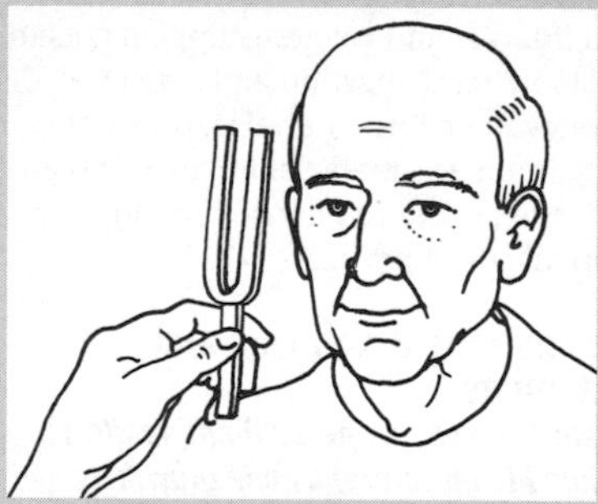

If his hearing is normal, he'll hear the air-conducted tone twice as long as the bone-conducted tone. However, if he hears the bone-conducted tone for as long as he hears the air-conducted tone or longer, he may have conductive hearing loss. A positive test result can also indicate sensorineural hearing loss because the inner ear's perception of sound waves by air or bone conduction is compromised.

such as straining, bending, or heavy lifting; and to avoid contact with anyone who has an upper respiratory tract infection.

- Teach the patient and a family member how to change the external ear dressing (eye or gauze pad) and care for the incision. Stress the importance of protecting the ears against cold.
- Emphasize the need to complete the prescribed antibiotic regimen and to return for scheduled follow-up care, which includes removing the packing. Point out that hearing may be masked by packing and dressing as well as by swelling from the operation. Inform the patient that he may not detect noticeable improvement in his hearing until 1 to 4 weeks after surgery.
- Before discharge, instruct the patient to avoid loud noises and sudden pressure changes, such as those that occur while diving or flying, until healing is complete (usually within 6 months). Advise him against blowing his nose for at least 1 week to prevent bacteria-contaminated air from entering the eustachian tubes.
- Advise the patient not to wet his head while showering and not to wash his hair for 2 weeks. (If this is unacceptable, suggest that dry shampoo can be used as long as none is allowed to enter the ears.) Then for the next 4 weeks, tell him to avoid getting water in his ears when washing his hair. Tell him not to swim for 6 weeks.
- Instruct the patient to avoid straining during defecation and to prevent constipation by increasing fluids, if able, and eating a diet high in fiber.
- Provide information about hearing aids, if appropriate.

OXYGEN THERAPY

A patient needs oxygen therapy when hypoxemia is caused by a respiratory or cardiac emergency or an increase in metabolic function. In a respiratory emergency, oxygen administration enables the patient to reduce his ventilatory effort. When conditions, such as atelectasis or adult respiratory distress syndrome, impair diffusion, or when lung volume is decreased from alveolar hypoventilation, this procedure boosts alveolar oxygen levels.

In a cardiac emergency, oxygen therapy helps meet the increased myocardial workload as the heart tries to compensate for hypoxemia. Oxygen administration is particularly important for a patient whose myocardium is already compromised — from a myocardial infarction or a cardiac arrhythmia.

When metabolic demand is high — as in cases of massive trauma, burns, or high fever — oxygen administration supplies the body with enough oxygen to meet its cellular needs. This procedure also increases oxygenation in the patient with a reduced blood oxygen-carrying capacity, possibly from carbon monoxide poisoning or sickle cell crisis.

The adequacy of oxygen therapy is determined by arterial blood gas (ABG) analysis, oximetry monitoring, and clinical examinations. The patient's disease, physical condition, and age will help determine the most appropriate method of administration.

Supplies

- Oxygen source (wall unit, cylinder, liquid tank, or concentrator)
- Flowmeter
- Adapter, if using a wall unit, or a pressure-reduction gauge, if using a cylinder
- Sterile distilled water
- OXYGEN PRECAUTION sign
- Appropriate oxygen delivery system (nasal cannula, simple mask, partial rebreather mask, or nonrebreather mask for low-flow and variable oxygen concentrations; Venturi mask, aerosol mask, tracheostomy collar, T tube, tent, or

oxygen hood for high-flow and specific oxygen concentrations)

- Small-diameter and large-diameter connection tubing
- Gauze pads and tape (for oxygen masks)
- Jet adapter for Venturi mask (if adding humidity)
- Optional: oxygen analyzer, sterile humidity bottles and adapters, pulse oximetry monitor, Bipap machine (may be used for patients with chronic lung problems)

Implementation

- Check the oxygen outlet port to verify flow. Pinch the tubing near the prongs to ensure that an audible alarm will sound if the oxygen flow stops.
- Assess the patient's condition. In an emergency, verify that he has an open airway before administering oxygen.
- Check the patient's room to make sure it's safe for oxygen administration. Whenever possible, replace electrical devices with nonelectric ones and post a NO SMOKING sign in the patient's room. Oxygen supports combustion and the smallest spark can cause a fire.
- Place an OXYGEN PRECAUTION sign over the patient's bed and on the door to his room.
- Assist in placing the oxygen delivery device on the patient. Make sure it fits properly and is stable.
- Monitor the patient's response to oxygen therapy. Check his ABG values during initial adjustments of oxygen flow. Once the patient is stabilized, you may use pulse oximetry instead. Check the patient frequently for signs of hypoxia, such as decreased level of consciousness, increased heart rate, arrhythmias, restlessness, perspiration, dyspnea, use of accessory muscles, yawning or flared nostrils, cyanosis, and cool, clammy skin.

Key point **Because some older patients don't become cyanotic when hypoxic, you'll need to evaluate other signs.**

- When monitoring a patient's response to a change in oxygen flow, check the pulse oximetry monitor or measure ABG values 20 to 30 minutes after adjusting the flow. In the interim, monitor the patient closely for any adverse response to the change in oxygen flow.
- Observe the patient's skin integrity to prevent skin breakdown on pressure points from the oxygen delivery device. Wipe moisture or perspiration from the patient's face and from the mask as needed.
- If the patient will be receiving oxygen at a concentration above 60% for more than 24 hours, watch carefully for signs of oxygen toxicity. Remind the patient to cough and breathe deeply to prevent atelectasis. Also, to prevent serious lung damage, measure ABG values repeatedly to determine whether high oxygen concentrations are still necessary.
- Never administer oxygen at more than 2 L/minute by nasal cannula to a patient with chronic lung disease unless you have a specific order to do so. That's because some patients with chronic lung disease become dependent on a state of hypercapnia and hypoxia to stimulate their respirations; therefore, supplemental oxygen could cause them to stop breathing. However, long-term oxygen therapy of 12 to 17 hours daily may help patients with chronic lung disease sleep better, survive longer, and have a reduced incidence of pulmonary hypertension.

Complications

High concentrations of oxygen over a prolonged period can cause damage to the airway and lungs. Respiratory arrest is a possible complication if oxygen concentrations are too high for the patient with chronic obstructive pulmonary disease.

Patient teaching

- To ensure the patient's cooperation, describe the procedure to him and explain why he needs oxygen.
- Tell the patient and his family that the no-smoking policy must be enforced.
- Instruct the patient to notify staff members if his breathing difficulty worsens.
- Before discharging a patient who'll receive home oxygen therapy, make sure you know the types of oxygen therapy, the kinds of services that are available to him, and the service schedules offered by local home suppliers. Together with the physician and the patient, choose the device best suited to the patient.
- If the patient is to receive transtracheal oxygen therapy, teach him how to properly clean and care for the catheter. Tell him to keep the skin surrounding the insertion site clean and dry to prevent infection.
- No matter which device the patient uses, you'll need to evaluate his and his caregiver's ability and motivation to administer oxygen therapy at home. Make sure they understand the reason the patient is receiving oxygen and the safety guidelines for administering oxygen. Teach them how to properly use and clean the equipment and supplies and to care for skin in contact with the oxygen device.
- If your patient will be discharged with oxygen for the first time, make sure his health insurance covers home oxygen. If it doesn't, find out what criteria he must meet to obtain coverage and inform him of the requirement. Without a third-party payer, the patient may not be able to afford home oxygen therapy.

Documentation

When oxygen therapy is initiated, record the date and time of oxygen administration; the type of delivery device; the oxygen flow rate, the patient's vital signs, skin color, respiratory effort, and breath sounds; and any patient or family teaching.

During therapy, record the patient's vital signs, skin color, and response to therapy as well as any changes in his condition and pulse oximetry.

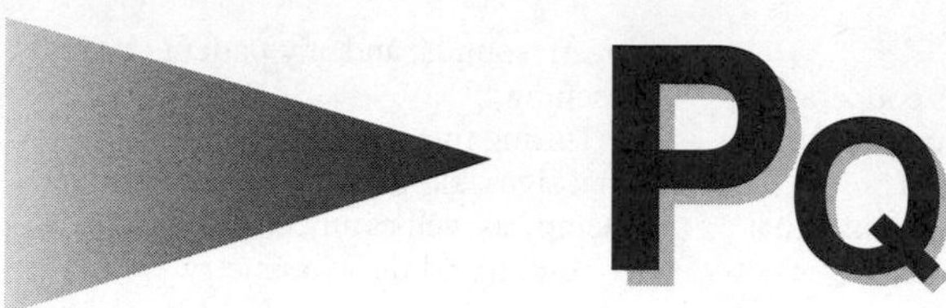

Pacemaker insertion

Designed to operate for 3 to 20 years, permanent pacemakers are self-contained devices that use electrical impulses to regulate cardiac rhythm. The surgeon implants the device in a pocket beneath the patient's skin. This is usually done in the operating room or cardiac catheterization laboratory. Nursing responsibilities involve monitoring the electrocardiogram (ECG) and maintaining sterile technique.

Candidates for permanent pacemakers include patients with myocardial infarction and persistent bradyarrhythmias and patients with complete heart block or slow ventricular rates caused by congenital or degenerative heart disease or cardiac surgery. Patients who suffer Stokes-Adams attacks as well as those with Wolff-Parkinson-White syndrome or sick sinus syndrome may also benefit from permanent pacemaker implantation.

Today, permanent pacemakers function in the demand mode, allowing the patient's heart to beat on its own but preventing it from falling below a preset rate. Pacing electrodes can be placed in the atria, in the ventricles, or in both chambers (called atrioventricular sequential or dual chamber pacemakers). The most common pacing modes are VVI for single-chamber pacing and DDD for dual-chamber pacing. (See *Understanding pacemaker codes.*)

A biventricular pacemaker is also available for patients with heart failure. This device differs from a standard pacemaker in that it has three leads instead of one or two. One lead is placed in the right atrium and the others are placed in each of the ventricles, where they simultaneously stimulate the right and left ventricle. This allows the ventricles to coordinate their pumping action and makes the heart more efficient.

Supplies

- Sphygmomanometer
- Stethoscope
- ECG monitor with oscilloscope and strip-chart recorder
- Sterile dressing tray
- Shaving supplies
- Sterile gauze dressing
- Hypoallergenic tape
- Antibiotics
- Analgesics
- Sedatives
- Emergency resuscitation equipment
- Sterile gown and mask
- I.V. line for emergency medications

Implementation

Before the procedure, ensure that the patient or a responsible family member signs a consent form, and ask the patient if he's allergic to anesthetics or iodine.

Preoperative care

- If ordered, shave the patient's chest from the axilla to the midline and from the clavicle to the nipple line on the side selected by the physician.
- Establish an I.V. line at a keep-vein-open rate so that you can administer emergency drugs if the patient experiences a ventricular arrhythmia.

▶ Obtain baseline vital signs and a baseline ECG.
▶ Provide sedation as ordered.

In the operating room

▶ If you'll be present to monitor arrhythmias during the procedure, put on a gown and mask.
▶ Connect the ECG monitor to the patient, and run a baseline rhythm strip. Make sure the machine has enough paper to run additional rhythm strips during the procedure. Leave the monitor screen on throughout the procedure.
▶ After preparing the site, the physician, guided by a fluoroscope and using a transvenous approach, passes the electrode catheter through the cephalic or external jugular vein and positions it under the trabeculae in the apex of the right ventricle. He then attaches the catheter to the pulse generator, inserts this into a pocket of subcutaneous tissue in the patient's chest wall, and sutures it closed, leaving a small outlet for a drainage tube.

Postoperative care

▶ Monitor the patient's ECG to check for arrhythmias and to ensure correct pacemaker functioning.
▶ Also monitor the I.V. flow rate; the I.V. line is usually kept in place for 24 to 48 hours postoperatively to allow for emergency treatment of arrhythmias.
▶ Check the dressing for signs of bleeding and infection (swelling, redness, or exudate). The physician may order prophylactic antibiotics for up to 7 days after the procedure.
▶ Change the dressing at least once every 24 to 48 hours, or according to the physician's orders and your health care facility's policy. If the dressing becomes soiled or the site is exposed to air, change the dressing immediately, regardless of when you last changed it.
▶ Check the patient's vital signs and level of consciousness (LOC) every 15 minutes for the first hour, every hour for

Understanding pacemaker codes

A permanent pacemaker is commonly identified by a three-letter code referring to how it's programmed.

First letter
(chamber that's paced)
A = atrium
V = ventricle
D = dual (both chambers)
O = not applicable

Second letter
(chamber that's sensed)
A = atrium
V = ventricle
D = dual (both chambers)
O = not applicable

Third letter
(how pulse generator responds)
I = inhibited
T = triggered
D = dual (inhibited and triggered)
O = not applicable

Examples of two common programming codes

DDD
Pace: atrium and ventricle
Sense: atrium and ventricle
Response: inhibited and triggered
This is a fully automatic, or universal, pacemaker.

VVI
Pace: ventricle
Sense: ventricle
Response: inhibited
This is a demand pacemaker, inhibited.

the next 4 hours, every 4 hours for the next 48 hours, and then once every shift. Confused, older patients with second-degree heart block won't show immediate improvement in LOC.

Key point **Watch for signs and symptoms of a perforated ventricle, with resultant cardiac tamponade: persistent hiccups, distant heart sounds, pulsus paradoxus, hypotension with narrow pulse pressure, increased venous pressure, cyanosis, distended neck veins, decreased urine output, restlessness, or complaints of fullness in the chest. If any of these develop, notify the physician immediately.**

Complications

Insertion of a permanent pacemaker places the patient at risk for certain complications, such as infection, lead displacement, a perforated ventricle, cardiac tamponade, lead fracture and disconnection, and pacemaker syndrome. Pacemaker syndrome consists of fatigue, dizziness, syncope, and distressing pulsations in the neck and chest. It can be associated with adverse hemodynamic effects.

Patient teaching

- Explain the procedure to the patient and his family, and answer any questions they may have.
- Provide and review literature from the manufacturer or the American Heart Association so the patient and family can learn about the pacemaker and how it works. Emphasize that the pacemaker merely augments the patient's natural heart rate.
- Provide the patient with an identification card that lists the pacemaker type and manufacturer, serial number, pacemaker rate setting, date implanted, and the physician's name.
- Teach the patient the signs of pacemaker malfunction.

Documentation

Document the type of pacemaker used, the serial number and manufacturer's name, pacing rate, date of implantation, and physician's name. Note whether the pacemaker successfully treated the patient's arrhythmias, and include other pertinent observations such as the condition of the incision site. Also document your patient teaching measures.

PAIN MANAGEMENT

When a person feels severe pain, he typically seeks medical help not only because he wants relief, but also because he believes the pain signals a serious problem. This perception produces anxiety, which in turn increases the patient's pain. To assess and manage pain properly, the nurse must depend on the patient's subjective description in addition to measurement by objective tools. (See *Pain and older people*.)

Interventions used to manage pain may include pharmacologic measures, emotional support, comfort measures, and cognitive techniques to distract the patient. Severe pain usually requires an opiate analgesic. Invasive measures, such as patient-controlled analgesia (PCA) and epidural analgesia, may also be required.

When selecting interventions to help a patient manage pain, consider the following:

- Choose pharmacologic interventions that are appropriate for the patient's level of pain.
- Anticipate adverse effects from drug use, especially with an older patient, and treat them aggressively.
- Provide timely and thorough assessments of the patient's status to determine the optimal approach to achieving comfort.
- Acknowledge and address the impact of psychosocial factors on the patient's perception of pain and its meaning.

Pain and older people

Pain is usually initiated by sensory stimuli, then individualized by a person's memory, expectations, emotions, and behavior. Your patients' perception of pain and psychological response to it are complex. The widespread belief that aging brings decreased pain sensitivity or increased pain tolerance lacks scientific support, yet older people have been known to present with painless myocardial infarctions and intra-abdominal catastrophes. It's unclear whether these clinical observations result from deficient pain reporting or age-related changes in pain receptors, nerve transmission, or central nervous system processing.

Incidence and causes

Some studies indicate that 25% to 50% of community-dwelling older people suffer important pain problems, compared to 45% to 80% of nursing home residents. Most pain complaints from nursing home residents are due to arthritis and musculoskeletal problems — particularly degenerative arthritis and lower back pain.

Cancer is a source of severe pain among older people, and they suffer disproportionately from painful peripheral vascular disease, herpes zoster, temporal arteritis, and polymyalgia rheumatica. Other common sources of pain are leg cramps, headaches, and diabetic neuropathies.

Consequences of pain

Psychosocial and economic consequences of pain also strongly affect your patients. Depression, decreased socialization, sleep disturbances, impaired ambulation, and increased health care needs and costs are all associated with pain. Deconditioning, gait disturbances, falls, slow rehabilitation, polypharmacy, cognitive dysfunction, and malnutrition are exacerbated by pain. Pain is a complication that can disrupt treatment goals and diminish your patients' quality of life.

Assessing pain in older patients

Adequate pain assessment is a challenge because your patients' multiple concurrent illnesses, underreporting of pain, and cognitive impairment may be factors. An accurate assessment involves asking your patient about pain, believing his responses, and taking his pain complaints seriously.

Lack of an accurate pain history can compound the problem. Approximately 3% to 15% of community-dwelling older people and 50% of nursing home residents have substantial cognitive impairment or dementia. Because of this, pain assessment instruments, such as visual analog scales, word descriptor scales, facial scales, and numerical scales — while helpful among younger patients — haven't been validated in older patients. However, ongoing research indicates that most patients with mild to moderate cognitive impairment can report pain intensity.

- Use a multidisciplinary approach to manage the patient's pain.
- Communicate a sense of empathy and caring to the patient in pain.

Supplies

- Patient's medication record and chart
- Pain assessment tool or scale
- Oral hygiene supplies
- Water
- Nonnarcotic analgesic (such as aspirin or acetaminophen)
- Optional: PCA device, mild narcotic (such as oxycodone or codeine), strong narcotic (such as morphine), and transdermal patch (such as fentanyl)

Implementation

▶ Explain to the patient how pain drugs work together with other pain management therapies to provide relief. Also explain that management aims to keep pain at the lowest acceptable level to permit optimal bodily function.

▶ Assess the patient's pain by asking key questions and noting his response to the pain. For instance, ask him to describe the duration, severity, and source of his pain. Look for physiologic or behavioral clues to the pain's severity. Tailor your questions to the patient's cognitive level, and allow sufficient time for the older patient to respond. (See *How to assess pain*.)

▶ Work with the patient and a family member or friend to develop a care plan, choosing interventions appropriate to the patient's lifestyle. These may include prescription and nonprescription drugs, emotional support, comfort measures, cognitive techniques, and education about pain and its management.

▶ Emphasize the importance of maintaining good bowel elimination habits, respiratory function, and mobility because pain can exacerbate problems in these areas.

▶ Implement your care plan. Remember that individuals respond to pain differently, so what works for one person might not work for another.

Drug administration

▶ Administer drugs orally whenever possible. Check the appropriate drug information for each drug you administer.

▶ Begin with a nonnarcotic analgesic, such as acetaminophen or aspirin, every 4 to 6 hours as ordered.

▶ If the patient needs more relief than a nonnarcotic analgesic provides alone or in combination with other nonsteroidal anti-inflammatory drugs, administer a mild narcotic (such as oxycodone or codeine) as ordered.

▶ If the patient needs still more pain relief, administer a stronger narcotic (such as morphine) as prescribed.

Drug alert The following analgesics have proved to be particularly dangerous for older adults and should be avoided: meperidine, pentazocine, propoxyphene, and methadone. Transdermal fentanyl should be initiated in low doses until the effects are determined.

▶ Administer the drug 30 minutes before any activity or procedure to ensure its effectiveness.

▶ Monitor closely for adverse effects due to age-related changes affecting the pharmacokinetics and pharmacodynamics of the drug.

▶ If ordered, teach the patient to use a PCA device, which can help the patient manage his pain and decrease his anxiety.

Emotional support

▶ Show your concern by spending time talking with the patient. He may be anxious and frustrated because of his inability to manage his pain. Such feelings worsen the pain.

▶ Make sure the patient understands the drug regimen.

Comfort measures

▶ Reposition the patient every 2 hours to reduce muscle spasms and tension and to relieve pressure on bony prominences. Use pillows and supports to provide support and cushioning. Elevating the head of the bed may help — for example, by reducing the pull on an abdominal incision, thereby diminishing pain. If appropriate, elevate a limb to reduce swelling, inflammation, and pain.

▶ Give the patient a back massage to help relax tense muscles.

▶ Use lotion or emollients to lubricate the older patient's dry skin.

▶ Perform passive range-of-motion exercises to prevent stiffness and further loss of mobility, to relax tense muscles, and to provide comfort.

▶ Provide oral hygiene. Keep a fresh glass of water at the bedside. Offer your

How to assess pain

To assess pain properly, consider both the patient's descriptions and your own observations of his physical and behavioral responses. During your assessment, keep in mind the age-related changes in the older patient.

Start by asking the following series of key questions. Bear in mind that the older person's responses are shaped by his prior experiences, selfimage, and beliefs about his condition. Allow him adequate time to process your questions and respond.

- Where is the pain located? How long does it last? How often does it occur?
- What does the pain feel like? (Have the patient describe it.)
- What relieves the pain or makes it worse?
- How do you usually get relief from it?

Ask the patient to rank his pain on a scale of 0 to 10, with 0 denoting lack of pain and 10 denoting the worst pain level. This helps the patient verbally evaluate pain therapies.

Observe the patient's behavioral and physiologic responses to pain. Physiologic responses may be sympathetic or parasympathetic.

Behavioral responses

Behavioral responses include altered body position, moaning, sighing, grimacing, crying, restlessness, withdrawal, muscle twitching, and immobility.

Sympathetic responses

Sympathetic responses are commonly associated with mild to moderate pain and include pallor, elevated blood pressure, dilated pupils, skeletal muscle tension, dyspnea, tachycardia, and diaphoresis.

Parasympathetic responses

Parasympathetic responses are commonly associated with severe, deep pain and include pallor, decreased blood pressure, bradycardia, nausea and vomiting, weakness, dizziness, and loss of consciousness.

patient a favorite beverage, such as apple juice, because many drugs tend to dry the mouth.

▶ Wash the patient's face and hands.

Cognitive therapy

▶ Help the patient enhance the effect of analgesics by using such techniques as distraction, guided imagery, deep breathing, and relaxation. You can easily use these "mind-over-pain" techniques at the bedside. Choose whichever method the patient feels most comfortable with. If possible, start these techniques when the patient feels little or no pain. If pain persists, begin with short, simple exercises. Before beginning, dim the lights, remove the patient's restrictive clothing, and eliminate noise from the environment.

▶ When using distraction, have the patient recall an interesting or pleasant experience or focus his attention on an enjoyable activity. For instance, he can use music as a distraction by turning on the radio when the pain begins. Have him close his eyes and concentrate on listening, raising or lowering the volume as his pain increases or subsides. Note, however, that distraction is usually effective only against brief pain episodes lasting less than 5 minutes and that the effects last only as long as the distracting activity.

▶ When using guided imagery, help the patient concentrate on a peaceful, pleasant image. Encourage him to focus on the details of the image he's selected by asking how it looks, sounds, smells, tastes, and feels. The positive emotions evoked by this exercise minimize pain.

▶ When using deep breathing, have the patient stare at an object and then slowly inhale and exhale as he counts aloud to maintain a comfortable rate and rhythm. Have him concentrate on the rise and fall of his abdomen. Encourage him to feel more and more weightless with each breath while he concentrates on the rhythm of his breathing or on any restful image.

▶ When using muscle relaxation, have the patient focus on a particular muscle group. Then ask him to tense the muscles and note the sensation. After 5 to 7 seconds, tell him to relax the muscles and concentrate on the relaxed state. Have him note the difference between the tense and relaxed states. After he tenses and relaxes one muscle group, have him proceed to another and another until he has included his entire body.

▶ Provide the patient with instructions for performing these techniques at home.

Complications

The most common adverse effects of analgesics include respiratory depression (the most serious), sedation, constipation, nausea, and vomiting.

Patient teaching

▶ Teach the patient about his prescribed drugs and their adverse effects.

▶ Tell him about alternative measures to relieve pain.

▶ Remind the patient that the results of cognitive therapy improve with practice. Help him through the initial sessions.

Special considerations

▶ Evaluate your patient's response to pain management. If he's still in pain, reassess him and alter your care plan as appropriate. Use the pain management techniques that work best for the patient.

▶ During periods of intense pain, the patient's ability to concentrate diminishes. If your patient experiences such pain, help him to select a cognitive technique that's simple to use. Once he selects a particular technique, encourage him to use it consistently.

Documentation

Document each step of the nursing process. Describe the subjective information you elicited from the patient, using his own words. Note the location, quality, and duration of the pain and any precipitating factors.

Record your nursing diagnoses, and include the pain relief method selected. Summarize your actions and patient teaching and the patient's response. If the patient's pain wasn't relieved, note alternative treatments to consider the next time pain occurs. Also record any complications of drug therapy.

PANCREATITIS

An inflammation of the pancreas, pancreatitis occurs in acute and chronic forms. It's associated with biliary heart disease, alcoholism, trauma, and certain drugs. It can also be idiopathic. Acute pancreatitis generally resolves clinically and histologically but is serious in nature and has a 10% mortality.

The most common causes of pancreatitis are biliary tract disease and alcoholism, but the disorder can also result from abnormal organ structure, metabolic or endocrine disorders (such as hyperlipidemia or hyperparathyroidism), pancreatic cysts or tumors, penetrating peptic ulcers, or trauma (blunt or iatrogenic). This disorder can also develop after the use of certain drugs, such as glucocorticoids, sulfonamides, thiazides, and oral contraceptives.

Pancreatitis may be a complication of renal failure, kidney transplantation, openheart surgery, and endoscopic retrograde cholangiopancreatography (ERCP). Predisposing factors include heredity and, in some patients, emotional or neurogenic factors.

Regardless of the cause, pancreatitis involves autodigestion: The enzymes normally excreted by the pancreas digest pancreatic tissue. Chronic pancreatitis is progressive destruction and calcification of pancreatic tissue.

If pancreatitis damages the islets of Langerhans, diabetes mellitus may occur. Fulminant pancreatitis (which occurs late in chronic pancreatitis) causes massive hemorrhage and total destruction of the pancreas, resulting in diabetic acidosis, shock, or coma. Respiratory complications include adult respiratory distress syndrome, atelectasis, pleural effusion, and pneumonia. Proximity of the inflamed pancreas to the bowel may cause paralytic ileus. Other complications include GI bleeding, pancreatic abscess, pseudocysts and, rarely, cancer.

Signs and symptoms

- Intense epigastric pain centered close to the umbilicus and radiating to the back, between the 10th thoracic and 6th lumbar vertebrae; aggravated by eating fatty foods, consuming alcohol, or lying in a recumbent position
- Weight loss, with nausea and vomiting
- Decreased blood pressure, tachycardia, fever, dyspnea or orthopnea (signs of respiratory complications)
- Changes in behavior and sensorium (may be related to alcohol withdrawal or may indicate hypoxia or impending shock)
- Generalized jaundice, Cullen's sign (bluish periumbilical discoloration), and Turner's sign (bluish flank discoloration) on inspection
- Steatorrhea (sign of chronic pancreatitis)
- Tenderness, rigidity, and guarding on abdominal palpation
- Dull sound on percussion (may indicate pancreatic ascites)
- Absent or decreased bowel sounds (in paralytic ileus)

Diagnostic tests

- *Blood studies* revealing a serum amylase level above 180 Somogyi units/dl (130 U/L) and a serum lipase level above 80 U/L are the diagnostic hallmark of acute pancreatitis.
- *Urinalysis* reveals urinary amylase level above 80 amylase units/hour (17 U/hour).
- Supportive *laboratory blood studies* reveal elevated white blood cell count and serum bilirubin level. Many patients have hypocalcemia, which appears to be associated with the severity of the disease. Blood and urine glucose tests may reveal transient glucosuria and hyperglycemia. In chronic pancreatitis, significant laboratory findings include elevations in serum alkaline phosphatase, amylase, and bilirubin levels; transiently elevated serum glucose levels; and elevated lipid and trypsin levels in stools.
- *Abdominal and chest X-rays* detect pleural effusions and differentiate pancreatitis from other diseases that cause similar symptoms.
- *Computed tomography scan* and *ultrasonography* reveal an increased pancreatic diameter and identify pancreatic cysts and pseudocysts. Ultrasonography can also rule out gallbladder disease, which is a treatable cause of acute pancreatitis.
- *ERCP* shows the anatomy of the pancreas; identifies ductal system abnormalities, such as calcification or strictures; and differentiates pancreatitis from other disorders such as pancreatic cancer.

Treatment

The goals of treatment are to maintain circulation and fluid volume, to relieve pain, and to decrease pancreatic secretions. Emergency treatment for shock (the most common cause of death in early-stage pancreatitis) consists of vigorous I.V. replacement of electrolytes and proteins. Metabolic acidosis secondary to hypovolemia and impaired cellular perfusion requires vigorous fluid volume replacement. Blood transfusions may be needed if shock occurs. Food and fluids are withheld to allow the pancreas to rest and to reduce pancreatic enzyme secretion.

Acute pancreatitis

Nasogastric (NG) tube suctioning is usually required to decrease gastric distention and suppress pancreatic secretions. Prescribed medications may include low-dose meperidine to relieve abdominal pain (this drug causes less spasm at the ampulla of Vater than opiates such as morphine), antacids to neutralize gastric secretions, and histamine-2 receptor antagonists (such as cimetidine or ranitidine) to help decrease hydrochloric acid production.

Anticholinergics are given to reduce vagal stimulation, decrease GI motility, and inhibit pancreatic enzyme secretion. Total parenteral nutrition is used to maintain positive nitrogen balance. Pancreatic enzymes are administered if enzyme seceretion is impaired. Insulin is used to correct hyperglycemia, if present.

Once the crisis begins to resolve, oral low-fat, low-protein feedings are gradually implemented. Alcohol and caffeine are eliminated from the diet. If the crisis occurred during treatment with glucocorticoids or thiazide diuretics, these drugs are discontinued. If pancreatic abscess or pseudocyst occur, surgical drainage may be necessary. If biliary tract obstruction causes acute pancreatitis, a laparotomy may be required.

Chronic pancreatitis

Treatment depends on the cause. Nonsurgical measures are appropriate if the patient refuses or is not a suitable candidate for surgery. Measures to prevent and relieve abdominal pain are similar to those used in acute pancreatitis. Meperidine is usually the drug of choice, but it must be used cautiously in the older adult.

Treatments for related diabetes mellitus may include dietary modification, insulin replacement, or oral antidiabetic drugs. Malabsorption and steatorrhea are treated with pancreatic enzyme replacement.

Surgical intervention relieves abdominal pain, restores pancreatic drainage, and reduces the frequency of acute pancreatic attacks. Surgical drainage is required for an abscess or pseudocyst. If biliary tract disease is the underlying cause, cholecystectomy or choledochotomy is performed. A sphincterotomy is indicated to enlarge a pancreatic sphincter that has become fibrotic. To relieve obstruction and allow drainage of pancreatic secretions, pancreaticojejunostomy (anastomosis of the jejunum with the opened pancreatic duct) may be required.

Key nursing diagnoses and outcomes

Imbalanced nutrition: Less than body requirements related to malabsorption caused by pancreatic enzyme deficiency

Treatment outcomes: The patient will regain and maintain normal weight and will exhibit no signs or symptoms of malnutrition.

Ineffective protection related to loss of ability to control blood glucose levels naturally due to alpha- and beta-cell damage

Treatment outcomes: The patient will regain and maintain normal serum blood glucose levels and will exhibit no ketones in urine.

Chronic pain related to inflammatory process

Treatment outcome: The patient won't develop chronic pain.

Nursing interventions

- Administer meperidine (in lower doses for the older adult) or other analgesics, as ordered, and document the drugs' effectiveness.
- Maintain the NG tube for drainage or suctioning.

▶ In case of hypocalcemia, keep airway and suction apparatus handy and pad the side rails of the bed.
▶ Restrict the patient to bed rest, and provide a quiet and restful environment.
▶ Place the patient in a comfortable position that also allows maximal chest expansion such as Fowler's position.
▶ Assess the patient's level of pain. Evaluate his response to administered analgesics, and monitor for adverse reactions.
▶ Assess pulmonary status at least every 4 hours to detect early signs of respiratory complications.
▶ Monitor fluid and electrolyte balance, and report any abnormalities. Maintain an accurate record of intake and output. Weigh the patient daily and record his weight.
▶ Evaluate the patient's present nutritional status and metabolic requirements. Provide I.V. fluids and parenteral nutrition, as ordered. As soon as the patient can tolerate it, provide a diet high in carbohydrates, low in proteins, and low in fat.
▶ Monitor serum glucose levels, and administer insulin as ordered.
▶ Keep water and other beverages at the bedside, and encourage the patient to drink plenty of fluids.
▶ Don't confuse thirst caused by hyperglycemia (indicated by serum glucose levels up to 350 mg/dl and glucose and acetone in the urine) with dry mouth caused by NG intubation and anticholinergics.
▶ Watch for signs of calcium deficiency: tetany, cramps, carpopedal spasm, and seizures.
▶ Prepare the patient for surgery as indicated.
▶ If the patient has chronic pancreatitis, allow him to express feelings of anger, depression, and sadness related to his condition and help him to cope with these feelings.
▶ Counsel the patient to contact a self-help group, such as Alcoholics Anonymous, if needed or consult a psychiatrist, as indicated.

PATIENT TEACHING

▶ Emphasize the importance of avoiding factors that precipitate acute pancreatitis, especially alcohol.
▶ Refer the patient and a family member or friend to the dietitian. Stress the need for a diet high in carbohydrates and low in protein and fats. Caution the patient to avoid caffeinated beverages and irritating foods.
▶ Point out the need to comply with pancreatic enzyme replacement therapy. Instruct the patient to take the enzymes with meals or snacks to help digest food and to promote fat and protein absorption. Advise him to watch for and report any of the following adverse effects of enzyme therapy: nausea, abdominal cramping, and diarrhea.
▶ If the patient has chronic pain, teach a family member how to give I.M. injections as ordered.

PARKINSON'S DISEASE

One of the most common cripplers, Parkinson's disease is a slowly progressive, chronic, degenerative condition that characteristically causes progressive muscle rigidity, postural instability, bradykinesia, and resting tremors. As the person loses mobility, he may experience injury from falls and skin breakdown.

The cause of Parkinson's disease is unknown in most cases. Studies of the extrapyramidal brain nuclei (corpus striatum, globus pallidus, and substantia nigra) have established that a dopamine deficiency occurs. As a result of this deficiency, the excitative effect of acetylcholine is unchecked, causing symptoms of cholinergic excess, such as rigidity, tremors, bradykinesia, and postural instability.

Symptoms are commonly subtle. They occur in varying combinations and change as the disease progresses. Early symptoms, such as fatigue and generalized slowness, may be mistaken for signs of normal aging. Therefore, assessment requires a health history, physical examination findings, and diagnostic test results. Inquire about past medical conditions and obtain a thorough drug history to uncover possible causes of parkinsonian symptoms.

Parkinson's disease may occur after epidemic encephalitis. Trauma or ischemia may produce parkinsonian symptoms, as may long-term administration of certain drugs, such as phenothiazines and reserpine. Rarely, parkinsonian symptoms stem from exposure to toxins, such as manganese dust or carbon monoxide.

Signs and symptoms

- Fatigue when performing activities of daily living (ADLs) and muscle cramps in legs, neck, and trunk (in early stages)
- Characteristic slow, shuffling gait, stooped posture, and balance disturbances
- Slow movements (bradykinesia) or difficulty initiating simple movement (akinesia)
- Tremors (a classic sign) that typically begin in the fingers and may increase with stress or anxiety and decrease with purposeful movement and sleep
- Rigidity (a cardinal sign), which can involve any or all of the striated muscles (including "cogwheel" or "lead-pipe" rigidity); dysarthria and hypophonia from vocal cord rigidity
- Masklike facial expression, with fixed, wide-open eyes
- Drooling
- Constipation, urine retention, and dysphagia in later stages
- Secondary symptoms from autonomic nervous system involvement, including oily skin, increased perspiration, lacrimation, heat sensitivity, and postural hypotension
- Rapid mood swings or depression
- Cognitive disturbances, such as memory deficits or confusion (in severe disease)
- Rarely, oculogyric crisis (eyes fixed upward, with involuntary tonic movements) or blepharospasm (contraction of the orbicular muscle)

Diagnostic tests

- *Computed tomography scan* or *magnetic resonance imaging* may be performed to rule out other disorders such as intracranial tumors.
- *Urinalysis* may reveal reduced dopamine levels but usually has little value in identifying Parkinson's disease. Only an autopsy can definitively reveal a dopamine deficiency.

Treatment

Parkinson's disease has no cure, so the goal of treatment is to relieve symptoms and keep the patient mobile and functioning independently as long as possible.

Levodopa, a dopamine replacement drug, is effective during the first few years it's prescribed. The drug is given in increasing doses until signs and symptoms are relieved or adverse reactions appear. Because adverse reactions can be serious, levodopa is commonly given in combination with carbidopa to halt peripheral dopamine synthesis.

The patient may receive a bromocriptine additive to reduce the levodopa dose. When levodopa is ineffective or toxic, alternative drug therapy includes anticholinergics (such as trihexyphenidyl or benztropine) and anihistamines (such as diphenhydramine). The central anticholinergic and sedative effects of antihistamines also make them useful in decreasing tremors.

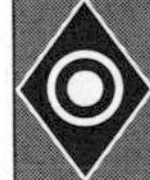

Drug alert Because of age-related changes affecting pharmacodynamics and pharmacokinetics, older patients receiving antiparkinsonian drugs are at increased risk for developing adverse reactions. Watch for ad-

verse psychiatric responses, such as anxiety and confusion, and for cardiac reactions, such as orthostatic hypotension and pulse irregularities. Be especially alert for eyelid twitching, an early sign of toxicity.

Anticholinergics may be used alone or in combination with levodopa to control tremors and rigidity. Amantadine, an antiviral agent, is used early in treatment to reduce rigidity, tremors, and akinesia. Selegiline, an enzyme-inhibiting agent, allows conservation of dopamine and enhances the therapeutic effect of levodopa. Tricyclic antidepressants may be given to decrease the depression that commonly accompanies the disease.

Oxidative stress theory research has caused controversy regarding drug therapy for Parkinson's disease. Although the levodopa and carbidopa combination has traditionally been a first-line drug for Parkinson's disease management, it has been associated with an acceleration of the disease process. Administering selegiline after levodopa and carbidopa may be more effective.

When drug therapy fails, stereotaxic neurosurgery is sometimes an effective alternative. In this procedure, electrical coagulation, freezing, radioactivity, or ultrasound destroys the ventrolateral nucleus of the thalamus to prevent involuntary movement. Such neurosurgery is more effective in young, otherwise healthy people with unilateral tremor or muscle rigidity. As with drug therapy, neurosurgery is a palliative measure that can only relieve symptoms.

Another medication, pramipexole, may be used alone or in conjunction with levodopa. Some data show it may delay the use of levodopa for nearly 2 years and, when used in combination with levodopa, is reduces the amount required.

Physical therapy helps the patient maintain normal muscle tone and function. This may include active and passive range-of-motion exercises, routine daily activities, walking, and baths and massage to help relax muscles.

Possible complications from Parkinson's disease are pressure ulcers and contractions. Older patients who suffer from malnourishment or fragile skin integrity may be at greater risk for these effects.

Key nursing diagnoses and outcomes

Impaired home maintenance management related to self-care deficits caused by neuromuscular dysfunction

Treatment outcomes: The patient will describe changes needed to promote maximum health and safety at home; seek and get help from family members, friends, and agencies to meet personal needs; and maintain an optimal level of health within the disease limitations.

Impaired physical mobility related to involuntary movement

Treatment outcomes: The patient will use appropriate safety precautions and will maintain functional mobility without injury.

Chronic low self-esteem related to involuntary movement and drooling

Treatment outcomes: The patient will acknowledge feelings of low self-esteem, seek help in raising self-esteem, and demonstrate an increase in self-esteem.

Nursing interventions

- Provide emotional and psychological support to your patient and his family members. Listen to their specific concerns and answer their questions.
- Encourage the patient to use coping skills. Help him identify social activities that he can continue to participate in; then encourage him to participate to help bolster self-esteem and prevent depression.
- Promote the patient's independence by asking him to participate in care-related decisions. Help him identify ADLs that he can perform, and teach him nec-

essary self-care skills. Provide positive reinforcement. Make sure that all caregivers are aware of the patient's capabilities. Allow sufficient time for the patient to complete his care. Assist him with self-care in later stages of illness when disability is more profound.

- Assess the patient's nutritional status, and monitor his body weight. Observe for conditions that can hinder adequate nutritional intake, such as difficulty swallowing, because of tremors or depression. Consult with the dietitian, physical therapist, physician, or occupational therapist, as needed, to plan an effective nutritional program.
- Keep suction equipment available in case of aspiration. Offer semisolid foods if the patient has difficulty swallowing. Provide supplementary feedings or small, frequent meals to increase caloric intake, if needed.
- Help establish a regular bowel elimination routine by encouraging the patient to drink at least 2qt (2 L) of liquids daily (unless contraindicated), eat high-fiber foods, exercise daily, and establish a regular time for elimination. Also, make sure he has an elevated toilet seat to ease sitting.
- Provide assistive devices as appropriate. For example, to help the patient turn himself in bed, tie a rope to the foot of the bed and extend it to the patient so that he can grasp it and pull himself to a sitting position. Make sure the patient and caregiver demonstrate proper use of any assistive devices, such as a walker or cane.
- Ask the physical therapist to develop a program of daily exercises to increase muscle strength, decrease muscle rigidity, prevent contractures, and improve coordination. The program should include stretching and postural exercises, swimming, and stationary bicycling.
- Because fatigue may make the patient more dependent on others, provide rest periods between activities.
- Protect the patient from injury by raising the bed's side rails, as appropriate, and assisting him as necessary when he walks. Keep his environment free from clutter that could result in falls. Make sure he sits in chairs equipped with armrests and back supports.
- Provide frequent warm baths and massage to help relax muscles and relieve cramps.
- If the patient's speech is affected, consult with the speech therapist.
- If the patient experiences depression that isn't easily resolved without drug therapy, discuss the problem with the physician, who may prescribe antidepressants.
- Refer the patient and his family to the National Parkinson's Foundation; American Parkinson Disease Association, Inc.; Parkinson's Disease Foundation; United Parkinson's Foundation; and International Tremor Foundation.

PATIENT TEACHING

- Teach the patient and his family members about the disorder, its progressive nature, and all prescribed treatments.
- Explain the purpose, dosage, possible adverse effects, and precautions for all prescribed drugs. Tell the patient to notify the physician if any drugs lose their effectiveness or cause adverse reactions. Explain that the physician may need to adjust the dosage or change medications.
- Encourage the patient to exercise daily and to follow the planned physical therapy program. Teach him simple stretching exercises to promote flexibility.
- Explain the importance of daily bathing if the patient has oily skin and increased perspiration.
- Suggest that the patient wear clothing fitted with Velcro fasteners or zippers rather than buttons to make dressing easier.
- To decrease the risk of aspiration, instruct the patient to sit upright when eating.
- If appropriate, show the patient the best way to eat. Teach him to place food

on his tongue, close his lips, chew first on one side and then the other, then lift his tongue up and back and make a conscious effort to swallow. Tell his family members to allow plenty of time for meals.

- Show his family members how to prevent pressure ulcers and contractures by proper positioning.
- Explain household safety measures to the patient and his caregiver. For example, suggest installing hand rails in bathrooms, halls, and stairs. Instruct them to remove throw rugs to prevent falls.
- Teach the patient to walk with a wide based gait to improve his balance and prevent falls. Also, tell him to rise slowly to a sitting position and to change positions slowly.

PATIENT-CONTROLLED ANALGESIA

Patient-controlled analgesia (PCA) puts the patient in charge of relieving his own pain by letting him give himself boluses of a narcotic when his pain increases. When patients control their own analgesia, they use less narcotic and are sedated for less time than when they receive prescribed doses through another route. In addition, they tend to experience less pain and return to normal activities sooner.

Steadily improving technology has increased the popularity of PCA, which is usually administered I.V. An I.V. PCA pump can deliver small amounts of a narcotic at a slow, continuous rate. I.V. administration allows faster and more predictable drug absorption than I.M. administration.

Morphine is the most commonly prescribed drug for PCA, but many other drugs are also given, including hydromorphone, buprenorphine, and meperidine. The anesthesiologist determines the drug based on the patient's weight, age, and previous narcotics usage. He may establish a basal rate (the maximum amount the patient may receive hourly in continuous infusion). He'll also determine whether a bolus dose can be given and how often. Within these limits, the patient controls the amount of drug he receives.

Patients receiving PCA therapy need to be mentally alert and able to understand and comply with instructions and procedures. PCA is contraindicated in patients with limited respiratory reserve, a history of drug abuse, or a psychiatric disorder.

With PCA, the patient controls drug delivery by pressing a button on the pump. Before the device can be used, it must be programmed to deliver the specified dose at the correct time intervals. You can set up a pump to deliver PCA S.C. or I.V. (See *Initiating subcutaneous PCA therapy,* page 444.)

If the patient is using a pump that provides a continuous infusion, he can control incidental pain (from coughing, for example) or breakthrough pain. If he's receiving continuous infusion therapy at home, the pump should allow him to stop and start the infusion. If the patient is having steady pain that gradually increases or decreases or pain that's worse at one time or another, he should be able to regulate the hourly infusion rate. If he has sudden but brief increases in pain, he should be able to give himself bolus doses along with the infusion. However, if his pain is intermittent, he might not need a continuous infusion at all.

Supplies

- Patient's medication record and chart
- PCA device, including specified concentration of drug in solution
- I.V. line or S.C. site
- Alcohol
- Appropriate site dressing
- Gloves

Initiating subcutaneous PCA therapy

Subcutaneous (S.C.) patient-controlled analgesia (PCA) therapy is commonly used to manage chronic pain. This therapy can be administered through a number of routes such as the abdominal route shown below. If you're initiating PCA through this route, after cleaning the insertion site follow these steps:

- Insert a 27G butterfly needle or a commercial S.C. infusion needle into the patient's abdomen or into another area with accessible S.C. tissue.
- Cover the site with a dressing.
- Calculate the hourly S.C. dose the same way you would an I.V. dose, considering both the hourly infusion rate and the bolus doses.
- Monitor the patient's S.C. absorption of a drug, which depends on the patient's condition. The maximum volume per hour that a well-nourished and well-hydrated patient can usually absorb is 2 to 2.5 ml. If your patient can't absorb that much, you may need to increase the drug's concentration. The minimum volume per hour should be about 1 ml.
- Inspect the site twice per day for signs of irritation or development of cellulitis. If it becomes irritated, change to a new site as often as necessary and apply a corticosteroid cream two or three times per day. Otherwise, change the site weekly or according to your facility's policy.

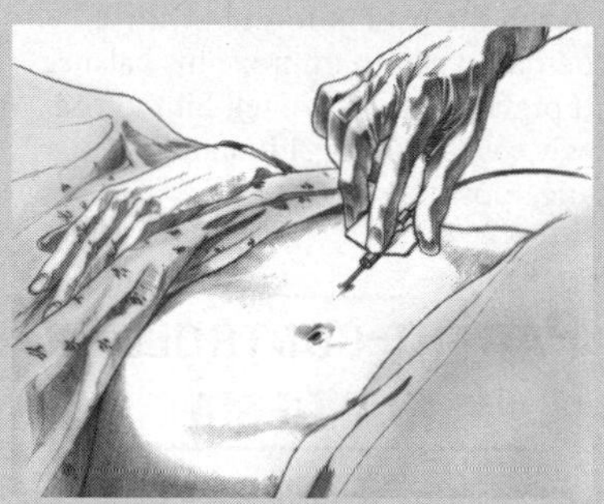

Implementation

▶ In conjunction with the physician, determine the initial trial bolus dose and a time interval between boluses. Program this information into the pump. Once these safety limits are set, the patient can push the button to receive a dose when he feels pain. You and the physician may decide to change the dose or the lockout interval after you see how the patient responds.

▶ To determine bolus doses for bolus-only PCA pumps, follow these guidelines: If the patient has only intermittent pain, simply estimate a dose and increase or decrease it until you determine the amount that relieves pain. Calculate the number of milligrams per dose and the total dose (or number of boluses) that he may receive per hour. When working with older patients, the rule of thumb is to start low and go slowly.

▶ To determine lockout intervals for bolus doses, follow these guidelines: For I.V. boluses (bolus only or bolus plus continuous infusion), set the lockout interval for 6 minutes or more. Typically, pain relief following an I.V. narcotic bolus takes 5 to 10 minutes. For S.C. boluses (bolus only or bolus plus continuous infusion), set the lockout interval for 30 minutes or more. Typically, pain relief following an S.C. bolus takes 15 to 60 minutes. For spinal boluses (bolus only or bolus plus continuous infusion), set the lockout interval for 60 minutes or more. Typically, pain relief following a spinal bolus takes 30 to 60 minutes.

▶ If the patient hasn't been receiving opiates, first give the drug until his pain is relieved (the loading dose). With morphine, for example, give 1 to 5 mg every 10 minutes until the pain subsides. Then set the pump's hourly infusion rate to equal the total number of milligrams per hour needed to control the pain.

▶ If you set the pump so that the patient can give himself bolus doses, decrease the hourly infusion rate. Check his response every 15 to 30 minutes for 1 to 2 hours after changing the settings.

▶ If you can program the pump to deliver a continuous infusion plus bolus doses, remember this rule of thumb: The initial total hourly dose shouldn't exceed the cumulative bolus doses per hour needed to relieve the patient's pain. For example, if the patient needs a total of 6 mg of morphine over 1 hour, you can begin therapy with a continuous infusion of 3 mg/hour, allowing bolus doses of 0.5 mg every 10 minutes (six boluses/hour). If the patient needs six or more boluses, check with the physician about increasing the hourly infusion rate.

▶ Before giving an opiate analgesic, review the patient's drug regimen.

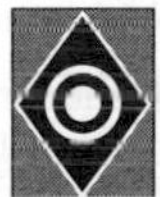

Drug alert **Because of age-related changes affecting pharmacokinetics and pharmacodynamics, the older patient is at risk for adverse effects and may require a smaller loading dose or bolus doses. Also, concurrent use of two central nervous system depressants can cause excessive drowsiness, oversedation, disorientation, and anxiety.**

▶ Use caution when programming the PCA pump. After changing the program, don't start the pump until another nurse has double-checked the new settings.

▶ Monitor vital signs according to facility policy such as every 2 hours for the first 8 hours after starting PCA. Check the pump at least twice per day to ensure adequate dosing of the pain medication.

▶ Because opiate analgesics can cause postural hypotension, guard against accidents. Keep the side rails raised on the patient's bed. If the patient is mobile, help him out of bed and assist him in walking. Encourage him to practice coughing and deep breathing to promote ventilation and prevent pooling of secretions, which could lead to respiratory difficulty.

▶ Watch for respiratory depression during PCA therapy. If the patient's respiratory rate declines to 10 or fewer breaths per minute, call his name and touch him. Tell him to breathe deeply. If he can't be roused or is confused or restless, notify the physician and prepare to give oxygen. If ordered, give a narcotic antagonist such as naloxone (which should be kept readily available). Respiratory depression during PCA isn't common because if a patient receives too much narcotic, he falls asleep and can't press the bolus button. Make sure family members or staff members don't give extra doses of the narcotic when a patient hasn't requested them.

▶ Evaluate the drug's effectiveness at regular intervals. Frequently assess the patient's level of comfort and reaction to the pain, according to your facility's policy. Is the patient getting relief? Is he developing a tolerance to the drug? Does the dosage need to be increased because of persistent or worsening pain? Although opiate analgesics should be given in the smallest effective dose over the shortest time period, they shouldn't be withheld or given in ineffective doses. These drugs lead to psychological dependence in fewer than 1% of hospitalized patients.

▶ If a patient has persistent nausea and vomiting during therapy, the physician may change the medication. If ordered, give the patient an antiemetic such as chlorpromazine. If anaphylaxis occurs, treat the symptoms and give another drug for pain relief, as ordered.

▶ To prevent constipation, give the patient a stool softener and, if necessary, a senna derivative laxative. Provide a high-fiber diet and encourage the patient to drink fluids. Regular exercise may also help. In case of urine retention, monitor the patient's intake and output.

Complications

The primary complication of PCA is respiratory depression. Other potential complications include anaphylaxis, nausea, vomiting, constipation, postural hypotension, and drug tolerance. Infiltration into subcutaneous tissue and catheter occlusion can also occur, which can cause the drug to back up into the primary I.V. tubing.

Patient teaching

- Your patient must understand how PCA works for therapy to succeed. In many cases, you're in the best position to teach him and members of his family about PCA. You might have to reinforce your teaching several times, especially with an older patient or one who's confused. Keep in mind that PCA isn't for everyone. A patient won't do well with this method if he can't understand it.
- When teaching your patient the techniques involved in PCA, emphasize that he'll be able to control his pain. Reassure him that the method is safe and effective but that he could experience mild discomfort.
- Home care patients must receive particularly good instructions. Include the patient's family members in your teaching session, if possible, and tell them to contact the physician whenever they suspect a problem.

Documentation

Always document the drug given, the amount (including boluses), the effectiveness of the treatment, any adverse reactions the patient experiences, and the patient's vital signs. Document your patient teaching measures.

PATIENT SELF-DETERMINATION

The Patient Self-Determination Act, passed in 1991, requires health care facilities to inform newly admitted patients of their right to accept or refuse treatment if they become gravely ill. The documents containing patients' wishes are called advance directives. The most common advance directives are living wills and durable powers of attorney, which designate a health care proxy who will make decisions in the event that the patient becomes unable to do so. The concept of self-determination, the right of a person to decide what will or won't happen to his body, has its origins in both constitutional (legal) rights and autonomy (ethical) rights. This concept is most commonly considered in cases involving death and dying, but it applies to all aspects of consent and refusal.

Competent adults have the right to refuse medical treatment unless the state can show that its interests outweigh that right. Examples of overriding state interests include protecting third parties, especially minor children; preserving life, especially that of minors and incompetents; and protecting society from the spread of disease. Competent adults may decide which treatments they will receive and which they will refuse. In some states, oral wishes are upheld by the judiciary. The court examines documentation of the patient's wishes and then determines whether the patient knew of a terminal condition when expressing these wishes or was talking in general terms about future care in case of terminal illness. The courts are reluctant to enforce generalities: Vague talk about potential future events usually carries little weight in court.

Important court cases

For years, legal experts have concluded that competent adults have the right to refuse medical treatment even if the refusal is certain to cause death — a view that's consistent with the trend in a majority of states to decriminalize suicide. But it wasn't until 1984 that an appellate court directly confronted this issue, when a clearly competent patient — who had a serious illness that was probably incurable but not necessarily terminal—refused necessary life-sustaining treatment.

Bartling v. Superior Court (1984) concerned the rights of a competent adult to have life-support equipment disconnected (over the objections of his physicians and the hospital) even though this action would hasten his death. Bartling, a severely emphysemic patient, entered the hospital for depression. While hospitalized, a tumor was noted on his X-ray. During the subsequent biopsy, his lung collapsed and a tracheostomy tube was inserted. The patient was dependent on a ventilator when the case was heard in court. Although Bartling died during the course of the appeal, the appellate court held that the "right of a competent adult to refuse medical treatment is a constitutionally guaranteed right which must not be abridged."

In *Bouvia v. Superior Court* (1986), the court addressed many of the same issues. Bouvia, a 28-year-old patient with severe cerebral palsy, sought removal of a nasogastric tube, which was inserted and maintained against her will to allow forced feedings. Here, the court wrestled not only with the right of a competent adult to refuse medical treatment, but also with the facility's obligation to serve the autonomous interests of individual patients. In *Bouvia,* those autonomous interests included medical support to prevent further pain and suffering during the dying process, so the patient received appropriate medications.

Incompetent patients present a totally different picture. The first court case to challenge the judiciary in this respect was the Karen Quinlan case (1976). In this case, Karen Quinlan's parents argued that unwanted life support violated their comatose daughter's constitutional right to privacy. The New Jersey Supreme Court allowed Quinlan's father to authorize the withdrawal of life support systems for her, arguing that: "The only practical way to prevent destruction of the (privacy) right is to permit the guardian and family of Karen to render their very best judgment...as to whether she would exercise it in these circumstances."

The decision was a difficult one to reach because Karen didn't meet the Harvard criteria for brain death. Although she was dependent on a respirator at the time of the court case, she did have some brain activity and some reflex movements. The decision also conflicted significantly with a precedent-setting New Jersey case that held that one should always save a life, even if the patient's objection to lifesaving procedures was based on religious beliefs (*John F. Kennedy Memorial Hospital v. Heston* [1971]).

The next significant decision in this area of the law was in the case of *Superintendent of Belchertown State School v. Saikewicz* (1977). This case concerned the issue of whether Mr. Saikewicz, a 67-year-old profoundly retarded resident of a state facility, should receive therapy for his newly diagnosed leukemia. The Massachusetts Supreme Court used the doctrine of *substituted judgment* (subjective determination of how a person would have chosen to exercise his right to refuse treatment if he were capable of making his wishes and opinions known) to decide what the patient would have wanted. Unlike the *Quinlan* decision, the *Saikewicz* decision met with general disfavor because the court rejected the notion that decisions to refuse treatment should be made by patients' families and physicians with the aid of ethics committees. Instead, it held that the decision to discontinue therapy "must reside with the judicial process and the judicial process alone."

In *Eichner v. Dillon* (1980), the court restricted the decision to terminate extraordinary life-support treatments to the patient who was terminally ill or in a "vegetative coma characterized as permanent or irreversible with an extremely remote possibility of recovery." However, it allowed family members or the legal guardian of the incompetent patient to request the right to terminate life-support treatments. In this case, the patient's religious superior, Father Eichner, requested the right to terminate treatment. The *Eichner* case combined the substituted judgment doctrine applied in the *Saikewicz* decision with the best interest test derived from the *Quinlan* case. (*Best interest* refers to personal preferences that were made known while a now-incompetent patient was rational and capable of stating preferences in case of a catastrophic event.) While not a perfect solution, the decision did soften the negative impact of the *Saikewicz* decision.

Finally, in *Cruzan v. Director, Missouri Department of Health* (1990), the court ruled that right-to-die issues should be decided on a state-by-state basis and that there should be little, if any, constitutional limit on what states may do. Since this decision, the states have given more latitude to family members, and the courts have struggled to find instances in which patients expressed, however fleetingly, their desires about sustaining life with artificial or life-support measures.

Two recent cases illustrate this trend. In *In re Fiori* (1995), a Pennsylvania court held that a hospital could terminate life-support treatment for a patient in a persistent vegetative state without a court order if the hospital obtained the consent of close family members and two physicians. The court limited this ruling to patients in a persistent vegetative state with no cognitive powers and no chance of recovery who never clearly expressed a preference for termination.

In *Grace Plaza of Great Neck, Inc. v. Elbaum* (1993), the court held that where doubt exists as to an incompetent patient's desired course of treatment, a judicial determination is necessary before life support can be terminated. The court further stated that proof of a patient's desires, as expressed in a living will or a prior statement, for example, should limit a health care provider's autonomy in denying termination of treatment.

Special considerations

The geriatric nurse should be familiar with the requirements of the federal Patient Self-Determination Act and should understand the laws regulating patient self-determination for the state in which she practices. The Patient Self-Determination Act requires health care providers to provide adult patients with written notice of state laws pertaining to their rights to refuse care and to develop advanced directives regarding their health care. It also requires health care providers to inform patients of institutional policies regarding advance directives.

The nurse should ask whether the patient has executed an advance directive and should document the response in the medical record. In addition, staff members may also need to be educated about advance directives. The nurse needs to ensure compliance with state laws about advance directives as well as maintain written policies and procedures implementing the requirements.

The geriatric nurse should ensure that the older patient has been provided the necessary information and the opportunity to execute an advance directive. Examine your own feelings and be supportive of your patient, even if you disagree with the choice he has made.

PEPTIC ULCER DISEASE

Occurring as circumscribed lesions in the mucosal membrane, peptic ulcers can develop in the lower esophagus, stomach, duodenum, or jejunum. The major forms are duodenal ulcer and gastric ulcer; both are chronic conditions resulting from contact of the mucosa with gastric juice (especially hydrochloric acid and pepsin).

Duodenal ulcers, which account for about 80% of peptic ulcers, affect the proximal part of the small intestine. These ulcers follow a chronic course characterized by remissions and exacerbations; 5% to 10% of patients develop complications that necessitate surgery. They occur most commonly in men between ages 20 and 50. About 4% of older adults admitted to the hospital with acute abdominal pain are diagnosed with peptic ulcer disease.

Gastric ulcers, which affect the stomach mucosa, are most common in middle-aged and older men, especially among the poor and undernourished and in chronic users of aspirin or alcohol.

Bacterial infection with *Helicobacter pylori* has been identified as the leading cause of peptic ulcer disease. Two other leading causes are the use of nonsteroidal anti-inflammatory drugs (NSAIDs) and pathologic hypersecretory states such as Zollinger-Ellison syndrome. (See *Causes of peptic ulcer,* page 450.)

Untreated peptic ulcers can lead to various complications. Erosion of the mucosa can cause GI hemorrhage, which can progress to hypovolemic shock, perforation, and obstruction. Obstruction may cause the stomach to distend with food and fluid and result in abdominal or intestinal infarction. Penetration, in which the ulcer crater extends beyond the duodenal walls into attached structures, such as the pancreas, biliary tract, liver, or gastrohepatic omentum, occurs fairly frequently with a duodenal ulcer.

Signs and symptoms

- Pain in the left epigastrium (described as sharp, gnawing, burning, boring, or aching) that's typically relieved by eating in duodenal ulcer, or triggered or aggravated by eating in gastric ulcer
- Feeling of fullness or distention
- Weight loss and loss of appetite
- Vomiting (rare)
- Pallor (anemia from blood loss)
- Epigastric tenderness on palpation
- Hyperactive bowel sounds on auscultation
- Hematemesis or melena
- Tachycardia and hypotension (from acute or chronic blood loss)
- Boardlike abdomen and rebound tenderness (if perforated)
- Patient history that reveals predisposing factors, such as smoking, use of aspirin or other medications, or associated disorders

Diagnostic tests

- *Barium swallow* or *upper GI and small-bowel series* may reveal the presence of an ulcer. Barium swallow is the initial test performed on a patient whose symptoms aren't severe.
- *Endoscopy* is the major diagnostic test for peptic ulcers. It confirms ulcer presence and permits biopsy and cytologic studies to rule out *H. pylori* or cancer.
- *Upper GI tract X-rays* reveal abnormalities in the mucosa.
- *Laboratory analysis* may detect occult blood in stools and anemia from blood loss.
- *Serologic testing* may reveal an elevated white blood cell count as well as antibodies to *H. pylori.*
- *Gastric secretory studies* show hyperchlorhydria.
- *Urea breath test* may detect active *H. pylori* infection.

Treatment

Bismuth and two other antimicrobial agents, usually tetracycline or amoxicillin and metronidazole, are given to eradicate *H. pylori*. Antacids are given to reduce gastric acidity. A histamine-2 receptor antagonist, such as cimetidine or ranitidine, is used in the short term (up to 8 weeks) to reduce gastric secretions.

Sucralfate, given for duodenal ulcers, forms complexes with proteins at the base of an ulcer, making a protective coating that prevents further digestive action of acid and pepsin. Antisecretor

Causes of peptic ulcer

Although more research is needed to unveil the exact mechanisms of ulcer formation, several causative factors are known.

Helicobacter pylori

How *H. pylori* produces an ulcer isn't clear, but 9 of 10 ulcers may be caused by this bacteria. *H. pylori* has been found to release a toxin that promotes mucosal inflammation and ulceration. Acid seems to be mainly a contributor to the consequences of the bacterial infection rather than the dominant cause.

Drug therapy

Salicylates and other nonsteroidal anti-inflammatory drugs (NSAIDs), reserpine, or caffeine may erode the mucosal lining. NSAIDs may cause a gastric ulcer by inhibiting prostaglandins (the fatty acids) — particularly the E-series prostaglandins. These substances, present in large quantities in the gastric mucosa, inhibit injury by stimulating secretion of gastric mucus and gastric and duodenal mucosal bicarbonate (a neutralizing agent). They also promote gastric mucosal blood flow, maintain the integrity of the gastric mucosal barrier, and help renew the epithelium after a mucosal injury.

Certain illnesses

Pancreatitis, hepatic disease, Crohn's disease, preexisting gastritis, and Zollinger-Ellison syndrome are associated with ulcer development. In Zollinger-Ellison syndrome, gastrinomas (gastrin-secreting islet cell tumors commonly found in the pancreas) stimulate gastric acid secretion. This large volume of acid eventually erodes the gastric mucosa and contributes to ulcer formation.

Blood type

For unknown reasons, gastric ulcers commonly strike people with type A blood. Duodenal ulcers tend to afflict people with type O blood, perhaps because these people don't secrete blood group antigens (mucopolysaccharides, which may serve to protect the mucosa) in their saliva and other body fluids.

Genetic factors

Duodenal ulcers are about three times more common in first-degree relatives of duodenal ulcer patients than in the general population.

Exposure to irritants

Like certain other drugs, alcohol inhibits prostaglandin secretion, triggering a mechanism much like the one caused by NSAIDs. Cigarette smoking also appears to encourage ulcer formation by inhibiting pancreatic secretion of bicarbonate. It may also accelerate the emptying of gastric acid into the duodenum and promote mucosal breakdown.

Trauma

Critical illness, shock, or severe tissue injury from extensive burns or from intracranial surgery may lead to a stress ulcer.

Normal aging

The pyloric sphincter may wear down in the course of aging, which permits the reflux of bile into the stomach. This appears to be a common contributor to the development of gastric ulcers in older people.

agents, such as misoprostol, may be used if the ulceration resulted from NSAID use that must be continued for another condition such as arthritis. Sedatives and tranquilizers, such as chlordiazepoxide and phenobarbital, may be used for patients with gastric ulcers.

Anticholinergics, such as propantheline, are used to inhibit the vagus nerve effect on the parietal cells and to reduce gastrin production and excessive gastric activity in duodenal ulcers. (These drugs are usually contraindicated in gastric ulcers; they prolong gastric emptying and can aggravate the ulcer.)

Standard therapy also includes rest and decreased activity to help reduce gastric secretions. Diet therapy may consist of eating six small meals daily (or small hourly meals) rather than three regular meals. Usually, diet therapy involves the elimination of foods that cause distress, including nicotine, caffeine, and alcohol. Some physicians allow small amounts of alcohol with meals.

If GI bleeding occurs, emergency treatment includes passage of a nasogastric tube to provide a cool saline or water lavage, possibly containing norepinephrine. Gastroscopy allows visualization of the bleeding site and coagulation by laser or cautery to control bleeding. This therapy allows surgery to be postponed until the patient's condition stabilizes.

Surgery is indicated for perforation, unresponsiveness to conservative treatment, suspected cancer, and other complications. The type of surgery chosen for peptic ulcers depends on the location andextent of the ulcer. Choices include bilateral vagotomy, pyloroplasty, and gastrectomy.

Patients with gastric ulcers should have a repeat endoscopy after 4 to 6 weeks of treatment to assess healing and test for gastric corrosions.

Key nursing diagnoses and outcomes

Imbalanced nutrition: Less than body requirements related to adverse GI effects

Treatment outcome: The patient will exhibit no signs or symptoms of nutritional deficiencies.

Deficient knowledge related to peptic ulcer

Treatment outcome: The patient will communicate an understanding of peptic ulcer disease and his prescribed treatment.

Risk for imbalanced fluid volume related to bleeding

Treatment outcome: The patient will maintain normal fluid volume balance.

Acute pain related to mucosal injury

Treatment outcome: The patient's pain will be alleviated.

Nursing interventions

- Administer medications as prescribed. Monitor their effectiveness and watch for adverse reactions.
- Provide six small meals per day or small hourly meals, as ordered. Advise the patient to eat slowly, chew thoroughly, and have small snacks between meals. Strive for a relaxed and comfortable atmosphere during meals.
- Assess the patient's nutritional status and the effectiveness of measures used to maintain it. Weigh the patient daily.
- Support the patient emotionally and offer reassurance.
- Schedule care so that the patient gets plenty of rest.
- Prepare the patient for surgery, as indicated.
- Assess for pain every 4 hours.
- Continuously monitor the patient for complications: hemorrhage (sudden onset of weakness, fainting, chills, dizziness, thirst, the desire to defecate, and passage of loose, tarry, or even red stools), perforation (acute onset of epigastric pain, followed by lessening of the pain and the onset of a rigid abdomen, tachycardia, fever, or rebound tenderness), obstruction (feeling of fullness or heaviness, copious vomiting of undigested food after meals), and penetration (pain radiating to the back, night distress). If any of the above occurs, notify the physician immediately.

PATIENT TEACHING

▶ Teach the patient about peptic ulcer disease, and help him to recognize its signs and symptoms. Explain scheduled diagnostic tests and prescribed therapies. Review symptoms associated with complications, and urge him to notify the physician if any of these occur.

▶ Teach the patient to observe for overt and occult signs of bleeding.

▶ Emphasize the importance of complying with the prescribed treatment regimen even after symptoms disappear.

▶ Review the proper use of prescribed medications, including the desired actions and possible adverse effects of each drug.

▶ Instruct the patient to take antacids 1 hour after meals. If he has cardiac disease or follows a sodium-restricted diet, advise him to take low-sodium antacids. Caution him that antacids may cause changes in bowel habits (diarrhea with magnesium-containing antacids, constipation with aluminum-containing antacids) or affect absorption of other medications (advise him not to take them simultaneously).

▶ Warn the patient to avoid aspirin-containing drugs, reserpine, ibuprofen, indomethacin, and phenylbutazone because they irritate the gastric mucosa. Also, advise against excessive intake of coffee and alcoholic beverages during exacerbations.

▶ Tell the patient to avoid nonprescription medications that contain corticosteroids, aspirin, or other NSAIDs such as ibuprofen. Explain that these drugs inhibit mucus secretion and leave the GI tract vulnerable to injury from gastric acid. Advise him to use alternative analgesics such as acetaminophen. If steroid drugs are essential, advise the patient to take them with an antacid. Caution him to avoid systemic antacids, such as sodium bicarbonate, because they can cause an acid-base imbalance.

▶ Encourage the patient to make appropriate lifestyle changes such as reducing stress.

▶ If the patient smokes, urge him to stop because smoking stimulates gastric acid secretion. Refer him to a smoking-cessation program.

▶ Teach the patient to avoid foods that cause pain such as those that contain caffeine, if possible.

PERIPHERAL VASCULAR DISEASE

Peripheral vascular disease, which results from a reduced blood supply to the tissues, can occur in the arterial or venous system. The onset can be gradual or sudden. Buildup of atherosclerotic plaque in the vessels or changes in the vessels resulting from diabetes will cause a gradual onset. A sudden onset occurs when the vessel suddenly becomes occluded, such as by a thrombus, an embolus, or a traumatic injury. In older adults, peripheral vascular disease typically occurs as arteriosclerosis obliterans, aneurysms, varicose veins, and deep vein thrombosis (DVT).

Arteriosclerosis obliterans, a thickening of the walls of the arterioles, is the most common type of peripheral vascular disease among older adults. In this disorder, the vessels become stiff and lose their elasticity because of the buildup of arteriosclerotic plaque.

Aneurysms are abnormal dilations of an arterial wall that occur most commonly in men over age 50. The weakened wall can rupture, become occluded, or be the source of emboli. Age-related atherosclerotic changes in the medial layer of the arterial wall are the most common cause of aneurysms in the leg vessels of older adults. Calcium, cholesterol, and other lipids accumulate in the arteries, and increased amounts of connective tissue and mucopolysaccharides are found in the intima. The resulting loss of elasticity causes the vessels to dilate and elongate.

Varicose veins are tortuous vessels engorged with blood. They usually begin in middle age and may eventually cause venous insufficiency or venous stasis ulcers, especially around the ankles. Primary varicose veins tend to run in families and affect both legs; they're twice as common in women as in men. They can result from congenital weakness of the valves or venous wall, from conditions that produce prolonged venous stasis. Secondary varicose veins usually occur in only one leg. They result from disorders of the venous system, such as deep vein thrombophlebitis, trauma, and occlusion.

DVT is thrombophlebitis of the deep veins. Clots form in one of the large veins, usually in a leg. Because it affects the veins that carry 90% of venous outflow from the legs, DVT is more serious than superficial vein thrombophlebitis. Studies indicate that up to 35% of hospitalized patients develop this disorder, which occurs more commonly in people with a sedentary lifestyle and those who have limited mobility because of an acute or chronic illness (especially with lower extremity fracture, joint replacement, or surgery). The incidence of deep subclavian vein thrombophlebitis is increasing as the use of subclavian vein catheters becomes more common. Superficial vein thrombophlebitis is usually self-limiting. It's also less likely to cause complications because superficial veins have fewer valves than deep veins.

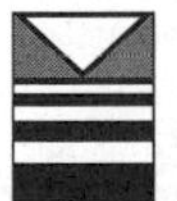

Key point Three factors — hypercoagulability, venous stasis, and endothelial damage — together cause thrombophlebitis. These factors are known as Virchow's triad.

Movement of blood through the veins is dependent on the pumping of the skeletal muscles through one-way valves. Any condition that results in decreased use of the skeletal muscles or that compromises the valves can lead to DVT. Risk factors include immobilization, decreased physical activity, venous damage, obesity, heart failure, polycythemia, thrombocytosis, dehydration, malignancy, hip fracture, and estrogen use. Once in place, DVT will further compromise the valves, contributing to the recurrent nature of this condition.

Although peripheral vascular disease can't be prevented, people can take steps to decrease the risk. (See *Living with peripheral vascular disease*.)

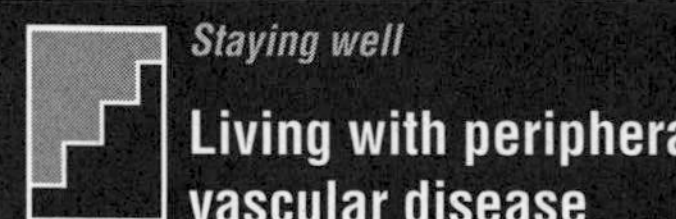

Staying well

Living with peripheral vascular disease

Peripheral vascular disease is commonly caused by atherosclerotic buildup within vessels. A diet with limited cholesterol intake, coupled with monitoring serum lipid levels and treating elevations, can limit this problem. Exercise increases circulation to the legs and should be started slowly after examination by a health care professional. Avoiding constrictive clothing and long periods of standing can limit varicose veins. Cigarette smoking is a major contributing factor to arterial insufficiency, so you should recommend a smoking cessation program to your patient to help prevent this process.

Signs and symptoms

Arteriosclerosis obliterans

- Intermittent claudication (pain with activity that subsides with rest); may progress to pain at rest in the older adult
- Cold feet and legs, edema, and trophic changes such as hair loss on the affected limb; thick toenails; dry, shiny, or atrophic skin; possibly ischemic ulcers on the toes and heels; dusky color when feet are in dependent position
- Possibly purple pregangrenous lesions or black, shriveled, and hard gangrenous lesions

Aneurysms

▶ Pain in the affected area (if the aneurysm is large enough to compress a nerve)
▶ Nonpulsating mass (if the artery is thrombosed)
▶ Pulsating mass in the upper thigh (with a femoral aneurysm)

Varicose veins

▶ Mild to severe leg symptoms, such as a heavy feeling that worsens in the evening and in warm weather; cramps at night; diffuse, dull aching after prolonged standing or walking; and fatigue (may be relieved by exercise, which improves venous return)
▶ Dilated, purplish, ropelike veins, particularly in the calf
▶ Nodules along affected veins and valve incompetence on palpation

Deep vein thrombosis

▶ New, rapidly occurring swelling of one limb with dependent edema (classic sign)
▶ Possible tenderness or a heavy, dull achiness in the involved extremity, commonly the calf (not affected by exercise)
▶ Possible fever, chills, and malaise
▶ Redness or swelling of the affected leg or arm
▶ Positive Homans' sign (pain in the affected calf) elicited by gentle dorsiflexion of the foot (reliablity is controversial)

Diagnostic tests

▶ *Arteriography* helps confirm the diagnosis and can disclose the type, location, and degree of an obstruction or aneurysm and the status of any collateral circulation.
▶ *Ultrasonography* determines the size of femoral and popliteal arteries and shows aneurysmal dilation, decreased blood flow distal to an arterial occlusion, or the presence or absence of venous backflow in deep or superficial veins. It's also the current diagnostic test of choice for DVT.
▶ *Computed tomography scan* confirms the size and location of an aneurysm. Segmental limb pressures and pulse volume measurements help evaluate the location and extent of an occlusion.
▶ *Photoplethysmography,* a noninvasive test, characterizes venous blood flow by noting changes in the skin's circulation. Venous outflow and reflux plethysmography can detect deep venous occlusion.
▶ *Ascending and descending venography* can demonstrate venous occlusion and patterns of collateral flow, but it's invasive and not routinely used.

Treatment

Arteriosclerosis obliterans

In mild, chronic occlusive disease, treatment usually consists of supportive measures. The physician may encourage the patient to quit smoking, to control hypertension, to reduce intake of cholesterol and saturated fats, to exercise mildly, and to provide foot and leg care. In more severe cases, drug therapy, surgery, or both may be necessary.

For persons with intermittent claudication caused by chronic arterial occlusive disease, pentoxifylline may be prescribed to improve blood flow through the capillaries. This drug is particularly useful for poor surgical candidates. Other prescribed drugs may include heparin to prevent emboli and dextran to reduce platelet adhesion and clot formation. Thrombolytics, such as urokinase, streptokinase, and alteplase, can dissolve clots and relieve the obstruction caused by a thrombus.

Acute arterial occlusive disease usually requires surgery—typically, embolectomy, thromboendarterectomy, or percutaneous transluminal coronary angioplasty. Intravascular stents may be placed in the iliac arteries.

Aneurysms

Aneurysms are usually repaired surgically.

Varicose veins

In mild or moderate forms, treatment may focus on self-care measures such as wearing elastic stockings; avoiding tight clothing and prolonged standing; elevating the legs; and walking or other exercise that promotes muscle contraction, minimizes venous pooling, and forces blood through the veins.

In severe cases, the physician may order custom-fitted, surgical-weight stockings with graduated pressure (highest at the ankle, lowest at the top). Stripping and ligation may be performed if the patient tires easily and has pain, heaviness, recurrent superficial thrombophlebitis, and external bleeding. For poor surgical risks, the physician may inject a sclerosing agent into small segments of affected veins.

Thrombophlebitis

Severe superficial vein thrombophlebitis may be treated with an anti-inflammatory drug (such as indomethacin), antiembolism stockings, warm compresses, and leg elevation.

For DVT, the physician may prescribe activity restrictions (bed rest with elevation of the affected arm or leg); drug therapy; application of warm, moist compresses to the affected area; and, in rare cases, surgery. Initial treatment usually includes anticoagulants (initially heparin, later warfarin).

For lysis of acute, extensive DVT, treatment may include streptokinase or urokinase, provided that the risk of bleeding doesn't outweigh the potential benefits of thrombolytic treatment.

Key nursing diagnoses and outcomes

Ineffective (peripheral) tissue perfusion related to narrowing or closure of peripheral arteries

Treatment outcome: The patient will regain adequate peripheral tissue perfusion.

Acute pain related to inflammation of peripheral veins

Treatment outcome: The patient will be free from pain when healing has occurred.

Nursing interventions

- ▶ Assess and record your patient's circulatory status, noting the location and quality of peripheral pulses in the affected leg.
- ▶ Administer prophylactic antibiotics, anticoagulants, and analgesics, as prescribed.
- ▶ If the patient is receiving anticoagulants, monitor coagulation times: activated partial thromboplastin time (APTT) for heparin therapy and prothrombin time (PT) and international normalized ratio (INR) for warfarin therapy. (Therapeutic values for APTT and PT are 1½ times the control; for the INR, a result between 2 and 3 is considered therapeutic.) Watch for signs and symptoms of bleeding, such as tarry stools, coffee-ground vomitus, bleeding gums, and ecchymoses. Also, monitor the patient for bleeding at I.V. sites.
- ▶ Remind the patient not to rub or massage the affected extremity. Place a cradle over the foot of the bed to keep the weight of the linens off the legs if needed.
- ▶ Measure and record the circumference of the affected arm or leg daily and compare it to measurements of the unaffected arm or leg. To ensure consistency, mark the skin where the measurement is taken.
- ▶ Assess the extremity daily for redness, tenderness, and signs of breakdown. Check the presence and status of peripheral pulses every 2 to 4 hours or as dictated by the patient's signs and symptoms.
- ▶ During an acute episode of DVT, enforce bed rest and elevate the affected limb until the episode subsides. After an acute episode, increase the patient's activities according to his tolerance level, and apply antiembolism stockings.

▶ To relieve limb pain caused by arterial occlusion, place the foot in a dependent position; limb elevation aggravates the pain. To ease pain caused by venous occlusion, elevate the limb.

▶ Provide clear and concise information about any impending surgery. Allow the patient to express his fears and anxieties about the disorder and about surgery, and provide emotional support. Encourage discussion about the impact the disorder will have on his life.

▶ Following surgery, carefully monitor the patient for early signs of thrombosis or graft occlusion, including severe pain, loss of pulse, or decreased skin temperature, sensation, and motor function. Monitor for signs of infection such as fever. Palpate distal pulses hourly for the first 24 hours and as ordered thereafter. Correlate your findings with those from the preoperative assessment. Mark the pulse sites on the patient's skin for future reference.

▶ Encourage the patient to walk to prevent venous stasis and thrombus formation. Administer a plasma volume expander such as dextran, as prescribed, to decrease platelet adhesion and prevent early graft closure.

▶ Observe the patient's behavior for nonverbal signs of pain. Administer analgesics, as prescribed, to alleviate pain.

PATIENT TEACHING

▶ Before surgery, teach the patient about surgical bypass and reconstruction of the artery. Review expected postoperative procedures, and answer any questions directly and honestly.

▶ After surgery, instruct the patient to report any indications of failure of the saphenous vein or prosthetic graft replacement, such as a faint or absent pulse, a pale or blue color in the leg or foot, or coldness to the touch in the leg or foot. If he has atherosclerosis, explain the risk for further arterial occlusions. Tell him to report the return of any preoperative symptoms, such as decreased motor function, evidence of leg ulcer or injury, pain in the extremity, or evidence of decreased blood flow to the affected area.

▶ Teach the patient how to care for his incision properly. Tell him to monitor the incision and report any drainage, redness, swelling, or tenderness in the area. Explain that persistent swelling may occur after popliteal artery resection. If antiembolism stockings are ordered, make sure they fit properly and demonstrate how to put them on. Emphasize the need to avoid constrictive clothing.

▶ If the patient is taking anticoagulants, emphasize the need to prevent bleeding. Instruct him to use an electric razor for shaving. Explain the importance of follow-up blood studies to monitor anticoagulant therapy. Caution against the use of tobacco and aspirin, and urge him to report evidence of bleeding, including bleeding gums, tarry stools, or bruising.

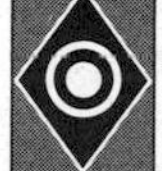

Drug alert Be aware that the excretion of pentoxifylline is slower in an older person, increasing the risk of drug toxicity. Stress the importance of reporting any adverse effects, such as headache, chest pain, dyspepsia, nausea, vomiting, bloating, flatus, and dizziness.

PERIPHERALLY INSERTED CENTRAL VENOUS CATHETER INSERTION AND CARE

For a patient who needs central venous (CV) therapy for 5 days to several months or who requires repeated venous access, a peripherally inserted central catheter (PICC) line may be the best option. The physician may order a PICC line for a patient who has suffered trauma or burns resulting in chest injury or who has respiratory compromise due to chronic obstructive pulmonary disease, a mediastinal mass, cystic fibrosis, or pneumothorax. In all of these conditions, a PICC line helps avoid complications that may occur with a CV line.

Made of silicone or polyurethane, a PICC is soft and flexible, with increased biocompatibility. It may range from 16G to 23G in diameter and from 16″ to 24″ (40.5 to 61 cm) in length. PICCs are available in single- and double-lumen versions, with or without guide wires. A guide wire stiffens the catheter, easing its advancement through the vein, but it can damage the vessel if used improperly.

PICC lines are being used increasingly for patients receiving home care. That's because they're easier to insert than other CV devices and provide safe, reliable access for drugs and blood sampling. A single catheter may be used for the entire course of therapy (approximately 1 to 140 days), resulting in greater convenience and reduced cost.

Infusions commonly given by PICC include total parenteral nutrition, chemotherapy, antibiotics, narcotics, analgesics, and blood products. PICC therapy works best when introduced early in treatment; it shouldn't be considered a last resort for patients with sclerotic or repeatedly punctured veins.

The patient receiving PICC therapy must have a peripheral vein large enough to accept the catheter. The physician or nurse inserts the PICC via the basilic, median antecubital, cubital, or cephalic vein. He then threads it to the superior vena cava or subclavian vein or to a noncentral site such as the axillary vein.

Supplies

- Catheter insertion kit
- Three alcohol swabs
- Three povidone-iodine swabs
- Povidone-iodine ointment
- 3-ml vial of heparin (100 units/ml)
- Latex injection port with short extension tubing
- Sterile and nonsterile measuring tape
- Vial of normal saline solution
- Sterile 2″ × 2″ and 4″ × 4″ gauze pads
- Tape
- Linen-saver pad
- Sterile drapes
- Tourniquet
- Sterile, transparent semipermeable dressing
- Two pairs of sterile gloves
- Gown
- Mask
- Goggles

Implementation

- Describe the procedure to your patient, and answer his questions.
- Gather the necessary supplies.

To insert a PICC

Note: Most regulating Boards require at least 8 hours of class time and three successful PICC insertions under the guidance of a preceptor before a nurse is considered PICC competent.

- Select the insertion site, and place the tourniquet on the patient's arm. Assess the antecubital fossa.
- If the patient will be receiving blood or blood products through the PICC line, use at least an 18G catheter.
- Remove the tourniquet.
- Determine catheter tip placement or the spot at which the catheter tip will rest after insertion. For placement in the subclavian vein, use the nonsterile measuring tape to measure the distance from the insertion site to the shoulder and from the shoulder to the sternal notch.
- For placement in the superior vena cava, measure the distance from the insertion site to the shoulder and from the shoulder to the sternal notch. Then add 3″ (7.6 cm).
- Have the patient lie in a supine position with his arm at a 90-degree angle to his body. Place a linen-saver pad under his arm.
- Open the PICC tray and drop the rest of the sterile items onto the sterile field.

Put on the sterile gown, mask, goggles, and gloves.

▶ Using the sterile measuring tape, cut the distal end of the catheter to the premeasured length. Cut the tip straight across to prevent the catheter from lying flush against the intima of the vein and possibly obstructing the infusion flow.

▶ Using sterile technique, withdraw 5 ml of the normal saline solution and flush the extension tubing and the latex cap.

▶ Remove the needle from the syringe. Attach the syringe to the hub of the catheter and flush.

▶ Prepare the insertion site by rubbing three alcohol swabs over it. Use a circular motion, working outward from the site about 6″ (15 cm). Repeat, using three povidone-iodine swabs. Pat the area dry with a sterile 4″ × 4″ gauze pad. Be sure not to touch the intended insertion site.

▶ Take off your gloves. Then apply the tourniquet about 4″ (10 cm) above the antecubital fossa.

▶ Put on a new pair of sterile gloves. Then place a sterile drape under the patient's arm and another on top of his arm. Drop a sterile 4″ × 4″ gauze pad over the tourniquet.

▶ Stabilize the patient's vein. Insert the catheter introducer at a 10-degree angle, directly into the vein.

▶ After successful vein entry, you should see a blood return in the flashback chamber. Without changing the needle's position, gently advance the plastic introducer sheath until you're sure the tip is well within the vein.

▶ Carefully withdraw the needle while holding the introducer still. To minimize blood loss, try applying finger pressure on the vein just beyond the distal end of the introducer sheath.

▶ Using sterile forceps, insert the catheter into the introducer sheath, and advance it into the vein. Remove the tourniquet using the 4″ × 4″ gauze pad.

▶ When you've advanced the catheter to the shoulder, ask the patient to turn his head toward the affected arm and place his chin on his chest. This will occlude the jugular vein and ease the catheter's advancement into the subclavian vein.

▶ Advance the catheter until about 4″ remains. Then pull the introducer sheath out of the vein and away from the introducer site.

▶ Grasp the blue tabs of the introducer sheath, and flex them toward its distal end to split the sheath.

▶ With the patient's arm below heart level, remove the syringe. Connect the capped extension set to the hub of the catheter.

▶ Ask the patient if he's having any pain associated with the therapy. If so, determine the pain's cause and take appropriate steps to alleviate it.

▶ Apply a sterile 2″ × 2″ gauze pad directly over the site and a sterile transparent semipermeable dressing over that. Leave this dressing in place for 24 hours.

▶ Assess the catheter insertion site through the transparent semipermeable dressing every 24 hours. Look at the catheter and check for any bleeding, redness, drainage, and swelling. Although bleeding is common for the first 24 hours after insertion, excessive bleeding after that period of time must be evaluated.

▶ After the initial 24 hours, apply a new sterile transparent semipermeable dressing. The gauze pad is no longer necessary. You can place Steri-Strips over the catheter wings. Flush with heparin solution.

To administer drugs

▶ With any CV line, be sure to check for blood return and flush with normal saline solution before administering a drug through a PICC line.

▶ Clamp the 7″ (17.8 cm) extension tubing, and connect the empty syringe to the tubing. Release the clamp and aspirate slowly to verify blood return.

Flush with 3 ml of normal saline solution; then administer the drug.

▶ After giving the drug, flush again with 3 ml of normal saline solution. (Also, remember to flush with the same solution between infusions of incompatible drugs or fluids.)

▶ A declotting agent, such as urokinase, can be used to clear a clotted PICC line by a physician or a PICC-certified nurse.

To change the dressing

▶ Change the dressing every 4 days for an inpatient and every 5 to 7 days for a home care patient. If possible, choose a transparent semipermeable dressing, which has a high moisture-vapor transmission rate. Use sterile technique.

▶ Wash your hands and assemble the necessary supplies. Position the patient with his arm extended away from his body at a 45- to 90-degree angle. Put on a sterile mask.

▶ Open a package of sterile gloves and use the inside of the package as a sterile field. Then open the transparent semipermeable dressing and drop it onto the field. Remove the old dressing by holding your left thumb on the catheter and stretching the dressing parallel to the skin. Repeat this step with your right thumb holding the catheter. Free the remaining section of the dressing from the catheter by peeling toward the insertion site from the distal end to the proximal end to prevent catheter dislodgment.

▶ Put on the sterile gloves. Clean the area thoroughly with three alcohol swabs, starting at the insertion site and working outward from the site. Repeat this step three times with povidone-iodine swabs and pat dry.

▶ Apply the dressing carefully. Secure the tubing to the edge of the dressing over the tape with ¼" adhesive tape.

To remove a PICC

▶ You'll remove a PICC when therapy is complete, if the catheter becomes damaged or broken and can't be repaired or, possibly, if the line becomes occluded. Measure the catheter after you remove it to ensure that the line has been removed intact and thus help prevent embolus formation in the catheter.

▶ Assemble the necessary equipment at the patient's bedside.

▶ Wash your hands and place a linen-saver pad under the patient's arm.

▶ Remove the tape holding the extension tubing. Open two sterile gauze pads on a clean, flat surface. Put on clean gloves. Stabilize the catheter at the hub with one hand. Without dislodging the catheter, use your other hand to gently remove the dressing by pulling it toward the insertion site.

▶ Next, gently tug on the PICC, it should come out easily. If you feel resistance, apply tension to the line by taping it down. Then try removing it again in a few minutes.

▶ Once you successfully remove the catheter, apply manual pressure to the site with a sterile gauze pad for 1 minute.

▶ Cover the site with the povidone-iodine ointment, and tape a new folded gauze pad in place. Dispose of used items properly, and wash your hands.

▶ Measure and inspect the catheter. If any part has broken off during removal, notify the physician immediately, and monitor the patient for signs of distress.

▶ For a hospital patient receiving intermittent PICC therapy, flush the catheter with 6 ml of normal saline solution and 6 ml of heparin (10 units/ml) after each use. For catheters that aren't being used, a weekly flush of 2 ml (1,000 units/ml) of heparin will maintain patency.

▶ PICC lines can remain in place for up to 12 months.

Complications

PICC therapy causes fewer and less severe complications than conventionally placed CV lines. Phlebitis, perhaps the most common complication, may occur during the first 48 to 72 hours after PICC insertion. It's more common in left-sided insertions and when a large-gauge catheter is used.

Air embolism, always a risk of venipuncture, poses less danger with PICCs than with traditional CV lines because the line is inserted below heart level. Some patients complain of pain at the catheter's insertion site, usually from chemical properties of the infused drug or fluid.

Catheter tip migration may occur with vigorous flushing. Patients receiving chemotherapy are most vulnerable to this complication because of frequent nausea and vomiting and subsequent changes in intrathoracic pressure. Catheter occlusion is a relatively common complication.

Patient teaching

▶ Teach the patient and his family about the PICC line and its care.

▶ Tell them which complications associated with PICC therapy to watch for.

Documentation

Document the entire procedure, including the size and type of catheter used, the insertion site, and any problems with catheter placement. Also document your patient teaching measures and ongoing site checks with each patient assessment.

PERITONEAL DIALYSIS

Like hemodialysis, peritoneal dialysis removes toxins from the blood of a patient with acute or chronic renal failure who doesn't respond to other treatments. But unlike hemodialysis, it uses the patient's peritoneal membrane as a semipermeable dialyzing membrane.

In this technique, a hypertonic dialyzing solution is instilled through a catheter inserted into the peritoneal cavity. (See *Catheters for peritoneal dialysis.*) Then, by diffusion, excessive concentrations of electrolytes and uremic toxins in the blood move across the peritoneal membrane and into the dialysis solution. Next, by osmosis, excessive water in the blood does the same. After an appropriate dwelling time, the dialysis solution is drained, taking toxins and wastes with it.

Peritoneal dialysis may be performed manually, by an automatic or semiautomatic cycler machine, or as continuous ambulatory peritoneal dialysis (CAPD). In manual dialysis, the nurse, the patient, or a family member instills dialyzing solution through the catheter into the peritoneal cavity, allows it to dwell for a specified time, and then drains it from the peritoneal cavity. Typically, this process is repeated for 4 to 8 hours at a time, five or six times per week.

The cycler machine requires aseptic setup and connection technique, and then it automatically completes dialysis.

CAPD is performed by the patient himself. He fills a special plastic bag with dialyzing solution and then instills the solution through a catheter into his peritoneal cavity. While the solution remains in the peritoneal cavity, the patient can roll up the empty bag, place it under his clothing, and go about his normal activities. After 4 to 8 hours of dwelling time, he drains the spent solution into the bag, removes and discards the full bag, and attaches a new bag and instills a new batch of dialyzing solution. He repeats the process to ensure continuous dialysis 24 hours a day, 7 days a week. As its name implies, CAPD allows the patient to be out of bed and active during dialysis and thus only minimally disrupts his lifestyle.

Some patients use CAPD in combination with an automatic cycler, in a treatment called continuous-cycling peritoneal dialysis (CCPD). In CCPD, the cycler performs dialysis at night while the patient sleeps and the patient performs cycling peritoneal dialysis in the daytime.

Peritoneal dialysis has several advantages over hemodialysis: It's simpler, less costly, and less stressful. What's more,

Catheters for peritoneal dialysis

The first step in any type of peritoneal dialysis is insertion of a catheter to allow instillation of dialyzing fluid. The surgeon may insert one of three different catheters, as described here.

Tenckhoff catheter

To implant a Tenckhoff catheter, the surgeon inserts the first 6¾″ (17 cm) of the catheter into the patient's abdomen. He then imbeds the next 2¾″ (7 cm) segment, which has a Dacron cuff at each end, subcutaneously. Within a few days after insertion, the patient's tissues grow around these Dacron cuffs, forming a tight barrier against bacterial infiltration. The remaining 3⅞″ (10 cm) of the catheter extends outside the abdomen and is equipped with a metal adapter at the tip to allow connection to dialyzer tubing.

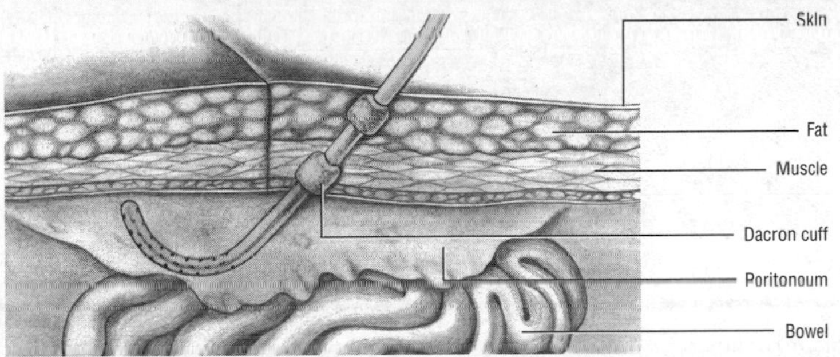

Flanged-collar catheter

To insert this kind of catheter, the surgeon positions its flanged collar just below the skin so that the device extends through the abdominal wall. He keeps the distal end of the cuff from extending into the peritoneum, where it could cause adhesions.

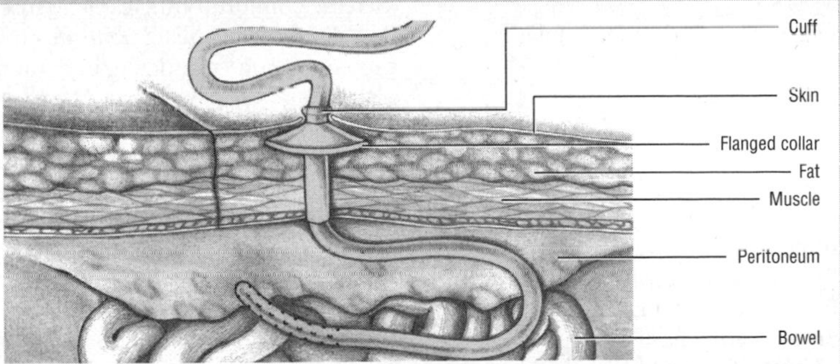

(continued)

Catheters for peritoneal dialysis *(continued)*

Column-disk peritoneal catheter

To insert a column-disk peritoneal catheter, the surgeon rolls up the flexible disk section of the implant, inserts it into the peritoneal cavity, and retracts it against the abdominal wall. The implant's first cuff rests just outside the peritoneal membrane; the second cuff rests just beneath the skin. Because the column-disk peritoneal catheter doesn't float freely in the peritoneal cavity, it keeps inflowing dialyzing solution from being directed at sensitive organs; this increases patient comfort during dialysis.

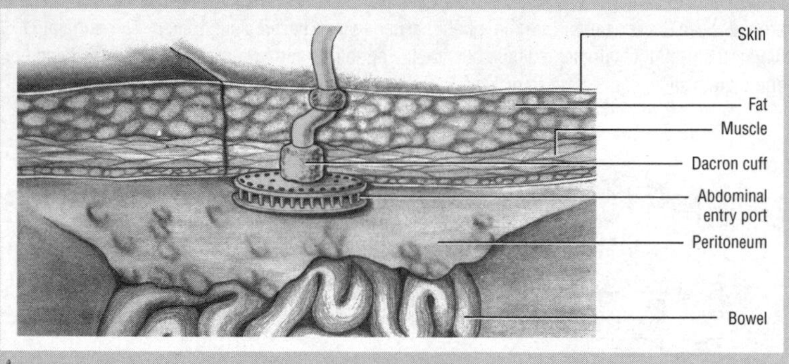

it's nearly as effective as hemodialysis while posing fewer risks.

Supplies

- Prescribed dialysate
- Warmer, heating pad, or water bath
- Masks
- Dialysis administration set with drainage bags
- Sterile gloves
- I.V. pole
- Sterile drape
- Peritoneal dialysis catheter
- Povidone-iodine solution (to prepare abdomen)
- Precut drain dressing
- Protective cap for catheter
- Small, sterile plastic clamp
- 4″ × 4″ gauze pads

Implementation

Before the procedure

- Explain the procedure to the patient if it's his first time.
- Before catheter insertion, take and record the patient's baseline vital signs and weight. (Be sure to check blood pressure in both the supine and standing positions.) Ask him to urinate to reduce the risk of bladder perforation and increase comfort during catheter insertion. If he can't urinate, perform straight catheterization, as ordered, to drain the bladder.
- While the patient is undergoing peritoneal catheter insertion, warm the dialysate to body temperature in a warmer, heating pad, or water bath. The dialysate may be a 1.5%, 2.5%, or 4.25% dextrose solution, usually with heparin added to prevent clotting in the catheter. The dialysate should be clear and colorless. Add any prescribed drugs at this time.
- Next, put on a surgical mask and prepare the dialysis administration set. Place the drainage bag below the patient to facilitate gravity drainage, and connect the outflow tubing to it. Then con-

nect the dialysis infusion lines to the bags or bottles of dialyzing solution, and hang the containers on an I.V. pole at the patient's bedside. Maintain sterile technique during solution and equipment preparation to avoid introducing pathogens into the patient's peritoneal cavity during dialysis.

▶ When the equipment and solution are ready, place the patient in the supine position, have him put on a surgical mask, and tell him to relax. Prime the tubing with solution, keeping the clamps closed, and connect one infusion line to the abdominal catheter.

▶ To test the catheter's patency, open the clamp on the infusion line and rapidly instill 500 ml of dialyzing solution into the patient's peritoneal cavity. Immediately unclamp the outflow line and let fluid drain into the collection bag; outflow should be brisk. Once you've established catheter patency, you're ready to start dialysis.

During the procedure

▶ To begin dialysis, open the clamps on the infusion lines and infuse the prescribed amount of dialyzing solution over 5 to 10 minutes. When the bottle is empty, close the clamps immediately to prevent air from entering the tubing.

▶ Allow the solution to dwell in the peritoneal cavity for the prescribed amount of time (usually between 10 minutes and 4 hours) so that excess water, electrolytes, and accumulated wastes can move from the blood through the peritoneal membrane and into the solution. After the prescribed dwelling time, open the outflow clamps and allow the solution to drain from the peritoneal cavity into the collection bag.

▶ Repeat the infusion-dwell-drainage cycle, using new solution each time, until you've instilled the prescribed amount of solution and completed the prescribed number of cycles.

▶ During dialysis, monitor the patient's vital signs every 10 minutes until they stabilize, then every 2 to 4 hours or as ordered. Report any abrupt or significant changes.

▶ Watch closely for developing complications. Peritonitis may be manifested by fever, persistent abdominal pain and cramping, slow or cloudy dialysis drainage, swelling and tenderness around the catheter, and an increased white blood cell count. If you detect any of these signs and symptoms, notify the physician and send a dialysate specimen to the laboratory for smear and culture.

▶ Observe the outflow drainage for blood. Keep in mind that drainage is commonly blood tinged after catheter placement but should clear after a few fluid exchanges. Notify the physician of bright-red or persistent bleeding.

▶ Watch for respiratory distress, which may indicate fluid overload or leakage of dialyzing solution into the pleural space. If it's severe, drain the patient's peritoneal cavity and call the physician.

▶ Periodically check the outflow tubing for clots or kinks that may be obstructing drainage. If you can't clear an obstruction, notify the physician.

▶ Have the patient change position frequently. Provide passive range-of-motion exercises, and encourage deep breathing and coughing. This will improve patient comfort, reduce the risk of skin breakdown and respiratory problems, and enhance dialysate drainage.

After the procedure

▶ When dialysis is completed, put on sterile gloves and clamp the catheter with a small, sterile plastic clamp. Disconnect the inflow line from the catheter, taking care not to dislodge or pull on the catheter, and place a sterile protective cap over the catheter's distal end.

▶ Apply povidone-iodine or antibiotic ointment to the catheter insertion site with a sterile gauze dressing, then place two split-drain dressings around the site and secure them with tape.

▶ Using sterile technique, change the catheter dressing every 24 hours or whenever it becomes wet or soiled.

▶ To help prevent fluid imbalance, calculate the patient's fluid balance at the end of each dialysis session or after every 8-hour period in a longer session. Include both oral and I.V. fluid intake as well as urine output, wound drainage, and perspiration. Record and report any significant imbalance, either positive or negative.
▶ Maintain adequate nutrition, and make sure the patient follows the prescribed diet. Keep in mind that the patient loses protein through the dialysis procedure and therefore requires protein replacement.
▶ Periodically check the patient's weight, and report any gain.
▶ If possible, introduce the patient to other patients on peritoneal dialysis to help him develop a support system. Arrange for periodic visits by a home care nurse to assess his adjustment to CAPD or cycling peritoneal dialysis.

Complications

Peritoneal dialysis can cause severe complications. The most serious one, peritonitis, is caused by bacteria entering the peritoneal cavity through the catheter or the insertion site. Other complications include catheter obstruction from clots, lodgment against the abdominal wall or kinking, hypotension, hypovolemia from excessive plasma fluid removal, pain, exit site and tunnel infections, insufficient flow of dialysate, and dialysate leakage.

Patient teaching

▶ For the first-time peritoneal dialysis patient, explain the purpose of the treatment and what he can expect during and after the procedure. Tell him that the physician will first insert a catheter into his abdomen to allow instillation of dialyzing solution; explain the appropriate insertion procedure.
▶ If the patient will perform CAPD or cycling peritoneal dialysis at home, make sure he thoroughly understands and can perform each step of the procedure. Normally, he'll go through a 2-week training program before beginning treatment on his own.
▶ Instruct the patient to wear a medical identification bracelet or carry a card identifying him as a dialysis patient. Also, tell him to keep the phone number of the dialysis center on hand at all times in case of an emergency.
▶ Tell the patient to watch for and report signs of infection and fluid imbalance. Make sure he knows how to take his vital signs to provide a record of response to treatment.
▶ Stress the importance of follow-up appointments with the physician and dialysis team to evaluate the success of treatment and detect any problems.

Documentation

Record the amount of dialysate infused and drained, any medications added to the solution, and the color and character of effluent. Also record the patient's daily weight and fluid balance. Use a peritoneal dialysis flowchart to compute total fluid balance after each exchange. Note the patient's vital signs and tolerance of the procedure and other pertinent observations.

PERITONITIS

An acute or chronic disorder, peritonitis is an inflammation of the peritoneum, the membrane that lines the abdominal cavity and covers the visceral organs. The inflammation may extend throughout the peritoneum or be localized as an abscess. Peritonitis commonly decreases intestinal motility and causes intestinal distention with flatus. Mortality is about 10%, with bowel obstruction the usual cause of death.

Although the GI tract normally contains bacteria, the peritoneum is sterile. In peritonitis, bacteria invade the peritoneum, usually as a result of inflammation and perforation of the GI tract due to a particular GI disorder (appendicitis, diverticulitis, peptic ulcer, volvulus, strangulated obstruction, abdominal neoplasm, or abdominal trauma). Peritonitis may also be caused by chemical inflammation after rupture of the bladder, perforation of a gastric ulcer, or released pancreatic enzymes.

In both bacterial and chemical inflammation, fluid containing protein and electrolytes accumulates in the peritoneal cavity and makes the transparent peritoneum opaque, red, inflamed, and edematous. Because the peritoneal cavity is so resistant to contamination, such infection is commonly localized as an abscess instead of disseminated as a generalized infection.

Peritonitis can lead to abscess formation, septicemia, respiratory compromise, bowel obstruction, and shock from third spacing of fluid into the peritoneal cavity.

Signs and symptoms

Early phase

- Vague, generalized abdominal pain or, in localized peritonitis, pain over a specific area (usually the inflammation site)
- Bowel sounds disclosed by auscultation

Later phase

- Increasingly severe and unremitting abdominal pain that may increase with movement and breathing; sometimes referred to the shoulder or thoracic area
- Abdominal distention, rigidity, and guarding
- Anorexia, nausea, and vomiting
- Inability to pass feces and flatus
- Fever (may not be present in older adult) and chills
- Tachycardia (in response to the fever)
- Hypotension
- Pain-avoiding behavior (lying very still in bed, often with knees flexed; shallow breathing; little movement)
- Decreased or absent bowel sounds on auscultation
- Rebound tenderness on palpation
- Tachypnea or dyspnea

Diagnostic tests

- *Blood studies* show leukocytosis (commonly a white blood cell count of more than 20,000/μl but may be less in an older adult)
- *Arterial blood gas analysis* reveals metabolic acidosis with respiratory compensation.
- *Abdominal X-rays* demonstrate edematous and gaseous distention of the small and large bowel. With perforation of a visceral organ, the X-ray shows air in the abdominal cavity.
- *Chest X-rays* may reveal elevation of the diaphragm.
- *Paracentesis* discloses the nature of the exudate and permits bacterial culture so appropriate antibiotic therapy can be instituted.
- *Computed tomography scan* of the abdomen or an abdominal and pelvic ultrasound may reveal abscess formation.

Treatment

To prevent peritonitis, early treatment of GI inflammatory conditions and preoperative and postoperative antibiotic therapy are important. After peritonitis develops, emergency treatment must combat infection, restore intestinal motility, and replace fluids and electrolytes.

Antibiotic therapy depends on the infecting organism but usually includes administration of cefoxitin with an aminoglycoside, or penicillin G and clindamycin with an aminoglycoside.

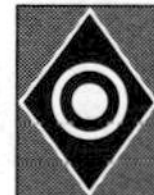

Drug alert Because many older adults have decreased renal function, they're at increased risk for nephrotoxicity from aminoglycoside therapy. Monitor renal function closely in these patients.

To decrease peristalsis and prevent perforation, the patient should receive nothing by mouth; instead, he requires supportive fluids and electrolytes parenterally.

Supplementary treatment includes administration of a narcotic analgesic such as morphine, nasogastric (NG) intubation to decompress the bowel, and possibly use of a rectal tube to facilitate the passage of flatus.

Surgery, which is necessary as soon as the patient's condition is stable enough to tolerate it, aims to control the source of the peritonitis. For example, an appendectomy may be performed for a ruptured appendix or a colon resection for a ruptured colon.

Peritoneal lavage may also be performed to remove the infected contents of the peritoneum and to prevent recurrent infection. Peritoneal lavage may be carried out laparoscopically.

Key nursing diagnoses and outcomes

Ineffective (GI) tissue perfusion related to inflammatory process

Treatment outcome: The patient will regain normal GI function with treatment.

Risk for imbalanced fluid volume related to excessive fluid loss into abdomen

Treatment outcome: The patient will maintain hemodynamic stability, as exhibited by normal vital signs.

Acute pain related to inflammatory process

Treatment outcomes: The patient will express feelings of comfort after analgesic administration and will comply with antibiotic therapy to alleviate inflammation and pain.

Nursing interventions

- Provide psychological support, and offer reassurance when appropriate.
- Administer prescribed medications, such as narcotic analgesics and antibiotics, as ordered. Monitor the patient for the desired effects of medications and possible adverse reactions to them.
- Maintain parenteral fluid and electrolyte administration, as ordered.
- Place the patient in semi-Fowler's position to help him breathe deeply with less pain and thus prevent pulmonary complications. Keep him on bed rest.
- Counteract mouth and nose dryness due to fever, dehydration, and NG intubation with regular hygiene and lubrication.
- Prepare the patient for surgery, as indicated. After surgery, monitor the patient for complications if appropriate.
- Assess fluid volume by checking mucous membranes, urine output, weight, vital signs, amount of NG tube drainage, and amount of I.V. infusion. Record intake and output, including NG tube drainage.
- If necessary, refer the patient to the social services department or a home health care agency that can help him obtain needed services during convalescence.

PATIENT TEACHING

- Teach the patient about peritonitis, what caused it, and necessary treatments.
- Review the proper use of prescribed medications, including correct administration, desired effects, and possible adverse effects.
- Provide preoperative teaching, and review postoperative care procedures.

PET THERAPY

Pets can combat loneliness in an elderly patient and help bridge the gap between the patient and the health care provider. Commonly used in long-term care facilities, pet therapy helps the older patient break through apathy and depression and improves interaction with others. Some facilities adopt a pet as a mascot for the facility and let the residents share responsibility for caring for it. Sharing responsibility for the pet builds a sense of community.

When compared with people who don't own pets, community dwelling elderly people who own pets have been found to have better activities of daily living levels, better exercise tolerance and lower serum cholesterol levels. In addition, they have fewer visits to the health care system. They also exhibit reduced stress and loneliness, enhanced emotional status, and better coping ability.

Implementation

- Select a pet that is well-behaved and has a good temperament. Pets that have gone through obedience training are ideal.
- Make sure the pet is cleared by a veterinarian and is up-to-date on his immunizations.
- If the pet is chosen as a mascot for the facility, have a responsible person make a schedule for residents who are interested in caring for the pet.
- The Delta Society, the national pet therapy organization, has branches in most major cities. Animals and owners must pass rigorous testing before being certified as a pet therapy team that can visit facilities. There's no charge for pet therapy through this organization.
- Allow the patient to play with and hold the pet. Encourage him to talk to the pet and reminisce about pets he once had. Provide as much time as he needs with the pet, if possible.

Special considerations

Ensure that the environment is appropriate for pet therapy. The facility should have an area where the pet can retreat and be kept out of the way of patients who are allergic to animals, have no interest in pets, or are afraid of them.

PLEURAL EFFUSION AND EMPYEMA

Normally, the pleural space contains a small amount of extracellular fluid that lubricates the pleural surfaces. However, if fluid builds up from either increased production or inadequate removal, pleural effusion results. An accumulation of pus and necrotic tissue in the pleural space results in empyema, a type of pleural effusion. Blood (hemothorax) and chyle (chylothorax) may also collect in this space.

The incidence of pleural effusion increases with heart failure (the most common cause), parapneumonia, cancer, and pulmonary embolism. (See *What causes pleural effusion?* page 468.) Pleural effusion may be transudative or exudative.

Empyema is usually caused by an infection in the pleural space. The infection may be idiopathic or may be related to pneumonitis, cancer, perforation, penetrating chest trauma, or esophageal rupture.

Signs and symptoms

- Dyspnea
- Pleuritic chest pain (in pleurisy)
- Fever and general feeling of malaise (in empyema)
- Trachea deviated away from the affected side
- Decreased tactile fremitus (with a large amount of effusion)
- Dullness over the effused area that doesn't change with respiration (on percussion)
- Diminished or absent breath sounds over the effusion; transitory pleural friction rub during both inspiration and expiration
- Patient history that shows underlying pulmonary disease (characteristically)

Diagnostic tests

- *Thoracentesis* allows analysis of aspirated fluid and may show the following:
  - Transudative effusion usually has a specific gravity below 1.015 and contains less than 3 g/dl of protein.
  - Exudative effusion has a ratio of protein in the fluid to serum of more than or equal to 0.5, pleural fluid lactate dehydrogenase (LD) of greater than or

What causes pleural effusion?

Transudative and exudative pleural effusions result from various disorders and conditions. Pleural effusion may also occur as a result of medications, such as chemotheraputic agents, sclerosing agents for esophageal varices, and other medications commonly used in elderly patients.

Transudative pleural effusion

An ultrafiltrate of plasma containing a low concentration of protein, a transudative pleural effusion may be caused by heart failure, hepatic disease with ascites, peritoneal dialysis, hypoalbuminemia, or disorders that increase intravascular volume.

The effusion stems from an imbalance of osmotic and hydrostatic pressures. Normally, the balance of these pressures in parietal pleural capillaries causes fluid to move into the pleural space; balanced pressure in visceral pleural capillaries promotes reabsorption of this fluid. However, when excessive hydrostatic pressure or decreased osmotic pressure causes excessive fluid to pass across intact capillaries, a transudative pleural effusion results.

Exudative pleural effusion

An exudative pleural effusion can result from tuberculosis, subphrenic abscess, pancreatitis, bacterial or fungal pneumonitis or empyema, cancer, parapneumonia, pulmonary embolism (with or without infarction), collagen disease (lupus erythematosus and rheumatoid arthritis), myxedema, intra-abdominal abscess, esophageal perforation, or chest trauma.

This type of effusion occurs when capillary permeability increases, with or without changes in hydrostatic and colloid osmotic pressures, allowing protein-rich fluid to leak into the pleural space.

equal to 200 IU, and a ratio of LD in pleural fluid to LD in serum of more than or equal to 0.6.

– Aspirated fluid in empyema contains acute inflammatory white blood cells and microorganisms and reveals leukocytosis.

– Fluid in empyema and rheumatoid arthritis — which can be the cause of an exudative pleural effusion — shows an extremely decreased pleural fluid glucose level.

– Pleural effusion that results from esophageal rupture or pancreatitis usually has fluid amylase levels higher than serum levels.

▶ A negative *tuberculin skin test* helps rule out tuberculosis as a cause.

▶ *Pleural biopsy* can help confirm tuberculosis or cancer, if thoracentesis doesn't provide a definitive diagnosis in exudative pleural effusion.

▶ Aspirated fluid may also be tested for lupus erythematosus cells, antinuclear antibodies, and neoplastic cells. Plus, it may be analyzed for color and consistency; acid-fast bacillus, fungal, and bacterial cultures; and triglycerides (in chylothorax).

Treatment

Depending on the amount of fluid present, symptomatic effusion may require thoracentesis to remove fluid or careful monitoring of the patient's own reabsorption of the fluid.

Chemical pleurodesis — the instillation of a sclerosing agent, such as tetracycline, bleomycin, or nitrogen mustard through the chest tube to create adhesions between the two pleura — can prevent recurrent effusions. Pleurectomy or pleural stripping is a surgical procedure that consists of stripping the parietal pleura away from the visceral pleura. This intensely inflammatory process causes an adhesion to form between the two layers, which prevents recurrent pleural effusions.

The patient with empyema needs one or more chest tubes inserted after thoracentesis. These tubes allow purulent material to drain. He may also need surgical treatment that includes decortication (removal of the thick coating over the lung) and rib resection to allow open drainage and lung expansion. He'll also require parenteral antibiotics and oxygen (if hypoxia is present).

Hemothorax requires drainage to prevent fibrothorax formation.

Key nursing diagnoses and outcomes

Risk for infection related to introduction of foreign object (thoracentesis needle, chest tube, or both) into chest cavity

Treatment outcome: The patient will remain free from infection, as evidenced by a normal temperature and white blood cell count.

Impaired gas exchange related to ineffective breathing pattern

Treatment outcome: The patient will maintain adequate ventilation with treatment.

Ineffective breathing pattern related to compromised lung expansion

Treatment outcome: The patient will regain his normal breathing pattern when the condition is eradicated.

Nursing interventions

- Prepare the patient for thoracentesis, as indicated, and reassure him throughout the procedure.
- Prepare the patient for chest tube insertion, as indicated.
- Provide meticulous chest tube care; if the patient has empyema, use sterile technique to change dressings around the tube insertion site.
- Ensure chest tube patency by watching for bubbles in the underwater-seal chamber. Record the amount, color, and consistency of any tube drainage.
- Keep petroleum gauze at the bedside in case of chest tube dislodgment.
- Don't clamp the chest tube; doing so may cause tension pneumothorax.
- If the patient has open drainage through a rib resection or intercostal tube, use secretion precautions. The patient will usually need weeks of such drainage to obliterate the empyema, so make home health nurse referrals if he'll be discharged with the tube in place.
- Administer oxygen and, in empyema, antibiotics, as ordered. Record the patient's response to these care measures, and monitor him for adverse reactions to the medications.
- Use an incentive spirometer to promote deep breathing, and encourage the patient to perform deep-breathing exercises to promote lung expansion.
- Monitor the patient's respiratory status frequently. Obtain arterial blood gas analysis if signs and symptoms of hypoxia develop.
- Throughout therapy, listen to the patient's fears and concerns and remain with him during periods of extreme stress and anxiety. Encourage him to identify care measures and actions that will make him comfortable and relaxed. Then try to perform these measures and encourage the patient to do so, too.
- After thoracentesis, watch for respiratory distress and signs of pneumothorax (sudden onset of dyspnea and cyanosis).

PATIENT TEACHING

- Explain all tests and procedures to the patient, and answer any questions he may have.
- Before thoracentesis, tell the patient to expect a stinging sensation from the local anesthetic and a feeling of pressure when the needle is inserted. Instruct him to tell you immediately if he feels uncomfortable or has trouble breathing during the procedure.
- If the patient developed pleural effusion because of pneumonia or influenza, tell him to seek medical attention promptly whenever he gets a chest cold.
- Teach the patient the signs and symptoms of respiratory distress. If any of these develop, tell him to notify his physician.

▶ Fully explain the drug regimen, including possible adverse effects. Emphasize the importance of completing the prescribed drug regimen.
▶ If the patient smokes, urge him to stop.

PNEUMONIA

An acute infection of the lung parenchyma that commonly impairs gas exchange, pneumonia can be classified in several ways. Based on microbiological etiology, it may be classified as viral, bacterial, fungal, protozoal, mycobacterial, mycoplasmal, or rickettsial in origin. Based on location, pneumonia may be classified as bronchopneumonia, lobular pneumonia, or lobar pneumonia. Bronchopneumonia involves distal airways and alveoli; lobular pneumonia, part of a lobe; and lobar pneumonia, an entire lobe.

The infection can also be classified as one of three types: primary, secondary, or aspiration pneumonia. Primary pneumonia results directly from inhalation or aspiration of a pathogen, such as a bacterium or a virus; it includes pneumococcal and viral pneumonia. Secondary pneumonia may follow initial lung damage from a noxious chemical or another insult (superinfection), or it may result from hematogenous spread of bacteria from a distant area. Aspiration pneumonia results from inhalation of foreign matter, such as vomitus or food particles, into the bronchi.

Pneumonia occurs in both sexes and at all ages. Older adults run a greater risk for developing it because their weakened chest musculature reduces their ability to clear secretions. Those in long-term care facilities are particularly susceptible. The infection carries a good prognosis for patients with normal lungs and an adequate immune system. However, bacterial pneumonia is the leading cause of death in debilitated patients. Pneumonia is also the leading cause of death from infectious disease in the United States.

The decreased immune response and decreased mobility of older people increase their likelihood of developing pneumonia. Other predisposing factors include chronic illness and debilitation, cancer (particularly lung cancer), abdominal and thoracic surgery, atelectasis, common colds and other viral respiratory infections, chronic respiratory disease, influenza, smoking, malnutrition, alcoholism, tracheostomy, exposure to noxious gases, aspiration, and immunosuppressive therapy. Aspiration pneumonia occurs in older or debilitated people, those receiving nasogastric (NG) tube feedings, and those with an impaired gag reflex, poor oral hygiene, or a decreased level of consciousness.

Bacterial pneumonia is the most common type of pneumonia found in older adults; viral pneumonia, the second most common type. In bacterial pneumonia, which can occur in any part of the lungs, an infection initially triggers alveolar inflammation and edema. Capillaries become engorged with blood, causing stasis. As the alveolocapillary membrane breaks down, alveoli fill with blood and exudate, resulting in atelectasis. In severe bacterial infections and in acute respiratory distress syndrome (ARDS), the lungs assume a heavy, liver-like appearance.

Viral infection, which typically causes diffuse pneumonia, first attacks bronchiolar epithelial cells, causing interstitial inflammation and desquamation. It then spreads to the alveoli, which fill with blood and fluid. In advanced infection, a hyaline membrane may form. As with bacterial infection, severe viral pneumonia may clinically resemble ARDS.

Impaired swallowing ability and a diminished gag reflex put older people at increased risk for aspiration pneumonia. These changes can occur after a cerebrovascular accident or any prolonged illness. In aspiration pneumonia, aspiration of gastric juices or food triggers similar inflammatory changes and also inactivates surfactant over a large area. Decreased surfactant leads to alveolar collapse. Acidic gastric juices may directly damage the airways and alveoli. Particles with the aspirated material may obstruct the airways and reduce airflow, which in turn leads to secondary bacterial pneumonia. (See *Understanding types of pneumonia,* page 472 to 474.)

Without proper treatment, pneumonia can lead to such life-threatening complications as septic shock, hypoxemia, respiratory failure, and ARDS. The infection can also spread within the patient's lungs, causing empyema or lung abscess. Or it may spread by way of the bloodstream or by cross-contamination to other parts of the body, causing bacteremia, endocarditis, pericarditis, or meningitis.

Signs and symptoms

- Fatigue
- Slight cough
- Pleuritic pain (may not be as severe as in a younger person)
- Rapid respiratory rate
- Tachycardia
- Fever (or, commonly in older patients, subnormal temperature)
- Shaking
- Productive cough (creamy yellow sputum suggesting staphylococcal pneumonia, green sputum denoting *Pseudomonas* infection, sputum that looks like currant jelly indicating *Klebsiella* infection, and clear sputum usually indicating no infection)
- Confusion, restlessness, and behavioral changes (from cerebral hypoxia)
- Dullness when you percuss (advanced pneumonia)
- Crackles, wheezing, or rhonchi over the affected lung area as well as decreased breath sounds and decreased vocal fremitus

Diagnostic tests

- *Chest X-rays* disclose infiltrates, confirming the diagnosis.
- *Gram stain* and *culture and sensitivity tests* show the bacterial cause of the infection. Because of age-related changes in the respiratory system, obtaining an adequate sputum specimen from an older adult is often more difficult.
- *Blood cultures* detect bacteremia and help determine the causative organism.
- *Blood studies* may reveal an elevated white blood cell (WBC) count in bacterial pneumonia and a normal or low WBC count in viral or mycoplasmal pneumonia. In some older adults, the WBC count may be in the normal range, even with bacterial pneumonia. Look for an elevated band count in the differential for a better indicator of bacterial infection.
- *Arterial blood gas* (ABG) *levels* vary, depending on the severity of the pneumonia and the underlying lung state.
- *Bronchoscopy* or *transtracheal aspiration* allows the collection of material for culture studies. Invasive procedures, however, pose a greater risk for the older adult, especially if he's frail or unable to cooperate.
- *Pulse oximetry* may show a reduced arterial oxygen saturation level.

Treatment

Antimicrobial therapy is based on the causative agent. The physician will choose the initial antimicrobial agent, depending on whether he believes the pneumonia to be community acquired or nosocomial. Once culture results are available, he may change the drug to match the sensitivity reports.

Supportive measures include a high-calorie diet and adequate fluid intake; bed rest; humidified oxygen therapy for hypoxia; bronchodilators, antitussives, and mechanical ventilation for respiratory failure; and analgesics to relieve pleuritic chest pain. A patient with severe pneumonia who is receiving mechanical venti-

Understanding types of pneumonias

This chart shows infections that can lead to viral or bacterial pneumonia. Included are the telltale respiratory signs and symptoms, tests to confirm the pneumonia, and typical treatment approaches.

Characteristics	Diagnostic tests	Treatment
Viral pneumonia		
Influenza ■ Signs and symptoms: cough (initially nonproductive; later, purulent sputum), marked cyanosis, dyspnea, high fever, chills, substernal pain and discomfort, moist crackles, frontal headache, myalgia ■ Poor prognosis, even with treatment; 50% mortality from cardiopulmonary collapse	■ *Chest X-ray:* diffuse bilateral bronchopneumonia radiating from hilus ■ *White blood cell (WBC) count:* normal to slightly elevated ■ *Sputum smears:* no specific organisms	■ Supportive treatment for respiratory failure includes endotracheal intubation and ventilator assistance; for fever, hypothermia blanket or antipyretics; for influenza A, amantadine.
Adenovirus ■ Insidious onset ■ Signs and symptoms: sore throat, fever, cough, chills, malaise, small amounts of mucoid sputum, retrosternal chest pain, anorexia, rhinitis, adenopathy, scattered crackles, rhonchi ■ Good prognosis; usually clears with no residual effects	■ *Chest X-ray:* patchy distribution of pneumonia; more severe than indicated by physical examination ■ *WBC count:* normal to slightly elevated	■ Treatment aims to relieve symptoms.
Measles (rubeola) ■ Signs and symptoms: fever, dyspnea, cough, small amounts of sputum, coryza, rash, cervical adenopathy	■ *Chest X-ray:* reticular infiltrates, sometimes with hilar lymph node enlargement ■ *Lung tissue specimen:* characteristic giant cells	■ Supportive treatment includes bed rest, adequate hydration, antimicrobials and, if necessary, assisted ventilation.
Chicken pox (varicella) ■ Present in 30% of adults with varicella ■ Signs and symptoms: characteristic rash, cough, dyspnea, cyanosis, tachypnea, pleuritic chest pain, and hemoptysis and rhonchi 1 to 6 days after onset of rash	■ *Chest X-ray:* bilateral, patchy, diffuse, nodular infiltrates; more extensive pneumonia than indicated by physical examination ■ *Sputum analysis:* predominant mononuclear cells and characteristic intranuclear inclusion bodies	■ Supportive treatment includes adequate hydration and, in critically ill patients, oxygen therapy.

Understanding types of pneumonia *(continued)*

Characteristics	Diagnostic tests	Treatment
Viral pneumonia *(continued)*		
Cytomegalovirus		
■ Difficult to distinguish from other nonbacterial pneumonia ■ In adults with healthy lung tissue, resembles mononucleosis and is generally benign; in immunocompromised hosts, varies from clinically inapparent to fatal infection ■ Signs and symptoms: fever, cough, shaking chills, dyspnea, cyanosis, weakness, diffuse crackle	■ *Chest X-ray:* in early stages, variable patchy infiltrates; in later stages, bilateral, nodular, and more predominant in lower lobes ■ *Percutaneous aspiration of lung tissue, transbronchial biopsy, or open-lung biopsy:* typical intranuclear and cytoplasmic inclusions on microscopic examination (virus can be cultured from lung tissue)	■ Supportive treatment includes adequate hydration and nutrition, oxygen therapy, and bed rest.
Bacterial pneumonia		
Streptococcus		
■ Caused by *Streptococcus pneumoniae* ■ Signs and symptoms: sudden onset of a single, shaking chill and sustained temperature of 102° to 104° F (38.9° to 40° C); often preceded by upper respiratory tract infection	■ *Chest X-ray:* areas of consolidation, often lobar ■ *WBC count:* elevated ■ *Sputum culture and Gram stain:* possibly gram-positive *S. pneumoniae*	■ Antimicrobial therapy with erythromycin begins after obtaining culture specimen but without waiting for results and continues for 7 to 10 days. Azithromycin, clarithryomycin, levofloxacin, and grepafloxacin are also effective.
Klebsiella		
■ More common in patients with chronic alcoholism, pulmonary disease, or diabetes ■ Signs and symptoms: fever, recurrent chills; cough producing rusty, bloody, viscous sputum (currant jelly); cyanosis of lips and nail beds from hypoxemia; shallow, grunting respirations	■ *Chest X-ray:* typically, but not always, consolidation in the upper lobe that causes bulging of fissures ■ *WBC count:* elevated ■ *Sputum culture and Gram stain:* possibly gram-negative *Klebsiella* cocci	■ Antimicrobial therapy consists of an aminoglycoside and, in serious infections, a cephalosporin.
Staphylococcus		
■ Commonly occurs in patients with viral illness, such as influenza or measles, and in those with cystic fibrosis ■ Signs and symptoms: fever of 102° to 104° F (38.9° to 40° C), recurrent shaking chills, bloody sputum, dyspnea, tachypnea, hypoxemia	■ *Chest X-ray:* multiple abscesses and infiltrates; frequently empyema ■ *WBC count:* elevated ■ *Sputum culture and Gram stain:* possibly gram-positive staphylococci	■ Antimicrobial therapy consists of nafcillin or oxacillin for 14 days if staphylococci are penicillinase-producing. ■ A chest tube drains empyema.

(continued)

Understanding types of pneumonia *(continued)*

Characteristics	Diagnostic tests	Treatment
Bacterial pneumonia *(continued)*		
Aspiration pneumonia ■ Results from vomiting and aspiration of gastric or oropharyngeal contents into trachea and lungs ■ Noncardiogenic pulmonary edema possible with damage to respiratory epithelium from contact with gastric acid ■ Subacute pneumonia possible with cavity formation ■ Lung abscess possible if foreign body present ■ Signs and symptoms: crackles, dyspnea, cyanosis, hypotension, tachycardia	■ *Chest X-ray:* areas of infiltrates (suggests diagnosis)	■ Antimicrobial therapy consists of penicillin G or clindamycin. ■ Supportive therapy includes oxygen therapy, suctioning, coughing, deep breathing, adequate hydration, and I.V. corticosteroids.

lation may need positive end-expiratory pressure to maintain adequate oxygenation.

Key nursing diagnoses and outcomes

Risk for infection related to potential for sepsis, lung abscess, and other complications

Treatment outcome: The patient will remain free from signs and symptoms of a second infection or cardiac dysfunction by complying with the prescribed treatment.

Impaired gas exchange related to acute infection of the lung parenchyma

Treatment outcomes: The patient will maintain a respiratory rate within 5 breaths of baseline and will regain and maintain normal ABG values.

Ineffective airway clearance related to thick sputum production

Treatment outcome: The patient will maintain a patent airway by coughing and expectorating sputum effectively.

Nursing interventions

▶ Administer prescribed antibiotics and other medications as ordered, and evaluate their effectiveness. Check the patient for adverse reactions.

▶ Monitor vital signs, and treat fever with analgesics.

▶ Assess the patient's respiratory status. Auscultate for breath sounds at least every 4 hours.

▶ Provide a quiet, calm environment with frequent rest periods.

▶ Monitor the patient's ABG levels, especially if he's hypoxic. Administer supplemental oxygen if the patient's partial pressure of oxygen in arterial blood falls below 60 mm Hg.

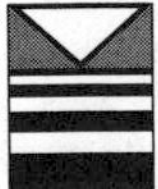

Key point If an older adult with pneumonia requires oxygen, administer it cautiously. High oxygen levels can depress the respiratory stimulus in the brain, reducing respiration and promoting carbon dioxide retention. Older patients have a diminished cough and gag reflex, weaker respiratory muscles, and a reduced maximum

breathing capacity. Because sedatives, cough suppressants, and narcotics suppress respiratory drive and the cough and gag reflex, their use is often contraindicated in these patients.

▶ Provide a high-calorie, high-protein diet of soft foods to offset the calories the patient uses to fight the infection. To improve intake, offer nutritional supplements between meals.

▶ If the patient is extremely debilitated, supplement oral feedings with NG tube feedings or parenteral nutrition. To prevent aspiration during NG tube feedings, elevate the patient's head, check the tube position, and administer the feeding slowly. Don't give large volumes at one time because this could cause vomiting.

▶ Listen to the patient's fears and concerns, and remain with him during periods of severe stress and anxiety. Encourage him to identify actions and care measures that promote comfort and relaxation.

▶ In severe pneumonia that requires endotracheal intubation or a tracheostomy with or without mechanical ventilation, provide thorough respiratory care and suction often, using sterile technique, to remove secretions.

▶ To control the spread of infection, dispose of secretions properly.

▶ Obtain blood cultures if appropriate.

▶ Obtain sputum specimens as needed. Use suction if the patient can't produce a specimen.

▶ Encourage incentive spirometry.

▶ Administer chest percussion to help mobilize secretions.

PATIENT TEACHING

▶ Explain all procedures (especially intubation and suctioning) to the patient and his family.

▶ Review the patient's medication regimen. Stress the need to take the entire course of drugs to prevent a relapse.

▶ Discuss ways to avoid spreading the infection to others. Remind the patient to sneeze and cough into tissues and to dispose of the tissues in a waxed or plastic bag. Advise him to wash his hands thoroughly after handling contaminated tissues

▶ Emphasize the importance of adequate rest to promote full recovery and prevent a relapse. Explain that the physician will inform the patient when he can resume full activity and return to work.

▶ Urge the patient to drink 2 to 3 qt (2 to 3 L) of fluid daily to maintain adequate hydration and keep mucus secretions thin for easier removal.

▶ Teach the patient and his family members about chest physiotherapy. Explain that postural drainage, percussion, and vibration help to mobilize and remove mucus from the patient's lungs.

▶ Teach the patient procedures and therapies for clearing lung secretions, such as deep-breathing and coughing exercises as well as home oxygen therapy. Explain pursed-lip breathing as a method to help control breathing.

▶ Encourage all bedridden and postoperative patients to perform deep-breathing and coughing exercises frequently. Position such patients properly to promote full aeration and drainage of secretions.

▶ Urge the patient to avoid irritants that stimulate secretions, such as cigarette smoke, dust, and significant environmental pollution. If necessary, refer him to community programs or agencies that can help him stop smoking.

▶ Advise the patient to avoid using antibiotics indiscriminately for minor infections. Doing so could result in upper airway colonization with antibiotic-resistant bacteria. If pneumonia develops, the organisms that produce the pneumonia may require treatment with more toxic antibiotics.

▶ Encourage the older patient to ask his physician about an annual influenza vaccination and a pneumococcal pneumonia vaccination. In addition, encourage him to eat well, get adequate rest and sleep, and avoid crowds and smoking to help prevent pneumonia.

Special considerations

Because older adults can tire easily when asked to take deep breaths, begin auscultation at the base of the lungs, and work toward the apex, alternating left to right. Normal breath sounds for older adults often include diminished breath sounds and some chronic, mild adventitious sounds.

POLYPHARMACY

An older person with multiple disorders or symptoms may take prescribed drugs from several physicians at once for acute or chronic ailments. He may also self-medicate with nonprescription drugs to relieve common complaints, such as indigestion, dizziness, constipation, and insomnia. This multiple-drug use, known as polypharmacy, is a serious problem in geriatric care. (See *Risk factors for polypharmacy*.)

Risk factors for polypharmacy

Many factors can contribute to polypharmacy in older adults. The more risk factors that exist, the greater the person's risk of polypharmacy. The most common risk factors include:

- advanced age
- multiple symptoms
- multiple medical conditions
- many prescriptions
- multiple physicians
- lack of a primary provider to coordinate therapy
- use of several pharmacies
- changes in drug regimen
- hoarding of medications
- self-treatment.

If the patient and his physicians fail to communicate and make adjustments regarding concurrent drug use, the patient may fall into a pattern of inappropriate and excessive drug use that puts him at risk for drug interactions and adverse reactions and confounds therapeutic goals. (See *Recognizing polypharmacy*.)

Advise the elderly patient to carry a list with him at all times of all prescription and nonprescription (over-the-counter) drugs and herbs that he may take on a regular basis. He should show this list to each health care provider.

Interactions

The drugs most commonly used by older patients are antihypertensives, cardiac drugs, and diuretics. A person who takes two or more drugs concurrently may experience any of the following reactions:

- indifference — no interactive effect
- potentiation — increased action resulting from the drug combinations
- antagonism — negation or reduction of effect of either drug
- synergism — a combined effect greater than the sum total of each individual drug's effects (rare).

Any of these effects can occur as a result of the altered drug metabolism characteristic of aging.

Adverse reactions

The risk of adverse drug reactions increases with each drug the patient takes. Common adverse reactions include confusion, dizziness, anorexia, incontinence, weakness, immobility, and rashes. The safest approach is to follow the "rule of five": No more than five drugs at the lowest dose should be prescribed.

Many prescription and nonprescription drugs can cause a one-time reaction or symptoms of substance abuse related to repeated overmedication or taking a large quantity one time only. Such drugs include anesthetics, analgesics, anticholinergics, anticonvulsants, antihistamines, antihypertensives, cardiovascular drugs, antimicrobials, antiparkinsonian agents, chemotherapeutic drugs, corticosteroids, GI preparations, muscle relaxants, nonsteroidal anti-inflammatory drugs, antidepressants, and disulfiram.

Nonprescription preparations that contain bromide can mimic a wide variety of psychiatric problems, including organic brain syndrome, because the bromide accumulates in the older person's body. Antihistamines and other drug classes can cause confusion.

Psychotropic and cardiovascular drugs, which are taken by 75% of nursing home residents, cause the most serious adverse drug reactions in older adults. For example, a patient who is taking an antihypertensive may suffer a hypertensive crisis from taking a nonprescription cold product.

Generic substitution adds a final element of unpredictability. The Food and Drug Administration's "20/20 rule" states that a generic drug must be shown to be equivalent to the proprietary drug in an amount plus or minus 20%. This means that a generic substitute may deliver 20% more or less than the therapeutic dose of the brand name product.

Special considerations

Misinterpretation of an elderly patient's symptoms can misdirect drug therapy. For example, exposure to heavy metals, rat poisons, or volatile substances (such as household gas and paint) may cause impaired cognition, hallucinations, delusions, and even seizures. A physician who fails to detect the underlying cause of these symptoms might prescribe drug therapy when simply removing the toxic substances would resolve the problem.

Recognizing polypharmacy

Because of your close contact with patients, you are the health care provider who is best able to recognize inappropriate use of multiple drugs. Suspect polypharmacy if your patient:

- takes several (usually 10 or more) drugs for no logical reason—for example, laxatives that aren't needed
- takes duplicate drugs, such as sleep aids and tranquilizers
- takes an inappropriate dosage
- uses contraindicated drugs
- uses drugs to treat adverse reactions.

POTASSIUM DEFICIENCY

A cation that's the dominant cellular electrolyte, potassium facilitates contraction of both skeletal and smooth muscles, including myocardial contraction. It figures prominently in nerve impulse conduction, acid-base balance, enzyme action, and cell membrane function. Because the normal serum potassium level has such a narrow range (3.5 to 5 mEq/L), a slight deviation in either direction can produce profound consequences.

Because many foods contain potassium, a potassium deficiency—known as hypokalemia—rarely results from a dietary deficiency. Instead, it usually results from excessive GI losses, as occur in vomiting, gastric suction, diarrhea, villous adenoma, or laxative abuse; chronic renal disease, with tubular potassium wasting; use of certain drugs, especially potassium-wasting diuretics, steroids, and certain sodium-containing antibiotics (such as carbenicillin); alkalosis or insulin effect, which causes potassium shifting into cells without

ECG changes in potassium deficiency

A deficiency of potassium can induce cardiac arrhythmias. In the solid-line waveform below, the solid line represents normal sinus rhythm, and the dotted line shows electrocardiogram (ECG) changes caused by potassium deficiency.

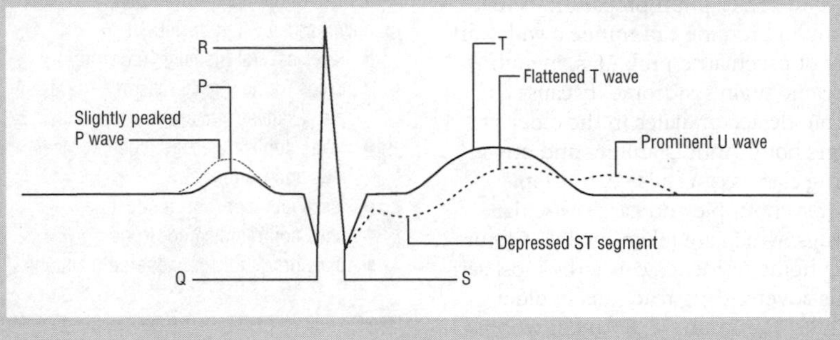

true depletion of total body potassium; prolonged potassium-free I.V. therapy; hyperglycemia; Cushing's syndrome; and severe serum magnesium deficiency.

Potassium imbalances may result in such complications as muscle weakness and flaccid paralysis and may also lead to cardiac arrest.

Signs and symptoms

- Nausea and vomiting
- Anorexia
- Abdominal distention
- Constipation
- Paralytic ileus
- Decreased peristalsis
- Neuromuscular weakness and hyporeflexia
- Dizziness, postural hypotension, and arrhythmias (from cardiovascular irregularities)
- Flaccid or respiratory paralysis

Diagnostic tests

- *Electrolyte studies* reveal potassium levels of less than 3.5 mEq/L.
- *Electrocardiogram* (ECG) readings reveal a depressed ST segment, slightly peaked P wave, flattened T wave, and a prominent U wave. (See *ECG changes in potassium deficiency*.)

Additional tests may be necessary to determine the cause of the deficiency.

Treatment

Treatment consists of increased dietary intake of potassium or oral supplements with potassium salts (preferably potassium chloride). Edematous patients with diuretic-induced hypokalemia should receive a potassium-sparing diuretic such as spironolactone.

Patients with GI potassium loss or severe potassium depletion require I.V. potassium replacement therapy. If hypocalcemia is also present, treatment should include calcium replacement. (See *Guidelines for I.V. potassium administration*.)

Key nursing diagnoses and outcomes

Imbalanced nutrition: Less than body requirements related to adverse GI effects

Treatment outcome: The patient will obtain relief from adverse GI effects when a normal serum potassium level is restored.

Decreased cardiac output related to arrhythmias

Treatment outcome: The patient will regain and maintain normal cardiac output, as exhibited by stable vital signs and a normal ECG.

Nursing interventions

▶ Administer I.V. potassium slowly and cautiously to prevent cardiac arrhythmias and vein irritation. Dilute potassium to a maximum of 1 mcg to 10 ml of dilutant; give slowly and never exceed 20 mcg/hour.

▶ If the patient is taking a liquid oral potassium supplement, have him sip it slowly to prevent GI irritation. Give the supplement with or after meals, with a full glass of water or fruit juice.

▶ Implement safety measures for the patient with muscle weakness or postural hypotension.

▶ Frequently monitor serum potassium and other electrolyte levels during potassium replacement therapy to avoid overcorrection leading to hyperkalemia.

▶ Assess intake and output carefully. Remember, the kidneys excrete 80% to 90% of ingested potassium. Never give supplementary potassium to a patient whose urine output is below 600 ml/day. Also, measure GI loss from suctioning or vomiting.

▶ Assess for abdominal distention, decreased bowel sounds, and constipation.

▶ Carefully monitor patients receiving cardiac glycosides because hypokalemia enhances their action. Assess for signs of digoxin toxicity (anorexia, nausea, vomiting, blurred vision, and arrhythmias).

▶ Monitor cardiac rhythm, and report any irregularities immediately.

PATIENT TEACHING

▶ To prevent hypokalemia, instruct patients (especially those taking diuretics) to include potassium-rich foods in their diets. Such foods include oranges, bananas, tomatoes, milk, dried fruits, apricots, peanuts, and dark green, leafy vegetables.

▶ Emphasize the importance of taking potassium supplements as prescribed, particularly if the patient is also taking cardiac glycosides or diuretics. If appropriate, teach the patient to recognize and report signs of digoxin toxicity such as pulse irregularities. Demonstrate the proper technique for assessing the patient's pulse.

▶ Make sure the patient can recognize signs of hypokalemia, including weakness and pulse irregularities. Tell him to report such signs to the physician.

Guidelines for I.V. potassium administration

I.V. replacement of potassium is necessary only if hypokalemia is severe or if the patient can't take supplements by mouth. Carefully monitor I.V. potassium replacement to prevent or lessen toxic effects. Follow these guidelines:

- I.V. infusion concentrations shouldn't exceed 40 mEq/L. The infusion rate shouldn't exceed 250 mEq/day, unless indicated.
- Use volumetric devices whenever concentrations of more than 40 mEq/L are infused.
- *Never* administer potassium by I.V. push or bolus; doing so may cause cardiac arrest.
- Monitor cardiac rhythm during rapid I.V. administration of potassium to avoid cardiac toxicity from inadvertent hyperkalemia. Report any irregularities immediately.
- Monitor the results of treatment by checking serum potassium levels and assessing for signs and symptoms of imbalance, such as muscle weakness and paralysis.
- Monitor the I.V. site for signs and symptoms of infiltration, phlebitis, or tissue necrosis.

POTASSIUM EXCESS

An elevated potassium level — known as hyperkalemia — usually results from reduced excretion by the kidneys. This may be caused by acute or severe chronic renal failure, oliguria due to shock or severe dehydration, or the use of potassium-sparing diuretics (such as triamterene) by patients with renal disease. Inadequate potassium excretion may also be due to hypoaldosteronism or Addison's disease.

Hyperkalemia may also result from failure to excrete excessive amounts of potassium infused I.V. or administered orally. Another cause is massive release of intracellular potassium, which can occur with burns, crushing injuries, severe infection, or acidosis.

Signs and symptoms

- Nausea
- Diarrhea
- Abdominal cramps
- Skeletal muscle weakness, or twitching
- Numbness and tingling
- Flaccid or respiratory paralysis
- Dizziness, postural hypotension, and arrhythmias (from cardiac irregularities)
- Irregular, unusually slow pulse

Diagnostic tests

- *Electrolyte studies* reveal potassium levels exceeding 5 mEq/L.
- *Electrocardiogram readings* reveal wide, flat P wave; prolonged PR interval; widened QRS complex; depressed ST segment; and tall, tented T wave. (See *ECG changes in potassium excess*.)

Additional tests may be necessary to determine the cause of the excess.

Treatment

Treatment consists of withholding potassium and administering a cation exchange resin orally or by enema. Sodium polystyrene sulfonate with 70% sorbitol produces exchange of sodium ions for potassium ions in the intestine.

In an emergency, rapid infusion of 10% calcium gluconate decreases myocardial irritability and temporarily prevents cardiac arrest but doesn't correct serum potassium excess; this therapy is contraindicated in patients receiving cardiac glycosides. Also, as an emergency measure, sodium bicarbonate I.V. increases pH and causes potassium to shift back into the cells.

Insulin and 10% to 50% glucose I.V. also move potassium back into cells. Infusions should be followed by dextrose 5% in water because infusion of 10% to 15% glucose will stimulate secretion of endogenous insulin. Hemodialysis and peritoneal dialysis also help remove excess potassium, but both are slow techniques.

Key nursing diagnoses and outcomes

Activity intolerance related to neuromuscular dysfunction

Treatment outcome: The patient will regain normal neuromuscular function with restoration of a normal serum potassium level.

Decreased cardiac output related to decreased ventricular filling time caused by the arrhythmia

Treatment outcome: The patient won't exhibit signs of decreased cardiac output, such as hypotension and altered tissue perfusion.

Nursing interventions

- Administer sodium polystyrene sulfonate orally or by retention enema. Encourage the patient to retain the enema for 30 to 60 minutes.
- Provide sufficient calories to prevent tissue breakdown and release of potassium into extracellular fluid.
- Implement safety measures for the patient with muscle weakness.

ECG changes in potassium excess

An excess of potassium can cause cardiac arrhythmias. In the waveform below, the solid line represents normal sinus rhythm, and the dotted line shows electrocardiogram (ECG) changes caused by potassium excess.

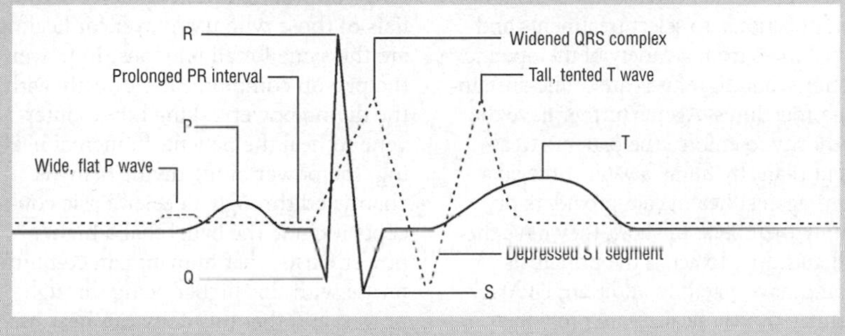

- If the patient needs a blood transfusion, infuse only fresh blood for patients with average to high serum potassium levels. Blood cell hemolysis that takes place in older blood releases potassium.
- Frequently monitor serum potassium and other electrolyte levels, and carefully record intake and output.
- Watch for signs of hypokalemia with prolonged use of sodium polystyrene sulfonate.
- Assess for clinical effects of hypoglycemia (muscle weakness, syncope, hunger, diaphoresis) with repeated insulin and glucose treatment.
- Monitor for and report cardiac arrhythmias.
- Assess for abdominal distention, intestinal cramping, and diarrhea.
- Watch for signs of hyperkalemia in predisposed patients, especially those with poor urine output and those receiving I.V. or oral potassium supplements.

PATIENT TEACHING

- To prevent hyperkalemia, tell patients who use salt substitutes containing potassium to discontinue them if urine output decreases.
- Make sure the patient can recognize signs of hyperkalemia, including weakness and pulse irregularities. Tell him to report such signs to the physician.

POWER OF ATTORNEY

Power of attorney is a common-law concept that allows one person (an agent) to speak for another (the principal). In early use, the power of attorney ended with the death or incapacity of the principal. To avoid this limitation, legislatures adopted the Uniform Durable Power of Attorney Act, which states that a durable power of attorney is valid even if the principal becomes incapacitated and legally incompetent.

The Durable Power of Attorney for Health Care (DPAHC), sometimes known as the Medical Durable Power of Attorney, allows a competent person to appoint a surrogate or proxy to make health care decisions for him in case he becomes incompetent to do so. With these statutes, family members and health care providers no longer need to guess whether the patient would have wanted his living will to be followed. Another person, under authority of the patient, may speak for the patient.

Under most DPAHC statutes, the agent a person chooses to make medical decisions for him has the right to ask questions, to select and remove physicians from the patient's care, to assess risks and complications, to select treatments and procedures from a variety of therapeutic options, and to refuse care or life-sustaining procedures. Agents further have the authority to enforce the patient's treatment plans by filing lawsuits or legal actions against health care providers or family members. In short, they have the full authority to act as the principals would have acted. In addition, DPAHC statutes protect health care providers from liability if they abide, in good faith, by the agent's decision.

Caution your patient to appoint agents who understand what he would want and are capable of making difficult decisions for him — typically, a spouse, relative, or friend. Encourage frank discussions regarding end-of-life care and living wills; this can prevent confusion and guilt among family members when an unforseen medical catastrophe occurs. Most states allow the patient to appoint a second or third agent, who would assume authority if the first person named was unable or unwilling to serve in this capacity. Without this latter provision, the patient's wishes might not be honored.

Special considerations

When presented with a DPAHC document, have your facility's legal counsel verify that the document meets state requirements. Competent older patients may be required to resign the document if the original form is deficient or doesn't fulfill state requirements.

PRAYER AND MENTAL HEALING

Individuals have used prayer and mental healing throughout the ages to seek assistance from a higher power for a wide range of problems. The underlying beliefs of those who use prayer for healing are the same for all religions. In prayer, the person communicates directly with the divine power, asking him to intervene to heal the patient. In mental healing, the power of the divine being is channeled through a healer. Basic concepts include the belief that a higher power exists, that humans can communicate with this higher being through prayer, and that this deity can hear human prayers and intervene in human affairs, including healing the sick. Most people who use prayer for healing view it as an adjunct to conventional medical treatment.

There are two main categories of mental healing. In type 1 healing, the healer enters into a spiritual level of consciousness where he views himself and the patient as a single being. No physical contact with the patient is necessary. Type 2 mental healing requires the healer to touch the patient in an attempt to transfer energy from the healer's hands to the diseased parts of the patient's body.

Implementation

- Provide the patient with privacy in a quiet, distraction-free environment.
- Facilitate the use of prayer and mental healing by asking the patient such questions as, "Is religion important to you?" and "Is it important in how you cope with your illness?"
- If religion is important to the patient, explore his religious practices with him to identify ways to incorporate them into his present situation.
- Determine whether the patient would like to discuss his faith with the facility chaplain or another clergy member.

Special considerations

- A patient who has attempted prayer and not seen the results he expected may express a sense of disappointment when the topic of spirituality is discussed. If this occurs and if possible, arrange for a clergy member to explore the patient's feelings with him.
- Some prayer rituals may be a lot for your health care facility to handle; however, you should continue to be sensitive to the patient's religious beliefs. Rites involving incense, large groups, or loud music and dance may require you to find a creative solution that allows your patient to engage in his religious beliefs but also respect the needs of other patients and your facility. For example, you could suggest that the patient be wheeled to an outside area of the facility if incense is involved or to a conference room off the unit during off-hours if noise or a large number of people is an issue.
- Be aware that ethical questions arise if prayer and mental healing are used without the patient's knowledge. Additionally, prayer and mental healing may be used to harm an individual instead of healing him.
- Advise your patient to consider prayer a complementary therapy, not a substitute for conventional medical care. If you have a patient whose religion advocates the use of prayer as the sole form of treatment, make sure he understands the consequences of foregoing conventional medical treatment so he can make an informed decision.

PRESBYCUSIS

Also known as sensorineural, senile, or progressive hearing loss, presbycusis is marked by bilateral, symmetrical dysfunction of the ear's sensory elements (hair cells) or neural structures (cochlear nerve fibers). The most common type of hearing loss in older people, presbycusis affects both men and women (men are usually more impaired than women of the same age). It usually affects high-frequency sounds, but this in itself does not interfere with understanding speech until the disorder affects those high frequencies involved in consonant discrimination.

Four types of presbycusis are known: sensory, neural, metabolic, and cochlear. *Sensory presbycusis* begins in middle age and progresses slowly. The loss of cochlear neurons parallels loss in the organ of Corti.

In *neural presbycusis,* which develops later in life, loss of cochlear neurons occurs without loss in the organ of Corti. This form of presbycusis progresses rapidly and may be accompanied by other signs of central nervous system (CNS) decline, including intellectual deterioration, memory loss, and loss of motor coordination.

Metabolic presbycusis tends to run in families, usually begins in middle age, and progresses slowly. *Cochlear conductive presbycusis* also starts in middle age and is related to alterations in the motion mechanism of the cochlear duct.

Although the exact cause is unknown, the incidence of sensorineural hearing loss rises with age. Noise exposure, high-cholesterol diet, hypertension, metabolic factors, and heredity are contributing factors. Vascular lesions resulting in hypoperfusion may aggravate age-related changes in the ear and CNS.

Signs and symptoms

- Difficulty understanding people with high-pitched voices, such as women and young children (sounds may seem annoying or overly loud)
- Difficulty hearing conversations in large groups or in places with a lot of background noise
- Difficulty differentiating the sounds "s" and "th"
- Viewing speech of others as mumbled or slurred
- Tinnitus in one or both ears

Diagnostic tests

▶ *Pure tone audiometry* is the definitive test for sensorineural hearing loss. It can also help identify the type of presbycusis. Sensory presbycusis produces an abrupt loss of high-frequency sound but preserves good word discrimination. Neural presbycusis produces a loss of high-frequency sound and poor word discrimination. Metabolic presbycusis results in a flat threshold of audibility with normal speech discrimination until speech volume falls below 50 dB. Cochlear conductive presbycusis produces a bilaterally symmetrical, linearly descending threshold of audibility with speech discrimination better at steeper thresholds.

Treatment

Treatment for sensorineural hearing loss usually involves a hearing aid, which can increase the volume of sound transmitted to the hearing organs. Hearing aids are available in different forms: behind-the-ear aid, in-the-ear aid, eyeglass hearing aid, and body hearing aid.

Behind-the-ear aids, used for mild to moderate hearing loss, are easy to conceal, comfortable to wear, and have no long wires. They're also durable, and some models are equipped with a telephone pickup device.

In-the-ear aids fit directly into the ear canal and are supported by the outer ear. These aids are lightweight, easy to conceal, and lack external wires or tubes. However, they're suitable only for mild hearing loss because they provide less amplification than other types.

Eyeglass aids are also used for mild to moderate hearing loss. They're similar to behind-the-ear aids, except that the hearing unit is built into the arm of an eyeglass frame. A short length of tubing connects the hearing aid to the earmold. The frame can carry a signal from one ear to the other, so it's good for amplification in both ears. The eyeglass frame conceals the aid and hides the wires connecting the microphone and receiver. Bone-conduction hearing aids are also available in the eyeglass style.

In body hearing aids, the microphone, amplifier, and battery lie in a single case, which attaches to clothing or is carried in a pocket. The external receiver attaches directly to the earmold and connects to the amplifier by a long wire. This aid is the most powerful type, so it's usually used for severe hearing loss.

A cochlear implant may benefit severely deaf individuals. This surgically inserted device, which stimulates the auditory nerve, consists of an external microphone, a transmitter, and an implanted receiver. The transmitter receives signals from the microphone and sends them to the receiver located near the auditory nerve. The signals travel along an implanted wire to the nerve.

Key nursing diagnoses and outcomes

Disturbed sensory perception (auditory) related to hearing loss

Treatment outcome: The patient will adjust his lifestyle to the hearing loss to maintain safety and function adequately.

Anxiety related to diminished hearing

Treatment outcomes: The patient will express his concerns over his hearing loss and will develop coping methods to relieve anxiety.

Nursing interventions

▶ When speaking to a patient with hearing loss, stand directly in front of him, with the light on your face, and speak slowly and distinctly in a low tone. Avoid shouting.

▶ When approaching the patient, move to within his visual range and elicit his attention by raising your arm or waving; touching him may be unnecessarily startling.

▶ Carefully explain all diagnostic tests and health care facility procedures. The patient may depend totally on visual clues, so make sure he's in an area where he can observe unit activities and see people approaching.

- Suggest adjustments for the hearing impaired to improve functioning and maintain safety such as having an amplified telephone.
- Allow the patient to express his feelings about his hearing loss. Provide emotional support and encouragement if the patient is learning how to use a hearing aid.
- Make sure other caregivers are aware of the patient's handicap and his established method of communication (such as writing on a pad, using a message board, or signing).
- Rephrase statements in shorter, simpler sentences if you're misunderstood.
- Encourage family members to adjust communication to the patient's abilities and to be sure to include him in conversations such as by clueing him in about the topic of conversation whenever possible.

PATIENT TEACHING

- Teach the patient the importance of regular hearing evaluations. Stress that hearing loss, although an inconvenience, is often treatable.
- If appropriate, explain the components of a hearing aid, the different types available, and their advantages and disadvantages. Teach the patient how to care for his hearing aid and how to solve common problems.
- Advise the patient to look at the person speaking to them and to concentrate on his lip movements as well as his voice.
- Encourage family members to enunciate clearly and use adjunctive measures, such as a communication board if appropriate, to improve the patient's understanding of what they're saying.
- Teach the patient alternative methods of communication if hearing loss can't be corrected, such as writing on a pad or signing.
- Encourage the patient to admit hearing difficulties to others (such as store clerks and bank tellers) so that they can improve their method of communication.
- Encourage the patient to turn off the radio or television during conversations to eliminate background nosie.
- When dining in restaurants, tell the patient to choose a seat away from crowded or noisy areas.

Special considerations

As with other forms of hearing loss, sensorineural hearing loss can cause embarrassment and may lead to withdrawal from social activities. Profound isolation can have both psychological and physical effects.

PRESSURE ULCER PREVENTION

As a health care provider, you play a key role in maintaining the older patient's skin integrity, promoting comfort by averting dryness and itching, and preventing pressure ulcers, a major complication.

Because your patient's skin condition largely depends on his overall health, you'll need to help him maintain optimal nutrition and hydration. You may also need to provide additional guidance in personal hygiene and in protecting his skin from harsh environmental conditions.

As their name implies, pressure ulcers result when pressure — applied with great force for a short period of time or with less force over a longer period — impairs circulation, depriving tissues of oxygen and nutrients. Left untreated, ischemic areas can progress to tissue breakdown and infection.

Most pressure ulcers develop over bony prominences, where friction and shearing force combine with pressure to break down skin and underlying tissues. Common sites include the sacrum, coccyx, ischial tuberosities, and greater

Pressure ulcers: Who's at risk?

Older people are at greatest risk for developing pressure ulcers, especially those with the following conditions:

- circulation
- diabetes mellitus
- malnutrition
- immunosuppression
- dehydration
- incontinence
- significant obesity or thinness
- paralysis
- diminished pain awareness
- history of corticosteroid therapy
- previous pressure ulcers
- chronic illness that requires bed rest
- mental impairment (possibly related to coma, altered level of consciousness, sedation, confusion, or use of restraints)
- impaired mobility.

trochanters. Other sites include the skin over the vertebrae, scapulae, elbows, knees, and heels in bedridden and relatively immobile patients. (See *Pressure ulcers: Who's at risk?*)

Preventing pressure ulcers is crucial in older adults because the ulcers take longer to heal, thereby increasing the patient's risk of infection and other complications.

Supplies

▶ Turning sheet
▶ Pillows
▶ Optional: pressure-reducing device, such as a special mattress or mattress overlay

Implementation

▶ Assess the older person closely for risk factors; use an appropriate assessment tool, such as the Braden Scale, to determine his risk of developing pressure ulcers.
▶ Turn and reposition the patient every 1 to 2 hours unless contraindicated. For older persons who can't turn themselves or who are turned on a schedule, use pressure-reducing devices, such as a special mattress or mattress overlay made of air, gel, foam, or water.
▶ Post a turning schedule at the patient's bedside. Adapt position changes to the patient's situation.
▶ Lift the patient rather than sliding him because sliding increases friction and shear. Use a turning sheet and get help from coworkers if necessary.
▶ Use pillows to position your patient and increase his comfort. Try to keep sheets free of wrinkles, which can increase pressure and cause discomfort. (See *Positioning the patient in bed.*)
▶ Avoid placing the patient directly on his trochanter. Instead, position him on his side, at an angle of 30 to 60 degrees.
▶ Except for brief periods, avoid raising the head of the bed more than 30 degrees to prevent shearing pressure.
▶ As appropriate, perform active and passive range-of-motion exercises to relieve pressure and promote circulation.
▶ To promote blood flow to compressed tissues, a patient confined in a chair or wheelchair should shift his weight every half hour. If the patient needs your help, sit next to him and help him shift his weight to one buttock for 60 seconds; then repeat the procedure on the other side. Provide him with pressure-relieving cushions, as appropriate. However, avoid seating the patient on a rubber or plastic doughnut, which can increase localized pressure at vulnerable points.
▶ Adjust or pad appliances, casts, or splints, as needed, to ensure proper fit and to prevent increased pressure and impaired circulation.
▶ If the patient's condition permits, recommend a diet that includes adequate calories, proteins, and vitamins. Diet

Positioning the patient in bed

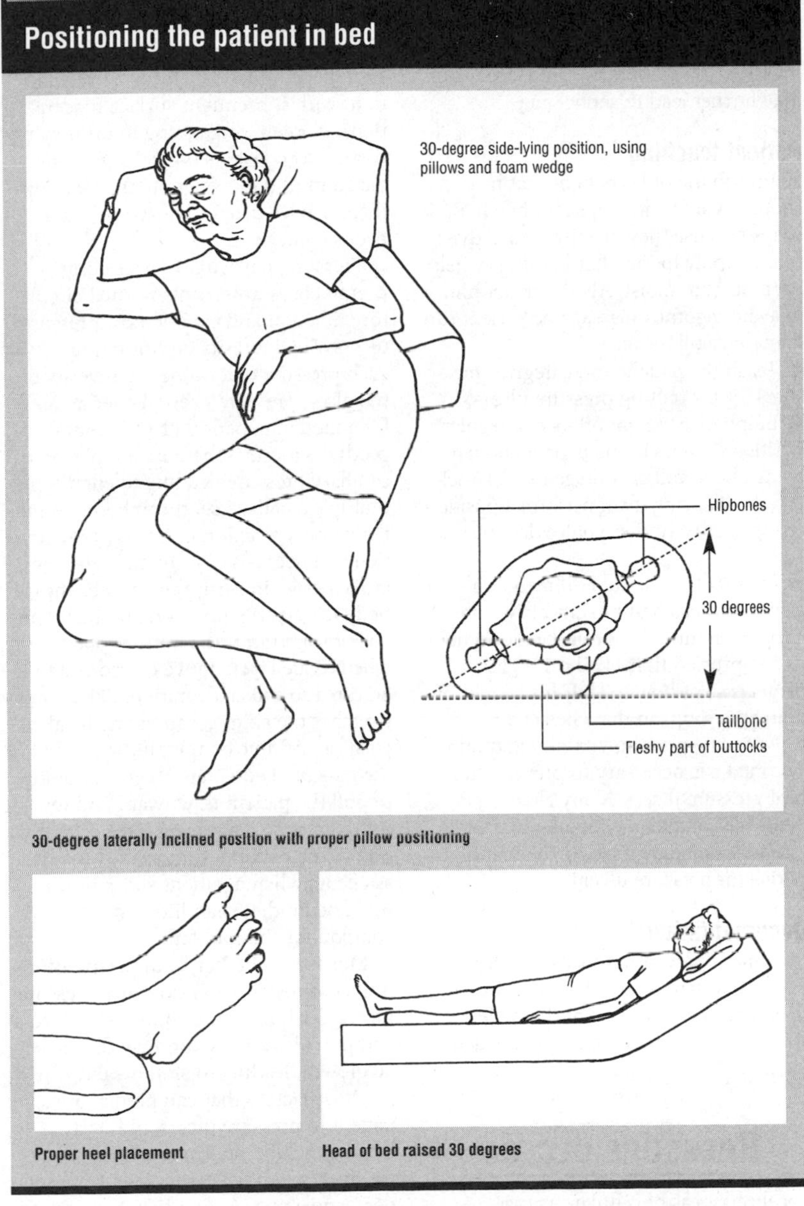

30-degree laterally inclined position with proper pillow positioning

Proper heel placement

Head of bed raised 30 degrees

therapy may involve a consultation with a dietitian, food supplements, enteral feeding, or total parenteral nutrition.

▶ If the patient is incontinent or develops diarrhea, clean and dry his soiled skin. Then apply a protective moisture barrier to prevent skin maceration.

Complications

If prevention measures fail, the pressure ulcers that develop can lead to bacterial invasion and secondary infection, which may further lead to septicemia.

Patient teaching

- Inform the older patient that he should avoid heat lamps and harsh soaps because they dry the skin. Advise him to apply lotion after bathing to help keep his skin moist. Also, instruct him to avoid vigorous massage because it can damage capillaries.
- Teach the patient and caregiver measures for preventing pressure ulcers.
- Emphasize the importance of regular position changes to the patient and family members, and encourage their participation by having them perform a position change correctly after you've demonstrated how.
- Instruct the patient confined to a chair or wheelchair to shift his weight every 30 minutes to promote blood flow to compressed tissues. Show a paraplegic patient how to shift his weight by doing push-ups in the wheelchair.
- Adequate protein, vitamin, and mineral intake is necessary to prevent and heal pressure ulcers. Many elderly patients have inadequate intake of these essential elements, placing them at higher risk for pressure ulcers.

Documentation

Document prevention measures provided, such as frequency of turning the patient, and the condition of the patient's skin. Also document any patient teaching.

PRESSURE ULCERS

Localized areas of cellular necrosis, pressure ulcers usually occur in the skin and subcutaneous tissue over bony prominences, particularly the sacrum, ischial tuberosities, greater trochanter, heels, malleoli, and elbows. These ulcers — also called decubitus ulcers, pressure sores, and bedsores — may be superficial, caused by local skin irritation (with subsequent surface maceration), or deep, originating in underlying tissue. Deep lesions typically go undetected until they penetrate the skin; by then, they've usually caused subcutaneous damage.

Pressure, particularly over bony prominences, interrupts normal circulatory function and causes most pressure ulcers. The intensity and duration of such pressure determine the severity of the ulcer; pressure exerted over an area for a moderate period (1 to 2 hours) produces tissue ischemia and increased capillary pressure, leading to edema and multiple small-vessel thromboses. An inflammatory reaction gives way to ulceration and necrosis of ischemic cells. Necrotic tissue, in turn, predisposes the body to bacterial invasion and infection.

Shearing force, the force applied when tissue layers move over one another, can also cause ulcerations. This force stretches the skin, compressing local circulation. As an example, if the head of the patient's bed is raised, gravity tends to pull the patient downward and forward, creating a shearing force. The friction of the patient's skin against the bed, as occurs when a patient slides himself up in bed rather than lifting his hips, compounds the problem.

Moisture, whether from perspiration or incontinence, can also cause pressure ulcers. Such moisture softens skin layers and provides an environment for bacterial growth, leading to skin breakdown.

Other factors that can predispose a patient to pressure ulcers and delay healing include poor nutrition, diabetes mellitus, paralysis, cardiovascular disorders, and aging. Added risks include obesity, insufficient weight, edema, anemia, poor hygiene, and exposure to chemicals.

Signs and symptoms

▶ Shiny, erythematous changes over the compressed area in early, superficial lesions (caused by localized vasodilation when pressure is relieved)
▶ Small blisters or erosions and ultimately necrosis and ulceration (when superficial erythema has progressed)
▶ Inflammation and, eventually, infection, leading to further necrosis
▶ Foul-smelling, purulent discharge seeping from a lesion that has penetrated the skin from beneath
▶ Black eschar around and over the lesion because infected, necrotic tissue prevents healthy granulation of scar tissue

Diagnostic tests

▶ *Wound culture and sensitivity testing* of the ulcer exudate identify the infective organisms.
▶ *Blood studies* for serum protein and serum albumin may be ordered to determine severe hypoproteinemia.

Treatment

Successful management of pressure ulcers involves relieving pressure on the affected area, keeping the area clean and dry, and promoting healing. Devices, such as pads, mattresses, and special beds, may be used to relieve pressure. However, turning and repositioning are still necessary. A diet high in protein, iron, and vitamin C can help promote healing.

Other treatments depend on the ulcer stage. (See *Stages of pressure ulcers*, page 490.) Stage 1 treatment aims to increase tissue pliability, stimulate local circulation, promote healing, and prevent skin breakdown. Specific measures include the use of hydrocolloids, lubricating sprays, moisturizing lotions, skin sealants, and transparent films. Adjunctive therapies inlude electrical stimulationg, nutritional support, support surface, and ultrasound, which may be used in all stages to enhance wound healing.

For stage 2 ulcers with light or moderate exudate or drainage, dressings include collagen, composites, foams, hydrogel wafers, moist impregnated gauzes and specialty absorptives.

For stage 3 or 4 ulcers, therapy aims to promote wound drainage, absorb any exudate, and promote healing. Dressings include collagen, foams (fillers), hydrocolloids (pastes, fillers), hydrogels (amorphores, gauze), moist impregnated packing gauzes and wound fillers. If necrosis is present, alginates are also effective. Debridement and hyperbaric oxygen therapy are included as adjuvant therapy.

Debridement of necrotic tissue may be necessary to allow healing. One method is to apply open wet dressings and allow them to dry on the ulcer. Removal of the dressings mechanically debrides exudate and necrotic tissue. Occasionally, pressure ulcers require debridement using surgical, mechanical, or chemical techniques. In severe cases, skin grafting may be necessary.

Key nursing diagnoses and outcomes

Impaired skin integrity related to decreased blood flow

Treatment outcome: The patient will regain normal skin integrity.

Risk for infection related to impaired skin integrity

Treatment outcome: The patient will remain free from infection.

Deficient knowledge related to pressure ulcers

Treatment outcome: The patient will communicate an understanding of the care required for the existing pressure ulcer and of measures to prevent further ulcers.

Nursing interventions

▶ During each shift, check the patient's skin for changes in color, temperature, and sensation. Examine an existing ulcer

Stages of pressure ulcers

To protect the patient from pressure ulcer complications, learn to recognize the four stages of ulcer formation.

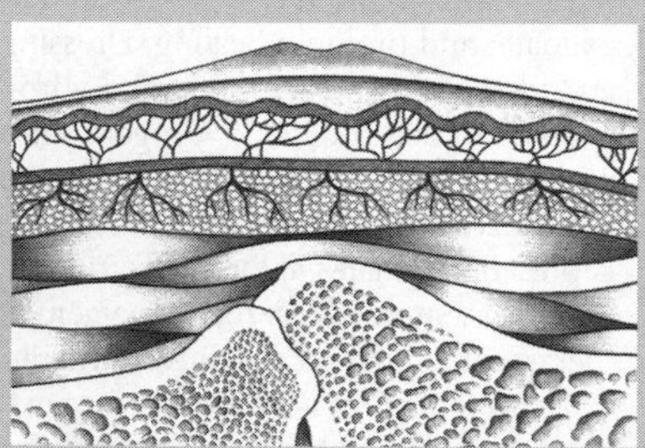

Stage 1

In stage 1, the skin stays red for 5 minutes after removal of pressure and may develop an abrasion of the epidermis. (A black person's skin may look purple.) The skin also feels warm and firm. The sore is usually reversible if you remove pressure.

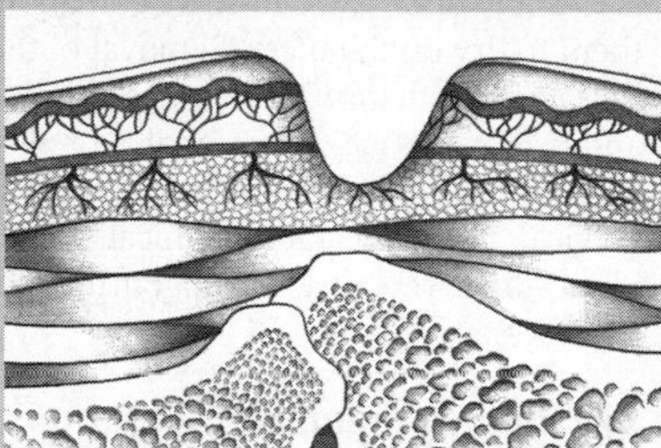

Stage 2

In stage 2, breaks appear in the skin, and discoloration may occur. Penetrating to the subcutaneous fat layer, the sore is painful and visibly swollen. If pressure is removed, the sore may heal within 1 to 2 weeks.

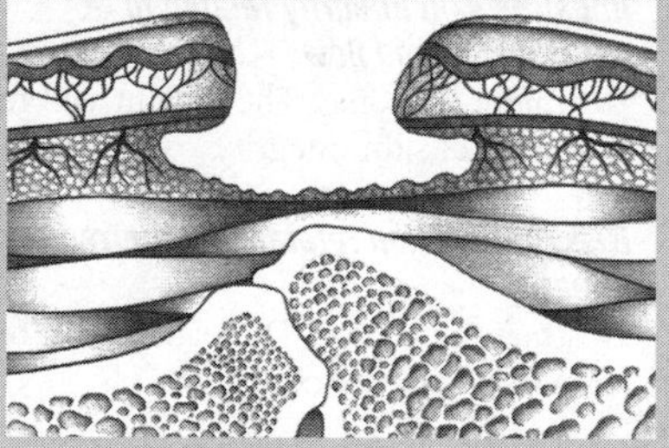

Stage 3

In stage 3, a hole develops that oozes foul-smelling yellow or green fluid. Extending into the muscle, the ulcer may develop a black leathery crust or eschar at its edges and eventually at the center. The ulcer isn't painful, but healing may take months.

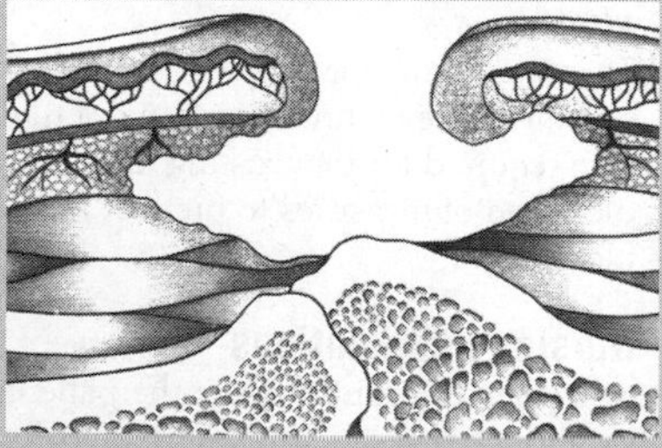

Stage 4

During stage 4, the ulcer destroys tissue from the skin to the bone and becomes necrotic. Findings include foul drainage and deep tunnels that extend from the ulcer. Months or even a year may elapse before the ulcer heals.

for any change in size or degree of damage.

▶ Reposition the patient at least every 2 hours around the clock. Minimize the effects of shearing force by using a footboard and not raising the head of the bed more than 30 degrees. Keep the patient's knees slightly flexed for short periods.

▶ Perform passive range-of-motion (ROM) exercises, or encourage the patient to do active exercises if possible.

▶ To prevent pressure ulcers in an immobilized patient, use pressure-relief aids on his bed.

▶ Give the patient meticulous skin care. Keep his skin clean and dry without using harsh soaps. Rub moisturizing lotions into the skin thoroughly to prevent maceration of the skin surface. Change bed linens frequently for a diaphoretic or incontinent patient.

▶ If the patient is incontinent, offer him a bedpan or commode frequently. A urinary or fecal incontinence device may be necessary. Use only a single layer of padding for urine and fecal incontinence because excessive padding increases perspiration, which leads to maceration. Excessive padding may also wrinkle, irritating the skin.

▶ Treat pressure ulcers as ordered by the wound care specialist.

▶ Encourage adequate food and fluid intake to maintain body weight and promote healing. Consult the dietitian to provide a diet that promotes granulation of new tissue. Encourage the debilitated patient to eat frequent, small meals that include protein and calorie-rich supplements. Assist the weakened patient with meals.

▶ Monitor the patient for infection at the ulcer site.

▶ Because anemia and elevated blood glucose levels may lead to skin breakdown, monitor hemoglobin and blood glucose levels and hematocrit.

PATIENT TEACHING

▶ Explain the function of pressure-relief aids and topical agents, and demonstrate their proper use.

▶ Teach the patient and a family member position-changing techniques and active and passive ROM exercises.

▶ Stress the importance of good hygiene. Teach the patient to avoid skin-damaging agents, such as harsh soaps, alcohol-based products, tincture of benzoin, and hexachlorophene.

▶ As indicated, explain debridement procedures and prepare the patient for skin graft surgery.

▶ Teach the patient and his family to recognize and record signs of healing. Explain that treatment typically varies according to the stage of healing.

▶ Encourage the patient to eat a well-balanced diet and consume an adequate amount of fluids, explaining their importance in promoting healthy skin. Point out dietary sources rich in vitamin C, which aids wound healing, promotes iron absorption, and helps in collagen formation.

PRIVACY

Although the United States Constitution doesn't formally sanction a right to privacy, the earliest articles proposing such a basic right were published in 1890. Since that time, a series of Supreme Court decisions (*Roe v. Wade,* 1973; *Griswald v. Connecticut,* 1965; *Eisenstadt v. Baird,* 1972; and *In re Quinlan,* 1976) have carved out such rights.

Today, the concept of privacy as it relates to health care includes several issues: a patient's right to information about his health status, his freedom from unwanted intrusion by health care workers, and his freedom from disclosure of private facts by health care personnel. Legislative changes also greatly affect the way medical records and privacy issues are handled.

How can you uphold your patient's right to privacy? In general, by maintaining the confidentiality of his health-related information and providing sufficient information for the patient and his family members to make realistic, competent decisions about health care.

Special considerations

To help your patient make informed health care decisions, make sure he and his family understand his illness, the goals of his planned treatment, and his ultimate prognosis. Develop a care plan that incorporates the patient's goals and wishes. Make sure the nursing diagnoses you select meet your patient's goals and expectations.

By involving the patient in decision making about his care, interventions, risks, and outcomes, you not only keep the patient informed about his care, but also reduce the chance that he or his family will take legal action if the ultimate outcome is less than expected.

The courts have consistently held that nurses possess a vital and legally enforceable role as patient advocate. This role includes ensuring open communication with the patient and giving the patient decision-making power regarding his care. Providing patients with adequate information, in terms they can comprehend, from which they can make sound decisions about their health care ensures that you are serving as your patient's advocate.

Finally, keep in mind that your patient has the right to see or obtain a copy of his health records. When it comes to other, unrelated people, however, it's up to you to keep his health records private. You should reveal information about his health only with his consent or when required by law.

PROSTATE CANCER

The most common neoplasm in men over age 40, prostate cancer is a leading cause of cancer death in men. Prostate cancer has highest incidence among Blacks and lowest among Asians. Incidence appears to be unaffected by socioeconomic status or fertility. Adenocarcinoma is the most common form; only seldom does prostate cancer occur as a sarcoma.

Slow-growing prostate cancer seldom produces signs and symptoms until it's well advanced. When primary prostatic lesions spread beyond the prostate gland, they typically invade the prostatic capsule and spread along the ejaculatory ducts in the space between the seminal vesicles or perivesicular fascia. When prostate cancer is treated in its localized form, the 5-year survival rate is 70%; after metastasis, it's under 35%. Death usually results from widespread bone metastasis.

The primary risk factor for prostate cancer is age (seldom found in men under age 40). Endocrine factors also play a role. Androgens are known to be necessary for tumor growth. Progressive disease can lead to spinal cord compression, deep vein thrombosis, and pulmonary emboli.

Signs and symptoms

- Usually, no signs or symptoms in early disease
- Dysuria, nocturia, urinary frequency, complete urine retention, or hematuria
- Edema of the scrotum or leg (in advanced disease)
- Back or hip pain (may signal bone metastasis)
- On palpation, nonraised, firm, nodular mass with a sharp edge (in early disease) or a hard lump (in advanced disease)

Diagnostic tests

▶ *Digital rectal examination,* recommended yearly by the American Cancer Society for men over age 40, is the standard screening test.

▶ *Blood tests* may reveal elevated levels of prostate-specific antigen (PSA); although most men with metastasized prostatic cancer have an elevated PSA level, this finding also occurs with other prostatic diseases.

▶ *Transrectal prostatic ultrasonography* may be used for patients with abnormal digital rectal examination and PSA test findings.

▶ *Biopsy* is the definitive diagnostic test.

▶ *Bone scan* and *excretory urography* may determine the disease's extent.

▶ *Magnetic resonance imaging* and *computed tomography scans* can help define the tumor's extent.

Treatment

Therapy varies according to the cancer stage and may include prostatectomy, radiation therapy, hormonal therapy, orchiectomy (removal of the testes) to reduce androgen production, and hormonal therapy with synthetic estrogen (diethylstilbestrol). Radical prostatectomy is usually effective for localized lesions without metastasis. Transurethral resection of the prostate may be performed to relieve an obstruction in metastatic disease.

Radiation therapy may cure locally invasive lesions in early disease and may relieve bone pain from metastatic skeletal involvement. It may also be used prophylactically for patients with tumors in regional lymph nodes. Alternatively, brachytherapy or implantation of radioactive seeds or pellets into the prostate may be recommended because it permits increased radiation to reach the prostate but minimizes the surrounding tissues' exposure to radiation.

If hormonal therapy, surgery, and radiation therapy aren't feasible or successful, chemotherapy may be used. Chemotherapy for prostatic cancer (combinations of cyclophosphamide, doxorubicin, fluorouracil, cisplatin, etoposide, and vindesine) offers limited benefits. Researchers continue to seek the most effective chemotherapeutic regimen.

Key nursing diagnoses and outcomes

Impaired urinary elimination related to functional changes in lower urinary system

Treatment outcome: The patient will regain a normal urinary elimination pattern once prostate cancer has been treated.

Anxiety related to diagnosis

Treatment outcome: The patient will cope with the diagnosis without showing signs of severe anxiety.

Chronic pain related to metastasis to bone

Treatment outcome: The patient will become pain-free with eradication of prostate cancer.

Nursing interventions

▶ Encourage the patient to express his fears and concerns, including those about changes in his sexual identity. Offer reassurance when possible.

Cultural diversity **Individuals from some cultual groups may use folk or home remedies. For example, Polish Americans, especially those who have recently immigrated to the United States, may treat urination problems with a tea made from pumpkin seeds. Many individuals seek out "natural cures" and use over-the-counter preparations to alleviate their problems. This may delay medical treatment. During the patient history, ask the patient about any home remedies he may have used.**

▶ Administer ordered analgesics and provide comfort measures to reduce pain. Evaluate the patient's pain level and the effectiveness of administered analgesics. Encourage the patient to identify care measures that promote his comfort and relaxation.
▶ Monitor the patient's urinary system for dysfunction. Measure intake and output.
▶ Encourage the patient undergoing radiation to drink at least eight 8-oz glasses of fluid daily.
▶ Watch for the common adverse effects of radiation to the prostate: proctitis, diarrhea, bladder spasms, and urinary frequency. Internal radiation of the prostate almost always results in cystitis in the first 2 to 3 weeks of therapy. Administer analgesics and antispasmodics to decrease his discomfort.
▶ Prepare the patient for surgery as indicated.
▶ Monitor for complications of surgery. A radical prostatectomy may cause incontinence (2%), urethral stricture (8%), and erectile dysfunction (94%).
▶ Watch for adverse reactions (hot flashes, decreased libido, erectile dysfunction, and gynecomastia) in a patient receiving hormonal therapy with luteinizing hormone-releasing hormone analog agonists. During the first 2 to 4 weeks of therapy, symptoms of bone pain may increase because of "the flare phenomenon"—an increase in testosterone production that occurs at the beginning of hormonal therapy. Administer increased amounts of analgesics during this period, as needed.

PATIENT TEACHING

▶ Prepare the patient for the type of surgery he'll be having.
▶ If appropriate, discuss the adverse effects of pelvic radiation therapy, such as diarrhea, urinary frequency, nocturia, bladder spasms, rectal irritation, and tenesmus.
▶ Encourage the patient to maintain as normal a lifestyle as possible during recovery.
▶ When appropriate, refer the patient to the social services department, local home health care agencies, hospices, and prostate cancer support organizations.

PROSTATECTOMY

Prostatectomy, the partial or total surgical removal of the prostate, is used to treat prostate cancer and benign prostatic hyperplasia (BPH) when drug therapy and other treatments are ineffective. Depending on the disease, one of four approaches is used. Transurethral resection of the prostate (TURP), the most common approach, involves insertion of a resectoscope into the urethra to remove tissue with a wire loop and electric current. TURP may be used to treat a moderately enlarged prostate and as a palliative measure in prostate cancer to remove an obstruction.

Open surgical methods are used to treat benign growths and prostate cancer if the prostate is too large for TURP. Open approaches include suprapubic, retropubic, and perineal prostatectomy, a radical prostatectomy using the perineal approach. (See *Comparing types of prostatectomy,* pages 496 and 497.) Total or partial prostatectomy is also an option for men with significantly obstructive BPH; it's performed to remove diseased or obstructive tissue and restore urine flow through the urethra. Radical prostatectomy is a treatment option for early stages of prostate cancer. When the cancer is in its later stages, the prostate can't be resected and only palliative measures, such as TURP, are used to remove obstructions.

Implementation

▶ In TURP, the patient is placed in the lithotomy position and anesthetized. The surgeon then introduces a resectoscope into the urethra and advances it to the prostate. After instilling a clear irrigating solution and visualizing the obstruction, he uses the resectoscope's cutting loop to resect prostatic tissue and restore the urethral opening.

▶ In suprapubic prostatectomy, the patient is placed in the supine position and given a general anesthetic. The surgeon begins by making a horizontal incision just above the symphysis pubis. After instilling fluid into the bladder to distend it, he makes a small incision in the bladder wall to expose the prostate. He then shells the obstructing prostatic tissue out of its bed with his finger. After clearing the obstruction and ligating all bleeding points, he usually inserts a suprapubic drainage tube and a Penrose drain.

▶ In retropubic prostatectomy, the patient is placed in the supine position and anesthetized. The surgeon makes a horizontal suprapubic incision and approaches the prostate from between the bladder and the pubic arch. He then makes another incision in the prostatic capsule and removes the obstructing tissue. After controlling any bleeding, he usually inserts a suprapubic tube and a Penrose drain. This allows for pelvic lymph node dissection, which is necessary to stage prostate cancer.

▶ In perineal prostatectomy, the patient is anesthetized and placed in an exaggerated lithotomy position in which the knees are drawn up against the chest and the buttocks are slightly elevated. The surgeon makes an inverted U-shaped incision in the perineum and then removes the entire prostate and the seminal vesicles. He anastomoses the urethra to the bladder and closes the incision, leaving a Penrose drain in place. This approach is safer in patients who are obese or who have had previous lower abdominal or pelvic surgery.

Complications

Complications of prostatectomy include hemorrhage, infection, urine retention, erectile dysfunction, and incontinence.

Key nursing diagnoses and outcomes

Disturbed body image related to incontinence

Treatment outcomes: The patient will demonstrate skill in managing incontinence and will express positive feelings about himself.

Risk for infection related to drains and catheters left in place

Treatment outcome: The patient will remain free from signs and symptoms of infection.

Sexual dysfunction related to erectile dysfunction

Treatment outcome: The patient will identify treatment options to restore erectile ability or alternative sexual practices that are satisfying and acceptable to him and his partner.

Nursing interventions

Your main responsibilities in caring for a prostatectomy patient are patient teaching and monitoring for postoperative complications.

Before surgery

▶ Review the planned surgery, and encourage the patient to ask questions. Provide straightforward answers to help clear up any misconceptions he may have.

▶ Offer emotional support. Encourage the patient to express his fears, and help to allay them by emphasizing the positive aspects of the surgery, such as improved urination and prevention of further complications.

▶ Because some types of prostatectomy can result in erectile dysfunction, you may need to arrange for sexual counseling to help the patient and his partner cope with this often devastating complication.

▶ If the patient is scheduled for TURP, explain that this procedure often causes retrograde ejaculation but otherwise doesn't impair sexual function.

Comparing types of prostatectomy

Procedure and indications	Advantages and disadvantages
Transurethral resection of the prostate (TURP) ■ Benign prostatic hyperplasia (BPH) ■ Moderately enlarged prostate ■ Prostate cancer, as a palliative measure to remove obstruction	■ Safer and less painful and invasive than other prostate procedures ■ Doesn't require surgical incision ■ Short hospital stay ■ Little risk of erectile dysfunction ■ Risk of urethral stricture and delayed bleeding ■ Not a curative surgery for prostate cancer ■ May result in retrograde ejaculation
Perineal prostatectomy ■ Prostate cancer ■ BPH, if the prostate is too large for TURP and the patient is no longer sexually active	■ Allows direct visualization of gland ■ Permits drainage by gravity ■ Low mortality and decreased incidence of shock ■ High incidence of erectile dysfunction and incontinence ■ Risk of damage to rectum and external sphincter ■ Restricted operative field
Retropubic prostatectomy ■ BPH, if the prostate is too large for TURP ■ Prostate cancer, if total removal of gland is necessary	■ Allows direct visualization of gland ■ Avoids bladder incision ■ Short convalescent period ■ Patient may retain sexual function ■ Can't be used to treat associated bladder pathology ■ Increased risk of hemorrhage from prostate venous plexus
Suprapubic prostatectomy ■ BPH, if the prostate is too large for TURP ■ Bladder lesions	■ Allows exploration of wide area, for example, into lymph nodes ■ Simple procedure ■ Requires bladder incision ■ Hemorrhage control difficult ■ Urine leakage common around suprapubic tube ■ Prolonged and uncomfortable recovery

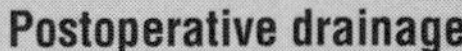

Postoperative drainage

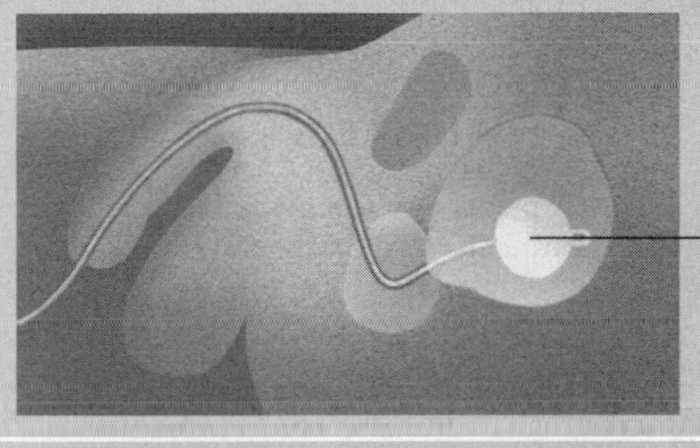

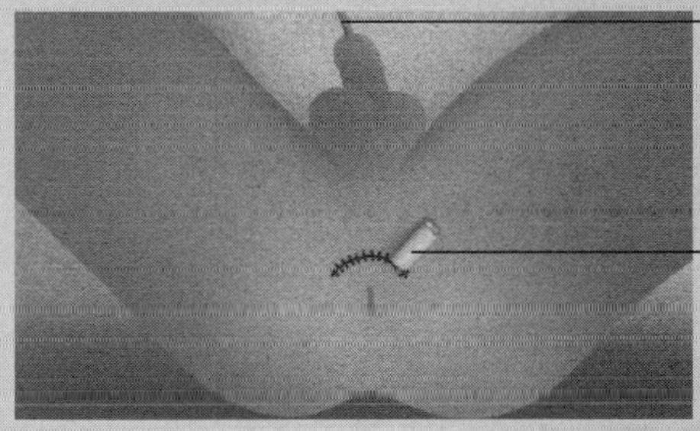

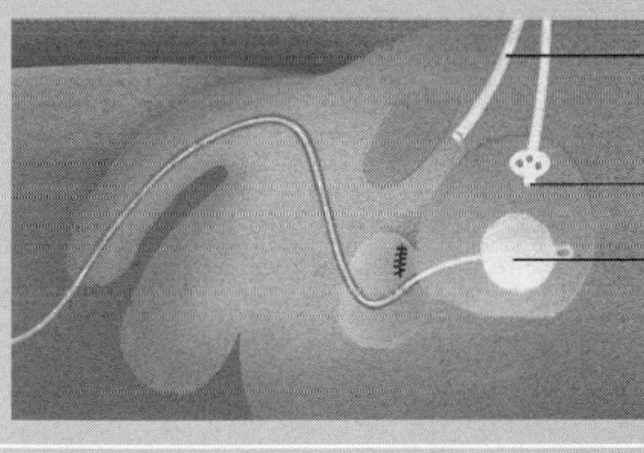

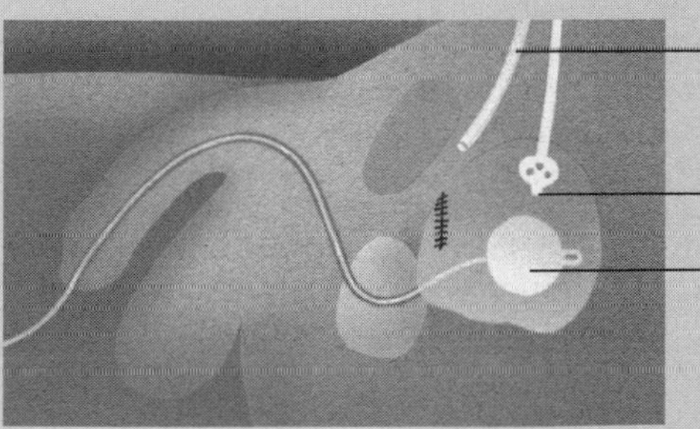

▶ Before surgery, administer an enema. Explain to the patient that he may have a catheter in place for several days to several weeks to ensure proper urine drainage and healing.

▶ Make sure the patient or a responsible family member has signed a consent form.

After surgery

▶ Monitor the patient's vital signs closely, looking for indications of hemorrhage and shock. Frequently check the incision site (if present) for signs of infection, and change dressings as necessary. Also, watch for and report signs of epididymitis: fever, chills, groin pain, and a tender, swollen epididymis.

▶ Record the amount and nature of urine drainage. Maintain indwelling urinary catheter patency through intermittent or continuous irrigation, as ordered. Watch for catheter blockage from kinking or clot formation, and correct as necessary.

▶ Maintain the patency of the suprapubic tube, if inserted, and monitor the amount and character of drainage. Drainage should be amber or slightly blood tinged; report any abnormalities. Keep the collection container below bladder level to promote drainage, and keep the skin around the tube insertion site clean and dry.

▶ Expect and report frank bleeding the first day after surgery. If bleeding is venous, the physician may increase the traction on the catheter or increase the pressure in the catheter's balloon end. If bleeding is arterial (bright red, with numerous clots and increased viscosity), it may need to be controlled surgically.

▶ As ordered, administer antispasmodics to control painful bladder spasms and analgesics to relieve incisional pain. Offer sitz baths to reduce perineal discomfort. Never administer drugs rectally after a total prostatectomy.

▶ Watch for signs of dilutional hyponatremia: altered mental status, muscle twitching, and seizures. If these occur, raise the bed's side rails to prevent injury, notify the physician, draw blood for serum sodium levels, and prepare hypertonic saline solution for possible I.V. infusion.

▶ Offer emotional support to the patient who has had a perineal prostatectomy because this procedure usually causes erectile dysfunction. Try to arrange for psychological and sexual counseling during the recovery period.

PATIENT TEACHING

▶ Tell the patient to take his prescribed medications as ordered. Suggest sitz baths for perineal discomfort.

▶ Tell the patient to drink ten 8-oz glasses of water a day and to urinate at least every 2 hours until his urine is clear and healing is complete. Advise him to notify the physician promptly if he has difficulty urinating.

▶ Explain that after catheter removal, he may experience transient urinary frequency and dribbling. Reassure the patient that he'll gradually regain control over urination. Teach him Kegel exercises to tighten the perineum and speed the return of sphincter control. Suggest that he avoid caffeine-containing beverages, which cause mild diuresis.

▶ Reassure the patient that slightly bloodtinged urine normally occurs for the first few weeks after surgery. However, tell him to report bright red urine or persistent hematuria.

▶ Tell the patient to immediately report any signs of infection, such as fever, chills, and flank pain.

▶ Warn the patient not to have sexual relations, lift anything heavier than 10 lb (4.5 kg), perform strenuous exercise (short walks are usually permitted), take long car trips, or drive a car until the physician gives permission. Explain that performing these activities too soon after surgery can cause bleeding.

▶ Urge the patient to keep all follow-up appointments and to have a yearly examination.

PULMONARY EDEMA

Marked by an accumulation of fluid in extravascular spaces of the lung, pulmonary edema is a common complication of cardiac disorders. It may occur as a chronic condition, or it may develop quickly and rapidly become fatal.

Pulmonary edema usually results from left-sided heart failure caused by arteriosclerotic, cardiomyopathic, hypertensive, or valvular heart disease. It stems from either of two mechanisms: increased pulmonary capillary hydrostatic pressure or decreased colloid osmotic pressure. Normally, the two pressures are in balance; when this balance changes, pulmonary edema results.

If pulmonary capillary hydrostatic pressure increases, the compromised left ventricle requires increased filling pressures to maintain adequate output; these pressures are transmitted to the left atrium, pulmonary veins, and pulmonary capillary bed. This forces fluids and solutes from the intravascular compartment into the interstitium of the lungs. As the interstitium overloads with fluid, fluid floods the peripheral alveoli and impairs gas exchange.

If colloid osmotic pressure decreases, the natural pulling force that contains intravascular fluids is lost — nothing opposes the hydrostatic force. Thus, fluid flows freely into the interstitium and alveoli, resulting in pulmonary edema.

Other factors that may predispose the patient to pulmonary edema include barbiturate or opiate poisoning, heart failure, infusion of excessive volumes of I.V. fluids or an overly rapid infusion, impaired pulmonary lymphatic drainage (from Hodgkin's disease or obliterative lymphangitis after radiation), and inhalation of irritating gases. Pulmonary edema is also linked to mitral stenosis and left atrial myxoma (which impair left atrial emptying), pneumonia, and pulmonary veno-occlusive disease.

Acute pulmonary edema may progress to respiratory and metabolic acidosis, with subsequent cardiac or respiratory arrest.

Signs and symptoms

▶ Persistent cough, possibly with frothy, bloody sputum
▶ Reports of a recent cold
▶ Dyspnea on exertion, paroxysmal nocturnal dyspnea, or orthopnea
▶ Labored respirations
▶ Restlessness and anxiety
▶ Neck vein distention
▶ Sweaty, cold, and clammy skin
▶ On auscultation, crepitant crackles and a diastolic (S_3) gallop or, in severe disease, wheezing (as alveoli and bronchioles fill with fluid), rhonchi and, ultimately, decreased or absent breath sounds

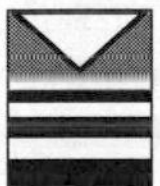

Key point If you detect inspiratory crackles, rhonchi, dry cough, or dyspnea, notify the physician immediately. Chest X-ray results may not be available until 24 hours after you've assessed the patient. Don't wait for X-ray findings if you suspect pulmonary edema.

▶ Decreased level of consciousness, worsening tachycardia, falling blood pressure, diminished breath sounds, thready pulse, and decreased cardiac output (in advanced stages)

Diagnostic tests

▶ *Arterial blood gas* (ABG) *analysis* usually shows hypoxia with variable partial pressure of carbon dioxide in arterial blood, depending on the patient's degree of fatigue. ABG results may also identify metabolic acidosis.
▶ *Chest X-rays* show diffuse haziness of the lung fields and, usually, cardiomegaly and pleural effusion.

- *Pulse oximetry* may reveal decreasing arterial oxygen saturation levels.
- *Pulmonary artery catheterization* identifies left-sided heart failure (indicated by elevated pulmonary artery wedge pressure). These findings help to rule out adult respiratory distress syndrome, in which wedge pressure usually remains normal.
- *Electrocardiography* may disclose evidence of previous or current myocardial infarction.

Treatment

High concentrations of oxygen can be administered by nasal cannula or mask. (Typically, the patient with pulmonary edema doesn't tolerate a mask.) If the patient's arterial oxygen levels remain too low, assisted ventilation can improve oxygen delivery to the tissues and usually improves his acid-base balance.

A bronchodilator, such as aminophylline, may decrease bronchospasm and enhance myocardial contractility. Diuretics, such as furosemide, ethacrynic acid, and bumetanide, increase urination, which helps to mobilize extravascular fluid.

Drug alert Older patients receiving diuretics require close observation because they're more susceptible to drug-induced diuresis. Excessive diuresis promotes rapid dehydration, leading to hypovolemia, hypokalemia, hyponatremia, and circulatory collapse.

Positive inotropic agents, such as cardiac glycosides, dobutamine, and milrinone lactate, enhance contractility. Pressor agents may be given to enhance contractility and to promote vasoconstriction in peripheral vessels. Antiarrhythmics may also be given, particularly to treat arrhythmias related to decreased cardiac output.

Arterial vasodilators, such as nitroprusside or nitroglycerin, can decrease peripheral vascular resistance, preload, and afterload. Morphine may reduce anxiety and dyspnea and dilate the systemic venous bed, promoting blood flow from pulmonary circulation to the periphery.

Key nursing diagnoses and outcomes

Anxiety related to inability to breathe comfortably

Treatment outcome: The patient will perform stress-reduction techniques to decrease anxiety.

Excess fluid volume related to fluid accumulation in lungs

Treatment outcome: The patient will regain and maintain a normal fluid balance with treatment.

Impaired gas exchange related to fluid accumulation in lungs

Treatment outcome: The patient will regain normal gas exchange with alleviation of pulmonary edema.

Nursing interventions

- Offer reassurance to the patient, who may be frightened by his inability to breathe normally. Provide emotional support.
- Place the patient in high Fowler's position to enhance lung expansion.
- Administer medications as ordered and note their effectiveness. Administer nitroprusside in dextrose 5% in water by I.V infusion. During administration, protect the solution from light by wrapping the bag with aluminum foil. Discard the unused solution after 24 hours. Monitor thiocyanate levels.
- Monitor the patient's vital signs frequently (every 5 to 15 minutes with nitroprusside and every 15 to 30 minutes with nitroglycerin). Watch for arrhythmias in patients receiving cardiac glycosides and for respiratory depression in those receiving morphine.
- Monitor the patient's intake and output.

▶ Evaluate serum electrolyte levels to assess kidney function and potassium level specifically for possible depletion from diuretics.

▶ Administer oxygen as ordered, and watch for complications.

▶ Assess respiratory status for increasing signs of distress.

▶ Monitor ABG values and pulse oximetry for oxygenation and signs of acidosis.

▶ If a pulmonary artery catheter is in place, monitor pulmonary end-diastolic and artery wedge pressures.

PATIENT TEACHING

▶ Explain all procedures to the patient and his family. Be sure to explain that pulmonary edema is a critical situation and may require emergency measures.

▶ Emphasize the importance of reporting early signs of fluid overload, such as swelling of lower extremities and dyspnea on exertion.

▶ Explain the reasons for sodium restrictions. List high-sodium foods and drugs.

▶ Review all prescribed medications with the patient. If he's taking digoxin, show him how to monitor his own pulse rate and warn him to report signs of toxicity. Encourage consumption of potassium-rich foods to lower the risk of toxicity and cardiac arrhythmias. If he's taking a vasodilator, teach him the signs of hypotension and emphasize the need to avoid alcohol. Explain to the patient to change positions slowly to minimize the effects of ortostatic hypotension, and prevent falling.

▶ Urge the patient to comply with the prescribed drug regimen to avoid future episodes of pulmonary edema.

▶ Discuss ways to conserve physical energy.

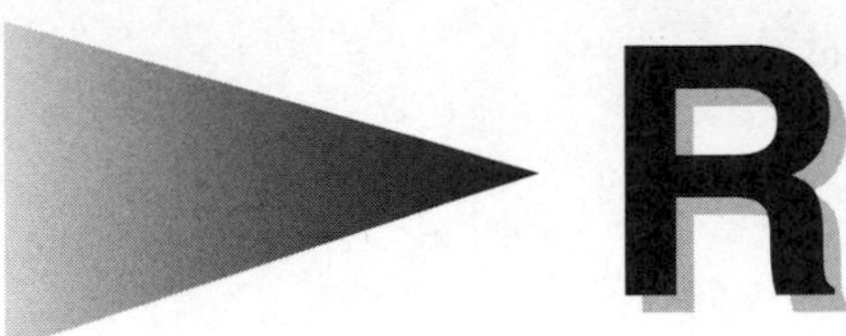

Radiation Therapy

About 60% of all cancer patients are treated with some form of external radiation therapy. Also called radiotherapy, this treatment delivers X-rays or gamma rays directly to the cancer site.

Radiation dosages are based on the type, stage, and location of the tumor as well as on the patient's size, condition, and overall treatment goals. Doses are given in increments, usually three to five times a week, until the total dose is reached.

The goals of radiation therapy include *cure,* in which the cancer is completely destroyed and not expected to recur; *control,* in which the cancer does not progress or regress, but is expected to progress at some later time; or *palliation,* in which radiation is given to relieve symptoms (such as bone pain, seizures, bleeding, and headache) caused by the cancer.

Radiation therapy may be augmented by chemotherapy, brachytherapy (radiation implant therapy), or surgery as needed.

External beam radiation therapy is delivered by machines that aim a concentrated beam of high-energy particles (photons and gamma rays) at the target site. Two types of machines are commonly used: units containing cobalt or cesium as radioactive sources for gamma rays, and linear accelerators that use electricity to produce X-rays. Linear accelerators produce high energy with great penetrating ability. Some (known as orthovoltage machines) produce less powerful electron beams that may be used for superficial tumors.

Supplies

- Radiation therapy machine
- Film badge or pocket dosimeter

Implementation

- Check to see that the radiation oncology department has obtained informed consent.
- Review the patient's clinical record for recent laboratory and imaging results, and alert the radiation oncology staff to any abnormalities or pertinent results (such as myelosuppression, paraneoplastic syndromes, oncologic emergencies, and tumor progression).
- Transport the patient to the radiology department.
- The patient begins by undergoing simulation (treatment planning), in which the target area is mapped out on his body using a machine similar to the radiotherapy machine. Then the target area is tattooed or marked in ink on his body to ensure accurate treatments.
- The physician and radiation oncologist determine the duration and frequency of treatments, depending on the patient's body size, the size of the area to be radiated (sometimes referred to as the port), the extent and location of cancer, and the treatment goals.
- During the actual session, the patient is positioned on the treatment table beneath the machine. Treatments last from a few seconds to a few minutes.

▶ After treatment is complete, the patient may return home or to his room.

Complications

Adverse effects arise gradually and diminish gradually after treatments. They may be acute, subacute (accumulating as treatment progresses), chronic (following treatment), and long-term (arising months to years after treatment). Adverse effects are localized to the area of treatment, and their severity depends on the total radiation dosage, underlying organ sensitivity, and the patient's overall condition.

Common acute and subacute adverse effects include altered skin integrity, altered GI and genitourinary function, altered fertility and sexual function, altered bone marrow production, fatigue, and alopecia.

Long-term complications may include radiation pneumonitis, neuropathy, skin and muscle atrophy, telangiectasia, fistulas, altered endocrine function, and secondary cancers.

Other complications of radiation therapy include headache, xerostomia, dysphagia, stomatitis, nausea and vomiting, heartburn, diarrhea, and cystitis.

Patient teaching

▶ Explain the treatment to the patient and his family to reduce anxiety and promote cooperation. Reassure the patient that he won't feel anything during the treatment and won't be radioactive afterward.

▶ Review the treatment goals and discuss the range of potential adverse effects and interventions to minimize them. Tell the patient to report any long-term adverse effects.

▶ Explain to the patient that the full benefit of radiation treatments may not occur until several weeks or months after treatment begins.

▶ Teach the patient and a family member proper skin care techniques and how to manage any complications of treatment.

▶ Emphasize the importance of keeping follow-up appointments with the physician.

▶ Inform the patient and his family members about local cancer services. Refer the patient to a support group such as a local chapter of the American Cancer Society.

Documentation

Record radiation precautions taken during treatment; the duration of the procedure and the patient's tolerance of it; grading of adverse effects, any interventions used to alleviate those effects, and the effectiveness of the interventions; teaching given to the patient and family and their responses to it; discharge plans and teaching; and referrals to local cancer services, if any.

RECTAL MEDICATION ADMINISTRATION

Medications that are administered rectally are usually in the form of suppositories or ointments. A rectal suppository is a small, solid, medicated mass, usually cone-shaped, with a cocoa butter or glycerin base. It may be inserted to stimulate peristalsis and defecation or to relieve pain, vomiting, and local irritation. Rectal suppositories commonly contain drugs that reduce fever, induce relaxation, interact poorly with digestive enzymes, or have a taste too offensive for oral use. The suppositories melt at body temperature and are absorbed slowly.

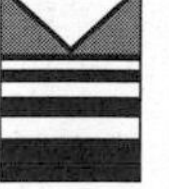

Key point Because insertion of a rectal suppository may stimulate the vagus nerve, this procedure is contraindicated in elderly patients with cardiac disease. Suppositories may also be contraindicated in patients who have had recent rectal or prostate surgery

How to administer a rectal suppository or ointment

When you insert a suppository, direct its tapered end toward the side of the rectum so it contacts the membranes, encouraging absorption of the medication.

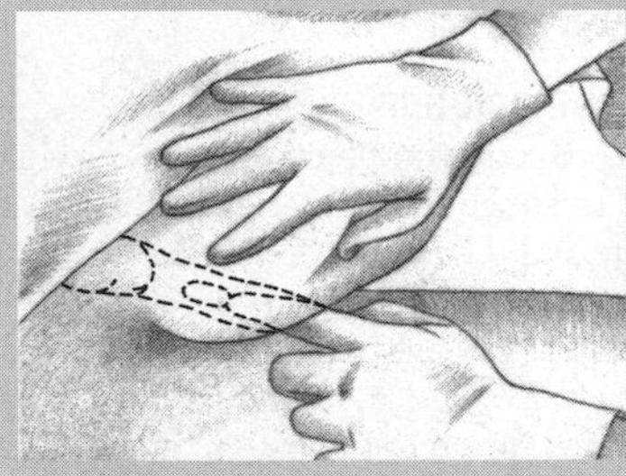

When you apply an ointment, be sure to lubricate the applicator to minimize pain on insertion. Direct the applicator tip toward the patient's umbilicus.

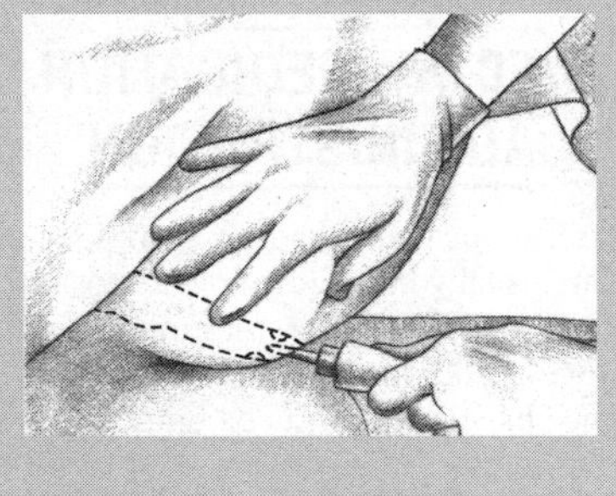

because of the risk of local trauma or discomfort during insertion.

An ointment is a semisolid medication used to produce local effects. It may be applied externally to the anus or internally to the rectum. Rectal ointments commonly contain drugs that reduce inflammation or relieve pain and itching.

Supplies

- Rectal suppository or tube of ointment and ointment applicator
- Patient's medication record and chart
- 4″ × 4″ gauze pads
- Gloves
- Water-soluble lubricant
- Optional: bedpan

Implementation

- Store rectal suppositories in the refrigerator until needed to prevent softening and possibly decreased effectiveness of the drug. A softened suppository is also difficult to handle and insert. To harden it again, hold the suppository (in its wrapper) under cold running water.
- Verify the order on the patient's medication record by checking it against the physician's order.
- Wash your hands with warm soap and water.
- Confirm the patient's identity by asking his name and checking the name, room number, and bed number on his wristband.
- Explain the procedure and the purpose of the drug to the patient.
- Provide privacy.

Inserting a rectal suppository

- Place the patient on his left side in Sims' position. Drape him with the bedcovers to expose only the buttocks.
- Put on gloves. Remove the suppository from its wrapper, and lubricate it with water-soluble lubricant.
- Lift the patient's upper buttock with your nondominant hand to expose the anus.
- Instruct the patient to take several deep breaths through his mouth to help relax the anal sphincters and reduce anxiety or discomfort during insertion.
- Using the index finger of your dominant hand, insert the suppository, tapered end first, about 3″ (7.5 cm), until you feel it pass the internal anal sphincter. Try to direct the tapered end toward the side of the rectum so it contacts the membranes. (See *How to administer a rectal suppository or ointment.*)
- Ensure the patient's comfort. Encourage him to lie quietly and, if applicable, to retain the suppository for the appropriate length of time. A suppository administered to relieve consti-

pation should be retained as long as possible (at least 20 minutes) to be effective. Press on the anus with a gauze pad if necessary until the urge to defecate passes.

▶ Because the intake of food and fluid stimulates peristalsis, a suppository used to relieve constipation should be inserted about 30 minutes before mealtime to help soften the feces in the rectum and facilitate defecation. A medicated retention suppository should be inserted between meals.

▶ Make sure the patient's call button is handy, and watch for his signal because he may be unable to suppress the urge to defecate. For example, a patient with proctitis has a highly sensitive rectum and may not be able to retain a suppository for long. If the patient has difficulty retaining the suppository, place him on a bedpan.

▶ Discard the used equipment.

Applying an ointment

▶ To apply externally, wear gloves or use a gauze pad to spread the drug over the anal area.

▶ To apply internally, attach the applicator to the tube of ointment and coat the applicator with water-soluble lubricant.

▶ Expect to use approximately 1″ (2.5 cm) of ointment. To gauge how much pressure to use during application, try squeezing a small amount from the tube before you attach the applicator.

▶ Lift the patient's upper buttock with your nondominant hand to expose the anus.

▶ Instruct the patient to take several deep breaths through his mouth to relax the anal sphincters and reduce anxiety or discomfort during insertion.

▶ Gently insert the applicator, directing it toward the umbilicus.

▶ Slowly squeeze the tube to eject the drug.

▶ Remove the applicator, and place a folded 4″ × 4″ gauze pad between the patient's buttocks to absorb excess ointment.

▶ Disassemble the tube and applicator. Recap the tube, and clean the applicator thoroughly with soap and warm water.

Complications

Incomplete drug absorption may occur if the patient can't retain the medication or if the rectum contains feces. Irritation of the mucosal tissues and pain may result if the patient has hemorrhoids or if the drug is irritating.

Patient teaching

▶ If the patient will have to use suppositories at home, teach him the proper procedure for rectal drug administration. Assess the patient's manual dexterity and ability to complete the task. If appropriate, enlist the help of a family member or caregiver.

▶ Inform the patient that the suppository may discolor his next bowel movement. Anusol suppositories, for example, can give feces a silver-gray pasty appearance.

Documentation

Record the administration time, the dose, and the patient's response. Document your patient teaching.

REFUSAL OF TREATMENT

People have the right not only to consent to medical care, but also to refuse it. Any mentally competent adult may legally refuse treatment if he's fully informed about his medical condition and the likely consequences of his refusal. A person may refuse treatment even after having given consent initially. The patient or guardian need only notify the health care provider that the patient no longer wishes to continue the therapy.

In some circumstances, when the danger of stopping therapy poses too great a risk for the patient, the law allows the therapy to continue. For example, a postoperative patient can't refuse procedures that ensure a safe transition from anesthesia. Likewise, a patient can't refuse immediate care for life-threatening arrhythmias following a myocardial infarction if that refusal would worsen his condition (unless a valid living will is on file). After the arrhythmias have abated, the patient may refuse further treatment.

The right of refusal does have potential consequences. The patient or guardian must be informed that refusing treatment will likely cause the patient's physical condition to deteriorate and may hasten death. The right of refusal can also block third-party reimbursements, because some insurance policies have a clause that denies or limits reimbursement when a patient refuses procedures that would aid in diagnosing or reducing injury or illness.

Most cases of refusal of treatment involve patients with a terminal illness or their families who want to discontinue life support. However, patients may also cite freedom of religion in refusing medical care.

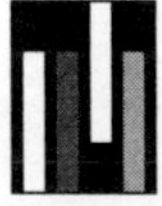

Cultural diversity **Cultural influences on treatment refusal are demonstrated by Jehovah's Witnesses and Christian Scientists, who may refuse treatment on religious grounds. Jehovah's Witnesses oppose blood transfusions based on their interpretation of a biblical passage that forbids "drinking" blood. Members of the Church of Christ, Scientist, reject all medical interventions, relying only on prayer to achieve healing.**

Special considerations

There are limitations on the patient's right to refuse therapy. The state may deny a patient's right of refusal in several instances. These state's rights exist to prevent crimes and protect the welfare of society as a whole. Limitations on refusal are designed to:

- preserve life if the patient doesn't have an incurable or terminal disease
- protect minor dependents
- prevent irrational self-destruction
- maintain the ethical integrity of health professionals by allowing the facility or other facility to treat the patient
- protect the public's health.

In cases filed to enforce the right to refuse care, the courts have attempted to balance the rights of the individual against those of society at large. In *Leach v. Akron General Medical Center* (1984), the court found that a patient has the right to refuse therapy based on a right to privacy. In this case, the patient was incompetent and the issue was whether to allow him to forgo life-sustaining treatment. In cases involving religious objections to treatment, the courts have generally upheld the right to refuse treatment based on the constitutionally protected right to religious freedom.

As a health care provider, you may have difficulty accepting a patient's decision to refuse treatment. But as a professional, you must respect that decision. If your patient refuses treatment, take the following steps:

- Tell him the risks involved in not undergoing the treatment.
- If the patient understands the risks but still refuses treatment, notify your supervisor and the physician.
- Record the patient's refusal in your nurses' notes.
- Ask the patient to complete a refusal of treatment release form. The signed form indicates that the appropriate treatment would have been given if the patient had consented. This form protects you, the physicians, and your facility from liability for not providing treatment.
- If the patient refuses to sign the release form, document this in your nurses' notes.

▶ Your facility may require the patient's spouse or closest relative to sign another refusal of treatment release form. Document whether the spouse or relative does so.

RESPIRATORY ACIDOSIS

This acid-base disturbance is characterized by reduced alveolar ventilation and manifested by hypercapnia (partial pressure of arterial carbon dioxide [$PaCO_2$] greater than 45 mm Hg). Respiratory acidosis can be acute (caused by sudden failure in ventilation) or chronic (resulting from long-term pulmonary disease). The prognosis depends on the severity of the underlying disturbance and the patient's general clinical condition.

Factors that predispose a patient to respiratory acidosis include:

▶ the use of drugs, such as narcotics, anesthetics, hypnotics, and sedatives, which depress the respiratory control center's sensitivity

▶ central nervous system (CNS) trauma, such as medullary injury, which may impair ventilatory drive

▶ chronic metabolic alkalosis, which may occur when respiratory compensatory mechanisms attempt to normalize pH by decreasing alveolar ventilation

▶ neuromuscular diseases, such as Guillain-Barré syndrome, myasthenia gravis, and poliomyelitis, in which respiratory muscles fail to respond properly to respiratory drive, reducing alveolar ventilation.

In addition, respiratory acidosis can be caused by an airway obstruction or parenchymal lung disease that interferes with alveolar ventilation or from chronic obstructive pulmonary disease (COPD), asthma, severe adult respiratory distress syndrome, chronic bronchitis, large pneumothorax, extensive pneumonia, or pulmonary edema.

Acute or chronic respiratory acidosis can produce shock and cardiac arrest.

Signs and symptoms

▶ Headache

▶ Dyspnea

▶ Diaphoresis

▶ Nausea and vomiting

▶ Bounding pulses on palpation

▶ Rapid, shallow respirations, tachycardia and, possibly, hypotension

▶ Altered level of consciousness (LOC), ranging from restlessness, confusion, and apprehension to somnolence

▶ Asterixis and depressed reflexes

Diagnostic tests

▶ *Arterial blood gas* (ABG) *analysis* confirms respiratory acidosis.

Key point **The following ABG values confirm respiratory acidosis: $PaCO_2$ above 45 mm Hg; pH typically below the normal range of 7.35 to 7.45; and bicarbonate (HCO_3^-) levels normal (22 to 26 mEq/L) in the acute acidosis but elevated (above 26 mEq/L) in chronic acidosis.**

Treatment

Effective treatment aims to correct the source of alveolar hypoventilation. If alveolar ventilation is significantly reduced, the patient may need mechanical ventilation until the underlying condition can be treated. This includes bronchodilators, oxygen, and antibiotics in COPD; drug therapy for conditions such as myasthenia gravis; removal of foreign bodies from the airway in cases of obstruction; antibiotics for pneumonia; dialysis to eliminate toxic drugs; and correction of metabolic alkalosis.

Dangerously low pH levels (less than 7.15) can produce profound CNS and cardiovascular deterioration, which may require administration of I.V. sodium bicarbonate. In chronic lung disease, elevated CO_2 levels may persist despite treatment.

Key nursing diagnoses and outcomes

Impaired gas exchange related to alveolar hypoventilation

Treatment outcomes: The patient will regain and maintain normal ABG values.

Ineffective breathing pattern related to rapid shallow respirations

Treatment outcomes: The patient will reestablish his respiratory rate within normal limits and will express a feeling of comfort with his breathing pattern.

Nursing interventions

- Be prepared to treat or remove the underlying cause such as an airway obstruction.
- Maintain adequate hydration by administering I.V. fluids.
- Give oxygen (only at low concentrations in patients with COPD) if the partial pressure of arterial oxygen drops.
- Give aerosolized or I.V. bronchodilators as prescribed, and monitor and record the patient's response to them.
- Start mechanical ventilation if hypoventilation can't be corrected immediately. Maintain a patent airway, and provide adequate humidification if acidosis requires mechanical ventilation. Continuously monitor ventilator settings if the patient requires intubation.
- Perform tracheal suctioning regularly and chest physiotherapy if ordered.
- Reassure the patient as much as possible, depending on his LOC. Allay the fears and concerns of family members by keeping them informed about the patient's status.
- Be alert for critical changes in the patient's respiratory, CNS, and cardiovascular function, and report such changes immediately. Also monitor and report variations in ABG levels and electrolyte status.
- To detect developing respiratory acidosis, closely monitor patients with COPD and chronic CO_2 retention for signs of acidosis. Also closely monitor all patients who receive narcotics and sedatives.

PATIENT TEACHING

- Instruct the patient who's recovering from a general anesthetic to turn and perform deep-breathing and coughing exercises frequently to prevent respiratory acidosis.
- Explain the reasons for ABG analysis.
- If the patient receives home oxygen therapy for COPD, stress the importance of maintaining the dose at the ordered flow rate. Teach the patient and a family member about home oxygen therapy use and safety measures.
- Alert the patient to possible adverse effects of prescribed drugs. Tell him to call the physician if any occur.

RESPIRATORY ALKALOSIS

Marked by a decrease in the partial pressure of arterial carbon dioxide ($Paco_2$) to less than 35 mm Hg and a rise in blood pH above 7.45, respiratory alkalosis is caused by alveolar hyperventilation. Uncomplicated respiratory alkalosis leads to a decrease in hydrogen ion concentration, which raises the blood pH. Hypocapnia occurs when the lungs eliminate more CO_2 than the body produces at the cellular level. In the acute stage, respiratory alkalosis is also called hyperventilation syndrome.

Factors that predispose a person to respiratory alkalosis include:

- compensation for metabolic acidosis
- heart failure
- central nervous system (CNS) injury to the respiratory control center
- extreme anxiety
- fever
- overventilation during mechanical ventilation
- pulmonary embolism
- salicylate intoxication (early).

Signs and symptoms

- Light-headedness
- Paresthesia
- Anxiety
- Rapid breathing
- Tetany, with visible twitching and flexion of the wrists and ankles; tachycardia; and deep, rapid breathing (in severe alkalosis)

In severe respiratory alkalosis, related cardiac arrhythmias may fail to respond to usual treatment. Some patients may have seizures.

Diagnostic tests

- *Arterial blood gas* (ABG) *analysis* confirms respiratory alkalosis and rules out compensation for metabolic acidosis. (See *Using ABG values to assess respiratory acid-base imbalances,* pages 510 and 511.)

Key point **The following ABG levels confirm respiratory alkalosis: $PaCO_2$ below 35 mm Hg; pH rising in proportion to fall in $PaCO_2$ in the acute stage but dropping toward normal (7.35 to 7.45) in the chronic stage; and bicarbonate (HCO_3^-) level normal (22 to 26 mEq/L) in the acute stage but decreased (less than 22 mEq/L) in the chronic stage.**

- *Serum electrolyte studies* may also be performed to detect metabolic acid-base disorders.

Treatment

Treatment attempts to eradicate the underlying condition — for example, by removing ingested toxins or by treating fever, sepsis, or CNS disorder. In severe respiratory alkalosis, the patient may need to breathe into a paper bag, which helps relieve acute anxiety and increase CO_2 levels. If respiratory alkalosis results from anxiety, sedatives and tranquilizers may help the patient.

Prevention of hyperventilation in patients receiving mechanical ventilation requires monitoring ABG levels and adjusting dead-space or minute volume.

Key nursing diagnoses and outcomes

Anxiety related to cause of respiratory alkalosis

Treatment outcomes: The patient will express feelings of anxiety and will exhibit a decrease in physical anxiety symptoms when respiratory alkalosis resolves.

Impaired gas exchange related to alveolar hyperventilation

Treatment outcomes: The patient will regain and maintain normal ABG values and will exhibit no signs or symptoms of severe respiratory alkalosis, such as cardiac arrhythmias and seizures.

Ineffective breathing pattern related to deep, rapid breathing

Treatment outcomes: The patient will regain a normal respiratory rate and pattern and will express a feeling of comfort with his breathing pattern.

Nursing interventions

- Provide supportive care for the underlying cause of respiratory alkalosis, as ordered.
- Stay with the patient during periods of extreme stress and anxiety. Offer reassurance and maintain a calm, quiet environment.
- If the patient is coping with anxiety-induced respiratory alkalosis, help him identify factors that precipitate anxiety. Also help him find coping mechanisms and activities that promote relaxation.
- Watch for and report changes in neurologic, neuromuscular, and cardiovascular functioning.
- Remember that twitching and cardiac arrhythmias may be associated with alkalemia and electrolyte imbalances. Monitor ABG and serum electrolyte levels closely. Report any variations immediately.

Using ABG values to assess respiratory acid-base imbalances

To help determine if a patient is experiencing a respiratory acid-base imbalance, follow the decision-tree steps below to interpret the patient's arterial blood gas (ABG) values.

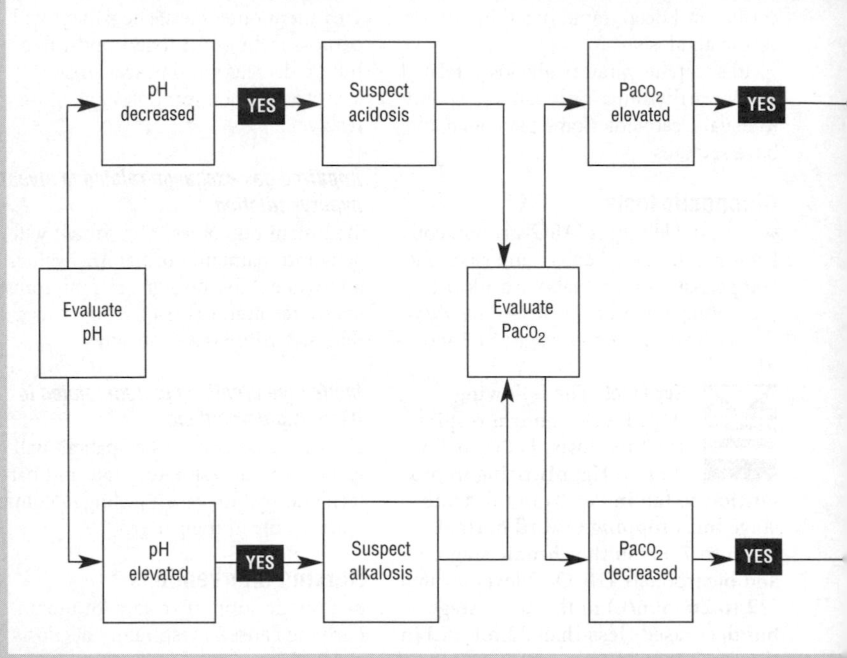

PATIENT TEACHING

- Explain all tests and treatments to the patient. Allow ample time to answer his questions.
- Teach the patient anxiety-reducing techniques, such as guided imagery, meditation, or yoga. Teach him how to counter hyperventilation with a controlled-breathing pattern.

RESTRAINT USE

The use of physical restraints to prevent patient falls has been the subject of considerable debate. Although preventing falls is important, studies have shown that restraints do not prevent serious injuries and can actually do more harm than good.

Restraining an elderly person to a bed or chair puts him at risk for a host of complications, including muscle weakness and atrophy, bone demineralization, loss of balance, pressure ulcers, orthostatic hypotension, hypostatic pneumonia, urine retention, constipation, decreased appetite, agitation, delirium, and depression. And the use of restraints often exacerbates the problem for which the patient was originally restrained, such as agitation or restlessness.

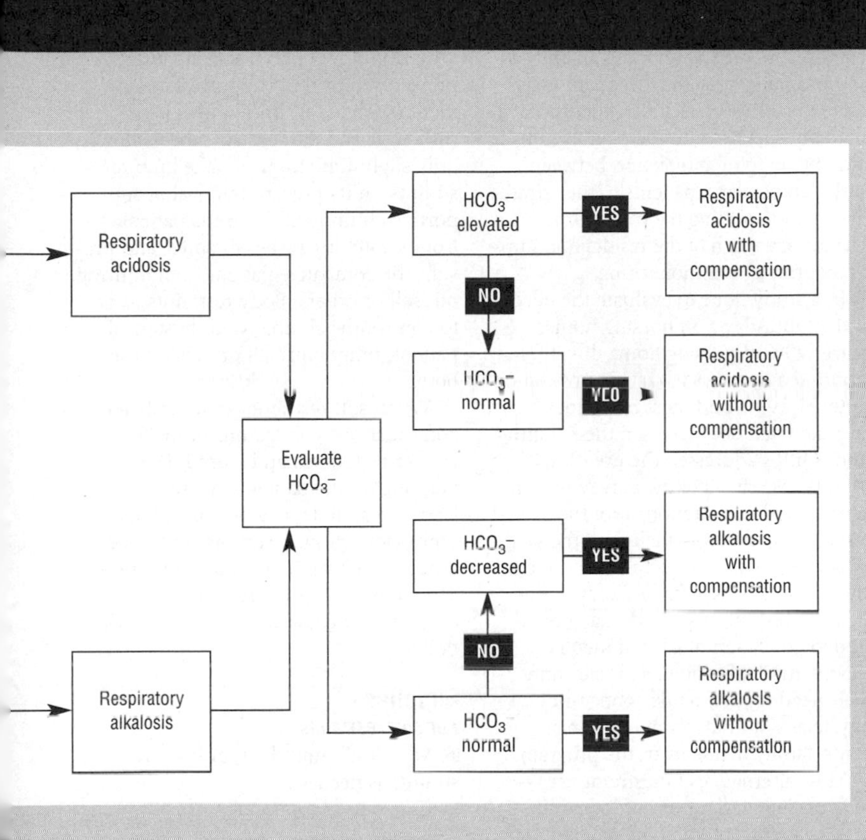

Of course, restraints are necessary at times, but they should be used only when all other alternatives have been tried and have failed.

The use of restraints is regulated by 1987 amendments to the Omnibus Budget Reconciliation Act (OBRA) of 1981, which state that nursing home residents have the right to be free from physical or chemical restraints that aren't required to treat "specific medical symptoms." All health care facilities have policies and procedures indicating when restraints are to be used and the nursing care that must be documented on restrained individuals. Because of the inappropriate use of restraints and the 1987 OBRA law, health care settings insist on securing a physician's order before applying restraints.

Alternatives to restraints

A newer trend in restraining patients is the use of a bed occupancy monitor to alert nursing staff immediately when the patient is no longer in bed. Although this device may not prevent the patient from falling, it does ensure rapid assistance. (Because some patients can successfully free themselves from all restraints, courts do consider how quickly and effectively the patient receives treatment after a fall.)

Other recommended alternatives to restraints include developing an ambulation program, providing frequent assistance to bathroom facilities, incorporating daily exercise into the plan of care, and encouraging interaction between staff members and patients. Other strategies include putting the call button within easy reach of the resident and implementing closer monitoring.

In a study done to evaluate the effect of the OBRA laws on nursing homes, nearly 90% of nursing home directors reported a decrease in restraint use since October 1990, and most respondents said they had not increased their staffing since OBRA addressed the use of restraints. Nearly all of the survey respondents noted that support from the facility's administration — including the facility owner, medical director, and director of nursing — was a major factor in decreasing restraint use. Other factors included education of all staff members, reassessment of residents to determine their need for restraints, cooperation of physicians, and involvement of residents' family members in the program.

Most alternatives to restraint use — such as daily indoor or outdoor walks with residents, saddle-type seats to prevent sliding out of chairs, and volunteers to assist residents — aren't difficult to implement. The most effective interventions are those that reflect regular and attentive monitoring as well as staff-patient interaction.

Making the transition to decreased restraint use requires an organized, planned effort to change attitudes, beliefs, practices, and policies within a health care facility. Cooperative effort at all levels can ultimately improve the quality of life for residents.

Types of restraints

Various types of soft restraints limit movement to prevent the confused, disoriented, or combative patient from injuring himself or others. Vest and belt restraints, used to prevent falls from a bed or a chair, permit full movement of arms and legs. Limb restraints, used to prevent removal of supportive equipment (such as I.V. lines, indwelling catheters, and nasogastric tubes) allow only slight limb motion. Like limb restraints, mitts prevent removal of supportive equipment, keep the patient from scratching rashes or sores, and prevent the combative patient from injuring himself or others. Body restraints, used to control the combative or hysterical patient, immobilize all or most of the body.

When soft restraints aren't sufficient and sedation is dangerous or ineffective, leather restraints can be used. Depending on the patient's behavior, leather restraints may be applied to all limbs (four-point restraints) or to one arm and one leg (two-point restraints). The duration of such restraint is governed by state law and by the facility's policy.

Supplies

For soft restraints

- Vest, limb, mitt, belt, or body restraint, as needed
- Gauze pads (optional)

For leather restraints

- Two wrist and two ankle leather restraints
- Four straps
- Key
- Large gauze pads to cushion each extremity

Implementation

- Obtain a physician's order for the restraint. The duration of the restraint order must be limited: 4 hours for adults, 2 hours for patients ages 9 to 17, and 1 hour for patients under age 9. The physician must see and evaluate the patient within 1 hour after the initiation of restraint use. The original order may be renewed only in accordance with these limits for up to a total of 24 hours. After the original order expires, a physician must see and evaluate the patient before a new order can be issued. A confused or combative patient should never be left unattended or unrestrained while you're attempting to secure the order.

- Before entering the patient's room, make sure the restraints are the correct size, using the patient's build and weight as a guide.
- If necessary, obtain adequate assistance to restrain the patient before entering his room. Enlist the aid of several coworkers and organize their effort, giving each person a specific task; for example, one person can explain the procedure to the patient and apply the restraints while the others immobilize the patient's arms and legs.
- Because the restrained patient has limited mobility, his nutrition, elimination, and positioning become your responsibility. To prevent pressure ulcers, reposition the patient regularly, and massage and pad bony prominences and other vulnerable areas.
- Never secure restraints to the side rails because someone might inadvertently lower the rail before noticing the attached restraint. This might jerk the patient's limb or body, causing him discomfort and trauma.
- Don't restrain a patient in the prone position. This position limits his field of vision, intensifies feelings of helplessness and vulnerability, and impairs respiration, especially if the patient has been sedated.
- If the patient is at high risk for aspiration, restrain him on his side.

Applying a vest restraint

- Assist the patient to a sitting position if his condition permits, and slip the vest over his gown. Crisscross the cloth flaps at the front, placing the V-shaped opening at the patient's throat. Never crisscross the flaps in the back because this may cause the patient to choke if he tries to squirm out of the vest.

Knots for securing soft restraints

When securing soft restraints, use knots that can be released quickly and easily, like those shown below. Use the reverse clove hitch to secure a limb restraint to a patient. Use the other three knots to secure a restraint to a bed frame. Remember, never secure restraints to the bed's side rails.

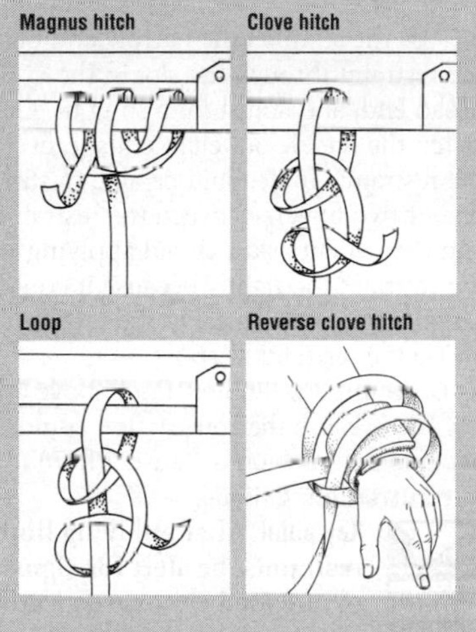

- Pass the tab on one flap through the slot on the opposite flap. Then adjust the vest for the patient's comfort. You should be able to slip your fist between the vest and the patient. Avoid wrapping the vest too tightly because it could restrict respiration.
- Tie all restraints securely to the frame of the bed, chair, or wheelchair and out of the patient's reach. Use a bow or a knot that can be released quickly and easily in an emergency. Never tie a regular knot to secure the straps. Leave 1″ to 2″ (2.5 to 5 cm) of slack in the straps to allow room for movement. (See *Knots for securing soft restraints*.)
- After applying the vest, check the patient's respiratory rate and breath sounds

regularly. Be alert for signs of respiratory distress. Also, make sure the vest hasn't tightened with the patient's movement. Loosen the vest frequently, if possible, so the patient can stretch, turn, and breathe deeply.

Applying a limb restraint

▶ Wrap the patient's wrist or ankle with gauze pads to reduce friction between the skin and the restraint, helping to prevent irritation and skin breakdown. Then wrap the restraint around the gauze pads.

▶ Pass the strap on the narrow end of the restraint through the slot in the broad end, and adjust for a snug fit. Or fasten the buckle or Velcro cuffs to fit the restraint. You should be able to slip one or two fingers between the restraint and the patient's skin. Avoid applying the restraint too tightly because it could impair circulation distal to the restraint.

▶ Tie the restraint as above.

▶ Don't apply a limb restraint above an I.V. site because the constriction could occlude the infusion or cause infiltration into surrounding tissue.

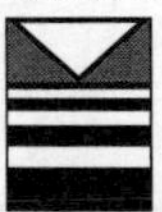

Key point After applying limb restraints, be alert for signs of impaired circulation in the extremity distal to the restraint. If the skin appears blue or feels cold, or if the patient complains of a tingling sensation or numbness, loosen the restraint. Perform range-of-motion (ROM) exercises regularly to stimulate circulation and prevent contractures and resultant loss of mobility.

Applying a mitt restraint

▶ Wash and dry the patient's hands.

▶ Roll up a washcloth or gauze pad, and place it in the patient's palm. Have him form a loose fist, if possible; then pull the mitt over it and secure the closure.

▶ To restrict the patient's arm movement, attach the strap to the mitt and tie it securely, using a bow or a knot that can be released quickly and easily in an emergency.

▶ When using mitts made of transparent mesh, check hand movement and skin color frequently to assess circulation. Remove the mitts regularly to stimulate circulation, and perform passive ROM exercises to prevent contractures.

Applying a belt restraint

▶ Center the flannel pad of the belt on the bed. Then wrap the short strap of the belt around the bed frame and fasten it under the bed.

▶ Position the patient on the pad. Then have him roll slightly to one side while you guide the long strap around his waist and through the slot in the pad.

▶ Wrap the long strap around the bed frame and fasten it under the bed.

▶ After applying the belt, slip your hand between the patient and the belt to ensure a secure but comfortable fit. A loose belt can be raised to chest level; a tight one can cause abdominal discomfort.

Applying leather restraints

▶ Position the patient supine on the bed, with each arm and leg securely held down to minimize combative behavior and to prevent injury to the patient and others. Immobilize the patient's arms and legs at the joints (knee, ankle, shoulder, and wrist) to minimize his movement without exerting excessive force.

▶ Apply pads to the patient's wrists and ankles to reduce friction between his skin and the leather, preventing skin irritation and breakdown.

▶ Wrap the restraint around the gauze pads. Then insert the metal loop through the hole that gives the best fit. Apply the restraints securely but not too tightly. You should be able to slip one or two fingers between the restraint and the patient's skin. A tight restraint can compromise circulation; a loose one can slip off or move up the patient's arm or leg, causing skin irritation and breakdown.

▶ Thread the strap through the metal loop on the restraint, close the metal loop, and secure the strap to the bed frame, out of the patient's reach.

▶ Lock the restraint by pushing in the button on the side of the metal loop, and tug it gently to make sure it's secure. Once the restraint is secure, a coworker can release the arm or leg. Flex the patient's arm or leg slightly before locking the strap to allow room for movement and prevent frozen joints and dislocations.

▶ Place the key in an accessible location at the nurse's station.

▶ After applying leather restraints, observe the patient regularly to provide emotional support and to reassess the continued need for restraints.

▶ Check the patient's pulse rate and vital signs at least every 2 hours. Remove or loosen the restraints one at a time, every 2 hours, and perform passive ROM exercises if possible. Watch for signs of impaired peripheral circulation, such as cool, cyanotic skin.

▶ To unlock the restraint, insert the key into the metal loop, opposite the locking button. This releases the lock, and the metal loop can be opened.

Complications

Restraints have the potential for serious adverse effects and harm. Physical restraints can cause skin breakdown, decreased peripheral circulation, impaired respiratory status, strangulation, neurologic damage, and death. Chemical restraints may cause increased drowsiness, respiratory distress, hemodynamic instability, decreased competence and judgment, and confusion.

Patient teaching

▶ Tell the patient what you're about to do, and describe the restraints to him.

▶ Assure him that restraints are being used to protect him from injury rather than to punish him.

Documentation

Key point When using restraints, it's vital to follow your facility's policy and procedure and to document why and how the patient was restrained, how patient safety needs were met while restraints were in use, and why restraint was continued or discontinued.

Document the type of behavior that required the restraints (including ineffective means of restraint that were used earlier), the exact type of restraints used, the date and time of application, and the patient's response to the restraints.

Also record patient safety factors, including vital signs, skin integrity, circulation in the restrained extremities, respiratory status, nutrition and elimination needs, and elevation of the patient's head before feeding. Include in the documentation the need for continued restraints and periodic assessments to ascertain when restraints may be removed.

RETINAL DETACHMENT

In retinal detachment, separation of the retinal layers creates a subretinal space that fills with fluid. Twice as common in men as in women, retinal detachment usually involves only one eye but may occur in the other eye later. Though it rarely heals spontaneously, a detached retina can usually be reattached successfully with surgery. The prognosis depends on the area of the retina affected. Untreated retinal detachment may result in severe vision impairment and possibly blindness.

Retinal detachment may be primary or secondary. A primary detachment occurs spontaneously because of a change in the retina or the vitreous, whereas a secondary detachment results from another problem, such as intraocular inflammation or trauma. The most common cause of retinal detachment is a hole or tear in the retina. This hole allows the liquid vitreous to seep between the retinal layers and separate the sensory retinal layer from its choroidal blood supply. In adults, retinal detachment usually results from degenerative changes related to aging (which cause a spontaneous tear). Predisposing factors include myopia, cataract surgery, and trauma.

Additionally, retinal detachment may result from fluid seeping into the subretinal space as an effect of inflammation, tumors, or systemic disease. Detachment may also result from traction placed on the retina by vitreous bands or membranes (resulting from proliferative diabetic retinopathy, posterior uveitis, or a traumatic intraocular foreign body, for example). It can also be inherited, usually in association with myopia.

Signs and symptoms

- Initially, complaints of seeing floating spots and recurrent light flashes
- As detachment progresses, gradual, painless vision loss described as looking through a veil, curtain, or cobweb

Diagnostic tests

- *Direct ophthalmoscopy* after full pupil dilation shows folds or discoloration in the usually transparent retina.
- *Indirect ophthalmoscopy* can detect retinal tears.
- *Ocular ultrasonography* may be performed to examine the retina if the patient has an opaque lens.

Treatment

Depending on the detachment's location and severity, treatment may include restricting eye movements to prevent further separation until surgical repair can be made. A hole in the peripheral retina may be treated with cryotherapy. A hole in the posterior retina may respond to laser therapy.

To reattach the retina, scleral buckling may be performed. In this procedure, the surgeon places a silicone plate or sponge over the reattachment site and secures it in place with an encircling band. The pressure exerted gently pushes the choroid and retina together. Scleral buckling may be followed by replacement of the vitreous with silicone, oil, air, or gas.

Key nursing diagnoses and outcomes

Anxiety related to potential for loss of vision in affected eye

Treatment outcomes: The patient will cope with anxiety by being involved in decisions about his care and will display fewer physical symptoms of anxiety.

Disturbed sensory perception (visual) related to loss of vision

Treatment outcome: The patient will compensate for vision loss by using adaptive devices.

Deficient diversional activity related to activity restrictions used to prevent further retinal detachment

Treatment outcomes: The patient will identify activities that he can do safely and will express a positive attitude about activity restrictions.

Nursing interventions

- Monitor the patient's degree of vision loss.
- Assess the patient's ability to perform activities of daily living (ADLs) and instrumental ADLs in response to his vision changes.
- Provide encouragement and emotional support to decrease anxiety caused by vision loss.
- Prepare the patient for surgery by cleaning his face with a mild (no-tears) shampoo. Give antibiotics and cycloplegic or mydriatic eyedrops as ordered.

▶ Postoperatively, position the patient as directed (the position will vary according to the surgical procedure). To prevent increasing intraocular pressure (IOP), administer antiemetics as indicated. Discourage any activities that would raise IOP. Assess the patient for persistent pain and report it if present. Give prescribed analgesics as needed.
▶ In macular involvement, keep the patient on bed rest (with or without bathroom privileges) to prevent further retinal detachment.
▶ To reduce edema and discomfort following laser therapy, apply ice packs and administer acetaminophen, as ordered, for headache.
▶ If the patient receives a retrobulbar injection, apply a protective eye patch because the eyelid will remain partially open.
▶ After removing the protective patch, give cycloplegic and steroidal or antibiotic eyedrops, as ordered. Apply cold compresses to decrease swelling and pain.
▶ Observe for slight localized corneal edema and periorbital congestion, which may follow laser therapy.

PATIENT TEACHING

▶ Explain to the patient undergoing laser therapy that the procedure may be done in same-day surgery. Warn him that he may have blurred vision for several days afterward.
▶ Instruct him to rest and to avoid driving, bending, heavy lifting, or any other activities that increase IOP for several days after eye surgery. Discourage activities that could cause the patient to bump his eye.
▶ Encourage leg and deep-breathing exercises to prevent complications of immobility.
▶ Show the patient having scleral buckling surgery how to instill eyedrops properly. After surgery, remind him to lie in the position recommended by the physician.
▶ Advise the patient to wear sunglasses if he develops photosensitivity.
▶ Instruct the patient to take acetaminophen as needed for headaches and to apply ice packs to his eye to reduce swelling and alleviate discomfort.
▶ Review the signs of infection, emphasizing those requiring immediate attention.

RHEUMATOID ARTHRITIS

A chronic, systemic, symmetrical inflammatory disease, rheumatoid arthritis primarily attacks peripheral joints and surrounding muscles, tendons, ligaments, and blood vessels. Spontaneous remissions and unpredictable exacerbations mark the course of this potentially crippling disease.

Rheumatoid arthritis occurs worldwide, affecting more than 6.5 million people in the United States alone. The disease strikes women three times more often than men. Although it can occur at any age, the peak onset period for women is between ages 35 and 50.

Rheumatoid arthritis usually requires lifelong treatment and, sometimes, surgery. In most patients, the disease follows an intermittent course and allows normal activity, although 10% suffer total disability from severe articular deformity, associated extra-articular symptoms (such as pericardial friction rub and shortness of breath), or both. The prognosis worsens with the development of nodules, vasculitis, and high titers of rheumatoid factor.

What causes the chronic inflammation characteristic of rheumatoid arthritis isn't known, but various theories point to infectious, genetic, and endocrine factors. A genetically susceptible person may develop abnormal or altered immunoglobulin (Ig) G antibodies when exposed to an antigen. Because the body doesn't recognize these altered IgG antibodies as "self," the person forms an antibody known as rheumatoid factor against them. By aggregating into complexes, rheumatoid factor generates inflammation.

Eventually, the cartilage damage caused by the inflammation triggers further immune responses, including complement activation. Complement, in turn, attracts polymorphonuclear leukocytes and stimulates the release of inflammatory mediators, which exacerbates joint destruction.

More is known about the pathophysiology of rheumatoid arthritis than about its causes. If unarrested, joint inflammation occurs in four stages. First, synovitis develops from congestion and edema of the synovial membrane and joint capsule. Formation of pannus — thickened layers of granulation tissue — marks the onset of the second stage. Pannus covers and invades cartilage and eventually destroys the joint capsule and bone.

The third stage is characterized by fibrous ankylosis — fibrous invasion of the pannus and scar formation that occludes the joint space. Bone atrophy and misalignment cause visible deformities and disrupt the articulation of opposing bones, causing muscle atrophy and imbalance and, possibly, partial dislocations or subluxations. In the fourth stage, fibrous tissue calcifies, resulting in bony ankylosis and total immobility.

Pain associated with movement may restrict active joint use and cause fibrous or bony ankylosis, soft tissue contractures, and joint deformities. Between 15% and 20% of patients develop Sjögren's syndrome with keratoconjunctivitis sicca. Rheumatoid arthritis can also destroy the odontoid process, part of the second cervical vertebra. Rarely, spinal cord compression may occur, particularly in patients with long-standing deforming rheumatoid arthritis.

Signs and symptoms

- Initially, insidious onset of nonspecific symptoms (fatigue, malaise, anorexia, persistent low-grade fever, weight loss, and vague articular symptoms, such as joint swelling and stiffness that occurs after inactivity)
- Later in the disease, localized articular symptoms, frequently in the fingers at the proximal interphalangeal, metacarpophalangeal, and metatarsophalangeal joints; usually occur bilaterally and symmetrically and may extend to the wrists, elbows, knees, and ankles
- Joint stiffness (after inactivity, especially on rising in the morning), tenderness and pain (at first only with movement, but eventually even at rest), and diminished joint function; eventually, joint deformities and contractures, especially if active disease continues
- Rheumatoid nodules on pressure areas such as the elbows (most common extra-articular finding)
- Spindle-shaped fingers (from marked edema and congestion in the joints); may become fixed in a characteristic swan neck deformity (hyperextension of the proximal interphalangeal joint with fixed flexion of the distal interphalangeal joint) or in a boutonniere deformity (persistent flexion of the proximal interphalangeal joint with hyperextension of the distal interphalangeal joint); hands appear foreshortened
- Stiff, weak, or painful muscles
- Tingling paresthesia in the fingers (from synovial pressure on the median nerve from carpal tunnel syndrome)
- Numbness or tingling in the feet or weakness or loss of sensation in the fingers (with peripheral neuropathy)
- Pain on inspiration (with pleuritis), shortness of breath (with pulmonary nodules or fibrosis), or pericardial friction rub (with pericarditis)
- Lesions, leg ulcers, and multiple systemic complications (with vasculitis)
- Eye redness (with scleritis or episcleritis)
- Upper motor neuron disorder, such as a positive Babinski's sign and weakness (with spinal cord compression)

Diagnostic tests

The criteria developed by the American Rheumatism Association can serve as guidelines to establish a diagnosis. However, failure to meet these criteria—particularly early in the disease—doesn't exclude the diagnosis. Although no test definitively diagnoses rheumatoid arthritis, the following are useful:

▶ *X-rays* show bone demineralization and soft-tissue swelling in early stages. Later, they help determine the extent of cartilage and bone destruction, erosion, subluxations, and deformities. They also show the characteristic pattern of these abnormalities, particularly symmetrical involvement, although no particular pattern is conclusive for rheumatoid arthritis.

▶ *Rheumatoid factor test* is positive in 75% to 80% of patients, as indicated by a titer of 1:160 or higher. Although the presence of rheumatoid factor doesn't confirm rheumatoid arthritis, it does help determine the prognosis; a patient with a high titer usually has more severe and progressive disease with extra-articular manifestations.

▶ *Synovial fluid analysis* shows increased volume and turbidity, but decreased viscosity and complement (C3 and C4) levels. The white blood cell count often exceeds 10,000/µl.

▶ *Serum protein electrophoresis* may show elevated serum globulin levels.

▶ *Erythrocyte sedimentation rate* (ESR) is elevated in 85% to 90% of patients. Because an elevated ESR frequently parallels disease activity, this test may help monitor the patient's response to therapy (as may a C-reactive protein test).

▶ *Complete blood count* usually shows moderate anemia and slight leukocytosis.

Treatment

Treatment requires a multidisciplinary approach to reduce pain and inflammation, preserve functional capacity, resolve pathologic processes, and bring about improvement. Salicylates, particularly aspirin, are the mainstay of therapy because they decrease inflammation and relieve joint pain. Nonsteroidal anti-inflammatory drugs (such as indomethacin, fenoprofen, and ibuprofen) may also be used for pain and inflammation.

Drug therapy may also include antimalarials (hydroxychloroquine), gold salts, penicillamine, or corticosteroids (prednisone). Immunosuppressants, such as cyclophosphamide, methotrexate, and azathioprine, may be used in the early stages of the disease. (See *Drug therapy for rheumatoid arthritis,* pages 520 and 521.)

Supportive measures include increased sleep (8 to 10 hours every night), frequent rest periods between daily activities, and splinting to rest inflamed joints (although, like corticosteroid therapy, immobilization can cause osteoporosis). A physical therapy program includes range-of-motion exercises and carefully individualized therapeutic exercises to forestall the loss of joint function as well as application of heat to relax muscles and relieve pain. Moist heat (hot soaks, paraffin baths, whirlpools) usually works best for patients with chronic disease. Ice packs may be used during acute episodes.

Surgical interventions include metatarsal head and distal ulnar resectional arthroplasty and insertion of a Silastic prosthesis between the metacarpophalangeal and proximal interphalangeal joints. Arthrodesis (joint fusion) may bring about stability and relieve pain but may also decrease joint mobility. Synovectomy (removal of destructive, proliferating synovium, usually in the wrists, fingers, and knees) may be used to halt or delay the course of the disease. Osteotomy (the cutting of bone or excision of a wedge of bone) may realign joint surfaces and redistribute stresses. Tendons that rupture spontaneously need surgical repair. Tendon transfers

(Text continues on page 522.)

Drug therapy for rheumatoid arthritis

Drug and adverse effects	Nursing interventions
aspirin Prolonged bleeding time; GI disturbances, including nausea, dyspepsia, anorexia, ulcers, and hemorrhage; hypersensitivity reactions ranging from urticaria to anaphylaxis; salicylism (mild toxicity: tinnitus, dizziness; moderate toxicity: restlessness, hyperpnea, delirium, marked lethargy; and severe toxicity: coma, seizures, severe hyperpnea)	■ Don't use in patients with GI ulcers, bleeding, or hypersensitivity. ■ Give with food, milk, an antacid, or a large glass of water to reduce adverse GI effects. ■ Monitor salicylate levels. ■ Teach the patient to reduce the dose, one tablet at a time, if tinnitus occurs. ■ Teach the patient to watch for signs of bleeding, such as bruising, melena, and petechiae.
cyclosporine Nephrotoxicity (increase in blood uea nitrogen [BUN] and serum creatinine levels), hypertension, bone marrow suppression, nausea, vomiting, paresthesia, bone pain	■ Avoid use in patients with preexisting hypertension or renal disease. ■ Monitor blood pressure closely. ■ Monitor blood urea nitrogen (BUN) and serum creatinine levels. ■ Be aware that levels may be increased by other medications metabolized by the liver.
fenoprofen, ibuprofen, naproxen, piroxicam, sumac, and tolmetin Prolonged bleeding time; central nervous system abnormalities (headache, drowsiness, restlessness, dizziness, tremors); GI disturbances, including hemorrhage and peptic ulcer; increased BUN and liver enzyme levels	■ Don't use in patients with renal disease or in asthmatics with nasal polyps. ■ Use cautiously in patients with GI disorders or cardiac disease and in patients allergic to other nonsteroidal anti-inflammatory drugs. ■ Give with milk or food to reduce adverse GI effects. ■ Tell the patient that the therapeutic effect may be delayed for 2 to 3 weeks. ■ Monitor renal, hepatic, and auditory function in long-term therapy. Stop the drug if abnormalities develop.
gold (oral and parenteral) Dermatitis, pruritus, rash, stomatitis, nephrotoxicity, blood dyscrasias, nitritoid crisis and, with oral form, GI distress and diarrhea	■ Observe for nitritoid crisis (flushing, fainting, sweating). ■ Check the patient's urine for blood and albumin before each dose. If you get a positive result, withhold the drug and notify the physician. ■ Stress the need for regular follow-up examinations, including blood and urine testing. ■ To avoid local nerve irritation, mix the drug well and give an I.M. injection deep in the buttock. ■ Advise the patient not to expect an improvement for 3 to 6 months. ■ Instruct the patient to report rash, bruising, bleeding, hematuria and oral uclers.

Drug therapy for rheumatoid arthritis *(continued)*

Drug and adverse effects	Nursing interventions
hydroxychloroquine Blood dyscrasias, GI irritation, corneal opacities, keratopathy or retinopathy	■ Don't use in in patients with retinal or visual field changes. ■ Use cautiously in patients with hepatic disease, alcoholism, glucose-6-phosphate dehydrogenase deficiency, or psoriasis. ■ Perform a complete blood count and liver function tests before therapy and during chronic therapy. Patients should also have regular opthalmologic examinations. ■ Give the drug with food or milk to reduce adverse GI effects. ■ Warn the patient that dizziness may occur.
methotrexate Bone marrow suppression; stomatitis, nausea, and vomiting; alopecia; tubular necrosis, cirrhosis, hepatic fibrosis, and hyperuricemia; pulmonary infiltrates; diarrhea, possibly leading to hemorrhagic enteritis and intestinal perforation	■ If adverse GI reactions occur, you may need to stop the drug, as ordered. ■ Administer antiemetics, as ordered, to control nausea and vomiting. ■ Report rash, redness, or ulcerations in the mouth and pulmonary adverse reactions, which may signal serious complications. ■ Monitor the patient's serum uric acid, serum creatinine, and BUN levels during therapy. As ordered, reduce the dose if BUN levels reach 20 to 30 mg/dl or serum creatinine levels reach 1.2 to 2 mg/dl. Stop the drug, as ordered, if BUN levels exceed 30 mg/dl or serum creatinine levels exceed 2 mg/dl.
prednisone Hyperglycemia, hypertension, fluid retention, weight gain, acne, cataracts, indigestion, muscle weakness, osteoporosis, mental status changes, insomnia, psychosis	■ Advise the patient not to stop taking the drug suddenly because this can lead to adrenal insufficiency. ■ Monitor blood glucose levels and blood pressure.
sulfasalazine Nausea, vomiting, abdominal pain, rash, bone marrow suppression, headache, hypersensitivity reaction.	■ Don't give this drug to patients with known sulfa allergy. ■ Monitor the patient's CBC, UA, and liver enzyme levels. ■ Caution the patient not to take the drug at same time as antacids, which interfere with its absorption.

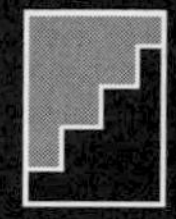

Staying well

Living with rheumatoid arthritis

Rheumatoid arthritis is a chronic disorder that may require your patient to make major lifestyle changes. These suggestions may prevent disease progression and will help your patient live more comfortably with this disorder:

- Advise the patient to maintain an erect posture when standing, walking, and sitting.
- Tell the patient to sit in chairs with high seats and armrests; she'll find it easier to get up from a chair if her knees are lower than her hips. If she doesn't own a chair with a high seat, recommend putting blocks of wood under the legs of a favorite chair. Suggest that she obtain an elevated toilet seat.
- Instruct the patient to pace daily activities, resting for 5 to 10 minutes out of each hour and alternating sitting and standing tasks.
- Stress the importance of adequate sleep and correct sleeping posture. Tell her to sleep on her back on a firm mattress and to avoid placing a pillow under her knees, which encourages flexion deformity.
- Stress the importance of wearing shoes with proper support.
- Tell the patient to avoid putting undue stress on joints and to use the largest joint available for a given task; to support weak or painful joints as much as possible; to avoid flexion and instead use extension; to hold objects parallel to the knuckles as briefly as possible; to always use her hands toward the center of her body; and to slide—not lift—objects whenever possible. Enlist the aid of an occupational therapist to teach the patient how to simplify activities and protect arthritic joints.
- Suggest dressing aids, such as a long-handled shoehorn, a reacher, elastic shoelaces, a zipper pull, and a buttonhook, and helpful household items, such as easy-open drawers, a hand-held shower nozzle, hand rails, and grab bars. The patient who has trouble maneuvering her fingers into gloves should wear mittens. Tell her to dress while in the sitting position whenever possible.

may prevent deformities or relieve contracture. Joint reconstruction or total joint arthroplasty may be necessary in advanced disease.

Key nursing diagnoses and outcomes

Ineffective role performance related to crippling effects of rheumatoid arthritis

Treatment outcome: The patient will learn to function in her usual roles as much as possible.

Impaired physical mobility related to pain and joint deformities

Treatment outcome: The patient will achieve the highest level of mobility possible within the confines of the disease.

Acute pain related to joint inflammation

Treatment outcome: The patient will have decreased pain.

Nursing interventions

▶ Provide emotional support. Remember that the patient can easily become depressed, discouraged, and irritable. Encourage her to express her fears concerning dependency, disability, sexuality, body image, and self-esteem. Refer her to appropriate counseling, as needed.

- Monitor the duration of morning stiffness. Duration more accurately reflects the severity of the disease than does intensity.
- Check for rheumatoid nodules, pressure ulcers, and skin breakdown, especially if the patient is in traction or wearing splints. These can result from immobility, vascular impairment, corticosteroid treatment, and improper splinting. Provide meticulous skin care. Use lotion or cleansing oil — not soap — on dry skin.
- Administer analgesics as prescribed. Assess the effectiveness of administered drugs and watch for adverse reactions. Also use such pain relieving measures as heat packs, soaks, and rest.
- Make sure the patient adheres to the prescribed physical therapy program.
- Prepare the patient for joint replacement, as indicated.
- For more information on coping with rheumatoid arthritis, refer the patient to the Arthritis Foundation.

PATIENT TEACHING

- Explain the nature of rheumatoid arthritis. Make sure the patient and her family understand that rheumatoid arthritis is a chronic disease that may require major changes in lifestyle and that "miracle cures" don't work. (See *Living with rheumatoid arthritis.*)
- Encourage a balanced diet, but make sure the patient understands that special diets won't cure rheumatoid arthritis. Stress the need for weight control because obesity further stresses the joints.
- Encourage the patient to take hot showers or baths at bedtime or in the morning to reduce the need for analgesics.
- Discuss the patient's sexual concerns. If pain creates problems during intercourse, discuss trying alternative positions, taking analgesics beforehand, and using moist heat to increase mobility.
- Before discharge, make sure the patient knows how and when to take prescribed drugs and how to recognize possible adverse effects.

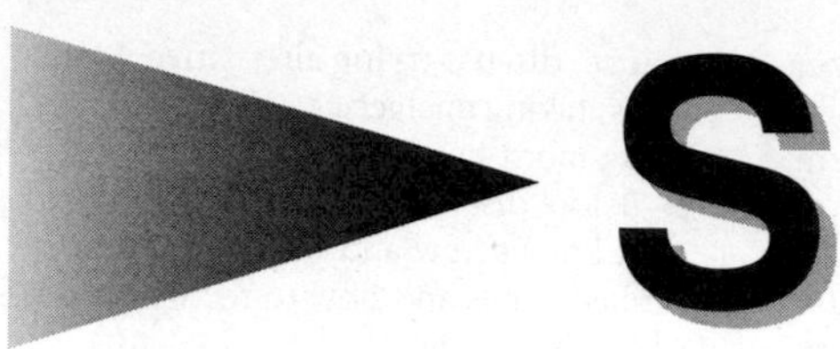

SEPTIC SHOCK

Characterized by low systemic vascular resistance (SVR) and elevated cardiac output, septic shock is thought to occur in response to infections that release microbes or one of the immune mediators. This disorder, which has a mortality as high as 25%, is usually a complication of another disorder or an invasive procedure. About 500,000 cases of septic shock occur in the United States annually.

Any pathogenic organism can cause septic shock. Gram-negative bacteria, such as *Escherichia coli, Klebsiella pneumoniae, Serratia, Enterobacter,* and *Pseudomonas,* are the most common causes, accounting for up to 70% of all cases. Opportunistic fungi cause about 3% of cases. Rare causative organisms include mycobacteria and some viruses and protozoa.

Many organisms that are normal flora on the skin or in the intestines are beneficial and pose no threat. But when they spread throughout the body by way of the bloodstream (gaining entry through any alteration in the body's normal defenses or through artificial devices that penetrate the body, such as I.V., intra-arterial, or urinary catheters and knife or bullet wounds), they can progress to overwhelming infection unless body defenses destroy them.

Initially, these defenses activate chemical mediators in response to the invading organisms. The release of these mediators results in low SVR and increased cardiac output. This is referred to as the hyperdynamic, or warm, phase of septic shock. Blood flow is unevenly distributed in the microcirculation, and plasma leaking from capillaries causes functional hypovolemia. Eventually, cardiac output falls and SVR increases. This is the hypodynamic, or cold, phase of septic shock, which leads to poor tissue perfusion and hypotension, resulting in multisystem organ failure and death.

Septic shock can occur in any person with impaired immunity, but older adults are at greatest risk. About two-thirds of septic shock cases occur in hospitalized patients, most of whom have an underlying disease. Those at high risk include patients with burns; chronic cardiac, hepatic, or renal disorders; diabetes mellitus; immunosuppression; malnutrition; stress; and excessive antibiotic use. Also at risk are patients who have had invasive diagnostic or therapeutic procedures, surgery, or traumatic wounds.

Complications of septic shock include disseminated intravascular coagulation, renal failure, heart failure, GI ulcers, and abnormal liver function.

Signs and symptoms

Early indicators

- Fever and chills (although 20% of patients may be hypothermic)

Hyperdynamic (or warm) phase

- Pink, flushed skin

- Altered level of consciousness (LOC) (agitation, anxiety, irritability, and shortened attention span)
- Rapid, shallow respirations
- Rapid, full, bounding pulse on palpation
- Normal or slightly elevated blood pressure
- Below-normal urine output

Hypodynamic (or cold) phase

- Pale, cold and clammy, and possibly cyanotic skin; may be mottled in peripheral areas
- Decreased LOC (possibly obtundation and coma)
- Rapid, shallow respirations
- Urine output of less than 25 ml/hour or absent
- Absent or rapid, weak, or thready pulse on palpation; may also be irregular if arrhythmias are present
- Hypotension (systolic pressure below 90 mm Hg or 50 to 80 mm Hg below the patient's previous level); crackles or rhonchi (with pulmonary congestion)

The patient history may include a disorder or treatment that can cause immunosuppression or invasive tests or treatments, surgery, or trauma.

Diagnostic tests

- *Blood cultures* are positive for the offending organism.
- *Complete blood count* indicates the presence or absence of anemia and leukopenia, severe or absent neutropenia, and usually the presence of thrombocytopenia.
- *Serum lactate dehydrogenase levels* are elevated with metabolic acidosis.
- *Urine studies* show increased specific gravity (more than 1.020), increased osmolality, and decreased sodium.
- *Arterial blood gas* (ABG) *analysis* demonstrates elevated blood pH and partial pressure of arterial oxygen and decreased partial pressure of arterial carbon dioxide with respiratory alkalosis in early stages.
- *Pulmonary artery pressure monitoring* with a thermodilution catheter reveals increased cardiac output and decreased SVR in the hyperdynamic phase, and decreased cardiac output and increased SVR in the hypodynamic phase.

Treatment

Identification and treatment of the underlying cause of septic shock is essential. If any I.V., intra-arterial, or urinary drainage catheters are in place, they should be removed and cultured. Aggressive antimicrobial therapy appropriate for the causative organism must be initiated immediately. Culture and sensitivity tests help determine the most effective antimicrobial.

Patients with who are at especially high risk for dying from sepsis may benefit from receiving the newly approved drug drotecogin alpha [activated]. Drugs should be discontinued or reduced in patients who are immunosuppressed because of drug therapy. Granulocyte transfusions may be used in patients with severe neutropenia.

Oxygen therapy should be initiated to maintain arterial oxygen saturation greater than 95%. Mechanical ventilation may be required if the patient goes into respiratory failure.

Colloid or crystalloid infusions are given to increase intravascular volume and raise blood pressure. After sufficient fluid volume has been replaced, diuretics such as furosemide can be given to maintain urine output above 20 ml/hour. If fluid resuscitation fails to increase blood pressure, a vasopressor (such as dopamine) can be started. A blood transfusion may be needed if the patient is anemic.

Cultural diversity Keep in mind that for religious reasons, Jehovah's Witnesses don't accept blood transfusions. An alternative therapy may be necessary.

Key nursing diagnoses and outcomes

Decreased cardiac output related to hypodynamic phase of septic shock

Treatment outcomes: The patient will regain and maintain adequate cardiac output, stable vital signs, and normal mental status.

Deficient fluid volume related to functional hypovolemia

Treatment outcomes: The patient will regain and maintain normal fluid and blood volume.

Risk for injury related to potential complications of septic shock

Treatment outcome: The patient will show no permanent adverse effects from septic shock.

Nursing interventions

- As ordered, remove any I.V., intra-arterial, or urinary drainage catheters, and send them to the laboratory to culture for the presence of the causative organism. New catheters can be placed in the intensive care unit.
- Record the patient's blood pressure, pulse, and respiratory rates every 1 to 5 minutes until they're stable. Record hemodynamic pressure readings as ordered, and monitor cardiac rhythm continuously. Systolic blood pressure less than 80 mm Hg usually results in inadequate coronary artery blood flow, cardiac ischemia, arrhythmias, and further complications of low cardiac output; below 70 mm Hg, inadequate kidney perfusion.
- Start an I.V. infusion with normal saline or lactated Ringer's solution, using a large-bore (14G to 18G) catheter, which allows easier administration of blood transfusions later.
- Administer appropriate antimicrobial drugs I.V. to achieve effective blood levels rapidly.
- Measure the patient's urine output hourly. Watch for signs of fluid overload, such as an increase in pulmonary artery wedge pressure. If urine output is less than 30 ml/hour, increase the fluid infusion rate. Notify the physician if urine output doesn't improve. He may order a diuretic to increase renal blood flow and urine output.
- Monitor ABG values. Administer oxygen as ordered to ensure adequate tissue oxygenation. Perform cardiopulmonary assessment frequently.
- Provide emotional support to the patient and his family.

PATIENT TEACHING

- Explain all procedures to the patient and his family to help relieve their anxiety.

SEXUALITY

It's a common misconception that advanced age makes a person physically and psychologically incapable of having sex or of maintaining a loving sexual relationship. Older people are commonly viewed as being sexual undesirable, disinterested in sex, and unable to perform functionally; however, most actually maintain sexual interest and activity well into their 70s and 80s.

Sexual responses and aging

Although research shows that older people experience sex-specific changes, such as decreased speed and duration of erection in men and diminished vaginal lubrication in women, it also shows that neither sexual response nor the capacity to experience orgasm decrease significantly with age. However, prolonged abstinence from sexual activity increases the risk of genital atrophy from disuse.

Besides physiologic changes, other factors that may inhibit sexual activity include cultural taboos, rigid moral principles, negative self-image, loss of privacy and independence, adverse drug effects, and illnesses, such as arthritis, neuropathy, and peripheral vascular disease. The fact that women typically live longer than men, leaving them without partners, also contributes to decreased sexual activity among older adults.

Many couples develop sexual problems later in life because they're uninformed about age-related physiological changes. For example, a man may perceive a diminishing ability to achieve an erection as evidence that he's becoming impotent; a woman may interpret this sign as evidence that the man no longer finds her attractive or that he's just too old for sex. Education regarding normal changes in sexual response may be necessary.

Nursing interventions

- Obtain a thorough assessment, but be sensitive to the patient's cultural background and moral values. If the patient is uncomfortable discussing sexual matters, respect his right not to do so and don't press the topic. The patient may broach the subject later, when he feels more comfortable.
- Ask about the patient's marital status and living arrangements to elicit information about partner availability. Also ask about the status of the relationship and the health of the partner.
- Determine whether the patient requires any screening, such as Papanicolaou testing, mammography, or prostate examination.
- Note past genitourinary or gynecological surgeries and infections as well as chronic illnesses, which can have a significant physical and psychosocial impact on sexual function.
- Carefully review the patient's medications. Many drugs adversely affect sexual function.

PATIENT TEACHING

- Suggest ways for the patient to increase his self-esteem, if appropriate.
- Provide information about sexuality and aging to increase the patient's knowledge and to dispel sexual myths. Discuss such points as the need for clitoral contact and stimulation to achieve orgasm in females and the need for more direct genital contact to achieve arousal and orgasm in older males.
- Explain to the patient that sexual performance may be impaired by consuming more than moderate amounts of alcohol.
- Suggest a variety of sexual activities other than intercourse than can help fulfill the patient's need for sexual contact (such as oral or manual genital stimulation, kissing, hugging, and handholding).
- Be sure to discuss human immunodeficiency virus and other sexually transmitted diseases, including risk factors and the importance of safer sex practices.
- Many nursing homes have policies that address such issues as cohabitation of husbands and wives, patient conduct, and privacy. Discuss sexual activity in the nursing home, if appropriate, and consult with the nursing home director as necessary.

SLEEP PATTERN DISTURBANCES

The importance of rest and sleep in maintaining physical health in older people is often discounted or ignored, particularly in institutional settings where routines are so important. Rest and sleep serve a restorative function both physiologically and psychologically. Physiologically, sleep rests body organs, conserves energy, preserves biorhythms, and restores mental alertness and neurologic efficiency. Psychologically, sleep reduces tension and fosters a feeling of well-being.

This restorative function is especially important to older people, who require more time to adjust to changes. Older people who are deprived of sleep may become forgetful, disoriented, or confused; cognitively impaired persons exhibit increased restlessness, wandering

Dealing with sleep disturbances

Difficulty falling or staying asleep is a common problem for older adults, whether they live at home or in a nursing home. If your patient has a sleep problem, advise him to:

- maintain the same daily schedule for waking, resting, and sleeping
- get up at his usual time even if his sleep has been disturbed or his bedtime changes temporarily
- establish a bedtime ritual and faithfully follow it
- exercise every day but avoid vigorous exercise at night
- limit naps to 1 to 2 hours per day, at the same time each day
- take a warm bath in the late afternoon or early evening
- eat a light snack of carbohydrates and fat before bed
- avoid caffeine-containing beverages and products, especially before bedtime
- practice relaxation methods, such as deep breathing, massage, listening to music, or reading relaxing material
- avoid alcoholic beverages or limit his intake to small amounts each day
- use the bed for sleep only
- if he's awake at night for longer than 30 minutes, get out of bed and engage in a nonstimulating activity such as reading.

behavior, and "sundowner syndrome" or "sundowning" (confusion, agitation, and disruptive behavior during late afternoon and early evening hours).

The quality of sleep may be affected by age-related changes, polypharmacy, and organic or mental disorders.

Sleep patterns in the elderly

Normal sleep consists of rapid eye movement (REM) and non-REM components. Non-REM sleep is subdivided into four stages: In stage I, dropping off to sleep, the person is easily aroused and doesn't realize he has been asleep. Muscle twitching or jerking signals relaxation during this stage. Stages II and III include progressively deeper sleep. In stage IV, the deepest level, arousal is difficult.

Stage IV sleep is essential for maintaining physiologic health. Sleep experts know that this stage is notably decreased in older people, but they haven't determined the effects of this decrease. Sleep patterns of older people are marked by frequent awakenings, diminished stage III and IV non-REM time, more time spent awake during the night as a whole, and more frequent daytime naps. Most healthy older adults report no symptoms related to these changes other than not getting enough sleep or sleeping poorly. Studies suggest that daytime napping may reduce nocturnal sleep time and quality in some older people. If indicated, advise your patients to monitor the effects of napping on their nighttime sleep and on their feelings of well-being during the day.

From stage IV, the person progresses to REM sleep. REM sleep occurs several times in the nightly sleep cycle but is most prominent in the early morning. In REM sleep, activity and vital signs accelerate, resulting in mounting excitement and tension release — manifested as tossing and turning, muscle twitching, and increased respiratory rate, heart rate, and blood pressure. Higher respiratory and heart rates may adversely affect patients who have chronic cardiopulmonary problems. Otherwise, REM sleep helps release tension and aids central nervous system metabolism. Lack of REM sleep has been shown to cause irritability and anxiety.

Assessing sleep patterns

A detailed assessment of a patient with a sleep disturbance includes direct observation, questioning the patient and family members about his sleep patterns, and possibly having the patient keep a sleep diary for 3 to 4 weeks. Sleep disorder laboratories may offer explicit analysis of the disruptive pattern.

You can learn the following through observation and direct questioning:

- how well the person sleeps at home
- bedtime and waking time
- bedtime rituals and preferred nighttime environment (amount of light and ventilation, room temperature, door open or closed, music, type of bedclothes)
- frequency and duration of awake time
- activities usually performed in the early evening hours
- food or fluids consumed shortly before bedtime
- leisure activities and hobbies
- drugs taken, including sleep aids
- tendency to sleep alone or with a partner
- perceived health status and satisfaction with life
- number of nightly trips to the bathroom.

If the patient will be keeping a sleep diary, ask him to record the following data:

- time that he wakes up
- time and amount of sleep medications taken (including repeated doses)
- episodes of disorientation or confusion
- frequency of need for pain drugs or of help with toileting
- time spent out of bed.

Special considerations

After determining the patient's sleep patterns, you can develop an individualized plan of care that balances the patient's needs with those of your facility.

- Keep staff-initiated noise (such as talking outside the patient's room) to a minimum, and adjust lighting appropriately.
- Late risers can complicate the morning schedule, but offering two sittings at breakfast may solve the problem.
- Care measures, such as comfortable positioning of patients who need assistance with mobility or activities of daily living, a backrub or massage, and soft music, can help induce sleep.
- If indicated, administer analgesics to a patient in pain.
- Teach the patient deep-breathing techniques, progressive relaxation exercises, and guided imagery to promote relaxation and sleep.
- Schedule all treatments and procedures during waking hours, and eliminate nighttime vital sign assessments as soon as the patient's condition permits.
- Consider administering sleep aids temporarily when other methods have failed. Commonly prescribed drugs used to induce sleep include the antihistamine diphenhydramine and the benzodiazepine temazepam. Melatonin may also improve sleep quality in some older patients. Monitor the patient for possible adverse reactions to these drugs (such as rebound insomnia, nightmares, and confusion).
- Regardless of setting, you can teach your patient certain helpful measures to promote healthy sleep. (See *Dealing with sleep disturbances*.)

SPECIALTY BEDS

Many different types of specialty beds are available to prevent complications of immobility, such as pressure ulcers and pneumonia. Among the most commonly used are the Clinitron therapy (air-fluidized) bed and the air-therapy bed. (See *Two types of specialty beds*, page 530.)

Two types of specialty beds

Specialty beds, such as the Clinitron therapy bed and the air-therapy bed, help prevent complications of immobility.

Clinitron therapy bed

Air-therapy bed

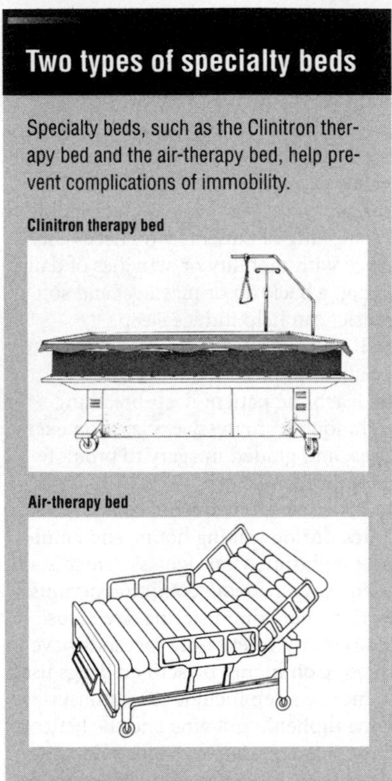

Clinitron therapy bed

Originally called the air-fluidized bed and designed for managing burns, the *Clinitron therapy bed* is now used for patients with various debilities. The bed is actually a large tub that supports the patient on a thick layer of silicone-coated microspheres of lime glass. A monofilament polyester filter sheet covers the microsphere-filled tub. Warmed air, propelled by a blower beneath the bed, passes through it. The resulting fluidlike surface reduces pressure on the skin sufficiently to avoid obstructing capillary blood flow, thereby helping to prevent pressure ulcers and to promote wound healing. The bed's air temperature can be adjusted to help control hypothermia and hyperthermia.

Small amounts of wound drainage can flow into the microspheres, eliminating the need for most dressings. In addition, use of this bed permits harmless contact between the bed's surface and grafted sites, promoting comfort and healing. Also, when the air pressure is turned off, the bed forms a firm surface that molds to the shape of the patient's body, allowing the nurse to move the patient or change his position.

The Clinitron therapy bed may be contraindicated for patients who can't mobilize and expel pulmonary secretions, because the lack of back support impairs productive coughing.

Air-therapy bed

Patients who have skin problems may benefit from an air-therapy bed instead of a Clinitron bed. This type of bed has air-filled compartments that can be inflated to varying degrees, thus providing different levels of support to different body parts.

Some air-therapy beds have a pulsating mode that can be programmed to deliver chest physiotherapy and a rotation mode that stimulates capillary blood flow, prevents venous stasis, increases peristalsis, and improves pulmonary hygiene. Some also come equipped with controls that help the nurse turn the patient when providing care. Because ordinary linen-saver pads block air flow, you'll need to use air-permeable pads that are available from the manufacturer.

Supplies

Clinitron therapy bed

- Clinitron therapy bed with microspheres (about 1,650 lb [750 kg])
- Filter sheet
- Flat sheet

Air-therapy bed

- Air-therapy bed
- Flat sheet
- Air-permeable linen-saver pads

Implementation

Clinitron therapy bed

▶ Normally, a manufacturer's representative or a trained health care professional prepares the bed for use. If you must help with the preparation, make sure the microspheres reach to within ½″ (1.3 cm) of the top of the tank. Then position the filter sheet on the bed with its printed side facing up. Match the holes in the sheet to the holes in the edge of the bed frame. Place the aluminum rails on the frame, with the studs in the proper holes. Depress the rails firmly, and secure them by tightening the knurled knobs to seal the filter sheet. Place a flat bed sheet over the filter sheet, and secure it with the elastic cord to prevent billowing. Turn on the air current to activate the microspheres. Then turn it off to ensure that the bed is working properly.

▶ With the help of three or more coworkers, transfer the patient to the bed using a lift sheet.

▶ Turn on the air pressure to activate the bed, and remove the lift sheet.

▶ Adjust the air temperature as necessary. Because the bed usually operates within 10° to 12° F (–11° to –12° C) of ambient air temperature, set the room temperature to 75° F (24° C). If microsphere temperature reaches 105° F (40.6° C), the bed automatically shuts off. It restarts automatically after 30 minutes.

▶ Monitor the patient's fluid and electrolyte status because the warm, dry air circulated by the Clinitron therapy bed increases evaporative water loss, possibly requiring modifications in oral or I.V. fluid intake. If the patient experiences excessive dryness of the upper respiratory tract, use a humidifier and mask, as ordered. Encourage coughing and deep breathing to help prevent pulmonary complications. After prolonged use of a Clinitron therapy bed, watch for hypocalcemia and hypophosphoremia.

▶ Cover any copiously draining wound with a porous dressing to absorb some of the drainage. Cover petroleum jelly or silver-based topical applications with an impervious dressing to minimize or prevent their absorption by the microspheres. Avoid using wet dressings or soaks because the excess fluid causes the microspheres to clump, impairing the fluid support effect. The bed restarts automatically if shut off for 30 minutes, so unplug it to perform longer procedures.

▶ To position a bedpan, roll the patient away from you, place the bedpan on the flat sheet, and push it into the microspheres. Then reposition the patient. To remove the bedpan, hold it steady and roll the patient away from you. Turn off the air pressure and remove the bedpan. Then turn the air on and reposition the patient.

▶ Don't wear a watch when handling the microspheres because they're small enough to penetrate the watch and damage the mechanism.

▶ Don't secure the filter sheet with pins or clamps, which may puncture the sheet and release microspheres. Take care to avoid puncturing the bed when giving injections. Repair any holes or tears with iron-on patching tape.

▶ Sieve the microspheres monthly or between patients to remove any clumped microspheres. Handle them carefully to avoid spills because they will make floors slippery and may cause falls.

▶ Treat a soiled filter sheet and clumped microspheres as contaminated items, and handle them according to your facility's policy.

▶ Change the filter sheet and operate the unit unoccupied for 24 hours between patients.

▶ Review the manufacturer's guidelines.

Air-therapy bed

▶ Normally, a manufacturer's representative prepares the bed for use.

▶ If the bed has a built-in scale, calibrate the scale using a sheet and the air-permeable linen-saver pad.
▶ With the help of three or more coworkers, transfer the patient to the bed using a lift sheet.
▶ If the bed can rotate, place the bed in the rotation mode at the settings determined by the manufacturer's representative. Note the patient's tolerance of rotation; you may have to decrease the angle of rotation if the patient can't tolerate the rotation.
▶ If the patient requires cardiopulmonary resuscitation (CPR) while on the air-therapy bed, simply put the bed in the CPR mode and begin resuscitation.

Complications

Bed malfunction could put the patient at risk for injury.

Patient teaching

▶ Explain and, if possible, demonstrate the operation of the Clinitron therapy bed for the patient. Tell him the reason for its use and that he'll feel as though he's floating on air. Then turn off the air pressure.
▶ If possible, show the patient the air-therapy bed and demonstrate its operation. Reassure him that the bed will hold him securely.

Documentation

Record changes in the patient's condition and his response to therapy in your progress notes. Note turning times and ongoing care on the flowchart. Document the condition of the patient's skin, including pressure ulcers and any other wounds. Finally, document your patient teaching.

SPEECH THERAPY

Speech is the means of using language in human interaction. An acute episode, such as a cerebrovascular accident or surgery, or a progressive neurologic disease, such as Parkinson's disease, can impair the patient's ability to speak.

Impairments in speech can be categorized into three groups: impairment in reception of verbal communication (for example, in patients who are unable to hear spoken words clearly), impairment of the speech-processing areas of the brain (for example, in patients with receptive or expressive aphasia), and impairment in the mechanics of speech (for example, in patients who have undergone a laryngectomy). If left untreated, impaired speech can lead to social isolation, decreased self-esteem, and depression. Therefore, speech therapy should be initiated as soon as the patient is able.

Implementation

▶ Ensure that a qualified speech therapist is involved early in the treatment plan. Speech therapists must possess a master's degree and be certified by the American Speech, Hearing, and Language Association.
▶ Observe and record the patient's speech and word recognition patterns.
▶ Use such communication tools as electromechanical boards, sentence structure boards, and computer programs.
▶ Explain situations, treatments, and any other pertinent information to the patient as if he understands. Normal speech is rehabilitative, even if the patient doesn't understand the words.
▶ Speak slowly; ask one question at a time and await a response. Ask yes or no questions if that is all the patient can respond to. Encourage the patient to articulate, even if his words convey no meaning.
▶ Use visual cues, objects, pictures, and gestures as well as words. Avoid patronizing and childish phrases.

Special considerations

▶ An aphasic patient may be especially prone to feelings of annoyance; remain calm and patient.

▶ Keep in mind that a patient with speech disorder isn't necesarily hard of hearing; use a normal voice when speaking.

SQUAMOUS CELL CARCINOMA

Arising from keratinizing epidermal cells, squamous cell carcinoma of the skin is an invasive tumor with the potential for metastasis. It occurs most commonly in fair-skinned white men over age 60. Outdoor employment and residence in a warm, sunny climate (such as the southern United States and Australia) greatly increase the risk of squamous cell carcinoma.

Lesions on sun-damaged skin tend to be less invasive and less likely to metastasize than lesions on unexposed skin. Notable exceptions are squamous cell lesions on the lower lip and the ears; these lesions are almost invariably markedly invasive metastatic lesions with a poor prognosis.

Predisposing factors associated with squamous cell carcinoma include overexposure to the sun's ultraviolet rays, X-ray therapy, ingestion of herbicides containing arsenic, chronic skin irritation and inflammation, exposure to local carcinogens (such as tar and oil), certain hereditary diseases (such as xeroderma pigmentosum and albinism), and the presence of premalignant lesions (such as actinic keratosis or Bowen's disease). Rarely, squamous cell carcinoma may develop on the site of smallpox vaccination, psoriasis, or chronic discoid lupus erythematosus.

Transformation from a premalignant lesion to squamous cell carcinoma may begin with induration and inflammation of the preexisting lesion. When squamous cell carcinoma arises from normal skin, the nodule grows slowly on a firm, indurated base. If untreated, this nodule eventually ulcerates and invades underlying tissues. Disease progression may lead to lymph node involvement and visceral metastasis, resulting in respiratory problems.

Signs and symptoms

▶ Scaly, keratotic lesions on the face, ears, and dorsa of the hands and forearms and on other sun-damaged skin areas; may have raised, irregular borders
▶ In late disease, lesions that grow outward (exophytic), are friable, and tend toward chronic crusting
▶ After metastasis, pain, malaise, anorexia, fatigue, and weakness

The patient history may reveal areas of chronic ulceration, especially on sun-damaged skin.

Diagnostic tests

▶ *Excisional biopsy* provides a definitive diagnosis of squamous cell carcinoma. Appropriate laboratory tests depend on systemic symptoms. (See *Staging squamous cell carcinoma*, page 534.)

Treatment

The size, shape, location, and invasiveness of the tumor and the condition of the underlying tissue determine the treatment method; a deeply invasive tumor may require a combination of techniques. All the major treatment methods have excellent cure rates. In most cases, the prognosis is better with a well-differentiated lesion than with a poorly differentiated one in an unusual location.

Depending on the lesion, treatment may consist of wide surgical excision; curettage and electrodesiccation, which offer good cosmetic results for smaller lesions; radiation therapy, which is generally used for older or debilitated patients; or chemosurgery, which is reserved for resistant or recurrent lesions.

Use of the chemotherapeutic agent fluorouracil typically results in complete healing within 1 to 2 months. This drug is available in various strengths (1%, 2%, and 5%) as a cream or solution. Local application causes immediate

Staging squamous cell carcinoma

Using the tumor, node, metastasis system, the American Joint Committee on Cancer has established the following staging system for squamous cell carcinoma.

Primary tumor

TX— Primary tumor can't be assessed
T0 — No evidence of primary tumor
Tis— Carcinoma in situ
T1— Tumor 2 cm or less in greatest dimension
T2— Tumor between 2 and 5 cm in greatest dimension
T3— Tumor more than 5 cm in greatest dimension
T4— Tumor invades deep extradermal structures (such as cartilage, skeletal muscle, or bone)

Regional lymph nodes

NX— Regional lymph nodes can't be assessed
N0— No evidence of regional lymph node involvement
N1— Regional lymph node involvement

Distant metastasis

MX— Distant metastasis can't be assessed
M0— No known distant metastasis
M1— Distant metastasis

Staging categories

Squamous cell carcinoma progresses from mild to severe as follows:
Stage 0— Tis, N0, M0
Stage I— T1, N0, M0
Stage II— T2, N0, M0; T3, N0, M0
Stage III— T4, N0, M0; any T, N1, M0
Stage IV— Any T, any N, M1

stinging and burning. Later effects include erythema, vesiculation, erosion, superficial ulceration, necrosis, and reepithelialization. The 5% solution induces the most severe inflammatory response but provides complete involution of the lesions with little recurrence. Fluorouracil treatment is continued until the lesions reach the ulcerative and necrotic stages (usually in 2 to 4 weeks). Then a corticosteroid preparation may be applied as an anti-inflammatory agent.

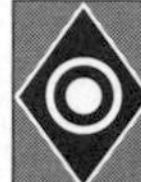

Drug alert Be careful to keep fluorouracil away from the eyes, scrotum, or mucous membranes. Warn the patient to avoid excessive exposure to the sun during the course of treatment because it intensifies the inflammatory reaction. A possible adverse effect of treatment is postinflammatory hyperpigmentation.

Key nursing diagnoses and outcomes

Body image disturbance related to skin lesions

Treatment outcome: The patient will express positive feelings about himself.

Impaired skin integrity related to skin lesions

Treatment outcome: The patient will regain skin integrity with the eradication of squamous cell carcinoma.

Deficient knowledge related to cause and treatment of diagnosis of squamous cell carcinoma

Treatment outcome: The patient will communicate an understanding of the treatment of squamous cell carcinoma and of skin-protection measures.

Nursing interventions

▶ Although disfiguring lesions are distressing, try to accept the patient as he is to increase his self-esteem and to promote a caring relationship.

▶ Listen to the patient's fears and concerns, and offer reassurance when appropriate. Remain with the patient during periods of severe stress and anxiety. Regularly evaluate the patient's degree of anxiety and acceptance of changes in body image.

▶ Accept the patient's perception of himself. Help the patient and his family set realistic goals and expectations.

▶ When you've determined that the patient is ready, involve him in making decisions related to his care. Provide positive reinforcement for the patient's efforts to adapt.

▶ Coordinate a consistent care plan for changing the patient's dressings. A standard routine helps the patient and his family members learn how to care for the wound.

▶ To promote healing and prevent infection, keep the wound dry and clean.

▶ Try to control odor with balsam of Peru, yogurt flakes, oil of cloves, or other odor-masking substances, even though they may be ineffective for long-term use. Topical or systemic antibiotics also temporarily control odor and eventually alter the lesion's bacterial flora.

▶ Provide periods of rest between procedures if the patient fatigues easily.

▶ Assess the patient for complications associated with squamous cell carcinoma.

▶ Monitor the patient for adverse effects of chemotherapy or radiation therapy, such as nausea, vomiting, diarrhea, and alopecia, and provide supportive care as indicated.

▶ Provide small, frequent meals consisting of high-protein, high-calorie foods if the patient is anorexic. Consult with the dietitian to incorporate foods that the patient enjoys into his diet.

PATIENT TEACHING

▶ Explain all procedures and treatments to the patient and his family. Encourage them to ask questions, and then answer them honestly.

▶ Instruct the patient to avoid excessive sun exposure to prevent a recurrence of cancer. Tell him to wear protective clothing (hats, long sleeves) whenever he's outdoors.

▶ Urge him to use a strong sunscreen—preferably with a skin protection factor of 15 or more—to protect his skin from ultraviolet rays. Advise him to apply sunscreen—as well as lipscreens to protect the lips from sun damage—30 to 60 minutes before sun exposure.

▶ Advise the patient to relieve local inflammation from topical fluorouracil with cool compresses or a corticosteroid ointment.

▶ Teach the patient to periodically examine his skin for precancerous lesions and to have them removed promptly.

▶ If appropriate, direct the patient and his family to hospital and community support services, such as social workers, psychologists, and cancer support groups.

STRESS

The health of an older person is a composite of the person's physical health, lifestyle, social support network, coping skills, and cognitive abilities. Age-related changes in social roles and health status effect the numbers and types of stressors experienced by older people. These changes may directly or indirectly influence the ways in which stress is handled.

Consider the life crises the older person typically faces: retirement, with accompanying loss of status and independence; loss of a spouse and other loved ones; sensory losses; and possibly disease, pain, surgery, dependence, and institutionalization. An older person may not exhibit stress in the traditional sense. Through his experience, he may have developed resources for dealing with stress. In some cases, what's stressful to a younger person may not be stressful to the older person because the older person has faced similar stressors or the stressor holds a lesser priority or sense of urgency than it does for the younger person.

Depending on the person's coping mechanisms, any one of these stressors could precipitate psychological problems. The cumulative effect could overwhelm even an emotionally strong, healthy person.

The following review will help you understand the losses and other stressful life events that older people face, how they respond to these losses, and how you can help them deal with these situations.

Loss of social supports

As adults reach advanced age, their social support network begins to break apart as friends die or move away. The strength and comfort these friends provided, which helped the individual to buffer or cope with loss, is no longer there. Such losses can be a catalyst to developing physical and mental illness in late life.

Other, less traditional losses may also result in a grieving process or progress to depression. These include the death of a pet, sale of a home, and admission to a long-term care facility. Even such seemingly minor events as ill-fitting dentures and having to give up driving have prompted serious suicide attempts in older adults.

Retirement

Many people define themselves by how they make their living; this self-image affects their lifestyle, friends, social network, and financial dealings. Retirement often precipitates changes in self-image as well as in spousal relationships and use of leisure time. Couples who enjoyed satisfying relationships while being separated for most of the working day may now need to adjust to being together for longer periods. As a result, troubled relationships may now become much more difficult. Lack of productive work and the absence of a social network outside the workplace often add to a negative outlook after retirement.

The earlier a person has prepared for retirement, the better his outlook and quality of life tend to be. If you have an older patient who's preparing for retirement, advise him to learn to:

- structure his leisure time
- plan to live within a limited budget
- get to know his spouse again, now that retirement approaches
- meet new friends outside of work, for example, through clubs, volunteer work, religious affiliations, and hobbies.

Widowhood

One of the most profound losses a person can experience is the death of a spouse. In addition, widowhood can seriously affect a person's financial status, social network, and physical and mental health. When the loss of a spouse occurs late in life, the person has a much greater risk of developing depression, anxiety, and substance abuse than a younger person because of decreased resiliency, a higher incidence of chronic illness, and the breakdown of social support networks. Older men have an even higher risk of developing physical and mental illness than older women.

Aside from the loss of companionship, the death of a spouse may leave unsettled issues that fester for years afterward. For example, unresolved guilt feelings related to infidelity, physical or substance abuse, or financial problems after widowhood can lead to serious mental illness, sometimes decades after the death of a spouse. Family and spousal caregivers especially may have such unresolved issues.

Make your older patient aware of counseling services, support groups, and other resources that are available to help him cope with the loss of a spouse.

Death of an adult child

Adult children are an important part of the older adult's social support network.

Certain ethnic groups, such as Jewish, Native American, and Asian families, place an especially high value on intergenerational relationships. The death of an adult child can be even more devastating to the older adult than the death of a spouse because parents expect their children to outlive them and be a support in old age. Refer an older patient who must cope with the loss of an adult child to an appropriate community resource, such as Interfaith, a clergyman, or a grief therapist.

Family estrangement

Older people may become estranged from family members for many reasons, such as drug or alcohol abuse and disagreements over religion, sexual orientation, choice of marriage partner, inheritance issues, or business dealings. Estrangement from grandchildren and great-grandchildren can be especially painful. As the years go by, an older person may yearn to reestablish family ties that were broken years before. Referring such a patient to family therapy can be very effective.

Changes in body image

Older adults may go through a grieving process and become depressed after their body image is changed by trauma, serious illness (such as stroke or coronary artery disease), surgery, or a decrease in functional ability. What's more, physical changes that impact lifestyle can be devastating to self-esteem and sexuality. You can assess your patient's response to a changed body image by encouraging discussion. If indicated, refer him to a psychotherapist for follow-up.

Financial loss

Many older people face serious financial hardships after retirement, especially if they must depend on Social Security as their primary or sole source of income. Also, older people today are especially vulnerable to financial scams. After experiencing serious economic hardship during the Depression in the 1930s, some older people have developed a lasting mistrust of financial institutions and may have large sums of money hidden in their homes. Con artists, aware of these possibilities, are adept at preying on older people. Some family members may also try to steal from their older relatives.

You may want to refer a vulnerable patient to a local senior center that offers financial counseling and information about crime prevention.

Special considerations

Patterns of coping with stress are learned behavior. Because mental health issues interfere with many aspects of life, older adults and their families can improve their quality of life by dealing with these issues. Many older people aren't referred for psychotherapy because of a mistaken belief that they would not benefit from it. A case worker or social worker can help reduce stress by implementing the services of community resources or psychological services.

SUBCUTANEOUS INJECTIONS

A drug moves into the bloodstream more rapidly when it's injected into the adipose (fatty) tissue beneath the skin than when it's given by mouth. Subcutaneous (S.C.) injection allows slower, more sustained drug infusion than I.M. injection; it also causes minimal tissue trauma and minimizes the risk of striking large blood vessels and nerves.

Drugs and solutions for S.C. injection are injected through a relatively short needle, using meticulous aseptic technique. The most common S.C. injection sites are the outer aspect of the upper arm, anterior thigh, loose tissue of the lower abdomen, buttocks, and upper back. S.C. injection is contraindicated in sites that are inflamed, edematous, scarred, or covered by a mole, birthmark, or other lesion. It may also be contraindicated in patients with impaired coagulation mechanisms.

Injection sites should be routinely rotated to prevent hypertrophy (thickening) of the skin and lipodystrophy (atrophy of tissue). Body sites shouldn't be used more than once every 6 to 7 weeks, if possible, to prevent hypertrophy and lipodystrohy. An exception to this is insulin injections, in which rotation of sites should be between like areas (arms-arms, thigh-thigh).

Supplies

- Patient's medication record and chart
- Prescribed drug
- Needle of appropriate gauge and length
- Gloves
- 1- to 3-ml syringe
- Alcohol pads
- Optional: insulin syringe, and insulin pump

Implementation

- Verify the order on the patient's medication record by checking it against the physician's order.
- Wash your hands.
- Check the label on the medication container against the order on the medication record.
- Confirm the patient's identity by asking his name and by checking the name, room number, and bed number on his wristband.
- Explain the procedure to the patient.
- Select a needle of the proper gauge and length. Usually, a 25G ⅝″ needle with a medium bevel works well for average-sized adults; obese individuals may require longer needles.
- If the drug is available in prefilled syringes, adjust the angle and depth of insertion according to needle length. If this isn't possible, you may have to transfer the drug to another syringe with an appropriately sized needle attached.
- Closely inspect the patient to determine the best injection site. With a decrease in body mass and loss of subcutaneous tissue, the deltoid area may not be an appropriate site for some older people. Rotate sites according to a schedule if the patient requires repeated injections. Use different areas of the body unless contraindicated by the specific drug. (Heparin, for example, should be injected only in certain sites.)
- Put on gloves.
- Position and drape the patient if necessary.
- Clean the injection site with an alcohol pad, beginning at the center of the site and moving outward in a circular motion. Allow the skin to dry before injecting the drug to avoid a stinging sensation from introducing alcohol into subcutaneous tissue.
- Loosen the protective needle sheath.
- With your nondominant hand, grasp the skin around the injection site firmly to elevate the subcutaneous tissue, forming a 1″ (2.5-cm) fat fold. Because the older patient has a decrease in subcutaneous tissue, you may need to grasp a larger area to obtain adequate tissue.
- Holding the syringe in your dominant hand, insert the loosened needle sheath between the fourth and fifth fingers of your other hand while still pinching the skin around the injection site. Pull back the syringe with your dominant hand to uncover the needle by grasping the syringe like a pencil. Don't touch the needle.
- Position the needle with its bevel up.
- Tell the patient he'll feel a prick as the needle is inserted.
- Insert the needle quickly in one motion at a 45-degree angle for an average-sized adult, a 90-degree angle for an obese adult, and an angle less than 45 degrees for a very thin adult. (See *Giving a subcutaneous injection*.)

- Release the patient's skin to avoid injecting the drug into compressed tissue and irritating nerve fibers.
- Pull back the plunger slightly to check for blood return. If no blood appears, begin injecting the drug slowly. If blood appears on aspiration, withdraw the needle, prepare another syringe, and repeat the procedure.
- Don't aspirate for blood return when giving insulin or heparin. It's not necessary with insulin and may cause a hematoma with heparin.
- After injection, remove the needle gently but quickly at the same angle used for insertion.
- Cover the site with an alcohol pad, and massage the site gently (unless you've injected a drug that contraindicates massage, such as heparin) to distribute the drug and facilitate absorption.
- Remove the alcohol pad, and check the injection site for bleeding or bruising. Because of vascular changes, older people are more subject to bruising and hematomas.
- Dispose of the injection equipment according to facility policy. To avoid needle-stick injuries, don't resheath the needle.

Giving a subcutaneous injection

Before giving the injection, elevate the subcutaneous tissue at the site by grasping it firmly.

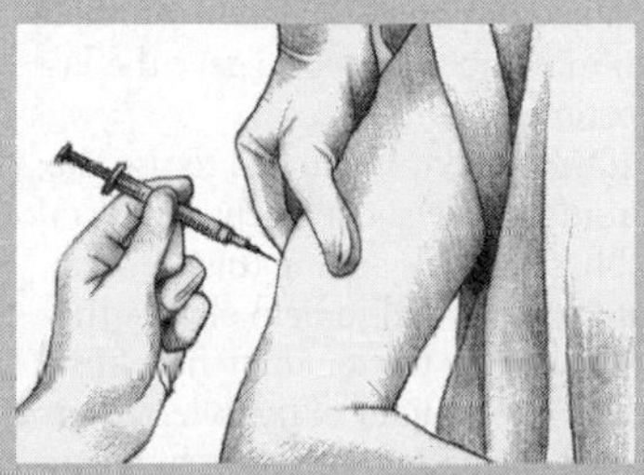

Insert the needle at a 45- or 90-degree angle to the skin surface, depending on needle length and the amount of subcutaneous tissue at the site. A thinner individual requires less of an angle (45 degrees). Some drugs, such as heparin, should always be injected at a 90-degree angle.

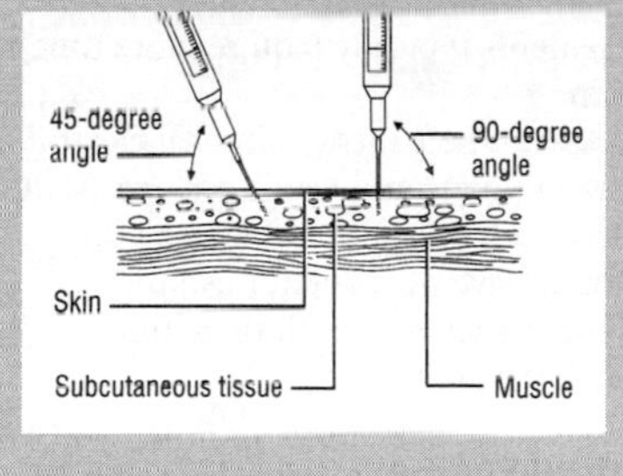

Special considerations

- Don't administer any injection within 2″ (5 cm) of a scar, a bruise, or the umbilicus.
- To establish more consistent blood insulin levels when giving insulin injections, rotate injection sites within anatomic regions.
- The preferred site for heparin injections is the lower abdominal fat pad, 2″ beneath the umbilicus, between the right and the left iliac crests. Injecting heparin into this area, which isn't involved in muscular activity, reduces the risk of local capillary bleeding. Always rotate the sites from one side to the other.

Complications

Concentrated or irritating solutions may cause formation of sterile abscesses. Repeated injections in the same site can cause lipodystrophy. A natural immune response, this complication can be reduced by rotating injection sites.

Patient teaching

- If the older person is to receive S.C. heparin injections at home, make sure that he and a caregiver can demonstrate the procedure for preparing and administering the injection. If the patient's vision is impaired, suggest using assistive devices, such as a scale magnifier or syringe-filling device.

▶ Encourage the patient to record the site used for heparin injection. Marking a body diagram and noting the date of the injection on the diagram will help him remember where he gave the last injection.

▶ If the patient is allowed to use the deltoid muscle site for heparin injections and has difficulty doing this, suggest that he use a wall to help elevate the subcutaneous tissue. Show him how to rotate the shoulder of the selected arm toward the body. Then have him lean against the wall so that the deltoid area is exposed, clean the site, and inject the drug.

▶ Encourage family members and friends to participate in learning how to perform S.C. injections.

▶ Assess the patient's readiness and ability to learn. Keep in mind that elderly patients typically require more time to learn.

▶ Assess the patient's physical capability to manipulate and read a syringe. Many clients can't see air bubbles, so you should have the patient push the plunger back and forth three times to purge the syringe.

Documentation

Record the date and time of the injection, the medication administered and the dose, the injection site and route, and the patient's reaction to the injection.

SUBDURAL HEMATOMA

Caused by blood leaking into the subdural space, a subdural hematoma can happen days or weeks after an injury and usually has an insidious onset. Because the presenting symptoms can mimic those associated with a cerebrovascular accident (CVA) or dementia, careful assessment is necessary.

The three types of subdural hematomas are classified by their onset. An *acute subdural hematoma* involves rapid onset of neurologic deterioration, occurring 3 to 6 hours after the injury. Mortality is usually greater than 50%, and survivors may have neurologic deficits. A *subacute subdural hematoma* has a slower course, with neurologic deterioration occurring gradually, 24 to 36 hours after the initial injury. The outcome for people with a subacute hematoma is more favorable than for those with an acute hematoma. A *chronic subdural hematoma* produces neurologic symptoms up to 6 weeks after the causative injury, which the patient usually forgets or deems insignificant. Without cerebral herniation, the outcome for chronic subdural hematoma is good; mortality is less than 10%.

A high incidence of subdural hematomas is found in elderly patients with gait or balance problems and anyone at risk for falls. Chronic subdural hematomas commonly occur in alcoholics, patients with seizure disorders, and patients with prolonged coagulation.

Most subdural hematomas occur when the patient's head hits a broad, hard object and the blow causes internal bleeding. Bleeding into the subdural space is either arterial or venous. Bleeding from an arterial source is usually severe and occurs with an acute trauma or, rarely, an aneurysm. Bleeding from large veins can also cause an acute hematoma. Subacute hematomas are commonly associated with slow venous bleeding.

In a chronic hematoma, the initial injury is small and usually doesn't produce any signs. As the hematoma develops, new capillaries form, which leak red blood cells and proteins. Local fibrinolysis prevents any further clot formation, leading to a cycle of clot lysis and reabsorption and minor bleeding. If bleeding occurs faster than reabsorption, a chronic subdural hematoma forms. This hematoma can grow quite large without causing any symptoms.

Key point An older person with cerebral atrophy can tolerate a larger subdural hematoma for a longer period of time than a younger person can before the hematoma causes neurologic changes. Therefore, a hematoma in an older patient can be very large before any symptoms are seen, even in an acute condition.

The outcome for a patient with a subdural hematoma depends on the length of time between injury and surgery, how quickly intracranial pressure (ICP) increases, and any associated intracranial damage. Complications include seizures and cerebral atrophy, which can lead to permanent neurologic deficits. In rapidly accumulating hematomas, brain stem herniation and death can occur as increased pressure and volume force the brain stem down into the base of the skull.

Signs and symptoms

- Weakness in one or more extremities
- Confusion and memory loss
- Difficulty speaking
- Gait or balance disturbances, ataxia
- Old bruise or scab over the site of a head injury
- Pupils of unequal size and reactions
- Aphasia
- Intense headache, vomiting, or visual deterioration from papilledema (acute); recurring headache (chronic)
- Changes in level of consciousness (LOC): in acute hematoma, rapid decline in LOC or coma; in subacute hematoma, slow deterioration in LOC; in chronic hematoma, periods of coherence and alertness alternating with periods of confusion and lethargy

The patient may report a recent fall or injury to the head (any time from a few hours to 3 days before the start of symptoms), or he may be unable to recall any injury.

Diagnostic tests

- *Computed tomography (CT) scan* visualizes the collection of blood below the dura.
- *Magnetic resonance imaging* yields the same image as a CT scan but may also allow visualization of the dura.
- *Angiography* is rarely used but may be indicated if the source of bleeding is suspected to be an aneurysm.

Treatment

Surgical evacuation is the required treatment in most cases. A craniotomy is usually performed for acute and subacute hematomas to evacuate the hematoma and identify and treat the cause of bleeding. Surgery for a chronic hematoma usually involves the creation of burr holes under local anesthesia. The hematoma is evacuated, and the area irrigated. A drain is commonly inserted intraoperatively to allow drainage of blood in the immediate postoperative period.

An older patient with a small chronic subdural hematoma may be monitored with frequent CT scans to check for resolution or expansion. If no expansion is seen, the hematoma is allowed to remain. Evacuation of a chronic hematoma in an older adult may be further complicated by decreased elasticity of the brain: If the fluid is present for any length of time, drainage leaves a space and the fluid reaccumulates.

Key nursing diagnoses and outcomes

Pain related to increased ICP

Treatment outcome: The patient will experience relief from pain after treatment.

Using the Glasgow Coma Scale

The Glasgow Coma Scale is used to assess a patient's level of consciousness (LOC). It was designed to help predict a patient's survival and recovery after a head injury. This scale minimizes subjective impressions in evaluating LOC.

The scale scores three observations: eye response, motor response, and verbal response to verbal stimuli. Each response receives a point value. If the patient is alert, can follow simple commands, and is completely oriented to person, place, and time, his score will total 15 points. If the patient is comatose, his score will total 7 or less. A score of 3, the lowest possible score, indicates deep coma and a poor prognosis. Many facilities display the Glasgow Coma Scale on neurologic flowsheets to show changes in the patient's LOC over time.

Observation	Response	Score
Eye response	Opens spontaneously	4
	Opens to verbal command	3
	Opens to pain	2
	No response	1
Motor response	Reacts to verbal command	6
	Reacts to painful stimulus:	
	■ Identifies localized pain	5
	■ Flexes and withdraws	4
	■ Assumes flexor position	3
	■ Assumes extensor posture	2
	No response	1
Verbal response	Is oriented and converses	5
	Is disoriented but converses	4
	Uses inappropriate words	3
	Makes incomprehensible sounds	2
	No response	1
TOTAL SCORE		3 to 15

Impaired (cerebral) tissue perfusion related to increased ICP due to bleeding

Treatment outcome: The patient will maintain or improve his current level of consciousness.

Nursing interventions

▶ Perform frequent neurologic assessments to detect changes in LOC, which may indicate expansion of the hematoma. Document LOC using the Glasgow Coma Scale to minimize the subjective impressions in your evaluation. (See *Using the Glasgow Coma Scale*.)

▶ Keep the call button within the patient's reach, and instruct him to use it if headache symptoms begin or increase.

▶ Administer analgesics as ordered. Use multiple pain-relief measures as requested by the older patient.

▶ Monitor the environment. Keep the room free from clutter.

▶ Monitor vital signs; increased blood pressure may cause increased ICP.

▶ Provide measures to help decrease ICP, such as keeping the head of the bed elevated, minimizing movement, and keeping the environment subdued.

▶ Prepare the patient for ordered diagnostic tests.
▶ If surgery is required, prepare the patient physically and emotionally.

After surgery

▶ Assess the patient's neurologic status to detect early signs of complications, especially increased ICP and cerebral ischemia.
▶ Monitor vital signs; assess for changes in respiratory patterns, which may be related to cerebral swelling or hematoma reaccumulation; and evaluate the patient for signs of infection.
▶ Monitor the amount and type of drainage accumulated in the drain.

PATIENT TEACHING

▶ Explain the nature of the disorder and the need for prompt treatment to help prevent complications. Also explain the purpose of diagnostic tests.
▶ Explain prescribed pain medications, including their purpose, actions, and potential adverse effects.
▶ Inform family members that the patient needs to remain calm and stress-free. Limit visitation and try to keep the atmosphere relaxed.
▶ Teach family members and the patient the techniques to decrease ICP, such as positioning, relaxation breathing, and maintaining a soothing atmosphere.
▶ Inform the patient about planned surgery. Clarify his risks and explain preoperative, postoperative, and follow-up home care.
▶ Tell the patient to be sure to notify the physician if he develops a headache.
▶ To prevent falls, instruct the patient to sit down and rest immediately if he experiences dizziness, disturbed balance, or weakness. To help prevent falls at home, suggest making minor changes such as installing a grab bar in the tub area.

SUCTIONING

The suctioning procedure removes secretions from the trachea or bronchi by means of a catheter inserted through the mouth, nose, tracheal stoma, tracheostomy tube, or endotracheal tube. Besides removing secretions, suctioning stimulates the cough reflex. This procedure helps maintain a patent airway to promote optimal exchange of oxygen and carbon dioxide and to prevent pneumonia that results from pooling of secretions. Performed as frequently as the patient's condition warrants, suctioning calls for strict aseptic technique.

Supplies

▶ Oxygen source (wall or portable unit and hand-held resuscitation bag with a mask, 15 mm adapter, or a positive end-expiratory pressure [PEEP] valve, if indicated)
▶ Wall or portable suction apparatus
▶ Collection container
▶ Connecting tube
▶ Suction catheter kit (or a sterile suction catheter, one sterile glove, one clean glove, and a disposable sterile solution container)
▶ 1-L bottle of sterile water or normal saline solution
▶ Sterile water-soluble lubricant (for nasal insertion)
▶ Syringe for deflating cuff of endotracheal or tracheostomy tube
▶ Waterproof trash bag
▶ Optional: sterile towel

Implementation

▶ Explain the procedure to the patient, even if he's unresponsive. Inform him that suctioning usually causes transient coughing or gagging, but that coughing is helpful for removal of secretions. If the patient has been suctioned previously, summarize the reasons for suctioning.
▶ Continue to reassure the patient throughout the procedure to minimize

anxiety, promote relaxation, and decrease oxygen demand.

▶ Choose a suction catheter of the appropriate size. The diameter should be no larger than half the inside diameter of the tracheostomy or endotracheal tube to minimize hypoxia during suctioning.

▶ Place the suction apparatus on the patient's overbed table or bedside stand. Position the table or stand on your preferred side of the bed to facilitate suctioning.

▶ Attach the collection container to the suction unit and the connecting tube to the collection container.

▶ Label and date the bottle of normal saline solution or sterile water.

▶ Open the waterproof trash bag.

▶ Assess the patient's vital signs, breath sounds, and general appearance to establish a baseline for comparison after suctioning.

▶ Review the patient's arterial blood gas and oxygen saturation levels if they're available.

▶ Evaluate the patient's ability to cough and deep-breathe because this will help move secretions up the tracheobronchial tree. If you'll be performing nasotracheal suctioning, check the patient history for a deviated septum, nasal polyps, nasal obstruction, nasal trauma, epistaxis, or mucosal swelling.

▶ Wash your hands.

▶ Unless contraindicated, place the patient in semi-Fowler's or high Fowler's position to promote lung expansion and productive coughing.

▶ Remove the top from the bottle of normal saline solution or sterile water. Then open the package containing the sterile solution container.

▶ Using strictly aseptic technique, open the suction catheter kit and put on the gloves. If using individual supplies, open the suction catheter and the gloves, placing the nonsterile glove on your nondominant hand and then the sterile glove on your dominant hand.

▶ Using your nondominant (nonsterile) hand, pour the normal saline solution or sterile water into the solution container.

▶ Place a small amount of water-soluble lubricant on the sterile area. Lubricant may be used to facilitate passage of the catheter during nasotracheal suctioning.

▶ Place a sterile towel over the patient's chest, if desired, to provide an additional sterile area.

▶ Using your dominant (sterile) hand, remove the catheter from its wrapper. Keep it coiled so it can't touch a nonsterile object. Using your other hand to manipulate the connecting tubing, attach the catheter to the tubing.

▶ Using your nondominant hand, set the suction pressure according to your facility's policy. Pressure is typically set between 80 and 120 mm Hg. Higher pressures don't enhance secretion removal and may cause traumatic injury. Occlude the suction port to assess suction pressure.

▶ Dip the catheter tip in the saline solution to lubricate the outside of the catheter and to reduce tissue trauma during insertion.

▶ With the catheter tip in the sterile solution, occlude the control valve with the thumb of your nondominant hand. Suction a small amount of solution through the catheter to lubricate the inside of the catheter, thus facilitating passage of secretions through it.

▶ For nasal insertion of the catheter, lubricate the tip of the catheter with the sterile, water-soluble lubricant to reduce tissue trauma during insertion.

▶ If the patient isn't intubated, or is intubated but isn't receiving supplemental oxygen or aerosol, instruct him to take three to six deep breaths to help minimize or prevent hypoxia during suctioning.

▶ If the patient isn't intubated but is receiving oxygen, evaluate his need for preoxygenation. If indicated, instruct him to take three to six deep breaths while using his supplemental oxygen. (If needed, the patient may continue to receive supplemental oxygen during suctioning by leaving his nasal cannula in one nostril or by keeping the oxygen mask over his mouth.)

▶ If the patient is being mechanically ventilated, preoxygenate him by using either a hand-held resuscitation bag or the sigh mode on the ventilator. To use the resuscitation bag, set the oxygen flow meter at 15 L/minute, disconnect the patient from the ventilator, and deliver three to six breaths with the resuscitation bag, as shown below.

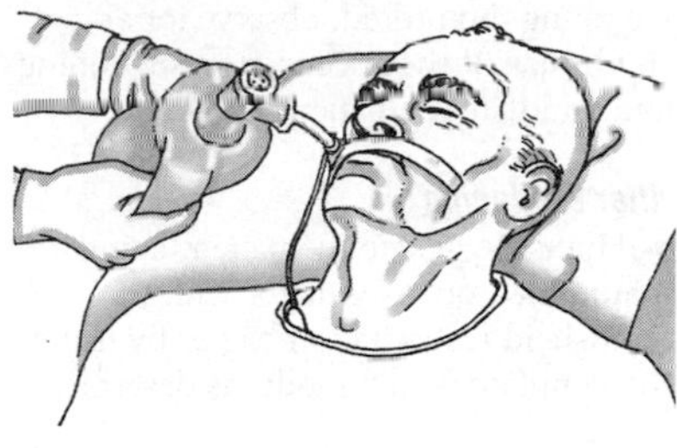

▶ If the patient is being maintained on PEEP, evaluate the need to use a resuscitation bag with a PEEP valve.

▶ To preoxygenate using the ventilator, first adjust the fraction of inspired oxygen (FIO_2) to 100%. Then either use the sigh mode or manually deliver three to six breaths. If you have an assistant for the procedure, the assistant can manage the patient's oxygen needs while you perform the suctioning.

Nasotracheal insertion in a nonintubated patient

▶ Disconnect the oxygen from the patient, if applicable.

▶ Using your nondominant hand, raise the tip of the patient's nose. Raising the nose into the sniffing position helps align the larynx and pharynx and may facilitate passing the catheter during nasotracheal suctioning. If the patient's condition permits, have an assistant extend the patient's head and neck above his shoulders. The patient's lower jaw may need to be moved up and forward. If the patient is responsive, ask him to stick out his tongue so he won't be able to swallow the catheter during insertion.

▶ Insert the catheter into the patient's nostril while gently rolling it between your fingers to help it advance through the turbinates.

▶ As the patient inhales, quickly advance the catheter as far as possible. Don't apply suction during insertion to avoid oxygen loss and tissue trauma.

▶ If the patient coughs as the catheter passes through the larynx, briefly hold the catheter still and then resume advancement when the patient inhales.

Insertion in an intubated patient

▶ In addition to the closed tracheal method, oxygen insufflation offers a new approach to suctioning. Oxygen insufflation suctioning uses a double-lumen catheter that allows oxygen insufflation during the suctioning procedure.

▶ Using your nonsterile hand, disconnect the patient from the ventilator.

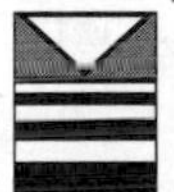

Key point **Studies show that instillation of normal saline solution into the trachea before suctioning may stimulate the patient's cough but doesn't liquefy the patient's secretions. Keeping the patient adequately hydrated and using bronchial hygiene techniques seems to have a greater effect on mobilizing secretions.**

▶ Using your sterile hand, gently insert the suction catheter into the artificial airway, as shown below.

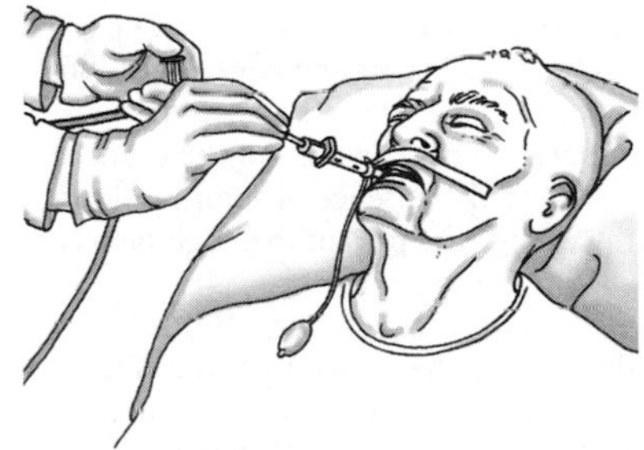

▶ Advance the catheter, without applying suction, until you meet resistance. If the patient coughs, pause briefly and then resume advancement.

Suctioning the patient

▶ After inserting the catheter, apply suction intermittently by removing and replacing the thumb of your nondominant hand over the control valve. Simultaneously use your dominant hand to withdraw the catheter as you roll it between your thumb and forefinger. This rotating motion prevents the catheter from pulling tissue into the tube as it exits, thus avoiding tissue trauma. Never suction more than 5 to 10 seconds at a time to prevent hypoxia.

▶ During suctioning, the catheter typically is advanced as far as the mainstem bronchi. However, because of tracheobronchial anatomy, the catheter tends to enter the right mainstem bronchus instead of the left. Using an angled catheter may help you guide the catheter into the left mainstem bronchus. Rotating the patient's head to the right seems to have a limited effect.

▶ If the patient is intubated, use your nondominant hand to stabilize the tip of the endotracheal tube as you withdraw the catheter, to prevent mucous membrane irritation or accidental extubation.

▶ If applicable, resume oxygen delivery by reconnecting the source of oxygen or ventilation and hyperoxygenating the patient's lungs before continuing to prevent or relieve hypoxia.

▶ Observe the patient, and allow him to rest for a few minutes before the next suctioning. The timing of each suctioning and the length of each rest period depend on his tolerance of the procedure and the absence of complications. Encourage the patient to cough between suctioning attempts.

▶ Observe the secretions. If they're thick, clear the catheter periodically by dipping the tip in the saline solution and applying suction. Normally, sputum is watery and tends to be sticky. Tenacious or thick sputum usually indicates dehydration. Watch for color variations. White or translucent color is normal; yellow indicates pus; green indicates retained secretions or *Pseudomonas* infection; brown usually indicates old blood; red indicates fresh blood; and a "red currant jelly" appearance indicates *Klebsiella* infection. When sputum contains blood, note whether it is streaked or well mixed. Also indicate how often blood appeared.

▶ If the patient's heart rate and rhythm are being monitored, observe for arrhythmias. If they occur, stop suctioning and ventilate the patient.

After suctioning

▶ Hyperoxygenate the patient being maintained on a ventilator with the hand-held resuscitation bag or by using the ventilator's sigh mode, as described earlier.

▶ Readjust the FIO_2 to the ordered settings.

▶ After suctioning the lower airway, assess the patient's need for upper airway suctioning. If the cuff of the endotracheal or tracheostomy tube is inflated, suction the upper airway before deflating the cuff with a syringe. Always change the catheter and sterile glove before resuctioning the lower airway to avoid introducing microorganisms into the lower airway.

▶ Discard the gloves and the catheter in the waterproof trash bag. Clear the connecting tubing by aspirating the remaining saline solution or water. Discard and replace suction equipment and supplies according to your facility's policy. Wash your hands.

▶ Auscultate lungs bilaterally and take vital signs, if indicated, to assess the procedure's effectiveness.

Complications

Because oxygen is removed along with secretions, the patient may experience hypoxemia and dyspnea. Anxiety may alter respiratory patterns. Cardiac arrhythmias can result from hypoxia and stimulation of the vagus nerve in the tracheobronchial tree. Tracheal or bronchial trauma can result from traumatic or prolonged suctioning.

Patients with compromised cardiovascular or pulmonary status are at risk for hypoxemia, arrhythmias, hypertension, or hypotension. Patients with a history of nasopharyngeal bleeding, who are taking anticoagulants, who've had a recent tracheostomy, or who have a blood dyscrasia are at an increased risk for bleeding as a result of suctioning. Use caution when suctioning patients who have increased intracranial pressure because it may increase pressure further.

If the patient experiences laryngospasm or bronchospasm (rare complications) during suctioning, disconnect the suction catheter from the connecting tubing and allow the catheter to act as an airway. Discuss with the patient's physician the use of bronchodilators or lidocaine to reduce the risk of this complication.

Patient teaching

- Explain the procedure and the reason for it to the patient.
- Tell him to call a nurse immediately if he feels short of breath or feels the need to be suctioned.

Documentation

Record the date and time of the procedure, the technique used, and the reason for suctioning. Note the amount, color, consistency, and odor (if any) of the secretions; any complications and the nursing action taken; and pertinent data regarding the patient's subjective response to the procedure. Also document your patient teaching.

SUICIDE

The risk of suicide in a depressed patient is very real. Depression is one of the strongest risk factors for attempted and completed suicides and may contribute to as many as 75% of all completed suicides. About 39% of successful suicides are committed by people over age 65, with the highest rate between ages 75 and 85. Suicide attempts in those over age 60 are five times more likely to be successful. The suicide rate for elderly men is seven times that for elderly women.

Risk factors for suicide include alcoholism, bereavement (especially within 1 year after a loss), loss of health, living alone, and the loss when a child marries and moves away.

Assessing the problem

Assess all depressed patients for self-destructive or suicidal tendencies. Not all depressed patients want to die, but a higher percentage of them commit suicide than patients with other diagnoses. Suicidal ideation can be disguised as indirect self-destructive behavior. For example, some older patients may refuse to eat or to comply with their medical regimen.

Assessing suicidal ideation involves specifically asking the patient whether he has thoughts of suicide and a plan for implementing it. Some patients have passive suicidal ideation — they have no plan or intent to commit suicide, but they do wish to be dead. Such patients must also be assessed to determine if they would ever do anything to hasten death. Don't worry that asking questions about suicide will make a patient begin thinking about it.

Taking action

As with a depressed patient, first report your concerns about potential suicide risk to the patient's physician for further

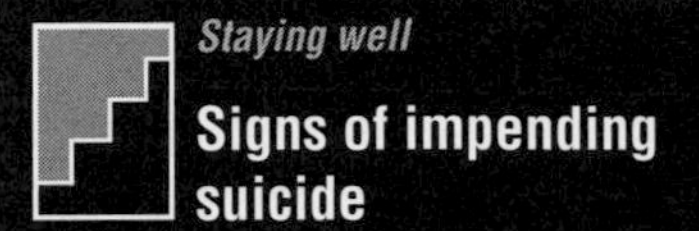

Staying well

Signs of impending suicide

Suicide among older adults rarely is an impulsive act; most suicide attempts are not empty gestures or threats.

Be alert for these warning signs of impending suicide:

- withdrawal
- social isolation
- signs of depression, which may include crying, fatigue, helplessness, poor concentration, reduced interest in sex and other activities, sadness, and weight loss
- farewells to friends and family members
- putting affairs in order
- giving away prized possessions
- expression of covert suicide messages and death wishes
- obvious suicide messages such as "I'd be better off dead."

medical evaluation and referral to a counselor or psychiatric practitioner. Any indication of suicidal ideation, regardless of how passive, should be assessed and taken seriously. In addition, teach family and friends to be on the lookout for warning signs of suicide. (See *Signs of impending suicide.*)

Patients at risk for suicide can be successfully treated through psychotherapy, drugs, support groups, and other methods. Help the patient see that he isn't alone. Assure him that even if he has no significant others in his personal life, caring and competent professionals are dedicated to seeing him through this low point.

If possible, encourage the patient to engage in physical activity to help release tension. Hobbies that require physical effort and activities such as walking, swimming, or gardening can be relaxing and provide a sense of accomplishment.

SURGICAL WOUND MANAGEMENT

When caring for a patient with a surgical wound, you perform procedures that help prevent infection by keeping pathogens out of the wound. Besides promoting patient comfort, such procedures also protect the skin surface from maceration and excoriation caused by contact with irritating drainage. They also allow you to measure wound drainage to monitor fluid and electrolyte balance.

The two primary methods used to manage a draining wound are dressing and pouching. Dressing is preferred unless caustic or excessive drainage is compromising the patient's skin integrity. In most cases, lightly seeping wounds with drains and wounds with minimal purulent drainage can be managed with packing and gauze dressings. Some wounds, such as those that become chronic, may require an occlusive dressing. A wound with copious, excoriating drainage calls for pouching to protect the surrounding skin. If your patient has a surgical wound, you must monitor him and choose the appropriate dressing.

Sterile technique should be ued during the initial dressing change; during later changes, sterile or aseptic technique (depending on wound type). The surgeon may order specific treatments or may consult wth a wound care specialist or enterostomal therapist to best determine wound treatment. The type of dressing depends on the wound characteristics and the goals of wound management. Be sure to change the dressing often enough to keep the skin dry. (See *Tailoring wound care to wound color.*)

Tailoring wound care to wound color

You can promote healing of any wound by keeping it moist, clean, and free of debris. If your patient has an open wound, you can assess how well it's healing by inspecting its color and then using the wound color to guide your specific management approach.

Red wound

Red, the color of healthy granulation tissue, indicates normal healing. When a wound begins to heal, a layer of pale pink granulation tissue covers the wound bed. As this layer thickens, it becomes beefy red.

Cover a red wound, keep it moist and clean, and protect it from trauma. Use a transparent dressing, a hydrocolloid dressing, or a gauze dressing moistened with sterile normal saline solution or impregnated with petroleum jelly or an antibiotic.

Yellow wound

Yellow is the color of exudate produced by microorganisms in an open wound. When a wound heals without complications, the immune system removes microorganisms. But if there are too many microorganisms to remove, exudate accumulates and becomes visible. Exudate usually appears whitish yellow, creamy yellow, yellowish green, or beige. Water content influences the shade: Dry exudate appears darker.

Clean a yellow wound and remove exudate, using high-pressure irrigation; then cover it with a moist dressing. Use absorptive products (for example, Debrisan beads and paste) or a moist gauze dressing with or without an antibiotic. You may also use hydrotherapy with whirlpool or high-pressure irrigation.

Black wound

Black, the least healthy color, signals necrosis. Dead, avascular tissue slows healing and provides a site for microorganisms to proliferate.

Debride a black wound. After removing dead tissue, apply a dressing to keep the wound moist and guard against external contamination. As ordered, use enzyme products, surgical debridement, hydrotherapy with whirlpool or high-pressure irrigation, or a moist gauze dressing.

Multicolored wound

If you note two or even three colors in a wound, classify the wound according to the least healthy color present. For example, if your patient's wound is both red and yellow, classify it as a yellow wound.

Supplies

- Waterproof trash bag
- Clean gloves
- Sterile gloves
- Gown and face shield or goggles, if indicated
- Sterile 4″ × 4″ gauze pads
- ABD pads, if indicated
- Sterile cotton-tipped applicators
- Sterile dressing set
- Topical medication, if ordered
- Adhesive or other tape
- Optional: shaving supplies; skin protectant, nonadherent pads, acetone-free adhesive remover or baby oil, sterile normal saline solution, graduated container

For a wound with a drain

- Sterile scissors
- Sterile 4″ × 4″ pads without cotton lining
- ABD pads
- Ostomy pouch or another collection bag

- Precut drain dressings
- Adhesive tape (paper or silk tape if the patient is hypersensitive)
- Surgical mask

Implementation

- Assemble all of the equipment in the patient's room.
- Explain the procedure to the patient to allay his fears and ensure his cooperation.
- Check the expiration date on each sterile package and inspect for tears.
- Open the waterproof trash bag, and place it near the patient's bed. Position the bag to avoid reaching across the sterile field or the wound when disposing of soiled articles.

Removing the old dressing

- Check the physician's order for specific wound care and drug instructions. Be sure to note the location of surgical drains to avoid dislodging them during the procedure.
- Identify the patient's allergies, especially to adhesive tape, topical solutions, or drugs.
- Medicate the patient for pain, if needed.
- Provide the patient with privacy, and position him as necessary. Expose only the wound site.
- Wash your hands thoroughly. Put on a gown and a face shield, if necessary. Then put on clean gloves.
- Loosen the soiled dressing by holding the patient's skin and pulling the tape or dressing toward the wound. This protects the newly formed tissue and prevents stress on the incision. Moisten the tape with acetone-free adhesive remover or baby oil, if necessary, to make the tape removal less painful (particularly if the skin is hairy). Don't apply solvents to the incision because they could contaminate the wound.
- Slowly remove the soiled dressing. If the gauze adheres to the wound, loosen the gauze by moistening it with sterile normal saline solution.
- Observe the dressing for the amount, type, color, and odor of drainage.
- Discard the dressing and gloves in the waterproof trash bag.

Caring for the wound

- Wash your hands. Establish a sterile field with all the equipment and supplies you'll need. If the physician has ordered ointment, squeeze the needed amount onto the sterile field. If you're using an antiseptic from a nonsterile bottle, pour the antiseptic cleaning agent into a sterile container so you won't contaminate your gloves. Then put on sterile gloves.
- Saturate the sterile gauze pads with the prescribed cleaning agent. Avoid using cotton balls because they may shed fibers in the wound, causing irritation, infection, or adhesion.
- If ordered, obtain a wound culture.
- Pick up the moistened gauze pad, and squeeze out the excess solution.
- Working from the top of the incision, wipe once to the bottom and then discard the gauze pad. With a second moistened pad, wipe from top to bottom in a vertical path next to the incision.
- Continue to work outward from the incision in lines running parallel to it. Always wipe from the clean area toward the less clean area (usually from top to bottom). Use each gauze pad for only one stroke to avoid tracking wound exudate and normal body flora from surrounding skin to the clean areas. Remember that the suture line is cleaner than the adjacent skin and the top of the suture line is usually cleaner than the bottom because more drainage collects at the bottom of the wound.
- Use sterile cotton-tipped applicators for efficient cleaning of tight-fitting wire sutures, deep and narrow wounds, or wounds with pockets. Remember to wipe only once with each applicator.

▶ If the patient has a surgical drain, clean the drain's surface last. Because moist drainage promotes bacterial growth, the drain is considered the most contaminated area. Clean the skin around the drain by wiping in half or full circles from the drain site outward.

▶ Clean all areas of the wound to wash away debris, pus, blood, and necrotic material. Try not to disturb sutures or irritate the incision. Clean to at least 1" (2.5 cm) beyond the end of the new dressing. If you aren't applying a new dressing, clean to at least 2" (5 cm) beyond the incision.

▶ Make sure that the edges of the incision are lined up properly, and check for signs of infection (heat, redness, swelling, and odor), dehiscence, or evisceration. If you observe such signs or if the patient reports pain at the wound site, notify the physician.

▶ Irrigate the wound as ordered.

▶ Wash the skin surrounding the wound with soap and water, and pat it dry using a sterile 4" × 4" gauze pad. Apply any prescribed topical medications.

▶ Apply a skin protectant, if needed.

▶ If ordered, pack the wound with gauze pads or strips folded to fit. Avoid using cotton-lined gauze pads because cotton fibers can adhere to the wound surface and cause complications. Pack the wound using the wet-to-damp method. Soaking the packing material in solution and wringing it out so it's slightly moist provides a moist wound environment that absorbs debris and drainage. Removing the packing will remove debris without disrupting new tissue. When packing a wound, don't pack it too tightly because this compresses adjacent capillaries and may prevent the wound edges from contracting. Avoid using overly damp packing because it slows wound closure from within and increases the risk of infection.

Applying a fresh gauze dressing

▶ Gently place sterile 4" × 4" gauze pads at the center of the wound, and move progressively outward to the edges of the wound site. Extend the gauze at least 1" (2.5 cm) beyond the incision in each direction, and cover the wound evenly with enough sterile dressings (usually two or three layers) to absorb all the drainage until the next dressing change. Use ABD pads to form outer layers, if needed, to provide greater absorbency.

▶ Secure the dressing's edges to the patient's skin with strips of tape to maintain the sterility of the wound site. Or secure the dressing with a T-binder or Montgomery straps to prevent skin excoriation, which may occur with repeated tape removal required by frequent dressing changes.

▶ Properly dispose of the solutions and trash bag, and clean or discard soiled equipment and supplies according to your facility's policy. If the patient's wound has purulent drainage, don't return unopened sterile supplies to the sterile supply cabinet because this could cause cross-contamination of other equipment.

Dressing a wound with a drain

▶ Use a precut drain sponge or tracheostomy dressing. If unavailable, prepare a drain dressing by using sterile scissors to cut a slit in a sterile 4" × 4" gauze pad. Fold the pad in half; then cut inward from the center of the folded edge. Don't use a cotton-lined gauze pad because cutting the gauze opens the lining and releases cotton fibers into the wound. Prepare a second pad the same way.

▶ Gently press one folded pad close to the skin around the drain so that the tubing fits into the slit. Press the second folded pad around the drain from the opposite direction so that the two pads encircle the tubing

▶ Layer as many uncut sterile 4″ × 4″ gauze pads or ABD pads around the tubing as needed to absorb expected drainage. Tape the dressing in place.

▶ If a sump drain isn't adequately collecting wound secretions, reinforce it with an ostomy pouch or another collection bag. Use waterproof tape to strengthen a spot on the front of the pouch near the adhesive opening; then cut a small "X" in the tape. Feed the drain catheter into the pouch through the "X" cut. Seal the cut around the tubing with more waterproof tape; then connect the tubing to the suction pump. This method frees the drainage port at the bottom of the pouch so you don't have to remove the tubing to empty the pouch. If you use more than one collection pouch for a wound or wounds, record drainage volume separately for each pouch. Avoid using waterproof material over the dressing because it reduces air circulation and promotes infection from accumulated heat and moisture.

Key point If the patient has two wounds in the same area, cover each wound separately with layers of sterile 4″ × 4″ gauze pads. Then cover both sites with an ABD pad secured to the patient's skin with tape. Don't use only an ABD pad to cover both sites because drainage quickly saturates a single pad, promoting cross-contamination.

▶ If your patient is sensitive to adhesive tape, use paper or silk tape because they are less likely to cause a skin reaction and will peel off more easily than adhesive tape. Use a surgical mask to cradle a chin or jawline dressing; this provides a secure dressing and avoids the need to shave the patient's hair.

Special considerations

▶ Because many physicians prefer to change the first postoperative dressing themselves to check the incision, don't change the first dressing unless you have specific instructions to do so. If you have no such order and drainage comes through the dressings, reinforce the dressing with fresh sterile gauze. Request an order to change the dressing, or ask the physician to change it as soon as possible. A reinforced dressing shouldn't be left in place longer than 24 hours because it's an excellent medium for bacterial growth.

▶ For the recent postoperative patient or a patient with complications, check the dressing every 30 minutes or as ordered. For the patient with a properly healing wound, check the dressing at least once every 8 hours. If the dressing becomes wet from the outside (for example, from spilled drinking water), replace it as soon as possible to prevent wound contamination.

Normal aging results in loss of thickness, elasticity, vascularity, and strength of skin tissue. As a result there's an increased risk of skin tears and tape irritations when removing adhesive from the skin of an older adult.Use paper tape, if available.

Complications

A major complication of a dressing change is an allergic reaction to an antiseptic cleaning agent, a prescribed topical medication, or adhesive tape. This reaction may lead to skin redness, rash, excoriation, or infection.

Patient teaching

▶ If the patient will be caring for a wound after discharge, teach him or a caregiver proper wound care, and ask for a return demonstration.

▶ Stress the importance of using aseptic technique. Teach the patient and caregiver how to examine the wound for signs of infection, and tell them to call the physician if they detect any.

▶ Provide written instructions for all procedures to be performed at home.

Documentation

Document the date, time, and type of wound management procedure; the amount of soiled dressing and packing removed; wound appearance (size, condition of margins, presence of necrotic tissue) and odor (if present); the type, color, consistency, and amount of drainage (for each wound); the presence and location of drains; any additional procedures, such as irrigation, packing, or application of a topical medication; the type and amount of new dressing or pouch applied; and the patient's tolerance of the procedure.

Record the color and amount of measurable drainage on the intake and output sheet. Also document your patient teaching.

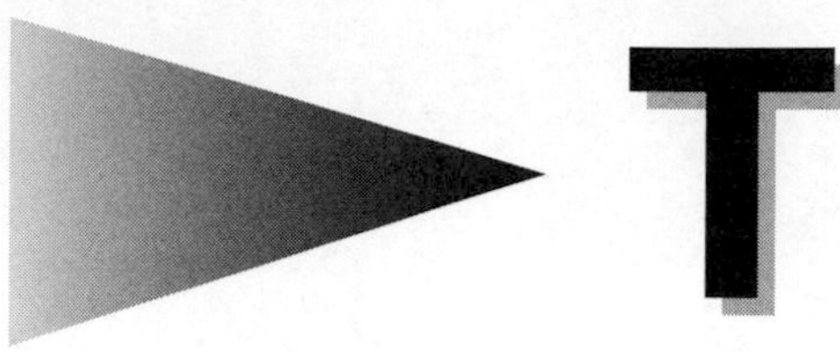

TEACHING THE ELDERLY ADULT

Teaching of older patients should be performed in a manner that promotes maximum understanding. Even with good directions, some elderly patients can become easily confused when more than one piece of information is involved. The better informed a patient is, the better he'll respond to a prescribed regimen. An adult learner brings his own life experience to the situation, which serves as a resource to the learning process. An effective teaching plan includes an assessment of the patient's learning needs, learning style, and barriers to learning as well as an assessment of the learning environment.

Supplies

- Pamphlets and booklets written in layman's terms, if available (make sure patient education materials cover the appropriate content, and are readable)

Implementation

- Give the patient an adequate verbal explanation supplemented by written instructions.
- Speak in language that matches the person's level of understanding, and deliver information in a slow, deliberate, and paced manner. Take into consideration any hearing or vision impairment.
- Be careful not to overload the individual with too much information at one time.
- It may take elderly patients longer to learn new materials. To enhance knowledge retention, you should avoid long teaching sessions; instead use several short sessions.
- Conduct teaching sessions when your patient has the most energy (in many cases, in the morning).
- Remember that group presentations may be cost effective, but they aren't always appropriate.
- If written information isn't available, develop a booklet or information sheet that meets the information needs of the patient, taking into account sight and memory changes as well as cognitive level. Information is best presented in a list of numbered items rather than in paragraph form.
- Encourage the patient to ask questions and express any fears or anxieties.
- Ask the patient to demonstrate the information taught, if appropriate.

Documentation

Note all information taught and the patient's understanding of the information.

TENS THERAPY

Transcutaneous electrical nerve stimulation (TENS) therapy is based on the gate-control theory of pain, which proposes that painful impulses pass through a "gate" in the brain when they've reached a critical threshold. A portable, battery-powered TENS device transmits painless electric current to peripheral nerves or directly to a painful area over relatively large nerve fibers. This treatment effectively alters the patient's perception of pain by blocking painful stimuli traveling over smaller fibers. Used for patients after surgery and those with chronic pain, TENS therapy reduces the need for analgesic drugs and may allow the patient to resume normal activities.

TENS therapy is successful for a variety of chronic pain conditions in older patients. Painful diabetic neuropathies, shoulder pain or bursitis, and fractured ribs respond to TENS therapy. Although some patients' pain has been relieved for years, the effectiveness of TENS usually diminishes with time and strong placebo effects have been associated with its use.

The success of TENS therapy depends on the appropriate placement of the electrodes and adjustment of the electric current. This involves meticulous searching, with the help of a trained physical therapist, to discover the best settings for an individual patient's optimum comfort.

Supplies

- TENS device
- Alcohol pads
- Electrodes
- Electrode gel
- Warm water and soap
- Leadwires
- Charged battery pack
- Battery recharger
- Adhesive patch or hypoallergenic tape

Implementation

- Wash your hands. Provide privacy. If the patient has never seen a TENS unit before, show him the device and explain the procedure.

Before TENS treatment

- With an alcohol pad, thoroughly clean the skin where the electrode will be applied. Then dry the skin using a patting motion.
- Apply electrode gel to the bottom of each electrode.
- Place the ordered number of electrodes on the proper skin area, leaving at least 2″ (5 cm) between them. Then secure them with the adhesive patch or hypoallergenic tape. Because the older patient's skin is often loose and thin, tape all sides evenly so the electrodes are firmly attached to the skin while ensuring that the patient's skin isn't damaged by securing the electrodes. To avoid interference with critical nerve function, never place the electrodes near the patient's eyes or over the nerves that innervate the carotid sinus or laryngeal or pharyngeal muscles. (See *Positioning TENS electrodes,* page 556.)
- If you must move the electrodes during the procedure, first turn off the controls. Follow the physician's orders regarding electrode placement and control settings. Incorrect placement of the electrodes will result in inappropriate pain control.
- Plug the pin connectors into the electrode sockets. To protect the cords, hold the connectors — not the cords themselves — during insertion.
- Turn the channel controls to the "off" position or to the position recommended in the operator's manual.
- Plug the leadwires into the jacks in the control box.
- Turn the amplitude and rate dials slowly, as the manual directs. (The patient should feel a tingling sensation.) Then adjust the controls on this device to the prescribed settings or to settings that are most comfortable. Most patients select stimulation frequencies of 60 to 100 Hz. Setting the controls too high can cause pain; setting them too low will fail to relieve pain. If the patient requires excessive levels of stimulation, contact the physician before continuing treatment.

Positioning TENS electrodes

In transcutaneous electrical nerve stimulation (TENS), electrodes placed around the peripheral nerves (or an incision site) transmit mild electrical pulses to the brain. The current is thought to block pain impulses. The patient can influence the level and frequency of his pain relief by adjusting the controls on the impulse generator.

Typically, electrode placement varies even though patients may have similar complaints. Electrodes can be placed in several ways:

- to cover the painful area or surround it, as with muscle tenderness or spasm or painful joints
- to "capture" the painful area between electrodes, as with incisional pain.

For the patient with peripheral nerve injury, place electrodes proximal to the injury (between the brain and the injury site) to avoid increasing pain. Placing electrodes in a hypersensitive area also increases pain. In an area lacking sensation, place electrodes on adjacent dermatomes.

The illustrations show combinations of electrode placement (black squares) and areas of nerve stimulation (shaded) for low back and leg pain.

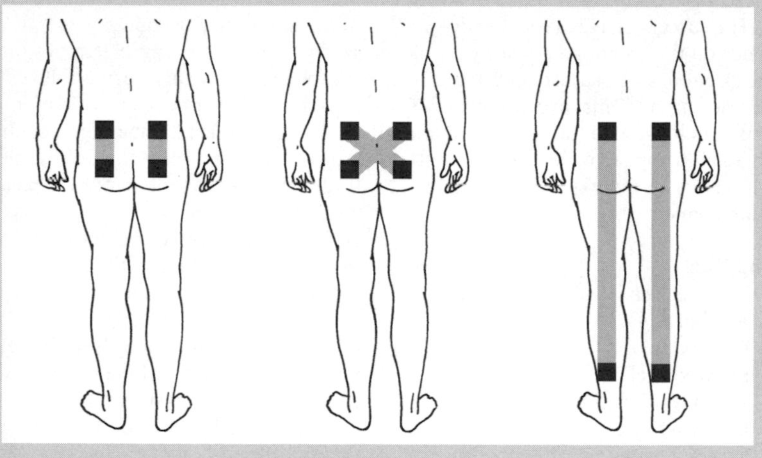

▶ Attach the TENS control box to part of the patient's clothing, such as a belt, pocket, or bra.

▶ To make sure the device is working effectively, monitor the patient for signs of excessive stimulation such as muscular twitches or signs of inadequate stimulation, which are signaled by the patient's inability to feel any mild tingling sensation. Question the patient about his feelings since the older patient may have diminished sensation.

After TENS treatment

▶ Turn off the controls and unplug the electrode leadwires from the control box.

▶ If you are to give another treatment soon, leave the electrodes in place; if not, remove them.

▶ Clean the electrodes with soap and water, and clean the patient's skin with alcohol pads and pat dry. (Don't soak the electrodes in alcohol because it will damage the rubber.)

- Monitor the site for signs of irritation and breakdown.
- Remove the battery pack from the unit and replace it with a charged battery pack.
- Recharge the used battery pack so it's always ready for use.
- If TENS is used continuously for postoperative pain, remove the electrodes at least daily to check for skin irritation, and provide skin care. If the patient is at high risk for skin irritation and breakdown, check the skin more often.

Complications

The patient may suffer skin irritation where the electrodes are taped and possible burns from the electrodes. There's also a danger of interference with pacemaker function and neural interference from TENS electrodes placed on the head or neck of patients with vascular disorders or seizure disorders.

Patient teaching

- If appropriate, let the patient study the operator's manual. Teach him how to place the electrodes properly and how to take care of the TENS unit.

Documentation

On the patient's medical record and the care plan, record the electrode sites and the control settings. Document the patient's tolerance of the treatment. Also evaluate pain control. Note your patient teaching.

THERAPEUTIC BATH

Also referred to as balneotherapy, a therapeutic bath combines water and additives to soothe and relax the patient, clean the skin, relieve inflammation and pruritus, and soften and remove crusts, scales, debris, and old drugs. Used primarily for their antipruritic and emollient effects, these baths coat irritated skin with a soothing, protective film. Because they constrict surface blood vessels, they also have an anti-inflammatory effect.

Antibacterial agents, such as acetic acid, potassium permanganate, or povidone-iodine, may be added to bath water to treat infected eczema, dirty ulcerations, furunculosis, and pemphigus. The addition of oatmeal powder, soluble cornstarch, or soybean complex to bath water creates a colloidal bath, which has a soothing effect and is used to treat generalized pruritus. Oil baths are useful for lubricating dry skin and easing eczematous eruptions. Sodium bicarbonate added to water produces an alkaline bath, which has a cooling effect and also helps relieve pruritus. A medicated tar bath may be used to treat psoriasis. The film of tar left on the skin works in combination with ultraviolet light to inhibit the rapid cell turnover characteristic of psoriasis.

A bedridden patient may benefit from a local soak with the therapeutic additive instead of a therapeutic tub bath.

Supplies

- Bathtub
- Bath mat
- Rubber mat
- Bath (utility) thermometer
- Therapeutic additive
- Measuring device
- Colander or sieve for oatmeal powder
- Two washcloths and two towels
- Hospital gown or loose-fitting cotton pajamas
- Lubricating cream or ointment (if ordered)

Implementation

- Check the physician's order and assess the patient's condition.
- Assemble supplies and draw the bath before bringing the patient to the bath area to prevent chilling him. Make sure the tub is clean and disinfected because

a patient with skin breakdown is particularly vulnerable to infection.

▶ Fill the tub with 6″ to 8″ (15 to 20 cm) of water, usually measuring 95° to 100° F (35° to 38° C). The treatment's purpose and the type of additive used will determine the water temperature. Cool to lukewarm water is used to relieve pruritus and when adding tar or starch. Warm baths are soothing, but water warmer than 100° F causes vasodilation, which could aggravate pruritus.

▶ If the patient is confined to bed, place the therapeutic additive in a basin of water at 95° to 100° F, and apply it with a washcloth, using light, gentle strokes.

▶ Measure the correct amount of therapeutic additive, according to the physician's order or package instructions. As the tub is filling, thoroughly mix the additive in the water. Add most substances directly to the water, but place oatmeal powder in a sieve or colander under the faucet to help it dissolve. Begin with 2 tablespoons of oatmeal powder; then add more powder or water as needed to regulate the thickness of the oatmeal bath.

▶ When giving a tar bath, wear a plastic apron or protective gown because tar preparations stain clothing.

▶ Explain the procedure to the patient and have him urinate. Wash your hands thoroughly, and then escort the patient to the bath area. Close the door to provide privacy and eliminate drafts.

▶ Check the water temperature with a bath thermometer. Help the patient undress, and assist him into the tub if necessary. Advise him to use the safety rails to prevent falls.

Cultural diversity Keep in mind that a patient's cultural background may affect his reaction to therapeutic bathing. For example, an older Japanese patient, who may be reluctant to use a shower, may gain extra comfort from a therapeutic bath because soaking baths are the preferred method of personal cleaning in Japan.

▶ Tell your patient that the bath may feel unpleasant at first because his skin is irritated, but assure him that the medication will soon coat and soothe his skin.

▶ Ask the patient to stretch out in the tub and submerge his body up to the chin. If he's capable, give him a washcloth to apply the bath solution gently to his face and other body areas that aren't immersed.

Key point If the patient is taking a tar bath, tell him to keep the bath solution out of his eyes because tar is an eye irritant.

▶ Warn the patient against scrubbing his skin to avoid further irritation.

▶ Add warm water to the bath as needed to maintain a comfortable temperature.

▶ Allow the patient to soak for 15 to 30 minutes. If you must stay with him, pull the bath curtain; this gives him some privacy and protects him from drafts. If you must leave the room, show the patient how to use the call button and ensure his privacy.

▶ After the bath, help the patient from the tub. Have him use the safety rails to prevent falls.

▶ Help him pat his skin dry with towels. Don't rub the skin because rubbing removes some solutes and oils clinging to the skin and produces friction, which increases pruritus and may injure the skin.

▶ Apply lubricating cream or ointment, if ordered, to help hold water in the newly hydrated skin.

▶ Provide a fresh hospital gown or loose-fitting cotton pajamas. Advise the patient to avoid wearing pajamas, underwear, or other clothing that isn't loose-fitting and made of cotton. Tight clothing and scratchy or synthetic materials can aggravate skin conditions by causing friction and increasing perspiration.

▶ Escort the patient to his room, and make sure he's comfortable.

▶ Drain the bath water, clean and disinfect the tub, and dispose of soiled materials properly. If you have given an oatmeal powder bath, drain and rinse the tub immediately or the powder will cake, making later removal difficult.

Complications

The heat generated by the bath may produce weakness or faintness. The therapeutic additive may lead to skin irritation.

Patient teaching

▶ Explain the procedure to the patient and describe its benefits.
▶ Instruct the patient to report any feelings of weakness, faintness, or skin irritation.

Documentation

Record the date, time, and duration of the bath. Note the water temperature, the type and amount of additive used, skin appearance before and after the bath, the patient's tolerance of the treatment, and the bath's effectiveness. Also document your patient teaching.

THORACOTOMY

A surgical incision into the thoracic cavity, a thoracotomy is done to locate and examine abnormalities, such as tumors, bleeding sites, or thoracic injuries; to perform a biopsy; or to remove diseased lung tissue. This procedure is commonly performed to remove part or all of a lung to spare healthy lung tissue from disease. Lung excision may involve pneumonectomy, lobectomy, segmental resection, or wedge resection.

A *pneumonectomy* is the excision of an entire lung. It's usually performed to treat bronchogenic cancer but may also be used to treat tuberculosis, bronchiectasis, or lung abscess. It's used only when a less radical approach can't remove all diseased tissue. After pneumonectomy, chest cavity pressures stabilize and, over time, fluid fills the cavity where lung tissue was removed, preventing significant mediastinal shift.

A *lobectomy* is the removal of one of the five lung lobes. Lobectomy can treat bronchogenic cancer, tuberculosis, lung abscess, emphysematous blebs or bullae, benign tumors, or localized fungal infections. After this surgery, the remaining lobes expand to fill the entire pleural cavity.

A *segmental resection* is the removal of one or more lung segments and preserves more functional tissue than lobectomy. It's commonly used to treat bronchiectasis. Remaining lung tissue needs to be reexpanded.

A *wedge resection* is the removal of a small portion of the lung without regard to segments. Wedge resection preserves the most functional tissue of all the surgeries but can treat only a small, well-circumscribed lesion. Remaining lung tissue needs to be reexpanded. (See *Understanding types of lung excision*, page 560.)

Other types of thoracotomy include:
▶ Exploratory thoracotomy is done to examine the chest and pleural space in evaluating chest trauma and tumors.
▶ Decortication is used to help reexpand the lung in a patient with empyema. It involves the removal or stripping of the thick, fibrous membrane covering the visceral pleura.
▶ Thoracoplasty is performed to remove part or all of one rib and reduce the size of the chest cavity. It decreases the risk of mediastinal shift when tuberculosis has reduced lung volume.

Implementation

▶ After the patient is anesthetized, the surgeon performs a thoracotomy using one of three approaches. In a posterolateral thoracotomy, the incision starts in the submammary fold of the anterior chest, is drawn below the scapular tip and along the ribs, and then is curved posteriorly and up to the spine of the scapula. Any type of lung excision calls

Understanding types of lung excision

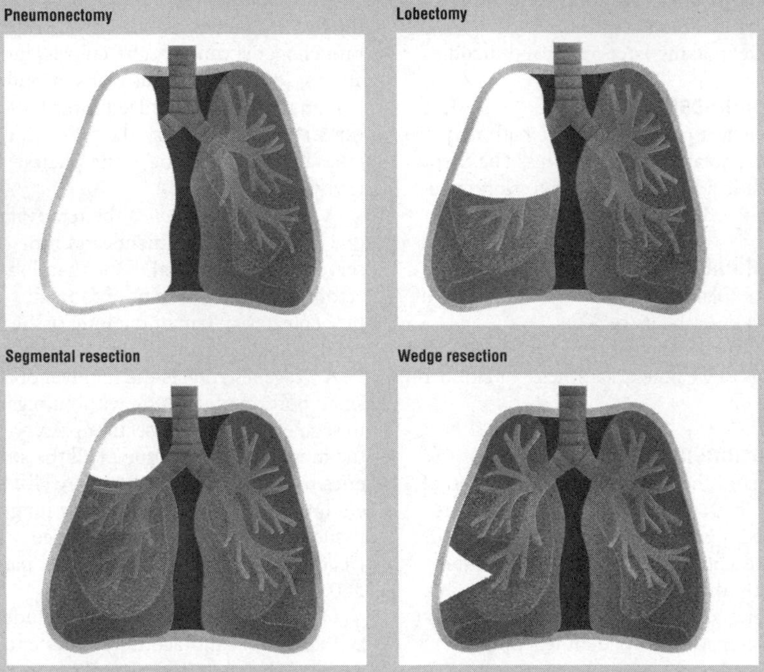

Pneumonectomy

Lobectomy

Segmental resection

Wedge resection

for a posterolateral incision through the fourth, fifth, sixth, or seventh intercostal space.

▶ In an anterolateral thoracotomy, the incision begins below the breast and above the costal margins, extending from the anterior axillary line and then turning downward to avoid the axillary apex. A median sternotomy involves a straight incision from the suprasternal notch to below the xiphoid process and requires that the sternum be transected with an electric or air-driven saw.

▶ Once the incision is made, the surgeon takes a biopsy, locates and ties off sources of bleeding, locates and repairs injuries within the thoracic cavity, or spreads the ribs and exposes the lung area for excision. If he's performing a pneumonectomy, he ligates and severs the pulmonary arteries. Next, he clamps the mainstem bronchus leading to the affected lung, divides it, and then closes it with nonabsorbable sutures or staples. He then removes the lung. To ensure airtight closure, he places a pleural flap over the bronchus and closes it. Then, he severs the phrenic nerve on the affected side, allowing it to reduce the size of the pleural cavity. After air pressure in the cavity stabilizes, he closes the chest.

▶ In a lobectomy, the surgeon resects the affected lobe and ligates and severs the appropriate arteries, veins, and bronchial passages. He may insert one or two chest tubes for drainage and to aid lung reexpansion.

▶ In a segmental resection, the surgeon removes the affected segment and ligates and severs the appropriate artery, vein, and bronchus. In a wedge resection, he clamps and excises the affected area and then sutures it. In both resections, he inserts two chest tubes to aid lung reexpansion.

▶ After completing the procedure requiring the thoracotomy, the surgeon closes the chest cavity and applies a dressing.

Complications

Hemorrhage, infection, and tension pneumothorax are possible. Additional complications include bronchopleural fistula and empyema. A lung excision may also cause a persistent air space that the remaining lung tissue doesn't expand to fill. Removal of up to three ribs may be necessary to reduce chest cavity size and allow lung tissue to fit the space.

Key nursing diagnoses and outcomes

Anxiety related to the surgical procedure

Treatment outcomes: The patient will identify and express feelings of anxiety, and demonstrate healthy coping behaviors and fewer physical signs of anxiety.

Impaired gas exchange related to mismatch between ventilation and perfusion as a result of a thoracotomy

Treatment outcome: The patient will show no signs or symptoms of respiratory distress.

Ineffective airway clearance related to pain caused by thoracotomy

Treatment outcomes: The patient will maintain a patent airway, and demonstrate effective deep-breathing and coughing exercises.

Nursing interventions

▶ Explain the thoracotomy procedure to the patient, and inform him that he'll receive a general anesthetic. Prepare him psychologically, according to his condition. A patient having a lung biopsy, for example, faces the fear of cancer as well as the fear of surgery and needs ongoing emotional support. In contrast, a patient with a chronic lung disorder, such as tuberculosis or a fungal infection, may view having a lung excision as a cure for his ailment.

▶ Inform the patient that, postoperatively, he may have chest tubes in place and may receive oxygen.

▶ If a pneumonectomy is to be performed, arrange for laboratory studies, as ordered. Tests to assess cardiac function may include pulmonary function tests, electrocardiography, chest X-ray, arterial blood gas analysis, bronchoscopy and, possibly, cardiac catheterization.

▶ Ensure that the patient or a responsible family member has signed a consent form.

▶ If the patient had a pneumonectomy, make sure he lies only on his operative side or his back until he's stabilized. This prevents fluid from draining into the unaffected lung if the sutured bronchus opens.

▶ If the patient has a chest tube in place, make sure it's functioning and monitor him for signs of tension pneumothorax, such as dyspnea, chest pain, an irritating cough, vertigo, syncope, or anxiety. If the patient develops any of these signs or symptoms, palpate his neck, face, and chest wall for subcutaneous emphysema and palpate his trachea for deviation from the midline. Auscultate his lungs for decreased or absent breath sounds on the affected side. Then percuss them for hyperresonance. If you suspect tension pneumothorax, notify the physician at once and help him to identify the cause.

▶ Provide analgesics, as ordered.

▶ Have the patient begin coughing, deep-breathing exercises, and incentive spirometry as soon as he's stabilized. Auscultate his lungs, place him in semi-Fowler's position, and have him splint his incision to facilitate coughing and deep breathing. Have him cough every 2 hours until his breath sounds clear.

▶ Perform passive range-of-motion (ROM) exercises the evening of surgery and two or three times daily thereafter. Progress to active ROM exercises.

PATIENT TEACHING

▶ Before surgery, teach him coughing and deep-breathing techniques. Explain that he'll use these after surgery to facilitate lung reexpansion. Also teach him how to use an incentive spirometer; record the volumes he achieves to provide a baseline.
▶ Tell the patient to continue his coughing and deep-breathing exercises when he returns home to prevent complications. Advise him to report any changes in sputum characteristics to his physician.
▶ Instruct the patient to continue performing ROM exercises to maintain mobility of his shoulder and chest wall.
▶ Tell the patient to avoid contact with people who have upper respiratory tract infections and to refrain from smoking.
▶ Provide the patient with instructions for wound care and dressing changes and refer him to home health care, as needed.

THROMBOLYTIC THERAPY

Thrombolytic drugs provide rapid correction of acute and extensive thrombotic disorders. The Food and Drug Administration has approved these drugs for treating certain thromboembolic disorders, such as acute pulmonary emboli and coronary thrombi. In addition, these drugs may be used to dissolve thrombi in arteriovenous catheters, thereby restoring blood flow. They're the drugs of choice to break down newly formed thrombi.

Thrombolytic drugs are given I.V. early in acute myocardial infarction to open an occluded coronary artery and to prevent primary or secondary thrombus formation in the vessels surrounding the necrotic area, thus minimizing myocardial damage. The goal (as outlined in the American Heart Association algorithm for ischemic chest pain) is to deliver a fibrolytic agent within 30 minutes of arrival to the emergency department. Thrombolytic drugs are also used to treat stroke.

Thrombolytic drugs work by converting plasminogen to the enzyme plasmin, which lyses thrombi, fibrinogen, and other plasma proteins.

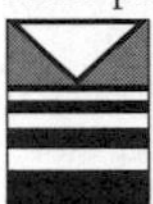

Key point Patients age 75 and older are at greater risk for cerebral hemorrhage because they're more apt to have preexisting cerebrovascular disease.

Implementation

▶ After I.V. catheter insertion, the thrombolytic agent is infused according to the manufacturer's directions.
▶ To dissolve a thrombus in an arteriovenous catheter, the physician infuses the desired amount of the drug into the catheter until the thrombus dissolves.

Complications

The major hazards of thrombolytic therapy are bleeding, delayed lysis, and reocclusion. As the myocardium becomes reperfused, arrhythmias may also occur.

Key nursing diagnoses and outcomes

Anxiety related to therapy and the potential for severe complications

Treatment outcome: The patient will show decreased physical signs of fear.

Decreased cardiac output related to reperfusion arrhythmias

Treatment outcome: The patient will regain or maintain an adequate cardiac output.

Risk for deficient fluid volume related to potential for bleeding

Treatment outcome: The patient will show no signs or symptoms of bleeding.

Nursing interventions

Before therapy

- Before thrombolytic therapy is given, draw serum samples for blood typing and crossmatching and for determination of prothrombin time and partial thromboplastin time.
- Obtain a baseline electrocardiogram (ECG), and obtain electrolyte, arterial blood gas, blood urea nitrogen, creatinine, and cardiac enzyme levels.
- Check subsequent findings against these baseline readings regularly throughout therapy.
- Start an adequate number of I.V. lines (usually at least four) and an indwelling urinary catheter.
- Before initiating thrombolytic therapy, obtain an MRI or CT scan of the brain to ensure that changes in mental status are the result of an occlusion and not cerebral hemorrhage.

During therapy

- At the start of therapy, watch for signs of hypersensitivity: hypotension, shortness of breath, wheezing, a feeling of tightness and pressure in the chest, and angioedema. Keep emergency resuscitation equipment readily available.
- Throughout therapy, continuously monitor the ECG and compare it with baseline readings to detect possible arrhythmias. Inform the physician of any abnormalities, and be prepared to administer lidocaine or procainamide, as ordered.
- Carefully assess the patient for signs of bleeding. Monitor him every 15 minutes for the first hour, every 30 minutes for the next 7 hours, and then once every 8 hours thereafter. If you detect bleeding, stop therapy and notify the physician. Ensure that packed red blood cells, whole blood, and aminocaproic acid are readily available to treat possible hemorrhage.
- Check the patient's vital signs frequently, and monitor pulses, color, and sensory function in the extremities every hour.
- Because the patient is prone to bruising during therapy, handle him gently and as little as possible. Keep invasive procedures and venipunctures to a minimum, use manual blood pressure cuffs, and pad the side rails of his bed to prevent injury.

After therapy

- Expect to administer anticoagulants to prevent recurrence of thromboses.

PATIENT TEACHING

- Explain the procedure to the patient and describe its benefits and risks.
- Instruct the patient to immediately report any bleeding, such as from puncture sites or gums or in stools.

TOPICAL MEDICATION ADMINISTRATION

Topical drugs are applied directly to the skin surface. They include lotions, pastes, ointments, creams, powders, shampoos, and aerosol sprays. The drug is absorbed through the epidermal layer into the dermis. The extent of absorption depends on the vascularity of the region. Except for nitroglycerin and certain supplemental hormone replacements, topical drugs are commonly used for local, rather than systemic, effects. Ointments have a fatty base, which is an ideal vehicle for such drugs as antimicrobials and antiseptics. Typically, topical drugs should be applied two or three times a day to achieve their therapeutic effect.

Supplies

- Patient's medication record and chart
- Prescribed drug
- Sterile tongue blades
- Gloves
- Sterile 4″ × 4″ gauze pads
- Transparent semipermeable dressing
- Adhesive tape
- Solvent (such as cottonseed oil)

Implementation

▶ Verify the order on the patient's medication record by checking it against the physician's order on the chart.

▶ Make sure the label on the drug agrees with the order. Read the label again before you open the container and as you remove the drug from the container.

▶ Explain the procedure thoroughly to the patient to reduce the patient's fear and promote cooperation.

▶ Confirm the patient's identity by asking his name and checking the name, room number, and bed number on his wristband.

▶ Provide privacy.

▶ Wash your hands to prevent cross-contamination, and put a glove on your dominant hand. Be sure to wear gloves to prevent absorption of the medication by your own skin.

▶ If the patient has an infectious skin condition, use sterile gloves.

▶ Help the patient assume a comfortable position that provides access to the area to be treated.

▶ Expose the area to be treated. Make sure the skin or mucous membrane is intact (unless the drug has been ordered to treat a skin lesion such as an ulcer). Application of a drug to broken or abraded skin may cause unwanted systemic absorption and result in further irritation.

▶ If necessary, clean the skin of debris, including crusts, epidermal scales, and old drugs. You may have to change the glove if it becomes soiled.

Applying a paste, cream, or ointment

▶ Open the container. Place the lid or cap upside down to prevent contamination of the inside surface.

▶ Remove a tongue blade from its sterile wrapper and cover one end with the drug from the tube or jar. Then transfer the drug from the tongue blade to your gloved hand.

▶ Apply the drug to the affected area with long, smooth strokes that follow the direction of hair growth. This technique avoids forcing the drug into hair follicles, which can cause irritation and lead to folliculitis. Avoid excessive pressure when applying the drug because it could abrade the skin.

▶ Don't apply too much ointment to any skin area. It may cause irritation and discomfort, stain clothing and bedding, and make removal difficult.

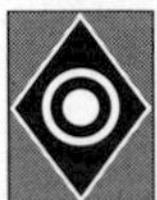

Drug alert Don't apply topical ointments to mucous membranes as liberally as you would to skin because mucous membranes are usually moist and absorb ointment more quickly than skin does. Never apply ointment to the eyelids or ear canal unless ordered. The ointment may congeal and occlude the tear duct or ear canal.

▶ To prevent contamination of the drugs, use a new tongue blade each time you remove medication from the container.

Removing an ointment

▶ Never apply drugs without first removing previous applications to prevent skin irritation from an accumulation of medication.

▶ To remove ointment, wash your hands and put on gloves; then rub solvent on them, and apply it liberally to the treated area in the direction of hair growth. Alternatively, saturate a sterile gauze pad with the solvent and use this pad to gently remove the ointment. Remove excess oil by gently wiping the area with the sterile gauze pad. Don't rub too hard to remove the drug because you could irritate the skin.

Applying other topical medications

▶ To apply shampoos, follow package directions.

▶ To apply aerosol sprays, shake the container, if indicated, to completely mix the drug. Hold the container 6″ to 12″ (15 to 30 cm) from the skin or follow the manufacturer's recommendation. Spray the drug evenly over the treatment area to apply a thin film.

- To apply powders, dry the skin surface, making sure to spread skin folds where moisture collects. Then apply a thin layer of powder over the treatment area.
- To protect applied medications and prevent them from soiling the patient's clothes, tape an appropriate amount of sterile gauze pad or a transparent semipermeable dressing over the treated area. If you're applying topical drugs to the patient's hands or feet, cover the site with white cotton gloves for the hands or terry cloth scuffs for the feet.
- Assess the patient's skin for signs of irritation, allergic reaction, or breakdown.

Complications

Skin irritation, rash, or allergic reaction to the topical medication may occur.

Skin changes that occur with aging can influence absorption. These changes include increased capillary fragility and permeability; increased melanocytes; and decreased subcutaneous fat, extracellular water, surface lipids, sebaceous gland activity, and blood supply.

Patient teaching

- Instruct the patient on the proper administration of the topical drug. Because an elderly patient may have diminished manual dexterity and movement, assess the patient's ability to handle the supplies if he's to apply a medication at home.

Documentation

Record the drug applied; the time, date, and site of application; and the condition of the patient's skin at the time of application. Note subsequent effects of the drug, if any. Document patient teaching measures and their effect.

TOTAL PARENTERAL NUTRITION

Total parenteral nutrition (TPN) is the parenteral administration of a solution of dextrose, proteins, electrolytes, vitamins, and trace elements in amounts that exceed the patient's energy expenditure and thereby achieve anabolism. Because this solution has about six times the solute concentration of blood, it requires dilution by delivery into a high-flow central vein to avoid injury to the peripheral vasculature. Typically, the solution is delivered to the superior vena cava through an indwelling subclavian vein catheter.

A patient may receive TPN for any of the following reasons:

- debilitating illness lasting longer than 2 weeks
- limited or no oral intake for longer than 7 days, such as in cases of multiple traumatic injuries, severe burns, or anorexia nervosa
- loss of 10% or more of pre-illness weight
- serum albumin level below 3.5 g/dl
- poor tolerance of long-term enteral feedings
- chronic vomiting or diarrhea
- continued weight loss despite adequate oral intake
- GI disorders that prevent or severely reduce absorption, such as bowel obstruction, Crohn's disease, ulcerative colitis, short bowel syndrome, cancer malabsorption syndrome, and bowel fistulas
- inflammatory GI disorders, such as pancreatitis and peritonitis
- excessive nitrogen loss resulting from wound infection, fistulas, or abscesses
- renal or hepatic failure.

Because TPN solution supports bacterial growth and the central venous (CV) line gives systemic access, contamination and sepsis are always a risk. Strict surgical asepsis is required during solution, dressing, tubing, and filter changes. Site care and dressing changes should be performed according to your facility's policy, usually at least three times weekly (once weekly for transparent dressings), and whenever the dressing becomes wet, soiled, or nonocclusive. Tubing and filter changes are performed every 24 to 48 hours, according to your facility's policy.

Supplies

- Infusion pump and sterile tubing
- Extension tubing
- Two pairs of sterile gloves
- Alcohol pads
- Cotton-tipped applicators, some soaked in an organic solvent and some soaked in povidone-iodine solution
- Bags or bottles of TPN solution
- 0.22-micron cellulose membrane filter (1.2 microns if solution contains lipid emulsions or albumin)
- 2″ × 2″ precut dressing
- Reflux valve
- Luer-lock connection or tape
- Time tape
- Transparent semipermeable dressing
- Intake and output record
- Optional: Sterile drape, mask

Implementation

- Remove the 1-L, 2-L, or 3-L bags or bottles of TPN solution from the refrigerator at least 1 hour before use. Giving the patient a chilled solution can cause him pain, hypothermia, venous spasm, and venous constriction.
- Double-check the contents of the solution and the physician's orders. Then observe the solution for cloudiness, turbidity, and particles and the container for cracks; if any of these are present, return the solution to the pharmacy.
- Explain the procedure to the patient and his family member, to reduce fear and promote cooperation.
- Always maintain strict aseptic technique when preparing and handling equipment.
- Connect, in sequence, the pump tubing, cellulose membrane filter (if applicable), and extension tubing. Tape the tubing connections or use the luer-lock connections, if available, to prevent accidental separation, which can lead to air embolism, exsanguination, and sepsis. Squeeze the drip chamber of the tubing before spiking the bag or bottle, turn it upright and, using strict aseptic technique, insert the tubing spike into the port of the TPN container and release the drip chamber. This prevents accidental dripping of TPN solution from a bottle (bags won't drip). Start the flow of solution to prime the tubing and remove air. Gently tap the tubing to dislodge air bubbles trapped in the Y ports.
- If necessary, attach a time tape to the TPN container to allow approximate measurement of fluid intake.
- Attach the set-up to the infusion pump, and prepare it according to the manufacturer's instructions.
- Administer the solution at the specified rate.
- When using a CV line for TPN, the following are contraindicated: infusion of blood or blood products, bolus injection of drugs, simultaneous administration of I.V. solutions, measurement of CV pressure, aspiration of blood for routine laboratory tests, addition of drug to a TPN solution container, and use of three-way stopcocks.
- Be alert for swelling at the catheter insertion site. This indicates extravasation of the TPN solution, which can cause necrosis. Check the catheter tubing for leaks from mechanical or chemical disruption.

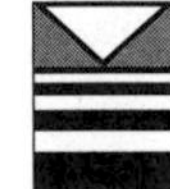

Key point Watch for signs and symptoms of air embolism: dyspnea, apprehension, chest pain, tachycardia, hypotension, cyanosis, seizures, loss of consciousness, and cardiopulmonary arrest. If you suspect air embolism, position the patient in left Trendelenburg's position to allow air to pass from the pulmonary artery, and administer supplemental oxygen. It may take several minutes for the air to dissipate.

▶ If required, put on a mask (especially if the patient is immunodeficient), and position the patient supine, with his head turned away from the catheter insertion site. If the facility's policy dictates and the patient can tolerate it, place a mask over his nose and mouth. Place a sterile drape over the patient if he's being mechanically ventilated.

▶ Put on gloves.

▶ Remove the dressing carefully, pulling the tape gently from the skin to minimize traumatic injury. Then inspect the skin for signs of infection and the catheter for leaks or other mechanical problems. Remove your gloves.

▶ Wash your hands, put on sterile gloves, and clean the catheter insertion site three times with alcohol pads or cotton-tipped applicators soaked in an organic solvent such as 70% alcohol. Work in a circular motion, moving from the insertion site outward to the edge of the adhesive border to avoid introducing contaminants from the unclean area.

▶ Working in a circular motion, as before, clean the insertion site and the catheter three times with cotton-tipped applicators soaked in povidone-iodine solution.

▶ Instruct the patient to perform Valsalva's maneuver or to hold his breath on deep inspiration as you change the I.V. tubing. If the patient is being mechanically ventilated, change the I.V. tubing immediately after the machine delivers a breath at peak inspiration. These measures increase intrathoracic pressure and prevent air embolism.

▶ Set the infusion pump at the ordered flow rate, and then start the infusion.

▶ Ensure that the junction of the catheter tubing is secure (you may use luer-lock connections), remove the contaminated gloves, and put on a sterile pair.

▶ Apply a precut dressing around the catheter, if desired, to avoid irritation from catheter placement directly on the skin.

▶ Apply a transparent semipermeable dressing over the insertion site; these allow visualization of the site. Remove your gloves.

▶ Write the catheter insertion date, the date of the dressing change, and your initials on a strip of tape and apply this to the dressing.

▶ Loop and tape the administration tubing (but not the filter) over the intact dressing to prevent tension on the catheter and its inadvertent removal if the tubing is pulled.

▶ Observe the patient for signs of thrombosis or thrombophlebitis, such as erythema and edema at the catheter insertion site; ipsilateral swelling of the arm, neck, or face; pain along the course of the vein; and other systemic manifestations. If such signs occur, notify the physician immediately; he may remove the catheter and start a heparin infusion at a peripheral site.

▶ Observe for catheter retraction from the vein, which may result from loosening of the sutures at the insertion site. Measure catheter length from the insertion site to the hub during dressing changes for verification.

Complications

Catheter-related sepsis is the most serious complication of TPN. Although uncommon, subclavian or jugular vein thrombosis can result from a malpositioned catheter and can precede septicemia. Air embolism, a potentially fatal complication, can occur during tubing replacement from inadvertent disconnection of the tubing or from undetected hairline cracks in the tubing. Extravasation of TPN solution can cause necrosis, with sequential sloughing of the epidermis and dermis.

Patient teaching

▶ Explain TPN to the patient and describe its benefits and risks.

▶ Tell the patient to call the nurse if the dressing becomes loose or soiled.

▶ Instruct the patient to report any pain or discomfort at the insertion site.
▶ Tell him to call the nurse immediately if the catheter becomes dislodged or the tubing becomes disconnected.

Documentation

Record the times of tubing, filter, and solution changes; the condition of the catheter insertion site; your observations on the patient's condition; and any complications and resulting treatments. Document patient teaching measures and their effect.

TRACHEOSTOMY CARE

Whether a tracheotomy is performed in an emergency situation or after careful preparation, as a permanent measure or as temporary therapy, tracheostomy care has consistent goals. Your care must ensure airway patency by keeping the tube free of mucus buildup, maintain mucous membrane and skin integrity, prevent infection, and provide psychological support.

The patient may have one of three types of tracheostomy tube — uncuffed, cuffed, or fenestrated. Tube selection depends on the patient's condition and the physician's preference.

The uncuffed tube, which may be plastic or metal, allows air to flow freely around the tracheostomy tube and through the larynx, reducing the risk of tracheal damage. It's a safer choice for children but increases the risk of aspiration in adults. The cuffed tube, made of plastic, is disposable. The cuff and the tube won't separate accidentally inside the trachea because the cuff is bonded to the tube. Also, a cuffed tube doesn't require periodic deflating to lower pressure because cuff pressure is low and evenly distributed against the tracheal wall. Although cuffed tubes may cost more than other tubes, they reduce the risk of tracheal damage. The plastic fenestrated tube permits speech through the upper airway when the external opening is capped and the cuff is deflated. It also allows easy removal of the inner cannula for cleaning. However, a fenestrated tube may become occluded.

Whichever tube is used, tracheostomy care should be performed using aseptic technique until the stoma has healed to prevent infection. For recently performed tracheotomies, use sterile gloves for all manipulations at the tracheostomy site. Once the stoma has healed, clean gloves may be substituted for sterile ones.

Supplies

For aseptic stoma and outer-cannula care

▶ Waterproof trash bag
▶ Two sterile solution containers
▶ Normal saline solution
▶ Hydrogen peroxide
▶ Sterile cotton-tipped applicators
▶ Sterile 4″ × 4″ gauze pads
▶ Sterile gloves
▶ Prepackaged sterile tracheostomy dressing (or 4″ × 4″ gauze pad)
▶ Equipment and supplies for suctioning and for mouth care
▶ Water-soluble lubricant or topical antibiotic cream
▶ Materials as needed for cuff procedures and for changing tracheostomy ties

For aseptic inner-cannula care

▶ Prepackaged commercial tracheostomy-care set or sterile forceps
▶ Sterile nylon brush
▶ Sterile 6″ (15-cm) pipe cleaners
▶ Sterile gloves
▶ A third sterile solution container
▶ Disposable temporary inner cannula (for a patient on a ventilator)

For changing tracheostomy ties

▶ 30″ (76-cm) length of tracheostomy twill tape
▶ Bandage scissors
▶ Sterile gloves
▶ Hemostat

For emergency tracheostomy tube replacement

- Sterile tracheal dilator or sterile hemostat
- Sterile obturator that fits the tracheostomy tube in use
- Extra sterile tracheostomy tube and obturator in appropriate size
- Suction equipment and supplies

Keep these supplies in full view in the patient's room at all times for easy access in case of emergency. Consider taping an emergency sterile tracheostomy tube in a sterile wrapper to the head of the patient's bed for easy access in an emergency.

For cuff procedures

- 5- or 10-cc syringe
- Padded hemostat
- Stethoscope

Implementation

- Assess the patient's condition to determine his need for care.
- Explain the procedure to the patient, even if he is unresponsive. Provide privacy.
- Wash your hands, and assemble all equipment and supplies in the patient's room.
- Check the expiration date on each sterile package, and inspect each package for tears.
- Open the waterproof trash bag, and place it next to you so you can avoid reaching across the sterile field or the patient's stoma when discarding soiled items.
- Establish a sterile field near the patient's bed (usually on the overbed table), and place equipment and supplies on it.
- Pour normal saline solution, hydrogen peroxide, or a mixture of equal parts of both solutions into one of the sterile solution containers; then pour normal saline solution into the second sterile container for rinsing. For inner-cannula care, you may use a third sterile solution container to hold the gauze pads and cotton-tipped applicators saturated with cleaning solution. If you'll be replacing the disposable inner cannula, open the package containing the new inner cannula while maintaining aseptic technique. Obtain or prepare new tracheostomy ties, if indicated.
- Place the patient in semi-Fowler's position (unless it's contraindicated) to decrease abdominal pressure on the diaphragm, thereby promoting lung expansion.
- Remove any humidification or ventilation device.
- Using aseptic technique, suction the entire length of the tracheostomy tube to clear the airway of any secretions that may hinder oxygenation.
- Reconnect the patient to the humidifier or ventilator, if necessary.

To clean a stoma and outer cannula

- Put on sterile gloves if you aren't already wearing them.
- With your dominant hand, saturate a sterile gauze pad with the cleaning solution. Squeeze out the excess liquid to prevent accidental aspiration. Then wipe the patient's neck under the tracheostomy tube flanges and twill tapes.
- Saturate a second pad and wipe until the skin surrounding the tracheostomy is cleaned. Use additional pads or cotton-tipped applicators to clean the stoma site and the tube's flanges. Wipe only once with each pad and then discard it to prevent contamination of a clean area with a soiled pad.
- Rinse debris and hydrogen peroxide (if used) with one or more sterile 4″ × 4″ gauze pads dampened in normal saline solution. Dry the area thoroughly with additional sterile gauze pads; then apply a new sterile tracheostomy dressing.
- Remove and discard your gloves.

To clean a nondisposable inner cannula

- Put on sterile gloves.
- Using your nondominant hand, remove and discard the patient's tracheostomy dressing. Then with the same

hand, disconnect the ventilator or humidification device and unlock the tracheostomy tube's inner cannula by rotating it counterclockwise. Place the inner cannula in the container of hydrogen peroxide.

▶ Working quickly, use your dominant hand to scrub the cannula with the sterile nylon brush. If the brush doesn't slide easily into the cannula, use a sterile pipe cleaner.

▶ Immerse the cannula in the container of normal saline solution and agitate it for about 10 seconds to rinse it thoroughly.

▶ Inspect the cannula for cleanliness. Repeat the cleaning process if necessary. If the cannula is clean, tap it gently against the inside edge of the sterile container to remove excess liquid and prevent aspiration. Don't dry the outer surface because a thin film of moisture acts as a lubricant during insertion.

▶ Reinsert the inner cannula into the patient's tracheostomy tube. Lock it in place and then gently pull on it to be sure it's positioned securely. Reconnect the mechanical ventilator. Apply a new sterile tracheostomy dressing.

▶ If the patient can't tolerate being disconnected from the ventilator for the time it takes to clean the inner cannula, replace the existing inner cannula with a clean one and reattach the mechanical ventilator. Then clean the cannula just removed from the patient and store it in a sterile container until the next time tracheostomy care is performed.

To care for a disposable inner cannula

▶ Put on clean gloves.

▶ Using your dominant hand, remove the patient's inner cannula. After evaluating the secretions in the cannula, discard it properly.

▶ Pick up the new inner cannula, touching only the outer locking portion. Insert the cannula into the tracheostomy and, following the manufacturer's instructions, lock it securely.

To change tracheostomy ties

▶ Obtain assistance from another nurse or a respiratory therapist because of the risk of accidental tube expulsion during this procedure. Patient movement or coughing can dislodge the tube.

▶ Wash your hands thoroughly and put on sterile gloves, if you're not already wearing them.

▶ If you're not using commercially packaged tracheostomy ties, prepare new ties from a 30″ (76-cm) length of twill tape by folding one end back 1″ (2.5 cm) on itself. Then, with the bandage scissors, cut a ½″ (1.3-cm) slit down the center of the tape from the folded edge.

▶ Prepare the other end of the tape in the same way.

▶ Hold both ends together and, using scissors, cut the resulting circle of tape so that one piece is approximately 10″ (25 cm) long and the other is about 20″ (51 cm) long.

▶ Assist the patient into the semi-Fowler's position, if possible.

▶ After your assistant puts on gloves, instruct her to hold the tracheostomy tube in place to prevent its expulsion during replacement of the ties. However, if you must perform the procedure without assistance, fasten the clean ties in place before removing the old ties to prevent tube expulsion.

▶ With the assistant's gloved fingers holding the tracheostomy tube in place, cut the soiled tracheostomy ties with the bandage scissors or untie them and discard the ties. Be careful not to cut the tube of the pilot balloon.

▶ Thread the slit end of one new tie a short distance through the eye of one tracheostomy tube flange from the underside; use the hemostat, if necessary, to pull the tie through. Then thread the other end of the tie completely through the slit end, and pull it taut so it loops firmly through the tube's flange. This avoids knots that can cause discomfort, tissue irritation, pressure, and necrosis at the patient's throat.

▶ Fasten the second tie to the opposite flange in the same manner.

▶ Instruct the patient to flex his neck while you bring the ties around to the side and tie them together with a square knot. Flexion produces the same neck circumference as coughing and helps prevent an overly tight tie. Instruct your assistant to place one finger under the tapes as you tie them to ensure that they're tight enough to avoid slippage but loose enough to prevent choking or jugular vein constriction. Placing the closure on the side allows easy access and prevents pressure necrosis at the back of the neck when the patient is recumbent.

▶ After securing the ties, cut off the excess tape with the scissors and instruct your assistant to release the tracheostomy tube.

▶ Make sure the patient is comfortable and can reach the call button easily.

▶ For the patient with traumatic injury, radical neck dissection, or cardiac failure, check tracheostomy-tie tension frequently because neck diameter can increase from swelling and cause constriction. Also frequently check the neonatal or restless patient because ties can loosen, possibly predisposing to tube misplacement.

To conclude tracheostomy care

▶ Replace any humidification device.

▶ Give mouth care, as needed, because the oral cavity can become dry and malodorous or develop sores from encrusted secretions.

▶ Observe soiled dressings and any suctioned secretions for amount, color, consistency, and odor.

▶ Properly clean or dispose of all equipment, supplies, solutions, and trash, according to your facility's policy.

▶ Remove and discard your gloves.

▶ Make sure the patient is comfortable and that he can easily reach the call button.

▶ Make sure all necessary supplies are readily available at the bedside.

▶ Repeat the procedure at least once every 8 hours or as needed. Change the dressing as often as necessary, whether or not you also perform the entire cleaning procedure, because a dressing wet with exudate or secretions predisposes the patient to skin excoriation, breakdown, and infection.

To deflate and inflate a tracheostomy cuff

▶ Read the cuff manufacturer's instructions because cuff types and procedures vary widely.

▶ Assess the patient's condition, explain the procedure to him, and reassure him. Wash your hands thoroughly.

▶ Help the patient into semi-Fowler's position, if possible, or place him in a supine position so secretions above the cuff site will be pushed up into the mouth if the patient is receiving positive-pressure ventilation.

▶ Suction the oropharyngeal cavity to prevent any pooled secretions from descending into the trachea after cuff deflation.

▶ Release the padded hemostat clamping the cuff inflation tubing, if a hemostat is present.

▶ Insert a 5- or 10-cc syringe into the cuff pilot balloon and very slowly withdraw all air from the cuff. Leave the syringe attached to the tubing for later reinflation of the cuff. Slow deflation allows positive lung pressure to push secretions upward from the bronchi. Cuff deflation may also stimulate the patient's cough reflex, producing additional secretions.

▶ Remove any ventilation device. Suction the lower airway through any existing tube to remove all secretions. Then return the patient to the ventilation device.

▶ Maintain cuff deflation for the prescribed period of time. Observe the patient for adequate ventilation, and suction as necessary. If the patient has difficulty breathing, reinflate the cuff immediately by depressing the syringe plunger very slowly. Inject the least amount of air necessary to achieve an adequate tracheal seal.

▶ When inflating the cuff, you may use the minimal-leak technique or the minimal occlusive volume technique to help gauge the proper inflation point.

▶ If you're inflating the cuff using cuff-pressure measurement, be careful not to exceed 25 mm Hg. If the pressure exceeds 25 mm Hg, notify the physician because you may need to change to a larger size tube, use higher inflation pressures, or permit a larger air leak. A cuff pressure of about 18 mm Hg is usually recommended.

▶ After you've inflated the cuff, if the tubing doesn't have a one-way valve at the end, clamp the inflation line with a padded hemostat (to protect the tubing) and remove the syringe.

▶ Check for a minimal-leak cuff seal. With minimal cuff inflation, you shouldn't feel air coming from the patient's mouth, nose, or tracheostomy site, and a conscious patient shouldn't be able to speak.

▶ Be alert for air leaks from the cuff itself. Suspect a leak if injection of air fails to inflate the cuff or increase cuff pressure, if you're unable to inject the amount of air you withdrew, if the patient can speak, if ventilation fails to maintain adequate respiratory movement with pressures or volumes previously considered adequate, or if air escapes during the ventilator's inspiratory cycle.

▶ Note the exact amount of air used to inflate the cuff to detect tracheal malacia if more air is consistently needed.

▶ Make sure the patient is comfortable and can easily reach the call button and communication aids.

▶ Properly clean or dispose of all equipment, supplies, and trash, according to your facility's policy.

▶ Replenish any used supplies, and make sure all necessary emergency supplies are at the bedside.

▶ Consult the physician about first-aid measures you can use for your tracheostomy patient should an emergency occur. Follow your facility's policy regarding procedure if a tracheostomy tube is expelled or if the outer cannula becomes blocked. If the patient's breathing is obstructed — for example, when the tube is blocked with mucus that can't be removed by suctioning or by withdrawing the inner cannula — call the appropriate code and provide manual resuscitation with a hand-held resuscitation bag or reconnect the patient to the ventilator. Don't remove the tracheostomy tube entirely because this may allow the airway to close completely. Use extreme caution when attempting to reinsert an expelled tracheostomy tube because of the risk of tracheal trauma, perforation, compression, and asphyxiation. Reassure the patient until the physician arrives (usually a minute or less in this type of code or emergency).

▶ Refrain from changing tracheostomy ties unnecessarily during the immediate postoperative period before the stoma track is well formed (usually 4 days), to avoid accidental dislodgment and expulsion of the tube. Unless secretions or drainage is a problem, ties can be changed once a day.

▶ Refrain from changing a single-cannula tracheostomy tube or the outer cannula of a double-cannula tube. Because of the risk of tracheal complications, the physician usually changes the cannula, with the frequency of change depending on the patient's condition.

▶ If the patient's neck or stoma is excoriated or infected, apply a water-soluble lubricant or topical antibiotic cream as ordered. Remember not to use a powder or an oil-based substance on or around a stoma because aspiration can cause infection and abscess.

▶ Replace all equipment, including solutions, regularly according to your facility's policy to reduce the risk of nosocomial infections.

Complications

The following complications can occur within the first 48 hours after tracheostomy tube insertion: hemorrhage at the operative site, causing drowning; bleeding or edema within the tracheal tissue, causing airway obstruction; aspiration of secretions; introduction of air into the pleural cavity, causing pneumothorax; hypoxia or acidosis, triggering cardiac arrest; and introduction of air into surrounding tissues, causing subcutaneous emphysema.

Secretions collected under dressings and twill tape can encourage skin excoriation and infection. Hardened mucus or a slipped cuff can occlude the cannula opening and obstruct the airway. Tube displacement can stimulate the cough reflex if the tip rests on the carina or can cause blood vessel erosion and hemorrhage. Just the presence of the tube or cuff pressure can produce tracheal erosion and necrosis.

Patient teaching

- If the patient is being discharged with a tracheostomy, start self-care teaching as soon as he's receptive. Teach the patient how to change and clean the tube.
- If he's being discharged with suction equipment (a few patients are), make sure he and a family member are knowledgeable and feel comfortable about using this equipment.

Documentation

Record the date and time of the procedure; type of procedure; the amount, consistency, color, and odor of secretions; stoma and skin condition; the patient's respiratory status; change of the tracheostomy tube by the physician; the duration of any cuff deflation; the amount of any cuff inflation; and cuff pressure readings and specific body position. Note any complications and the nursing action taken, any patient or family member teaching and their comprehension and progress, and the patient's tolerance of the treatment.

TRACHEOTOMY

The surgical creation of an opening into the trachea through the neck, tracheotomy is most commonly performed to provide an airway for the intubated patient who needs prolonged mechanical ventilation. It may also be performed to prevent an unconscious or paralyzed patient from aspirating food or secretions; to bypass upper airway obstruction caused by trauma, burns, epiglottitis, or a tumor; or to help remove lower tracheobronchial secretions in a patient who can't clear them.

Although endotracheal intubation is the treatment of choice in an emergency, tracheotomy may be used if intubation is impossible. For the laryngectomy patient, a permanent tracheotomy, in which the skin and the trachea are sutured together, provides the necessary stoma.

After creation of the surgical opening, a tracheostomy tube is inserted to permit access to the airway. Selection of a specific tube depends on the patient's condition and the physician's preference. (See *Comparing tracheostomy tubes*, page 574.)

Implementation

If the patient doesn't have an endotracheal tube in place, the physician inserts this tube with the patient under general anesthesia. Then the physician makes a horizontal incision in the skin below the cricoid cartilage and vertical incisions in the trachea. He places a tracheostomy tube between the second and third tracheal rings, and he may also place retraction sutures in the stomal margins to stabilize the opening. Finally, he inflates the tube cuff (if present), provides ventilation, suctions the airways, and provides oxygen by mist.

Complications

Tracheotomy can cause serious complications. Within 48 hours after surgery,

Comparing tracheostomy tubes

Tracheostomy tubes, made of plastic or metal, come in uncuffed, cuffed, or fenestrated varieties. Tube selection depends on the patient's condition and the physician's preference. Make sure you're familiar with the advantages and disadvantages of these commonly used tracheostomy tubes.

Tube type	Advantages	Disadvantages
Uncuffed (plastic or metal) 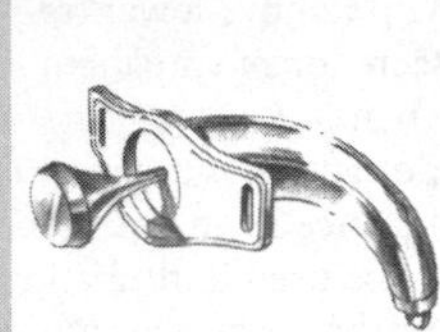	▪ Permits free flow of air around tube and through larynx ▪ Reduces risk of tracheal damage ▪ Allows mechanical ventilation in a patient with neuromuscular disease	▪ Lack of cuff increases the risk of aspiration. ▪ An adapter may be necessary for ventilation.
Plastic cuffed (low pressure and high volume) 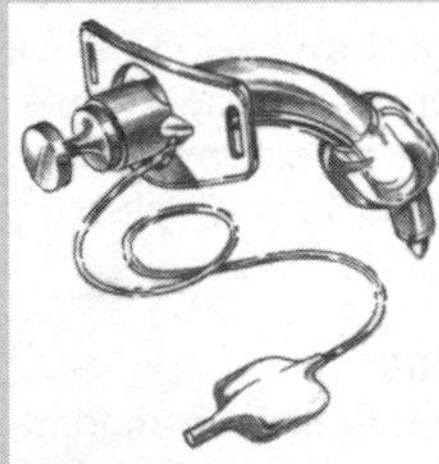	▪ Disposable ▪ Cuff bonded to tube; won't detach accidentally inside trachea ▪ Cuff pressure low and evenly distributed against tracheal wall; no need to deflate periodically to lower pressure ▪ Reduces risk of tracheal damage	▪ This tube may be costlier than other tubes.
Fenestrated 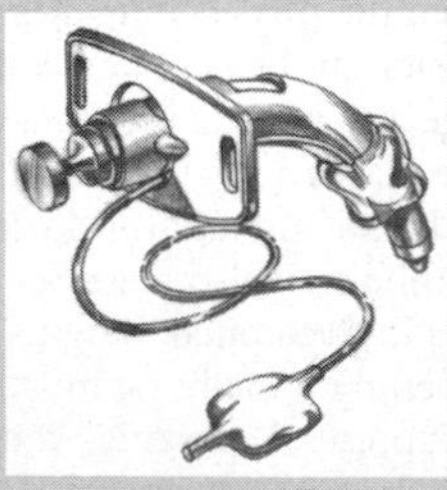	▪ Permits speech through upper airway when external opening is capped and cuff is deflated ▪ Allows breathing by mechanical ventilation with inner cannula in place and cuff inflated ▪ Inner cannula easily removed for cleaning	▪ Fenestration may become occluded. ▪ Inner cannula can become dislodged.

the patient may develop hemorrhage at the site, bleeding or edema within the tracheal tissue, aspiration of secretions, pneumothorax, or subcutaneous emphysema. After 48 hours, continued attention to sterile suctioning, careful cuff monitoring, and meticulous stoma care can reduce the risk of subsequent complications, such as stoma or pulmonary infection, ischemia and hemorrhage, airway obstruction, hypoxia, and arrhythmias.

Key nursing diagnoses and outcomes

Risk for infection related to removal of normal protective barrier with insertion of tracheostomy tube

Treatment outcome: The patient will remain free from all signs and symptoms of infection.

Impaired verbal communication related to inability to speak

Treatment outcomes: The patient will regain normal verbal ability when a temporary tracheostomy is removed, or will demonstrate the correct use of adaptive equipment if the tracheostomy is permanent.

Ineffective airway clearance related to accumulation of tracheobronchial secretions and inability to mobilize secretions

Treatment outcome: The patient will demonstrate equal bilateral breath sounds and clear lung fields on a chest X-ray.

Nursing interventions

Before surgery

- For an emergency tracheotomy, briefly explain the procedure to the patient (if possible), and quickly obtain supplies or a tracheotomy tray.
- For a scheduled tracheotomy, explain the procedure and the need for general anesthesia to the patient and a family member or friend. If possible, mention whether the tracheostomy will be temporary or permanent. As needed, discuss a communication system with the patient, such as a letter board, a magic slate, or flash cards, and have him practice using it so he can communicate comfortably while his speech is limited. If the patient will have a long-term or permanent tracheostomy, introduce him to someone who has undergone a similar procedure and has adjusted well to tube and stoma care.
- Ensure that samples for arterial blood gas (ABG) analysis and other diagnostic tests required by your facility have been collected and that the patient or a responsible family member has signed a consent form.

After surgery

- Auscultate breath sounds every 2 hours after tracheotomy, noting crackles, rhonchi, or diminished sounds. Turn the patient every 2 hours to prevent pooling of tracheal secretions. Note the amount, consistency, color, and odor of secretions. As ordered, provide chest physiotherapy to help mobilize secretions.
- Provide humidification to reduce the drying effects of oxygen on mucous membranes and to thin secretions. Expect to deliver oxygen through a T-piece connected to a nebulizer or heated cascade humidifier. Monitor ABG results and compare them with baseline values, to help determine if oxygenation and carbon dioxide removal is adequate. As ordered, also monitor the patient's oximetry values.
- Using sterile equipment and technique, suction the tracheostomy, as ordered, to remove excess secretions. Use a suction catheter no larger than half the diameter of the tracheostomy tube, and minimize oxygen deprivation and tracheal trauma by keeping the bypass port open while inserting the catheter. Once the catheter is in as far as it can be advanced, don't apply suction. Withdraw the catheter 1″ to 2″ (3 to 5 cm) and

then apply suction using a gentle twisting motion as you withdraw it to help minimize tracheal and bronchial mucosal irritation. Apply suction for no longer than 10 seconds at a time, and discontinue suctioning if the patient develops respiratory distress. Monitor for arrhythmias, which can occur if suctioning decreases the partial pressure of arterial oxygen below 50 mm Hg. Allow oxygen saturation to rise to 92% to 94%, if possible, before further suctioning is continued. Evaluate the effectiveness of suctioning by auscultating for breath sounds.

▶ A cuffed tube, usually inflated until the patient no longer needs controlled ventilation or is over the risk of aspiration, may cause tracheal stenosis from excessive pressure or incorrect placement. Prevent trauma to the interior tracheal wall by using pressures less than 25 cm H_2O (18 mm Hg) and the minimal-leak technique when inflating the cuff. Reduce the risk of trauma to the stoma site and internal tracheal wall by using lightweight corrugated tubing for the ventilator or nebulizer and providing a swivel adapter for the ventilator circuit.

▶ Make sure the tracheostomy ties are secure but not overly tight. Refrain from changing the ties unnecessarily until the stoma track is more stable, thereby helping to prevent accidental tube dislodgment or expulsion. Report any tube pulsation to the physician since this may indicate its proximity to the innominate artery, predisposing the patient to hemorrhage.

▶ Using sterile technique, change the tracheostomy dressing and check the color, odor, amount, and type of any drainage. Also check for swelling, erythema, and bleeding at the site, and report excessive bleeding or unusual drainage immediately.

▶ Keep a sterile tracheostomy tube (with obturator) at the patient's bedside, and be prepared to replace an expelled or contaminated tube. Also keep available a sterile tracheostomy tube (with obturator) that's one size smaller than the tube currently being used, since the trachea begins to close after tube expulsion, making insertion of the same size tube difficult.

PATIENT TEACHING

▶ Tell the patient discharged to home that he should notify his physician if he experiences any breathing problems, chest or stoma pain, or change in the amount or color of his secretions.

▶ Teach the patient and a family member how to care for the stoma and tracheostomy tube. Instruct him to wash the skin around his stoma with a moist cloth. Emphasize the importance of not getting water in his stoma. He should, of course, avoid swimming. When he showers, he should wear a stoma shield or direct the water below his stoma.

▶ Tell the patient to place a foam filter over his stoma in winter, thereby warming inspired air, and to wear a bib over the filter.

▶ Teach the patient to bend at the waist during coughing to help expel secretions. Tell him to keep a tissue handy to catch expelled secretions.

TRANSDERMAL MEDICATION ADMINISTRATION

Transdermal drugs are conveyed directly into the bloodstream from an adhesive disk or patch or a measured dose of ointment applied to the skin. This approach delivers drugs in a constant, controlled manner to provide a prolonged systemic effect. However, age-related changes in older persons, such as vascular changes resulting in a decreased blood supply, can affect drug absorption through the skin. Drugs available in transdermal form include nitroglycerin, used to control angina; estradiol for postmenopausal hormone replacement; clonidine, used to treat hypertension; nicotine, for smoking cessation; and fentanyl, a narcotic analgesic used to control chronic pain.

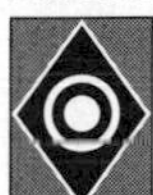

Drug alert Be especially watchful if fentanyl patches are prescribed for an older adult. Some older patients using the patch have died of overdoses, leading the manufacturer to advise restricting its use to those with severe chronic pain that can't be managed with less powerful analgesics.

Supplies

- Patient's medication record and chart
- Prescribed drug (disk or ointment)
- Application strip or measuring paper (for nitroglycerin ointment)
- Plastic wrap (optional for nitroglycerin ointment) or semipermeable dressing
- Adhesive tape
- Optional: gloves

Implementation

- Verify the order on the patient's drug record by checking it against the physician's order.
- Wash your hands and, if necessary, put on gloves.
- Check the label on the drug to make sure you'll be administering the correct drug in the correct dose.
- Explain the procedure to the patient to reduce fear and promote cooperation.
- Confirm the patient's identity by asking his name and checking the name, room number, and bed number on his wristband.
- Provide privacy.
- As needed, remove any previously applied drug.

Applying transdermal ointment

- Place the prescribed amount of ointment on the application strip or measuring paper, taking care not to get any on your skin.
- Apply the strip to any dry, hairless area of the body. Don't rub the ointment into the skin.
- Tape the application strip and ointment to the skin.
- If desired, cover the application strip with the plastic wrap, and tape the wrap in place.
- Before reapplying nitroglycerin ointment, remove the plastic wrap, application strip, and any remaining ointment from the patient's skin at the previous site.

Applying a transdermal disk

- Without touching the adhesive surface, remove the clear plastic backing.
- Apply the disk to a dry, hairless area — behind the ear, for example, as with scopolamine.

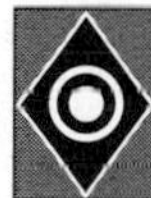

Drug alert Warn a patient using clonidine disks to check with his physician before using any over-the-counter cough preparations because these may counteract the effects of the drug.

- Store the drug as ordered.
- If you didn't wear gloves, wash your hands immediately after applying the disk or ointment to avoid absorbing the drug yourself.
- Reapply daily transdermal drugs at the same time every day to ensure a continuous effect, but alternate the application sites to avoid skin irritation. Avoid skin folds, scars, and any irritated skin areas.
- Instruct the patient to keep the area around the disk or ointment as dry as possible. If the strip or disk leaks or falls off, reapply a new one at a different site.
- Institute safety precautions to minimize the older adult's risk of falling as a result of orthostatic hypotension.

Complications

Skin irritation, such as pruritus or rash, may occur. The patient may also suffer adverse effects of the drug. For example, transdermal nitroglycerin may cause headaches and, especially in the older adult, postural hypotension. Scopolamine has various adverse effects; dry mouth and drowsiness are the most common. Transdermal estradiol carries an increased risk of endometrial cancer and thromboembolic disease. Clonidine may cause severe rebound hypertension, especially if withdrawn suddenly.

Drug alert When using clonidine and nitroglycerin, instruct the older adult to change positions slowly and to dangle his legs before getting out of bed to prevent orthostatic hypotension.

Patient teaching

- Explain the necessity of taking all prescribed drugs, and ensure that the patient and family members understand their intended effects.
- Teach the patient about proper administration of the transdermal drug.

Documentation

Record the type of drug, the dose, and the date, time, and site of application. Also note any adverse effects and the patient's response. Document your patient teaching measures and their effect.

TRANSFER TECHNIQUES

Transfer techniques are used when a patient can't change his position independently. General nursing considerations for transferring patients include the following: Use good body mechanics, avoid unnecessary strain to your lower back, and instruct the patient to assist as much as physically possible.

Transfer from bed to stretcher, one of the most common transfers, can require the help of one or more coworkers, depending on the patient's size and condition. Techniques for achieving this transfer include the straight lift, carry lift, lift sheet, and roller board.

In the *straight (or patient-assisted) lift*—used to move the very light patient or the patient who can assist transfer—the members of the transfer team place their hands and arms beneath the patient's buttocks and, if necessary, his shoulders. Other patients may require a *four-person straight lift,* detailed below. In the *carry lift,* team members roll the patient onto their upper arms and hold him against their chests. In the *lift sheet transfer,* they place a sheet under the patient and lift or slide him onto the stretcher. In the *roller board transfer,* two team members slide the patient onto the stretcher.

For the patient with diminished or absent lower-body sensation or one-sided weakness, immobility, or injury, transfer from bed to wheelchair may require partial support to full assistance—initially by at least two persons. Subsequent transfer of the patient with generalized weakness may be performed by one nurse.

Using a hydraulic lift to raise the immobile patient from the supine to the sitting position allows safe, comfortable transfer between bed and chair. It's indicated for the obese or immobile patient for whom manual transfer poses the potential for nurse or patient injury. Although most hydraulic lift models can be operated by one person, it's better to have two staff members present during transfer to stabilize and support the patient.

Supplies

Transfer from bed to stretcher

- Stretcher
- Roller board or lift sheet, if necessary

Transfer from bed to wheelchair

- Wheelchair with locks (or sturdy chair)
- Pajama bottoms (or robe)
- Shoes or slippers with nonslip soles
- Optional: transfer board (see *Teaching the patient to use a transfer board*)

Teaching the patient to use a transfer board

For the patient who can't stand, a transfer board allows safe movement from bed to wheelchair. To perform this transfer, take the following steps.

- First explain and demonstrate the procedure. Eventually, the patient may become proficient enough to transfer himself independently or with some supervision.
- Place the wheelchair parallel to and facing the foot of the bed. Lock the wheels, and remove the armrest closest to the patient. Make sure the bed is flat, and adjust its height so that it's level with the wheelchair seat.
- Help the patient to a sitting position on the edge of the bed, with his feet resting on the floor. Make sure the front edge of the wheelchair seat is aligned with the back of the patient's knees as shown in the illustration below. Although it's important that the patient have an even surface on which to transfer, he may find it easier to transfer to a slightly lower surface.

Positioning the board

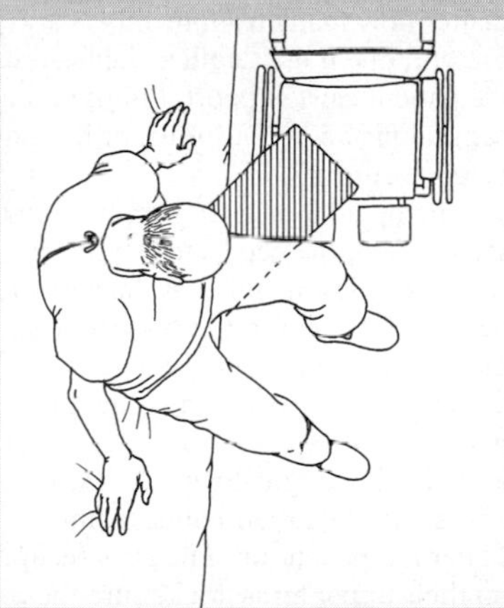

- Ask the patient to lean away from the wheelchair while you slide one end of the transfer board under him.
- Now, place the other end of the transfer board on the wheelchair seat, and help the patient return to the upright position.
- Stand in front of the patient to keep him from sliding forward. Tell him to push down with both arms, lifting his buttocks up and onto the transfer board. The patient then repeats this maneuver, edging along the board, until he's seated in the wheelchair. If the patient can't use his arms to help with the transfer, stand in front of him, put your arms around him, and — if he can — have him put his arms around you, as shown below. Don't allow the patient to put his arms around your neck. Gradually slide him across the board until he's safely in the chair.

Helping the patient

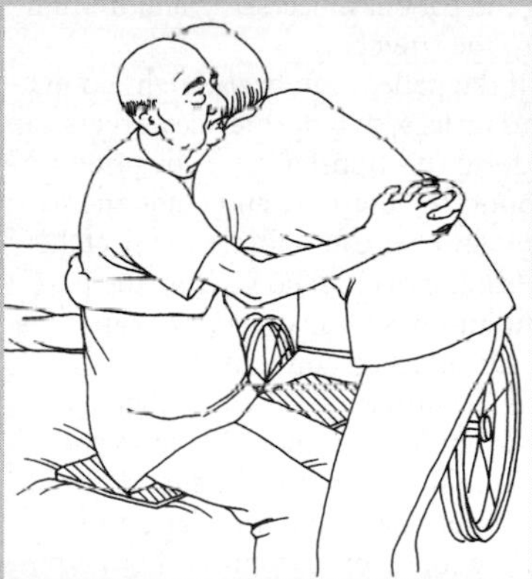

- Once the patient is in the chair, fasten a seat belt, if necessary.
- Then remove the transfer board, replace the wheelchair armrest, and reposition the patient in the chair. Use a safety belt, if indicated, and explain to the patient that it will help protect him from injury.

Transfer with a hydraulic lift

- Hydraulic lift, with sling, chains or straps, and hooks
- Chair or wheelchair

Implementation

- Inform the patient that you're going to move him and what technique will be used.
- Explain the procedure to the patient and demonstrate his role.
- If using a hydraulic lift, reassure the patient that it can safely support his weight and won't tip over.

Transfer from bed to stretcher

- Adjust the bed to the same height as the stretcher.
- Place the older adult in the supine position.
- When transferring a helpless or markedly obese patient from bed to stretcher, first lift and move the patient, in increments, to the edge of the bed. Then rest for a few seconds, repositioning the patient if necessary, and lift him onto the stretcher.
- If the patient can bear weight on his arms or legs, two or three coworkers can perform this transfer: One coworker can support the buttocks and guide the patient, another can stabilize the stretcher by leaning over it and guiding the patient into position, and a third can transfer any attached equipment.
- If a team member isn't available to guide equipment, move I.V. lines and other tubing first to make sure they're out of the way and not in danger of pulling loose, or disconnect tubes if possible.

Four-person straight lift

- Place the stretcher parallel to the bed, and lock the wheels of both to ensure the patient's safety.
- Stand at the center of the stretcher, and have another team member stand at the patient's head. The two other team members should stand next to the bed, on the other side — one at the center and the other at the patient's feet.
- Slide your arms, palms up, beneath the patient, while the other team members do the same. In this position, you and the team member directly opposite support the patient's buttocks and hips; the team member at the head of the bed supports the patient's head and shoulders; the one at the foot supports the patient's legs and feet.
- On a count of three, the team members lift the patient several inches, move him onto the stretcher, and slide their arms out from under him. Keep movements smooth to minimize patient discomfort and to avoid muscle strain by team members.

Four-person carry lift

- Place the stretcher perpendicular to the bed, with the head of the stretcher at the foot of the bed. Lock the bed and stretcher wheels to ensure the patient's safety.
- Raise the bed to a comfortable working height.
- If the patient is light, three coworkers can perform the carry lift; however, no matter how many team members are present, one must stabilize the head if the patient can't support it himself, has cervical instability or injury, or has undergone surgery.
- Line up all four team members on the same side of the bed as the stretcher, with the tallest member at the patient's head and the shortest at his feet. The member at the patient's head is the leader of the team and gives the lift signals.
- Tell the team members to flex their knees and slide their hands, palms up, under the patient until he rests securely on their upper arms. Make sure the patient is adequately supported at the head and shoulders, buttocks and hips, and legs and feet.
- On a count of three, the team members straighten their knees and roll the patient onto his side, against their

chests. This reduces strain on the lifters and allows them to hold the patient for several minutes if necessary.

▶ Together, the team members step back, with the member supporting the feet moving the farthest. The team members move forward to the stretcher's edge and, on a count of three, lower the patient onto the stretcher by bending at the knees and sliding their arms out from under the patient.

Four-person lift sheet transfer

▶ Position the bed, stretcher, and team members for the straight lift. Then instruct the team to hold the edges of the sheet under the patient, grasping them close to the patient to obtain a firm grip, provide stability, and spare the patient undue feelings of instability.

▶ On a count of three, the team members lift or slide the patient onto the stretcher in a smooth, continuous motion to avoid muscle strain and to minimize patient discomfort.

▶ Depending on the patient's size and condition, lift sheet transfer can require two to seven coworkers.

Roller board transfer

▶ Place the stretcher parallel to the bed, and lock the wheels of both to ensure the patient's safety.

▶ Stand next to the bed, and instruct a coworker to stand next to the stretcher.

▶ Reach over the patient and pull the far side of the bedsheet toward you to turn the patient slightly on his side. Your coworker then places the roller board beneath the patient, making sure the board bridges the gap between stretcher and bed.

▶ Ease the patient onto the roller board and release the sheet. Your coworker then grasps the near side of the sheet at the patient's hips and shoulders and pulls him onto the stretcher in a smooth, continuous motion. She then reaches over the patient, grasps the far side of the sheet, and logrolls him toward her.

▶ Remove the roller board as your coworker returns the patient to the supine position.

After all stretcher transfers

▶ Position the patient comfortably on the stretcher, apply safety straps, and raise and secure the side rails.

Transfer from bed to wheelchair

▶ Place the wheelchair parallel to the bed, facing the foot of the bed, and lock its wheels. Make sure the bed wheels are also locked. Raise the footrests to avoid interfering with the transfer.

▶ Check pulse rate and blood pressure with the patient supine to obtain a baseline. Then help him put on the pajama bottoms and slippers or shoes with nonslip soles to prevent falls.

▶ Raise the head of the bed and allow the patient to rest briefly to adjust to posture changes. Then bring him to the dangling position. Recheck pulse rate and blood pressure if you suspect cardiovascular instability. Don't proceed until the patient's pulse rate and blood pressure are stabilized to prevent falls.

▶ Tell the patient to move toward the edge of the bed and, if possible, to place his feet flat on the floor. Stand in front of the patient, blocking his toes with your feet and his knees with yours to prevent his knees from buckling.

▶ Flex your knees slightly, place your arms around the patient's waist, and tell him to place his hands on the edge of the bed. Avoid bending at your waist to prevent back strain.

▶ Ask the patient to push himself off the bed and to support as much of his own weight as possible. At the same time, straighten your knees and hips, raising the patient as you straighten your body.

▶ Supporting the patient as needed, pivot toward the wheelchair, keeping your knees next to his. Tell the patient to grasp the farthest armrest of the wheelchair with his closest hand.

▶ Help the patient lower himself into the wheelchair by flexing your hips and knees but not your back. Instruct him to reach back and grasp the other wheelchair armrest as he sits to avoid abrupt contact with the seat. Fasten the seat belt to prevent falls and, if necessary, check pulse rate and blood pressure to assess cardiovascular stability. If the pulse rate is 20 beats or more above baseline, stay with the patient and monitor him closely until it returns to normal because he is experiencing orthostatic hypotension.
▶ If the patient can't position himself correctly, help him move his buttocks against the back of the chair so the ischial tuberosities, not the sacrum, provide the base of support.
▶ Place the patient's feet flat on the footrests, pointed straight ahead. Then position the knees and hips with the correct amount of flexion and in appropriate alignment. If appropriate, use elevating leg rests to flex the patient's hips at more than 90 degrees; this position relieves pressure on the popliteal space and places more weight on the ischial tuberosities.
▶ Position the patient's arms on the wheelchair's armrests with shoulders abducted, elbows slightly flexed, forearms pronated, and wrists and hands in the neutral position. If necessary, support or elevate the patient's hands and forearms with a pillow to prevent dependent edema.
▶ If the patient starts to fall during transfer, ease him to the closest surface—bed, floor, or chair. Never stretch to finish the transfer. Doing so can cause loss of balance, falls, muscle strain, and other injuries—to you and the patient.
▶ If the patient has one-sided weakness, follow the preceding steps, but place the wheelchair on the patient's unaffected side. Instruct the patient to pivot and bear as much weight as possible on the unaffected side. Support the affected side because the patient will tend to lean to this side. Use pillows to support the hemiplegic patient's affected side to prevent slumping in the wheelchair.

Transfer with a hydraulic lift

▶ Because hydraulic lift models may vary in weight capacity, check the manufacturer's specifications before attempting patient transfer. Make sure the bed and wheelchair wheels are locked before beginning the transfer.
▶ Make sure the side rail opposite you is raised and secure. Then roll the patient toward you, onto his side, and raise the side rail. Walk to the opposite side of the bed and lower the side rail.
▶ Place the sling under the patient's buttocks with its lower edge below the greater trochanter. Then fanfold the far side of the sling against the back and buttocks.
▶ Roll the patient toward you onto the sling, and raise the side rail. Then lower the opposite side rail.
▶ Slide your hands under the patient and pull the sling from beneath him, smoothing out all wrinkles. Then roll the patient onto his back and center him on the sling.
▶ Place the appropriate chair next to the head of the bed, facing the foot.
▶ Lower the side rail next to the chair, and raise the bed only until the base of the lift can extend under the bed. To avoid alarming and endangering the patient, don't raise the bed completely.
▶ Set the lift's adjustable base to its widest position to ensure the highest level of stability. Then move the lift so that its arm lies perpendicular to the bed, directly over the patient.
▶ Connect one end of the chains (or straps) to the side arms on the lift; connect the other, hooked end to the sling. Face the hooks away from the patient to prevent them from slipping and to avoid the risk of their pointed edges injuring the patient. The patient may place his arms inside or outside the chains (or straps) or he may grasp them once the slack is gone, to avoid injury. (See *Using a hydraulic lift.*)

Using a hydraulic lift

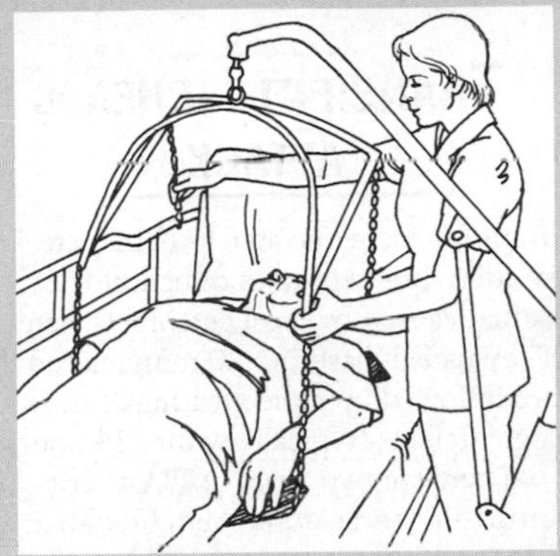

After placing the patient in a supine position in the center of the sling, position the hydraulic lift above him, as shown. Then attach the chains to the hooks on the sling.

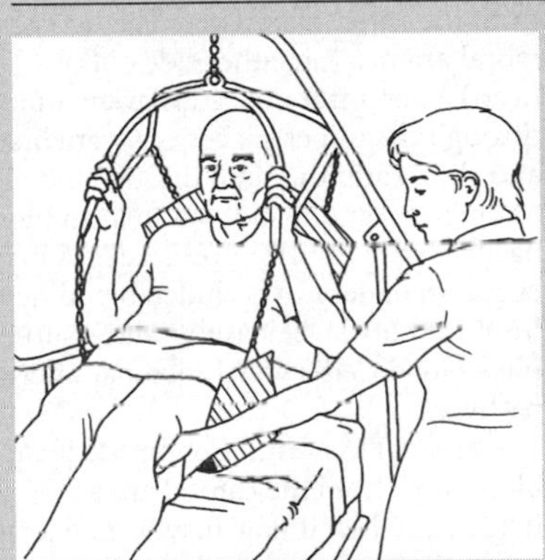

Turn the lift handle clockwise to raise the patient to the sitting position. If he's positioned properly, continue to raise him until he's suspended just above the bed, as shown.

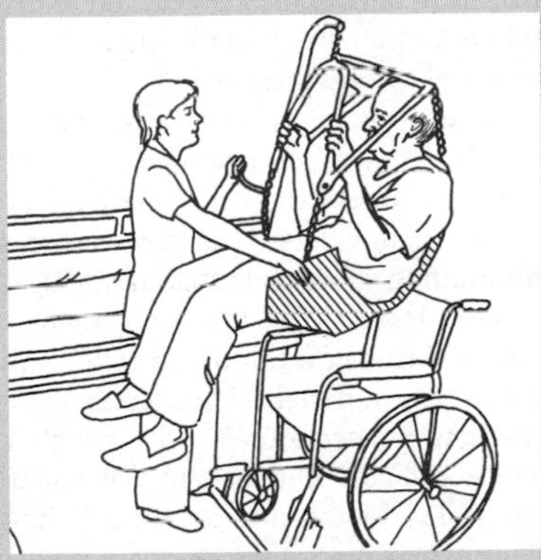

After positioning the patient above the wheelchair, turn the lift handle counterclockwise to lower him onto the seat, as shown. When the chains become slack, stop turning and unhook the sling from the lift.

▶ Tighten the turnscrew on the lift. Then, depending on the type of lift you're using, pump the handle or turn it clockwise until the patient has assumed a sitting position and his buttocks clear the bed surface by 1″ or 2″ (2.5 or 5 cm). Momentarily suspend the patient above the bed until he feels secure in the lift and sees that it can bear his weight.

▶ Steady the patient as you move the lift or, preferably, have another coworker guide the patient's body while you move the lift. Depending on the type of lift you're using, the arm should now rest in front or to one side of the chair.

▶ Release the turnscrew. Then depress the handle or turn it counterclockwise to lower the patient into the chair. While lowering the patient, push gently on his knees to maintain the correct sitting posture. After lowering the patient into the chair, fasten the seat belt to ensure his safety.

▶ Remove the hooks or straps from the sling, but leave the sling in place under the patient so you'll be able to transfer him back to the bed from the chair. Then move the lift away from the patient.

▶ To return the patient to bed, reverse the procedure.

Complications

Improper technique risks injury to the patient and staff.

Patient teaching

▶ Tell the patient to report any discomfort when he's being moved, so the transfer technique can be modified, if appropriate.

▶ Reassure the patient about his safety if he's anxious or fearful of falling out of the lift.

Documentation

Record the time, the type of transfer, and the extent of assistance. Note how the patient tolerated the activity. Complete other required forms, as necessary. Document any patient teaching measures and their effect.

TRANSIENT ISCHEMIC ATTACK

Transient ischemic attacks (TIAs) are sudden, brief episodes of neurologic deficit caused by focal cerebral ischemia. They usually last 5 to 20 minutes and are followed by rapid clearing of neurologic deficits (typically within 24 hours).

There are two types of TIAs: vertebrobasilar and carotid. Vertebrobasilar TIAs result from inadequate blood flow from the vertebral arteries. The two vertebral arteries (on either side of the head) extend from the subclavian artery, through the upper six cervical vertebrae, and then enter the skull through the foramen magnum and join to form the basilar artery. A vertebrobasilar TIA may occur secondary to occluded blood flow from the subclavian artery, which supplies blood to the vertebrobasilar arterial pathway.

Carotid TIAs result from inadequate blood flow from the carotid artery. Inadequate blood flow may be due to a narrowing or partial occlusion at the bifurcation of the common carotid artery where it branches into the internal and external carotid arteries.

TIAs occur most often in people over age 50. They affect men more commonly than women, and blacks have a higher risk than whites. TIAs may warn of an impending cerebrovascular accident (CVA). About 50% to 80% of patients who experience a thrombotic CVA have previously suffered a TIA. Accurately predicting when a CVA will occur after a TIA is difficult. One patient may suffer a single TIA followed by a CVA only hours later, whereas another patient, who may have had 50 TIAs, might not have a CVA for years.

TIAs may be caused by vascular disorders, such as extensive extracranial atherosclerosis, arteritis, and fibromuscular dysplasia, or blood disorders, such as hypercoagulability, polycythemia, and recurrent embolism. Any condition that lowers cerebrovascular blood flow, such as diminished cardiac output or subclavian steal syndrome (decreased supply of blood to the subclavian artery), can cause a TIA. Sometimes, a TIA can result from hyperextension and flexion of the head, for example, when a person falls asleep in a chair, impairing cerebral blood flow.

Signs and symptoms

- Dizziness
- Diplopia
- Dark or blurred vision
- Visual field deficits
- Ptosis
- Difficulty in speaking
- Difficulty in swallowing
- Unilateral or bilateral weakness
- Numbness in the fingers, arms, or legs (or all three sites)
- Staggering gait, or veering to one side
- Transient blindness in one eye
- Altered level of consciousness
- Numbness of the tongue
- Seizures
- Bruits on auscultation of the carotid artery
- Faint peripheral pulses on palpation
- Hypertension
- Possible history of frequent falls or a recent fall

Diagnostic tests

- *Oculoplethysmography* may indicate carotid occlusive disease by revealing delayed pulse arrival in one eye.
- *Carotid Doppler* or *transcranial Doppler study* may disclose blood flow disturbances.
- *Cerebral angiography* may be needed to confirm carotid stenosis or occlusion.
- *Digital subtraction angiography* may reveal carotid occlusion or severe carotid stenosis.
- *Magnetic resonance imaging* and *magnetic resonance arteriography* may provide additional information.

Treatment

TIAs significantly increase a person's risk of CVA and should be treated as quickly as possible. Aspirin is the preferred drug and is probably most helpful when the TIA is caused by emboli due to atherosclerotic plaque.

Warfarin may be prescribed, but prolonged therapy increases the risk of hemorrhagic complications. Short-term I.V. heparin may be ordered for patients suspected of having carotid or vertebrobasilar stenosis from thrombus formation. Dipyridamole and sulfinpyrazone are now only occasionally prescribed.

Surgery may be considered, primarily to treat carotid artery obstruction resulting from atherosclerosis or stenosis that isn't responsive to drug therapy, putting the patient at a greater risk for CVA. With vertebrobasilar TIAs (which usually don't lead to CVA), surgery is rarely performed because only the proximal vertebrobasilar arteries are surgically accessible. Surgical procedures include carotid endarterectomy and extracranial-intracranial bypass; however, the latter is controversial.

Recommended lifestyle changes to reduce risk factors may include weight loss, exercise, smoking cessation, and management of diabetes, hypertension, and hyperlipidemia.

Key nursing diagnoses and outcomes

Ineffective (cerebral) tissue perfusion related to lack of adequate oxygen supply to the brain

Treatment outcome: The patient will maintain or improve his current level of consciousness.

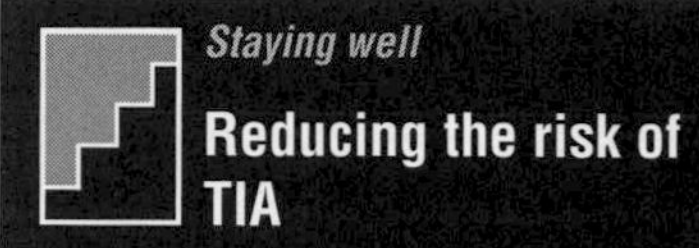

Staying well

Reducing the risk of TIA

Help the patient plan to reduce his risk of a future transient ischemic attack (TIA) by following these important guidelines:

- Work with the patient on a moderate exercise program.
- Refer the patient to a smoking cessation or weight loss program, if necessary.
- Discuss the need to comply with all treatments, which may include taking prescribed drugs to manage blood pressure, hyperlipidemia, or diabetes mellitus.
- Tell the patient to immediately report any neurologic symptoms, especially those lasting longer than 24 hours.
- Stress the need for keeping follow-up appointments.

Risk for injury related to decreased level of consciousness

Treatment outcome: The patient and his family members will develop strategies to maintain safety.

Nursing interventions

▶ Prepare the patient for ordered diagnostic tests. After invasive procedures, monitor him for complications.

▶ Monitor neurologic status and vital signs to detect TIA recurrence or progression to CVA.

▶ Administer ordered drugs, and assess for bleeding.

▶ Monitor the results of laboratory tests, including prothrombin time and international normalized ratio in patients receiving oral anticoagulants and partial thromboplastin time in patients receiving heparin. Also monitor the patient's hemoglobin level, hematocrit, and platelet count.

▶ Keep the call button near the patient, and instruct him to use it if he experiences any symptoms.

▶ Keep the bed's side rails raised at night and at other times, if warranted. Keep the patient's room free of clutter.

▶ If the patient fears a CVA, offer emotional support. Allow him to express his fears and concerns. Explain clearly the goals of treatment.

▶ If the patient requires surgery, prepare him physically and emotionally.

▶ Following surgery, assess the patient's neurologic status to detect early complications, especially increased intracranial pressure and cerebral ischemia. Also assess his vital signs. Expect to maintain his systolic blood pressure at 120 to 170 mm Hg to ensure cerebral perfusion. Also assess for airway obstruction, which may be related to excessive swelling in the neck, hematoma formation, or faulty head positioning.

PATIENT TEACHING

▶ Explain the nature of the disorder and the need for prompt treatment to help prevent a CVA. Also explain the purpose of diagnostic tests and the importance of keeping follow-up laboratory appointments.

▶ Inform the patient about prescribed drugs, including their purpose, action, dosage, route, possible adverse effects, and precautions. Tell the patient to be sure to notify the physician if bleeding occurs.

▶ To prevent falls, instruct the patient to sit down and rest immediately if dizziness, disturbed balance, or weakness occurs. To help prevent falls at home, suggest making minor changes, such as installing a grab bar in the tub area, removing clutter and throw rugs, and installing adequate lighting (especially on stairs and in bathrooms).

▶ Inform the patient about planned surgery. Clarify the risks, and explain preoperative, postoperative, and follow-up home care.

▶ Tell the patient that certain lifestyle changes will be necesary to prevent future TIAs. (See *Reducing the risk of TIA*.)

TUBERCULOSIS

An acute or chronic infection, tuberculosis (TB) is characterized by pulmonary infiltrates and by formation of granulomas with caseation, fibrosis, and cavitation. The American Lung Association estimates that active disease has increased by more than 20% in the past 5 years.

TB is twice as common in men as in women and four times as common in nonwhites as in whites. However, incidence is highest among people who live in crowded, poorly ventilated, unsanitary conditions, such as prisons, tenement houses, and homeless shelters.

TB results from exposure to *Mycobacterium tuberculosis* and sometimes other strains of mycobacteria. Transmission occurs when an infected person coughs or sneezes, spreading infected droplets.

When a person inhales these droplets, the bacilli lodge in the alveoli, causing irritation. The immune system responds by sending leukocytes, lymphocytes, and macrophages to surround the bacilli, and the local lymph nodes swell and become inflamed. If the encapsulated bacilli (tubercles) and the inflamed nodes rupture (as in an immunocompromised person), the infection contaminates the surrounding tissue and may spread through the blood and lymphatic circulation to distant sites.

After exposure to *M. tuberculosis*, roughly 5% of infected people develop active TB within 1 year; in the remainder, microorganisms cause a latent infection. The host's immunologic defense system usually destroys the bacillus or walls it up in a tubercle. But the live, encapsulated bacilli may lie dormant within the tubercle for years, reactivating later during the aging process to cause active infection.

The risk of TB is higher in older people who have close contact with a newly diagnosed TB patient, those who have had TB before, gastrectomy patients, and those affected with silicosis, diabetes, malnutrition, cancer, Hodgkin's disease, or leukemia. Drug and alcohol abusers, patients in mental institutions, and nursing home residents also have a higher incidence. The aging process weakens the immune system, further increasing the likelihood of tubercular infection in older people. The incidence is higher in people receiving treatment with immunosuppressants or corticosteroids and in those who have diseases that affect the immune system. (See *Who's at risk for TB?* page 588.)

TB can cause massive pulmonary tissue damage, with inflammation and tissue necrosis eventually leading to respiratory failure. Bronchopleural fistulas can develop from lung tissue damage, resulting in pneumothorax. The disease can also lead to hemorrhage, pleural effusion, and pneumonia. Small mycobacterial foci can infect other body organs, including the kidneys and the central nervous and skeletal systems.

Signs and symptoms

▶ Weakness and fatigue
▶ Anorexia
▶ Weight loss
▶ Blood-tinged sputum (less common initial sign in the older adult)
▶ Fever and night sweats (typical hallmarks of TB, may not be present in an older adult who exhibits a change in activity level or weight)
▶ Dullness (on percussion) over the affected area, a sign of consolidation or the presence of pleural fluid
▶ Crepitant crackles, bronchial breath sounds, wheezes, and whispered pectoriloquy

Who's at risk for TB?

The risk of tuberculosis (TB) is higher in the following:

- Black and Hispanic men between ages 25 and 44
- those in close contact with a newly diagnosed TB patient
- those who have had TB
- people with multiple sexual partners
- recent immigrants from Africa, Asia, Mexico, and South America
- gastrectomy patients
- people affected with silicosis, diabetes, malnutrition, cancer, Hodgkin's disease, or leukemia
- drug and alcohol abusers
- patients in mental institutions
- nursing home residents
- those receiving treatment with immunosuppressants or corticosteroids
- people with weak immune systems or diseases that affect the immune system, especially those with acquired immunodeficiency syndrome.

Diagnostic tests

▶ *Chest X-rays* show nodular lesions, patchy infiltrates (mainly in upper lobes), cavity formation, scar tissue, and calcium deposits. However, they may not help distinguish between active and inactive TB.

▶ *Tuberculin skin test* reveals that the person has been infected with TB at some point, but it doesn't indicate active disease. In this test, 5 tuberculin units (0.1 ml) of intermediate-strength purified protein derivative (PPD) are injected intradermally on the forearm, with results read in 48 to 72 hours. A positive reaction (equal to or more than a 10-mm induration) develops within 2 to 10 weeks after infection with the tubercle bacillus in both active and inactive TB. In older people, a two-step test should be performed. If the initial test is negative, it should be repeated in 1 week. If the response has waned, the second test will cause a conversion.

▶ The most definitive test is isolation of *M. tuberculosis* in the sputum, cerebrospinal fluid, urine, abscess drainage, or pleural fluid using *stains and cultures* that show heat-sensitive, nonmotile, aerobic, acid-fast bacilli.

▶ *Bronchoscopy* may be performed if the person can't produce an adequate sputum specimen. Several specimens may need to be tested to distinguish TB from other diseases that may mimic it (such as lung carcinoma, lung abscess, pneumoconiosis, and bronchiectasis).

▶ *Computed tomography scan* or *magnetic resonance imaging* allows the evaluation of lung damage or confirms a difficult diagnosis.

Treatment

Antitubercular therapy with daily oral doses of isoniazid, rifampin, and pyrazinamide (with ethambutol added in some cases) for at least 6 to 9 months usually cures TB. After 2 to 4 weeks, the disease is no longer infectious, and the patient can resume his normal activities while continuing to take the drug.

Drug alert Isoniazid (INH) must be used with caution in the older adult because the incidence of hepatic complications from the drug increases after age 35. INH prophylaxis in patients with a positive PPD test may not be indicated in the older adult because of the risk of hepatotoxicity. Monitor liver function very closely in the older adult receiving INH.

A person with atypical mycobacterial disease or drug-resistant TB may require second-line drugs, such as capreomycin, streptomycin, para-aminosalicylic acid, pyrazinamide, and cycloserine.

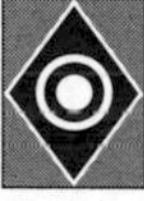

Drug alert The adverse effects of second-line drugs can be particularly hazardous to older adults. Para-

aminosalicylic acid can cause GI tract irritation, anorexia, nausea, vomiting, and diarrhea, which can lead to malnutrition. Streptomycin can damage the peripheral and central nervous systems, resulting in disequilibrium and hearing loss, which can compromise the person's safety.

Key nursing diagnoses and outcomes

Ineffective protection related to potential for recurrence and possible transmission of mycobacterial foci to other areas of the body

Treatment outcome: The patient will comply with the prescribed TB treatment to eradicate the infection and minimize the risk of other organs becoming infected.

Impaired gas exchange related to changes in pulmonary tissue

Treatment outcome: The patient will regain and maintain adequate ventilation.

Deficient knowledge related to TB

Treatment outcome: The patient will communicate an understanding of how TB is contracted and managed and how a recurrence can be prevented.

Nursing interventions

- Administer ordered antibiotics and antitubercular agents. Give isoniazid and ethambutol with food.
- Institute standard and airborne precautions. The Occupational Safety and Health Administration requires staff to wear a respirator with a high-efficiency particulate air filter when caring for the patient with TB. Isolate the infectious patient in a quiet, well-ventilated room until he's no longer contagious.
- Place a covered trash can nearby or tape a waxed bag to the bedside for used tissues. Tell the patient to wear a mask when he is outside his room.
- Make sure the patient gets plenty of rest. Provide for alternating periods of rest and activity to promote health as well as conserve energy and reduce oxygen demand.
- Provide the patient with well-balanced, high-calorie foods, preferably in small, frequent meals to conserve energy. (Small, frequent meals may also encourage the anorectic patient to eat more.) If the patient needs oral supplements, consult with the dietitian.
- Perform chest physiotherapy, including postural drainage and chest percussion, several times a day.
- Monitor the patient's respiratory status. Auscultate for breath sounds frequently.
- Provide written material about TB to the patient and family members.
- Because isoniazid can cause hepatitis or peripheral neuritis, monitor levels of aspartate aminotransferase and alanine aminotransferase.
- If the patient receives ethambutol, watch for signs of optic neuritis; report them to the physician, who probably will discontinue the drug. Assess the patient's vision monthly.
- If the patient receives rifampin, watch for signs of hepatitis, purpura, and a flu-like syndrome as well as other complications such as hemoptysis. Monitor liver and kidney function throughout therapy.
- Monitor the patient's compliance with treatment. An older person can have a very difficult time accepting the diagnosis of TB. Most older adults remember living in a time when people with TB were sent away to sanitariums for long periods of time. They may be unaware of new treatment methods and fearful of being institutionalized. Provide education on the treatment plan, and emphasize that treatment can be provided in the person's current living environment, once the initial infectious period has passed.

PATIENT TEACHING

- Visitors and facility personnel should wear masks in the patient's room.

▶ Teach the patient the signs and symptoms that require medical assessment: increased cough, hemoptysis, unexplained weight loss, fever, and night sweats.
▶ Advise anyone exposed to an infected patient to get a tuberculin test and, if ordered, a chest X-ray and prophylactic isoniazid.
▶ Show the patient and his family members how to perform postural drainage and chest percussion.
▶ Teach the patient coughing and deep-breathing techniques.
▶ Teach home oxygen administration and safety, if necessary.
▶ Teach the patient the adverse effects of his drug, and tell him to report reactions immediately.
▶ Emphasize the importance of regular follow-up examinations, and instruct the patient and his family members concerning the signs and symptoms of recurring TB. Stress the need to follow long-term treatment faithfully.
▶ Warn the patient taking rifampin that the drug will temporarily make his body secretions appear orange; reassure him that this effect is harmless.
▶ Explain standard and airborne precautions to the hospitalized patient. Before discharge, tell him that he must take precautions to prevent spreading the disease — such as wearing a mask around others until his physician tells him he's no longer contagious. He should tell all health care providers he sees, including his dentist and eye physician, that he has TB so that they can institute infection-control precautions.
▶ Teach the patient other specific precautions to avoid spreading the infection. Tell him to cough and sneeze into tissues and to dispose of the tissues properly. Stress the importance of washing his hands thoroughly in hot, soapy water after handling his own secretions. Also, instruct him to wash his eating utensils separately in hot, soapy water.
▶ Refer the patient to such support groups as the American Lung Association.

Special considerations

Changes in gastric secretions can cause the drugs prescribed for TB to be passed through the intestinal tract without being absorbed. Check the stools of older people for undissolved tablets.

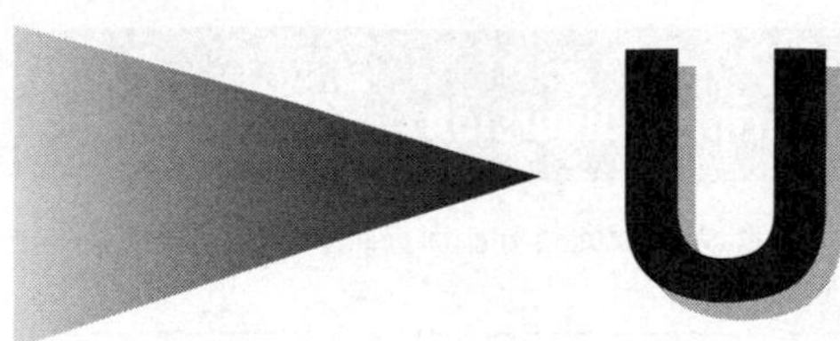

URINARY DIVERSION SURGERY

A urinary diversion provides an alternative route for urine excretion when pathology impedes normal flow through the bladder. Most commonly performed in patients who've undergone a cystectomy, diversion surgery also may be performed in patients with a congenital urinary tract defect; a severe, unmanageable urinary tract infection (UTI) that threatens renal function; an injury to the ureters, bladder, or urethra; an obstructive malignancy; or a neurogenic bladder.

There are several ways that urinary diversion surgery can be performed. Possible procedures include ileal conduit (also known as ureteroileal urinary conduit, ileal bladder, ileal loop, Bricker's procedure, and ureteroileostomy), continent internal ileal reservoir (also known as a Kock pouch), and orthotopic bladder replacement. (See *Reviewing selected types of urinary diversion*, page 592.)

Urinary diversions may be categorized as incontinent or continent. Incontinent diversions include the ileal conduit, ureterosigmoidostomy, and nephrostomy. With these types, urine flow is constant, and a permanent external collection device is required. Continent diversions include the Kock pouch and Indiana pouch. The advantage of these procedures is that an external collection bag isn't needed. However, there is the possibility of urine leakage

Ileal conduit, the most common urinary diversion, involves anastomosis of the ureters to a small portion of the ileum excised especially for the procedure, followed by the creation of a stoma from one end of the ileal segment. This resulting stoma is called a urostomy. It drains urine continuously and requires that the patient wear an external pouch at all times.

A ureterosigmoidostomy is an internal urinary diversion that redirects urine through the colon and then out the rectum. This detour into the colon causes two major complications: metabolic disorders (hyperchloremic acidosis) and pyelonephritis. To be a candidate for this procedure, the patient must have a competent internal sphincter because urine excretion will occur from the rectum, permanently. The drainage from the rectum will have the consistency of watery diarrhea, which can result in acidosis and electrolyte imbalances involving potassium, chloride, and magnesium. Pyelonephritis is caused by reflux of bacteria from the colon. This procedure isn't performed frequently.

Continent internal ileal reservoirs, such as the Kock pouch and Indiana pouch, are another type of urinary diversion. Following cystectomy, a segment of the small bowel or colon is used to create an internal pouch. For the Kock pouch, the ureters are then implanted into the sides of the pouch, with each ureter intussuscepted to create a nipple valve. The efferent ureter and nipple valve are brought to the skin surface of the anterior abdomen as a stoma

Reviewing selected types of urinary diversion

Types of urinary diversion include ileal conduit and continent internal ileal reservoir (Kock pouch or Indiana pouch).

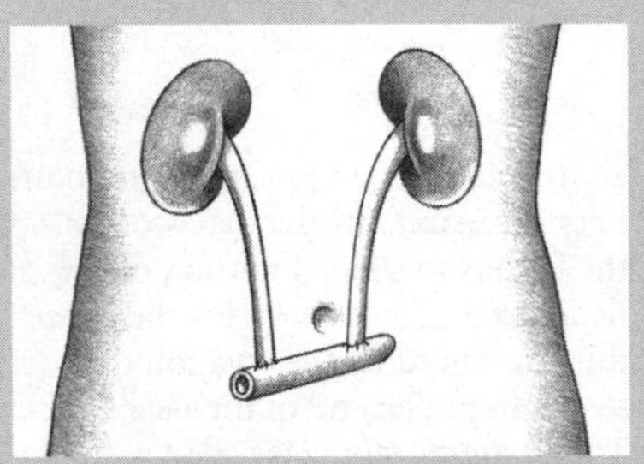

Ileal conduit

Both ureters are anastomosed to a small segment of ileum, one end of which is brought to the surface of the lower abdomen to form a stoma.

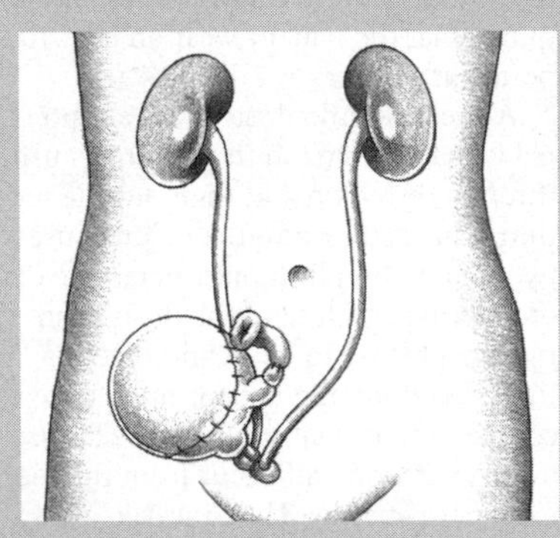

Continent internal ileal reservoir (Kock pouch)

An internal pouch is created from a segment of ileum. Both ureters are implanted into the sides of the pouch, and nipple valves are intussuscepted to them. One of the valves prevents backward flow of urine into the ureters from the pouch; the other valve is brought to the surface of the lower abdomen to form a stoma that is flush with the skin.

and prevent leakage of urine from the pouch. The afferent ureter and nipple valve prevent urine reflux.

Ureters are implanted differently in the Indiana pouch. They are tunneled through the tenia of the segment of colon used to construct the pouch.

Because the pouch is internal and can be trained to hold urine without leakage, it allows the patient to remain free of external appliances. It does, however, require the patient to catheterize the abdominal opening intermittently so as to empty the pouch.

The continent internal ileal reservoir has recently been modified so that the reservoir has both the ureters and urethra connected to it. This eliminates the need for a small opening in the abdominal wall and helps preserve the patient's body image. However, unless the lower portion of the bladder can be spared, continence depends solely on the urethra and external sphincter. Consequently, total bladder substitution is usually limited to men. Drainage of the internal pouch relies on passive emptying when the external sphincter is relaxed and on abdominal straining. If these techniques aren't sufficient, the patient must learn intermittent self-catheterization. Complications, such as tumor recurrence in the urethra and frequent nocturnal enuresis, can affect up to 50% of patients and are major drawbacks of the procedure.

Another possible procedure is a nephrostomy, which is a short-term technique that diverts urine away from an obstruction or lesion below the level of the renal pelvis.

Implementation

▶ The surgeon makes a midline or paramedial abdominal incision.

▶ To construct an ileal conduit, the surgeon excises a 6″ to 8″ (15- to 20-cm) segment of the ileum (also taking its mesentery to help preserve tissue viability) and then anastomoses the remaining ileal ends to maintain intestinal integrity. Next, he dissects the ureters from the bladder and implants them in the ileal segment. The surgeon then sutures one end of the ileal segment closed and brings the other end through the abdominal wall to form a stoma.

▶ To create a nephrostomy, the surgeon inserts a catheter into the renal pelvis either percutaneously or through a flank incision. This procedure is usually palliative because it carries a high risk of infection and calculus formation.

▶ The surgeon may create any one of a number of different types of continent internal ileal reservoirs (such as the Kock pouch or the Indiana pouch) using segments of the small bowel and colon. For example, if he decides to make a Kock pouch, he excises 24″ to 32″ (60 to 80 cm) of ileum and anastomoses the remaining ileal ends to maintain intestinal integrity. After shaping the isolated ileum segment into a pocket to serve as a bladder, he connects the Kock pouch to the urethra or uses an intussuscepted nipple valve to connect the pouch to the external skin of the anterior abdominal wall. He then constructs a second nipple valve at the other end of the pouch to prevent urine from flowing backward into the ureters. Finally, he implants the ureters at the site of the second nipple valve along with ureteral stents. The ureteral stents, which originate in the pelvis of the kidneys and extend through the ureter into the reservoir and out through the abdominal opening or separate stab wounds, are used to keep the ureters patent until they are no longer needed (usually 7 to 10 days postoperatively).

▶ Depending on the length, type of tubing used, and exit site, the stents may be placed to dependent drainage or may be contained with a pouching system. One or two drainage tubes are then inserted into the reservoir to maintain unobstructed drainage from the reservoir until healing has occurred and pouch integrity is confirmed.

Complications

Postoperative complications of urinary diversion surgery include skin breakdown around the stoma site, wound infection or wound dehiscence, urinary extravasation, ureteral obstruction, small-bowel obstruction, peritonitis, hydronephrosis, and stomal gangrene. Delayed complications include ureteral obstruction, stomal stenosis, pyelonephritis, renal calculi, and electrolyte disturbances. If chronic pyelonephritis occurs over a period of years, end-stage renal disease is possible. Also, the patient with a continent internal ileal reservoir may experience incontinence and, if the reservoir is connected to the urethra, frequent UTIs and tumor recurrence (if cystectomy was done due to bladder cancer).

Patients also commonly suffer psychological problems, such as depression and anxiety, related to altered body image and concern about lifestyle changes associated with the stoma and urine drainage. Even patients with a continent urinary reservoir attached to the urethra may still have a grief reaction to the loss of their natural bladder.

Key nursing diagnoses and outcomes

Disturbed body image related to presence of stoma

Treatment outcomes: The patient will acknowledge the change in body image, and will be able to perform self-care on his stoma without showing negative behavior.

Risk for infection related to potential for intraperitoneal leakage and greater exposure of the renal system to bacteria

Treatment outcome: The patient will communicate an understanding of how to prevent or reduce the risk of infection.

Impaired skin integrity related to urinary drainage from stoma

Treatment outcomes: The patient will communicate an understanding of how to manage his type of urinary diversion, and will demonstrate correct stoma care.

Nursing interventions

- Review the planned surgery with the patient, reinforcing the physician's explanations as necessary. Try using a simple anatomic diagram to enhance your discussion, and provide printed information from the United Ostomy Association or other sources, if possible and appropriate. Explain to the patient that he'll receive a general anesthetic and have a nasogastric (NG) tube in place after surgery.
- If appropriate, prepare the patient for the appearance and general location of the stoma. For example, if he's scheduled for an ileal conduit, explain that the stoma will be located somewhere in the lower abdomen, probably below the waistline.
- Ensure that the patient having a continent internal ileal reservoir understands that his substitute bladder won't function identically to the natural bladder. If the reservoir will be attached to the external skin, explain that the stoma will be flush with the skin of the anterior abdominal wall and that the exact location of the stoma is often decided during surgery.
- Review the enterostomal therapist's explanation of the urine collection device or catheterization procedure to be used after surgery. Reassure the patient that he'll receive complete training on how to manage urine drainage after he returns from surgery.
- If possible, arrange for a visit by a well-adjusted patient who's undergone the same type of urinary diversion as your patient. He can provide a firsthand account of the operation and offer some insight into the realities of ongoing care of urinary drainage. And, as appropriate, be sure to include the patient's family members in all aspects of preoperative teaching—especially if they'll be providing much of the routine care after discharge. Ensure that the patient or a responsible family member has signed a consent form.
- Before surgery, prepare the bowel to reduce the risk of postoperative infection from intestinal flora. As ordered, maintain the patient on a low-residue or clear liquid diet and administer a cleansing enema and an antimicrobial drug, such as erythromycin or neomycin. Other possible measures may include total parenteral nutrition or fluid replacement therapy for debilitated patients and prophylactic I.V. antibiotics.
- After the patient returns from surgery, monitor his vital signs every hour until they're stable. Carefully check and record urine output; report any decrease, which could indicate obstruction from postoperative edema or ureteral stenosis. Observe urine drainage for pus and blood; keep in mind that urine is often blood-tinged initially but should rapidly clear.
- Record the amount, color, and consistency of drainage from the incisional or stoma drain, ureteral stents (if present), and NG tube. Notify the physician of any urine leakage from the drain or suture line; such leakage may point to de-

veloping complications, such as hydronephrosis. Watch for signs of peritonitis (fever, abdominal distention and pain), which can develop from intraperitoneal urine leakage.

- Check dressings frequently and change them at least once each shift. (The physician will probably perform the first dressing change.) When changing dressings, check the suture line for redness, swelling, and drainage.
- Maintain fluid and electrolyte balance, and continue I.V. replacement therapy as ordered. Provide total parenteral nutrition, if necessary, to ensure adequate nutrition.
- Perform routine ostomy maintenance, as indicated. Make sure the collection device fits tightly around the stoma; allow no more than a ⅛″ (0.3-cm) margin of skin between the stoma and the device's faceplate. Regularly check the appearance of the stoma and peristomal skin. The stoma should appear bright red; if it becomes deep red or bluish, suspect a problem with blood flow and notify the physician. It should also be smooth; report any dimpling or retraction, which may point to stenosis. Check the peristomal skin for irritation or breakdown. Remember that the main cause of irritation is urine leakage around the edges of the collection device's faceplate. If you detect leakage, change the device, taking care to properly apply the skin sealer to ensure a tight fit.
- If the patient has a continent internal ileal reservoir, irrigate the drainage tube as ordered (usually every 2 to 8 hours) with about 60 ml of normal saline solution to maintain its patency. To avoid abdominal distention during the postoperative period and allow suture lines to heal, perform irrigation gently.
- If skin breakdown occurs, clean the area with warm water and pat it dry; then apply a light dusting of karaya powder and a thin layer of protective dressing. If you detect severe excoriation, notify the physician promptly.
- Provide emotional support throughout the recovery period to help the patient adjust to the stoma and collection pouch or to self-catheterization, as indicated. Assure him that the pouch shouldn't interfere with his lifestyle and that he can eventually resume all of his former activities.

PATIENT TEACHING

- Before the patient goes home, make sure he and his family members understand and can properly perform stoma care and change the ostomy pouch. With a continent internal ileal reservoir, be sure they can care for the pouch drainage tube until it's removed (usually 3 weeks postoperatively), empty the pouch correctly (using either passive emptying or intermittent self-catheterization), and irrigate the pouch as necessary.
- Instruct the patient and his family members to watch for and report signs of complications, such as fever, chills, flank or abdominal pain, and pus or blood in the urine.
- Tell the patient that he should be able to return to work soon after discharge; however, if his job requires heavy lifting, tell him to talk to his physician before resuming work. Explain that he can safely participate in most sports, even such strenuous ones as skiing, skydiving, and scuba diving. Do, however, suggest that he avoid contact sports, such as football and wrestling.
- If the patient expresses doubts or insecurities about his sexuality related to the stoma and collection device, refer him for sexual counseling.
- Stress the importance of keeping scheduled follow-up appointments with the physician and enterostomal therapist to evaluate reservoir function and stoma care and make any necessary changes in equipment. For instance, stoma shrinkage, which normally occurs within 8 weeks after surgery, may require a change in pouch size to ensure a tight fit.

▶ Refer the patient to a support group such as the United Ostomy Association.

URINARY INCONTINENCE

Urinary incontinence is never a normal sign of aging. It's always a symptom of an underlying problem. Millions of older adults suffer from some loss of voluntary control. Problems with urinary continence are called acute or persistent and can range from mild loss of bladder control to total incontinence. Acute incontinence occurs suddenly and is usually related to an acute illness. Common in hospitalized people, it usually ends once the illness is resolved. Acute incontinence can also be associated with drugs, treatments, and environmental factors.

Persistent incontinence is classified as urge incontinence, stress incontinence, overflow incontinence, and functional incontinence. Urge incontinence is a sudden strong desire to void accompanied by a leakage of urine. Stress incontinence is a sudden leakage of urine associated with activity such as laughing, sneezing, coughing, lifting, jumping, or bending. Overflow incontinence is a frequent, sometimes constant leakage of urine from a too-full bladder. Functional incontinence occurs with an intact lower urinary tract as the result of immobility or cognitive impairment. Several types of incontinence may coexist.

Many older adults accept incontinence as a part of the aging process and don't report problems. Women who've had children often accept stress incontinence as a normal consequence of aging and childbearing. Incontinence can be embarrassing or frustrating, making some older adults reluctant to discuss it. They may fear surgery or be unaware that treatment options exist. Also, older adults often feel that health care professionals aren't interested in the problem.

Advertising is in part responsible for perpetuating the idea that incontinence is an acceptable, normal part of aging, as noted in commercials that use active, youthful-looking people to sell incontinence products. The advertisements fail to mention that all incontinence should be investigated by a health care provider, who may be able to eliminate the cause. The media present a misleading message of hopelessness to the older person.

Incontinence is a leading cause of nursing home placement. The costs of incontinence care — supplies, laundry, and nursing care — are extremely high. Continence is a learned ability, requiring an intact genitourinary tract, competent sphincters, adequate cognitive and physical function, motivation, and an appropriate environment for toileting.

Causes of acute incontinence include confusion, dehydration, prescribed drugs, urethritis, and atrophic vaginitis. Infection, especially a symptomatic urinary tract infection (UTI), can also cause incontinence. Urinary incontinence can be caused by some endocrine imbalances, such as hypercalcemia and hyperglycemia. Restricted mobility or conditions that cause urine retention can precipitate urinary incontinence. Or it may result from depression in the older adult.

Urge incontinence is the result of involuntary bladder contractions. Irritation of the detrusor muscle (the external muscle coating the bladder) caused by local irritating factors such as infection, stones, tumor, or obstruction can lead to urge incontinence, as can hyperactivity of the detrusor muscle associated with cerebrovascular accident, suprasacral spinal disease, Parkinson's disease, dementia, and demyelinating disease.

Stress incontinence is caused by weakened anatomic support in the pelvic floor. Perinatal trauma, tissue weakening associated with aging, estrogen deficiency, pudendal nerve damage, and gynecologic trauma from surgery can cause weakening of the pelvic floor. Drugs, such as alpha-adrenergic blockers, analgesics, sedatives, and hypnotics can cause bladder outlet relaxation and incontinence.

Overflow incontinence occurs when the bladder becomes overdistended due to incomplete emptying. The aging adult often is unable to feel the full bladder. More common in men, overflow incontinence can be caused by an atonic or underactive detrusor muscle or obstruction. Diabetes and drugs that lead to urine retention — such as analgesics, psychotropics, alpha-adrenergic agonists, calcium channel blockers, and anticholinergic agents — can decrease activity of the detrusor. Anatomic obstruction can include prostatic hypertrophy, pelvic prolapse, stricture, tumor, or neurogenic conditions, such as multiple sclerosis or suprasacral lesions.

Functional incontinence is caused by disruption of a person's continence routine. Immobility and cognitive impairment are two common causes. The use of physical or chemical restraints or environmental barriers such as side rails can lead to functional incontinence in an older adult. Psychological issues, such as depression, regression, or bipolar disorders, are other causes. Clothing that is difficult to remove is also a cause of functional incontinence.

Not every patient with cognitive impairment is incontinent, so incontinence shouldn't automatically be expected or accepted in these individuals. It isn't uncommon to see mixed incontinence of two or more types in an individual — for example, a patient may suffer from stress incontinence and functional incontinence.

Signs and symptoms

- Reports of feeling the urge to void, with inability to reach the bathroom before urination begins
- Urgency, frequency, and nocturia
- Stress incontinence, characterized by leaking of small amounts of urine when laughing, sneezing, jumping, coughing, or bending
- Overflow incontinence, characterized by a poor or slow stream and the feeling of hesitancy or straining
- Functional incontinence, characterized by adequate urine volume and stream
- Poor hygiene or signs of infection
- Bladder located above the symphysis pubis

Diagnostic tests

- *Urinalysis* is used to look for bacteria, blood, and glucose in urine.
- *Uroflowmetry* is used to evaluate voiding pattern and to demonstrate bladder outlet obstruction by measuring the flow rate of the stream as the patient voids.
- *Cystometry* is used to assess the bladder's neuromuscular function by measuring the efficiency of the detrusor muscle reflex, intravesical pressure and capacity, and the bladder's reaction to thermal stimulation.
- *Excretory urography*, also called *intravenous pyelography*, is used to evaluate the structure and function of the kidneys, ureter, and bladder.
- *Voiding cystourethrography* is used to detect abnormalities of the bladder and urethra and to assess hypertrophy of the prostate lobes, urethral stricture, and the degree of compromise of a stenotic prostatic urethra (in men).
- *Retrograde urethrography*, used almost exclusively in men, aids diagnosis of urethral stricture and outlet obstruction.
- *External sphincter electromyography* measures electrical activity of the external urinary sphincter.
- *Rectal examination* of the male patient may reveal prostate enlargement or pain, possibly indicating benign prostatic hypertrophy or infection. The examination may also reveal an impaction that may be responsible for the incontinence.
- *Vaginal examination* may reveal vaginal dryness or atrophic vaginitis, indicating estrogen deficiency.
- *Postvoid residual catheterization* is used to determine the extent of bladder emp-

tying and the amount of urine left in the bladder after the patient has voided.

Treatment

Drug therapies match the cause of the incontinence. An antibiotic is prescribed if incontinence is caused by inflammation caused by bacterial infection. Anticholinergic drugs are used to improve bladder function and treat bladder spasms if detrusor muscle instability is suspected. Antispasmodic drugs are prescribed for detrusor hyperreflexia to suppress the bladder's smooth muscle activity. Estrogen, in either oral, topical, or suppository form, is used if atrophic vaginitis is present. Stress incontinence can sometimes be treated with antidepressant drugs.

Behavioral therapies include bladder training, habit and clock training, prompted voiding, and pelvic muscle exercises (Kegel exercises). The approach is selected to suit the patient's underlying problem. Habit and bladder training are well suited to the patient with urge incontinence. Pelvic floor exercises can be well utilized by the cognitively intact patient with stress incontinence. Behavioral interventions generally aren't selected for patients with incontinence secondary to overflow. Additional techniques, such as biofeedback and electrical stimulation, serve as adjuncts to behavioral therapy.

Habit training, helpful for patients with dementia or cognitive impairment, involves maintaining a rigid voiding schedule, usually every 2 to 4 hours. The patient's objective is to void before an accident occurs. Bladder retraining may be useful for the patient who has full cognitive function. It teaches the patient to resist the urge to void, gradually increasing bladder capacity and the intervals between voiding. As capacity increases, urgency and frequency decrease.

A pessary may be prescribed for the female patient with an anatomic abnormality, such as severe uterine prolapse or pelvic relaxation. The pessary is worn internally, like a contraceptive diaphragm, and stabilizes the bladder's base and the urethra, preventing incontinence during physical strain.

Short-term use of a condom catheter may be prescribed for the male patient to effectively help him avoid accidents. Sustained use of a condom should be avoided, as it can lead to UTI and skin irritation.

An artificial sphincter — consisting of a silicone cuffed sphincter with a pressure-regulating balloon and a bulb pump — may be inserted in the male patient after radical prostatectomy or in the female patient with stress incontinence that is unresponsive to other treatment. The cuff is placed around the bladder neck. The balloon holds the fluid that is used to inflate the cuff. The bulb pump is implanted in the scrotum or labia. As the bladder fills with urine, the pressure-sensitive cuff inflates to prevent urine from leaking around the bladder neck. The patient squeezes the pump to move fluid from the cuff into the pressurized balloon, allowing urination.

Surgical repair of the anterior vaginal wall or retropubic suspension of the bladder and urethra may be options for treatment of women with stress incontinence. Retropubic suspension restores the bladder and urethra to their proper intra-abdominal positions.

In men with urge incontinence resulting from prostatic hypertrophy, treatment may include transurethral resection of the prostate or open prostatectomy. Surgery may be used to remove obstructive lesions that cause urge or overflow incontinence.

Patients with overflow incontinence from urine retention may benefit from intermittent catheterization. Removing barriers, providing a well-lit environment, and giving frequent orientation to the bathroom's location will help the patient with functional incontinence.

Key nursing diagnoses and outcomes

Impaired urinary elimination related to underlying cause of urinary incontinence
Treatment outcome: The patient will regain continence.

Risk for impaired skin integrity related to urinary incontinence
Treatment outcome: The patient will maintain skin integrity.

Disturbed body image related to incontinence
Treatment outcome: The patient will communicate positive feelings about the change in body image.

Nursing interventions

▶ Explain all tests and procedures to your patient. Allow him to ask questions, and answer them honestly. Provide privacy for any discussions.
▶ Administer antibiotics and other drugs, as ordered.
▶ Orient the patient to the location of the bathroom and any call devices. Provide adequate lighting in the bathroom to help him avoid mishaps during the night. If he needs help to get to the bathroom, offer it every 2 hours or when he awakens.
▶ Explain bladder training routines and post the schedule. Assist the patient receiving bladder training in deep-breathing exercises to delay the urge to void. Give ample, positive reinforcement for all efforts toward continence.
▶ Provide frequent perineal care, and watch the aging adult for skin breakdown. Wash with mild soap and water, and pat the skin to dry it. Wash from the front to the back to avoid spreading contamination.
▶ Help the patient insert a pessary, as ordered. If intermittent catheterization is ordered, perform it on time and document the amount of urine returned.
▶ For the postoperative patient, record accurate intake and output measurements. Provide catheter care and ambulate him as soon as permitted.

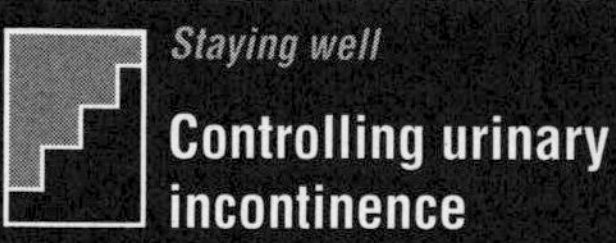

Staying well

Controlling urinary incontinence

Review the following information with your patient to help him control his urinary incontinence:

- Tell your patient that strong pelvic muscles can help prevent incontinence. Teach the female patient how to do Kegel exercises to strengthen muscles that control urine flow.
- Instruct the patient to limit or eliminate foods that irritate the bladder and cause urinary frequency, such as foods and beverages with caffeine (coffee, tea, cola, dark chocolate), alcohol, and the artificial sweetener aspartame. Explain that many prescription and nonprescription drugs also contain caffeine. Urge your patient to check food and drug labels carefully for this ingredient.
- Because urinary incontinence may stem from pressure on the bladder and the urethra due to constipation or fecal impaction, recommend a fiber-rich diet to help counter these conditions.

PATIENT TEACHING

▶ If the physician asks the patient to keep a record of fluid intake and voiding and incontinence episodes, advise him to review the record daily to make sure he's taking in at least eight 8-oz glasses (2,000 ml) of fluid daily. Explain that many incontinent patients consciously or unintentionally restrict fluids, which isn't the aim of treatment. Teach patients that a reduction in daytime fluid intake won't cure incontinence or the need to get up and void at night. If the patient is concerned about nocturia, suggest that he consume most fluids in the daytime and limit evening intake to small sips after 6 p.m.

▶ Teach the older person the actions and adverse effects of any drugs that are prescribed. If an antibiotic is ordered, stress the importance of taking all of the pills in the prescription.

▶ Describe all procedures and devices used to improve or manage urinary incontinence. (See *Controlling urinary incontinence,* page 599.) If habit training is in the treatment plan, be sure to include the patient's family members and other caregivers in your teaching. Stress the importance of keeping accurate records to help the physician monitor progress and adjust treatment. Direct the patient to urinate at the specified times, whether or not he feels the urge. If he needs to urinate at additional times, instruct him to do so immediately. Also tell him to urinate just before going to bed.

▶ If the patient is undergoing bladder retraining, demonstrate how to suppress the urge to void by breathing slowly and deeply. Encourage him to practice this procedure.

▶ Teach the patient with a pessary the correct technique for inserting and positioning the device. Also teach her to remove and clean it according to the physician's directions. Stress infection-prevention methods.

▶ Teach the male patient how to apply and wear a condom catheter, and point out ways to avoid complications such as contact dermatitis and penile maceration, ischemia, and obstruction.

▶ Review preoperative and postoperative instructions for the patient undergoing artificial sphincter implantation, including complications that may necessitate implant repair or removal. For example, the cuff or balloon can leak (uncommon) or trapped blood or other fluid contaminants can disable the bulb pump, impairing fluid passage to and from the cuff. Other complications include tissue erosion around the bulb or in the bladder neck or urethra, infection, inadequate occlusion pressure, and kinked tubing.

▶ Teach the patient and caregivers the correct technique for intermittent catheterization. Reassure them that although this procedure may seem difficult at first, practice makes it easier. Stress the importance of clean technique and tell them to report any signs of infection to the physician.

▶ For the woman undergoing surgical repair, explain that retropubic suspension restores the bladder and urethra to their proper intra-abdominal positions. Explain that the operation may be effective for only a short time in some women.

▶ For the male patient undergoing prostatic resection, explain the procedure and the preoperative and postoperative care.

▶ Discuss wearing protective pads and garments to augment habit training and bladder retraining. Mention that these absorbent devices boost comfort and confidence and allow the patient more mobility during treatment for urinary incontinence. Describe the different types available.

▶ Teach the patient how to prevent skin irritation and breakdown. After each incontinence episode, direct the patient to wash skin that's exposed to urine with mild soap and water. Instruct him to pat the area dry and then to apply a protective barrier cream.

URINARY TRACT INFECTION, LOWER

Lower urinary tract infections (UTIs) are the most common cause of bacterial sepsis in older adults. These infections are nearly 10 times more common in women than men — affecting 10% to 20% of all females at least once.

The two forms of lower UTI are cystitis (infection of the bladder) and urethritis (infection of the urethra). In adult males, lower UTIs typically are associated with anatomic or physiologic abnormalities and therefore need close evaluation. Most UTIs respond readily to treatment, but recurrence and resistant bacterial flare-ups during therapy are possible.

Weakened bladder muscles in women and enlarged prostates in men — changes associated with aging — can contribute to incomplete emptying of the bladder. Incontinence and the decreased ability of aging people to provide proper hygiene for themselves also increase the incidence of UTI by giving bacteria an entry route to the bladder. Older adults with chronic indwelling catheters are also at higher risk because the catheter provides an entry port for bacteria.

Most lower UTIs are caused by ascending infection by a gram-negative, enteric bacterium, such as *Escherichia coli, Klebsiella, Proteus, Enterobacter, Pseudomonas,* and *Serratia.* In a person with neurogenic bladder, an indwelling urinary catheter, or a fistula between the intestine and bladder, a lower UTI may result from simultaneous infection with multiple pathogens.

Studies suggest that infection results from a breakdown in local defense mechanisms in the bladder, which allows bacteria to invade the bladder mucosa and multiply. These bacteria can't be eliminated readily by normal urination.

Bacterial flare-up during treatment usually is caused by the pathogen's resistance to the prescribed antimicrobial therapy. Even a small number of bacteria (fewer than 10,000/ml) in a midstream urine specimen obtained during treatment casts doubt on the effectiveness of treatment.

In almost all patients, recurrent lower UTIs result from reinfection by the same organism or by some new pathogen. In the remaining patients, recurrence is associated with renal calculi, chronic bacterial prostatitis, or a structural anomaly that's a source of persistent infection.

The high incidence of lower UTI among females probably occurs because natural anatomic features facilitate infection. The female urethra is shorter than the male urethra (about 1″ to 2″ [2.5 to 5 cm] compared with 7″ to 8″ [18 to 20 cm]). It's also closer to the anus, allowing bacterial entry into the urethra from the vagina, perineum, or rectum, or from a sexual partner. In young men, release of prostatic fluid serves as an antibacterial shield. Men lose this protection around age 50 when the prostate gland begins to enlarge, resulting in a higher incidence of infection in older men.

Fecal matter, sexual intercourse, and instruments such as catheters and cystoscopes can introduce bacteria into the urinary tract and trigger infection. A narrowed ureter or calculi lodged in the ureter or bladder can obstruct urine flow. Slowed urine flow allows bacteria to remain and multiply, posing a risk of damage to the kidneys. Urinary stasis can promote infection, which, if undetected, can spread to the entire urinary system. In addition, because urinary tract bacteria thrive on sugars, diabetes is also a risk factor.

Vesicourethral reflux results when pressure inside the bladder (caused by coughing or sneezing) pushes a small amount of urine from the bladder into the urethra. When the pressure returns to normal, the urine flows back into the bladder, bringing bacteria from the urethra with it. In vesicoureteral reflux, urine flows from the bladder back into one or both ureters. The vesicoureteral valve normally shuts off reflux, but a damaged valve may not do its job.

Signs and symptoms

- Nausea, vomiting, and loss of appetite
- Bladder cramps or spasms
- Itching, a feeling of warmth during urination

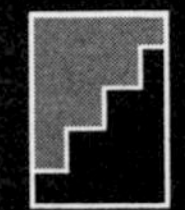

Staying well

Preventing lower UTIs

To help your patient prevent recurrent lower UTIs:

- Explain that fruit juices, especially cranberry juice, and oral doses of vitamin C may help acidify urine and enhance the action of some drugs. If the patient's condition allows, urge her to drink at least eight 8-oz (2,000 ml) glasses of fluid daily during treatment. More or less than this amount may alter the effects of antimicrobial drugs. Be aware that the aging adult may resist this suggestion because it causes her to make frequent trips, possibly up and down stairs, to urinate.
- Teach an older woman to carefully wipe the perineum from front to back and to thoroughly clean it with soap and water after bowel movements. If she is infection-prone, she should urinate immediately after sexual intercourse. Tell her never to postpone urination and to empty her bladder completely.
- Tell the male patient that prompt treatment of predisposing conditions, such as chronic prostatitis, helps prevent recurrent UTIs.

- Low back pain
- Chills
- Flank pain
- Foul-smelling urine
- Low-grade fever (may not occur in older patients)
- Male patient with a urethral discharge

Key point Often the first sign of lower UTI in an older adult is decreased alertness. The patient may not consider earlier symptoms significant.

Diagnostic tests

- *Microscopic urinalysis* showing red blood cell and white blood cell counts greater than 10 per high-power field suggests lower UTI.
- *Clean-catch urinalysis* revealing a bacterial count of more than 100,000/ml confirms UTI. Lower counts don't necessarily rule out infection, especially if the patient urinates frequently, because bacteria require 30 to 45 minutes to reproduce in urine. Clean-catch collection is preferred to catheterization, which can reinfect the bladder with urethral bacteria. However, catheterization may be the only option in an older patient.
- *Sensitivity testing* is used to determine the appropriate antimicrobial drug.
- *Voiding cystourethrography or excretory urography* may disclose congenital anomalies that predispose a person to recurrent UTI.

Treatment

Appropriate antimicrobials are the treatment of choice for most initial lower UTIs. A 7- to 10-day course of antibiotics is standard. Although studies suggest that a single dose or a 3- to 5-day regimen may be sufficient to render urine sterile, older patients may still need 7 to 10 days of antibiotics to fully benefit from treatment.

A repeat culture is done to rule out resistance. If the culture shows that urine isn't sterile after 3 days of antibiotic therapy, bacterial resistance probably has occurred, requiring a different antimicrobial.

A single dose of amoxicillin or co-trimoxazole may be effective for females with an acute, uncomplicated lower UTI. A urine culture taken 1 to 2 weeks later indicates whether the infection has been eradicated. Recurrent infections due to infected renal calculi, chronic prostatitis, or structural abnormalities may require surgery. Prostatitis also requires long-term antibiotic therapy. In older adults without these predisposing conditions, long-term, low-dose antibiotic therapy is the treatment of choice.

Because of the adverse GI and renal effects associated with antimicrobial therapy, asymptomatic UTIs are often left untreated.

Key nursing diagnoses and outcomes

Impaired urinary elimination related to inflammation of the lower urinary tract

Treatment outcome: The patient will regain and maintain normal urinary elimination.

Risk for infection related to high incidence of recurrent UTIs

Treatment outcome: The patient will remain free from recurrent UTIs as exhibited by a normal urinalysis and the absence of signs and symptoms of UTI.

Acute pain related to bladder spasms and cramps

Treatment outcome: The patient will become free from pain when the UTI is eliminated.

Nursing interventions

- Watch for GI disturbances from antimicrobial therapy. If ordered, give nitrofurantoin macrocrystals with milk or meals to prevent GI distress.
- If sitz baths don't relieve perineal discomfort, apply warm compresses sparingly to the perineum, but be careful not to burn the patient.
- Apply topical antiseptics on the urethral meatus, as necessary.
- Collect all urine specimens for culture and sensitivity testing carefully and promptly.

PATIENT TEACHING

- Explain the nature and purpose of antimicrobial therapy. Emphasize the importance of completing the prescribed course of therapy and strictly adhering to the ordered dosage.
- Familiarize the patient with prescribed drugs and their possible adverse effects. Suggest taking nitrofurantoin macrocrystals with milk or a meal to prevent GI distress. Warn the patient that phenazopyridine turns urine red-orange and stains clothing.
- Explain that an uncontaminated midstream urine specimen is essential for accurate diagnosis. Before collection, teach an older woman to clean the perineum properly and to keep the labia separated during urination.
- Suggest warm sitz baths for relief of perineal discomfort.
- Encourage the patient to wear cotton undergarments and avoid perfumed powders or bath oils.
- Explain to the patient practices that can help prevent future lower UTIs. (See *Preventing lower UTIs.*)

URINE SPECIMEN COLLECTION

A random urine specimen, usually collected as part of the physical examination or at various times during a stay in a health care facility, permits laboratory screening for urinary and systemic disorders as well as for drug screening. A clean-catch midstream specimen, once used only to confirm urinary tract infection, is now replacing random collection for many other purposes because it provides a virtually uncontaminated specimen without the need for bladder catheterization.

An indwelling catheter specimen — obtained either by clamping the drainage tube and emptying the accumulated urine into a container or by aspirating a sample with a syringe — requires aseptic technique to prevent catheter contamination and urinary tract infection. This method is contraindicated in patients who have recently undergone genitourinary surgery.

Supplies

For all specimens

- Gloves
- Label
- Laboratory request form

For a random specimen

- Bedpan or urinal with cover, if necessary
- Graduated container
- Specimen container with lid

For a clean-catch midstream specimen

- Basin
- Soap and water
- Towel
- Three sterile 2″ × 2″ gauze pads
- Povidone-iodine solution
- Sterile specimen container with lid
- Bedpan or urinal, if necessary

Commercial clean-catch kits containing antiseptic towelettes, sterile specimen container with lid and label, and instructions for use in several languages are widely used.

For an indwelling catheter specimen

- 20- or 30-ml syringe
- 21G or 22G 1½″ needle
- Tube clamp
- Sterile specimen cup with lid
- Alcohol pad

Implementation

- Explain the procedure to the patient and his family member, if necessary, to promote cooperation and prevent accidental disposal of specimens.
- Because the goal of a clean-catch midstream specimen is a virtually uncontaminated specimen, explain the procedure to the patient carefully. Provide illustrations to emphasize the correct collection technique, if possible.
- Inform the patient that you need a urine specimen for laboratory analysis.

Collecting a random specimen

- Provide privacy. Instruct the patient on bed rest to void into a clean bedpan or urinal, or ask the ambulatory patient to void into either one in the bathroom.
- Put on gloves. Then pour at least 120 ml of urine into the specimen container, and cap the container securely. If the patient's urine output must be measured and recorded, pour the remaining urine into the graduated container. Otherwise, discard the remaining urine. If you inadvertently spill urine on the outside of the container, clean and dry it to prevent possible cross-contamination.
- Label the specimen container with the patient's name and room number and the date and time of collection, attach the request form, and send it to the laboratory immediately. Delaying the specimen may alter test results.
- Clean the graduated container and urinal or bedpan, and return these to their proper storage. Discard disposable items.
- Wash your hands thoroughly to prevent cross-contamination.
- Offer the patient a washcloth and soap and water to wash his hands.

Collecting a clean-catch midstream specimen

- Tell the patient to remove all clothing from the waist down and to stand in front of the toilet as for urination or, if female, to sit far back on the toilet seat and spread her legs. Then have the patient clean the periurethral area (tip of the penis or labial folds, vulva, and urethral meatus) with soap and water and then wipe the area three times, each time with a fresh 2″ × 2″ gauze pad soaked in povidone-iodine solution or with the wipes provided in a commercial kit. Instruct the female patient to separate her labial folds with her thumb and forefinger. Tell her to wipe down one side with the first pad and discard it, to wipe the other side with the second pad and discard it and, finally, to wipe down the center over the urinary meatus with the third pad and discard it. Stress the importance of cleaning from front to back to avoid contaminating the genital area with fecal matter. For the uncircumcised male patient, emphasize the need to retract his foreskin to effectively clean the meatus and to keep it retracted during voiding.

▶ Tell the female patient to straddle the bedpan or toilet to allow labial spreading. She should continue to keep her labia separated with her fingers while voiding.

▶ Instruct the patient to begin voiding into the bedpan, urinal, or toilet because the urine stream washes bacteria from the urethra and urinary meatus. Then, without stopping the urine stream, the patient should move the collection container into the stream, collecting about 30 to 50 ml at the midstream portion of the voiding. The patient can then finish voiding into the bedpan, urinal, or toilet.

▶ Put on gloves before discarding the first and last portions of the voiding, and measure the remaining urine in a graduated cylinder for intake and output records, if necessary. Be sure to include the amount in the specimen container when recording the total amount voided.

▶ Take the sterile container from the patient, and cap it securely. Avoid touching the inside of the container or the lid. If the outside of the container is soiled, clean it and wipe it dry. Remove gloves and discard them properly.

▶ Wash your hands thoroughly to prevent cross-contamination. Tell the patient to wash his hands too.

▶ Label the container with the patient's name and room number, name of test, collection date and time, and suspected diagnosis, if known. If a urine culture has been ordered, note any current antibiotic therapy on the laboratory request form. Send the container to the laboratory immediately, or place it on ice to prevent specimen deterioration and altered test results.

Aspirating a urine specimen

If the patient has an indwelling urinary catheter in place, clamp the tube distal to the aspiration port for about 30 minutes. Wipe the port with an alcohol pad, and insert a needle with a 20- or 30-ml syringe into the port perpendicular to the tube, as shown below. Aspirate the required amount of urine, and expel it into the specimen container. Remove the clamp on the drainage tube.

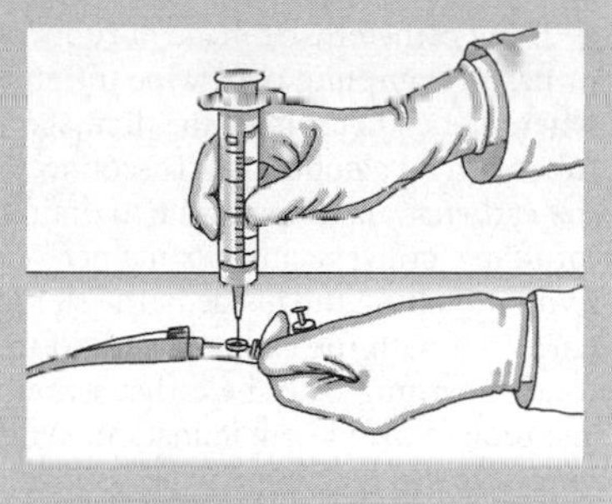

▶ Perform the procedure for the patient if he has difficulty with mobility or hand manipulation.

Collecting an indwelling catheter specimen

▶ About 30 minutes before collecting the specimen, clamp the drainage tube to allow urine to accumulate.

▶ Put on gloves. If the drainage tube has a built-in sampling port, wipe the port with an alcohol pad. Uncap the needle on the syringe, and insert the needle into the sampling port at a 90-degree angle to the tubing. Aspirate the specimen into the syringe. (See *Aspirating a urine specimen.*)

▶ If the drainage tube doesn't have a sampling port and the catheter is made of rubber, obtain the specimen from the catheter. Other types of catheters will leak after you withdraw the needle. To withdraw the specimen from a rubber catheter, wipe it with an alcohol pad just above the point where it connects to the drainage tube. Insert the needle into the rubber catheter at a 45-degree angle and withdraw the specimen. Never insert the needle into the shaft of the catheter because this may puncture the lumen leading to the catheter balloon.

- Transfer the specimen to a sterile container, label it, and send it to the laboratory immediately or place it on ice. If a urine culture is to be performed, be sure to list any antibiotic therapy on the laboratory request form.
- If the catheter isn't made of rubber or has no sampling port, wipe the area where the catheter joins the drainage tube with an alcohol pad. Disconnect the catheter, and allow urine to drain into the sterile specimen container. Avoid touching the inside of the sterile container with the catheter, and don't touch anything with the catheter drainage tube to avoid contamination. When you have the specimen, wipe both connection sites with an alcohol pad and join them. Cap the specimen container, label it, and send it to the laboratory immediately or place it on ice.

Key point Make sure you unclamp the drainage tube after collecting the specimen to prevent urine backflow that may cause bladder distention and infection.

Complications

Improper specimen collection could lead to misdiagnosis.

Patient teaching

- Explain to the patient the necessity for the specimen collection.

Documentation

Record the times of specimen collection and transport to the laboratory. Specify the test, and the appearance, odor, color, and any unusual characteristics of the specimen. If necessary, record the urine volume on the patient's intake and output records. Document patient teaching measures and their effect.

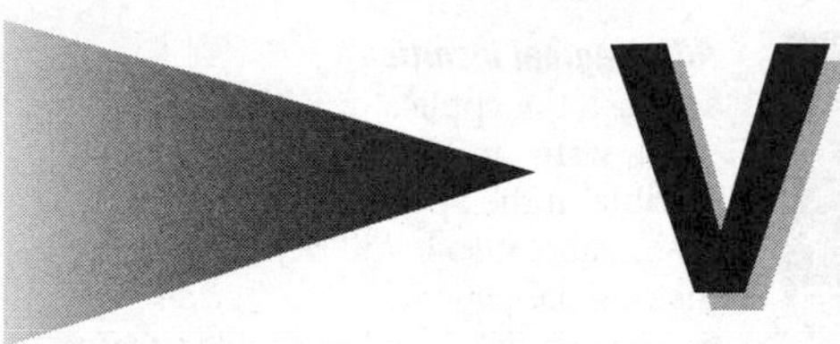

VAGINAL MEDICATION ADMINISTRATION

Vaginal medications are prepared as suppositories, creams, gels, and ointments. These drugs can be inserted as topical treatment for infection (particularly *Trichomonas vaginalis* and monilial vaginitis) or inflammation. Suppositories melt when they contact the vaginal mucosa, and their ingredients diffuse topically—as effectively as creams, gels, and ointments.

Vaginal drugs usually come with a disposable applicator that enables placement of the drug in the anterior and posterior fornices. Vaginal administration is most effective when the patient can remain lying down afterward to retain the drug. With reduced estrogen secretion, older women experience vaginal changes that increase their risk for atrophic vaginitis and infection, requiring vaginal treatment.

Supplies

- Patient's medication record and chart
- Prescribed drug
- Applicator, if necessary
- Gloves
- Water-soluble lubricant
- Small sanitary pad

Implementation

- If possible, plan to give vaginal drugs at bedtime, when the patient is recumbent.
- Verify the order on the patient's medication record by checking it against the physician's order.
- Confirm the patient's identity by asking her name and checking the name, room number, and bed number on her wristband.
- Provide privacy.
- Ask the patient to void.

How to insert a vaginal suppository

Place the suppository in the tip of an applicator. Then lubricate the applicator, hold it by the cylinder, and insert it into the vagina. To ensure the patient's comfort, direct the applicator down initially (toward the spine) and then up and back (toward the cervix), as shown here. When the suppository reaches the distal end of the vagina, depress the plunger.

Remove the applicator while the plunger is still depressed.

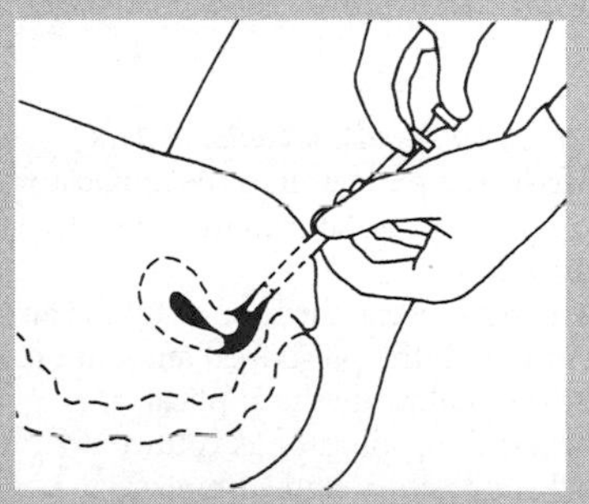

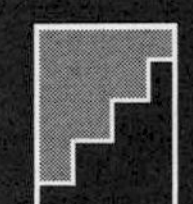

Staying well

Preventing vaginal infections

Discuss with the patient methods to reduce the occurrence of vaginal infections, such as:

- practicing good hygiene (using soap and water to clean after a bowel movement)
- voiding after sexual intercourse
- using a water soluble lubricant for sexual activity
- using barrier devices, such as a condom, to prevent the spread of sexually transmitted diseases.

▶ Ask the patient if she would rather insert the drug herself. If so, provide appropriate instructions. If not, proceed with the following steps.
▶ Help her into the lithotomy position.
▶ Expose only the perineum.

Inserting a suppository

▶ Remove the suppository from the wrapper, and lubricate it with water-soluble lubricant.
▶ Put on gloves and expose the vagina.
▶ With an applicator or the forefinger of your free hand, insert the suppository about 2″ (5 cm) into the vagina. (See *How to insert a vaginal suppository,* page 607.)

Inserting ointments, creams, or gels

▶ Insert the plunger into the applicator. Then fit the applicator to the tube of medication.
▶ Gently squeeze the tube to fill the applicator with the prescribed amount of the drug. Lubricate the applicator.
▶ Insert the applicator as you would a small suppository, and administer the drug by depressing the plunger on the applicator.

After vaginal insertion

▶ Wash the applicator with soap and warm water and store it, unless it is disposable. If the applicator can be used again, label it so it will be used only for the original patient.
▶ To keep the drug from soiling the patient's clothing and bedding, provide a sanitary pad.
▶ Help the patient return to a comfortable position, and advise her to remain in bed as much as possible for the next several hours.
▶ Wash your hands thoroughly.
▶ Refrigerate vaginal suppositories that melt at room temperature.

Complications

Vaginal drugs may cause local irritation.

Patient teaching

▶ Explain the procedure to the patient. Provide the rationale for the drug therapy as well as any possible adverse effects.
▶ Tell the patient to report any adverse effects promptly.
▶ Explain to the patient practices that may reduce her risk of future vaginal infections. (See *Preventing vaginal infections.*)

Documentation

Record the drug administered, the time, and the date. Note adverse effects and any other pertinent information. Document your patient teaching measures and their effect.

VALVULOPLASTY, BALLOON

Balloon valvuloplasty is used to enlarge the orifice of a heart valve that's stenotic because of a congenital defect, calcification, rheumatic fever, or aging. A physician performs valvuloplasty in a cardiac catheterization laboratory by inserting a balloon-tipped catheter through the femoral vein or artery, threading it into the heart, and repeatedly inflating it against the leaflets of the diseased valve.

Despite valvuloplasty's benefits, the treatment of choice for valvular heart disease remains surgery—either valve replacement or commissurotomy. But for those who are considered poor candidates for surgery, valvuloplasty offers an alternative.

Implementation

After preparing and anesthetizing the catheter insertion site, the physician inserts a catheter into the femoral artery (for left-heart valves) or femoral vein (for right-heart valves). He then passes the balloon-tipped catheter through this catheter and, guided by fluoroscopy, slowly threads it into the heart.

Next, he positions the deflated balloon in the valve opening and repeatedly inflates it with a solution containing normal saline and a contrast medium. As the balloon inflates, the valve leaflets split free from one another, permitting them to open and close properly and increasing the valvular orifice.

Valvuloplasty is considered a success if hemodynamic pressure decreases across the valve after balloon inflation. If it does, the physician removes the balloon-tipped catheter. However, he'll leave the other catheter in place, in case the patient needs to return to the laboratory for a repeat procedure.

Complications

Balloon valvuloplasty can worsen valvular insufficiency by misshaping the valve so that it doesn't close completely. Another serious complication is embolism caused by pieces of the calcified valve breaking off and traveling to the brain or lungs. In addition, valvuloplasty can cause severe damage to the delicate valve leaflets, requiring immediate surgery to replace the valve. Other complications include bleeding and hematoma at the arterial puncture site, arrhythmias, myocardial ischemia, myocardial infarction (MI), and circulatory defects distal to the catheter entry site.

Older patients with aortic disease frequently experience restenosis 1 to 2 years after undergoing valvuloplasty. Fortunately, the most serious complications of valvuloplasty—valvular destruction, MI, and calcium emboli— rarely occur.

Key nursing diagnoses and outcomes

Anxiety related to valvuloplasty

Treatment outcome: The patient will exhibit healthy behaviors to cope with anxiety.

Risk for injury related to complications of valvuloplasty

Treatment outcome: The patient will not sustain an injury as a result of valvuloplasty.

Risk for imbalanced fluid volume related to bleeding from insertion site during and after valvuloplasty

Treatment outcome: The patient will maintain normal vital signs and urine output.

Nursing interventions

Before the procedure

- Reinforce the physician's explanation of the procedure, including its risks and alternatives, to the patient. Restrict food and fluid intake for at least 6 hours before valvuloplasty, or as ordered.
- Explain that the patient will have an I.V. line inserted to provide access for any drugs. Mention that the patient's groin area will be shaved and cleaned with an antiseptic and that he'll feel a brief stinging sensation when a local anesthetic is injected.
- In simple and reassuring terms, explain that the physician will insert a catheter into an artery or vein in the groin area and that the patient may feel pressure as the catheter moves along the vessel. Also explain to the patient that he needs to be awake because the physi-

cian may need him to take deep breaths (to allow visualization of the catheter) and to answer questions about how he's feeling. Warn him that the procedure lasts up to 4 hours and that he may feel discomfort from lying flat on a hard table during that time.

▶ Ensure that the patient has signed a consent form.

▶ Make sure the results of routine laboratory studies and blood typing and crossmatching are available. Just before the procedure, palpate the bilateral distal pulses (usually the dorsalis pedis or posterior tibial pulses) and mark them with indelible ink. Take vital signs and assess color, temperature, and sensation in the patient's extremities to serve as a baseline for post-treatment assessment. Administer a sedative, as ordered.

▶ Once you've prepared the patient, place a 5-lb (2.3-kg) sandbag on his bed to be used later for applying pressure over the puncture site.

After the procedure

▶ When the patient returns to the critical care unit or postanesthesia area, he may be receiving I.V. heparin or nitroglycerin. He'll also have the sandbag placed over the cannulation site to minimize bleeding until the arterial catheter is removed. In addition, he will require continuous arterial and electrocardiogram monitoring.

▶ To prevent excessive hip flexion and migration of the catheter, keep the affected leg straight and elevate the head of the bed no more than 15 degrees. (At mealtime, you can elevate the head of the bed 15 to 30 degrees.) For the first hour, monitor vital signs every 15 minutes, then every 30 minutes for 2 hours, and then hourly for the next 5 hours. If vital signs are unstable, notify the physician and continue to check them every 5 minutes.

▶ When you take vital signs, assess peripheral pulses distal to the insertion site and the color, temperature, and capillary refill time of the extremity. If pulses are difficult to palpate because of the size of the arterial catheter, use a Doppler stethoscope. Notify the physician if pulses are absent.

▶ Observe the catheter insertion site for hematoma formation, ecchymosis, or hemorrhage. If an expanding ecchymotic area appears, mark the area to help determine the pace of expansion. If bleeding occurs, apply direct pressure and notify the physician.

▶ Following the physician's orders or your facility's protocol, auscultate regularly for murmurs, which may indicate worsening valvular insufficiency. Notify the physician if you detect a new or worsening murmur.

▶ Provide I.V. fluids at a rate of at least 100 ml/hour, or as ordered, to help the kidneys excrete the contrast medium. But be sure to assess for signs of fluid overload: distended neck veins, atrial and ventricular gallops, dyspnea, pulmonary congestion, tachycardia, hypertension, and hypoxemia.

▶ The physician will remove the catheter 6 to 12 hours after valvuloplasty. Afterward, apply a pressure dressing and assess vital signs according to the same schedule you used when the patient first returned to the unit.

PATIENT TEACHING

▶ Tell the patient that he can resume normal activity. Most patients with successful valvuloplasties experience increased exercise tolerance.

▶ Instruct the patient to call his physician if he experiences any bleeding or increased bruising at the puncture site or any recurrence of symptoms of valvular insufficiency, such as breathlessness or decreased exercise tolerance.

▶ Stress the need for regular follow-up visits with his physician.

VASCULAR ACCESS PORT MANAGEMENT

A vascular access device is surgically implanted under local anesthesia by a physician. The device consists of a silicone catheter attached to a reservoir, which is covered with a self-sealing silicone rubber septum. Such a device is used most commonly when an external central venous (CV) catheter isn't desirable for long-term I.V. therapy. The most common type of vascular access device is a vascular access port (VAP). One- and two-piece units with single or double lumens are available. (See *Understanding vascular access ports,* page 612.)

VAPs come in two basic types: top-entry and side-entry. The VAP reservoir can be made of titanium, stainless steel, or molded plastic. The type of port and catheter size to be used depends on the patient's therapeutic needs.

Implanted in a pocket under the skin, a VAP functions much like a long-term CV catheter, except that it has no external parts. The attached indwelling catheter tunnels through the subcutaneous tissue so the catheter tip lies in a central vein (the subclavian vein, for example). A VAP can also be used for arterial access or can be implanted into the epidural space, peritoneum, or pericardial or pleural cavity.

Typically, VAPs deliver intermittent infusions. Usually used for chemotherapy, a VAP can also deliver I.V. fluids, drugs, or blood products. You can also use a VAP to obtain blood samples.

VAPs offer several advantages, including minimal activity restrictions, few self-care measures for the patient to learn and perform, and few dressing changes (except when used to maintain continuous infusions or intermittent infusion devices). Implanted devices are easier to maintain than external devices. For instance, they require heparinization only once after each use (or periodically if not in use). They also pose less risk of infection because they have no exit site to serve as an entry for microorganisms.

Because VAPs create only a slight protrusion under the skin, many patients find them easier to accept than external infusion devices. However, because the device is implanted, the older person might find it more difficult to manage, particularly if he must administer drugs or fluids daily or frequently, or if his fine motor skills and manual dexterity are impaired. Some persons who fear or dislike needle punctures could be uncomfortable using a VAP and might require a local anesthetic. In addition, implantation and removal of the device requires surgery and hospitalization. The comparatively high cost of VAPs makes them worthwhile only for patients who require infusion therapy for at least 6 months.

Implanted VAPs are contraindicated in patients who have been unable to tolerate other implanted devices and in those who may develop allergic reactions. Be prepared to handle several common problems that could arise during infusion with a VAP, including an inability to flush the VAP, withdraw blood from it, or palpate it.

Supplies

- Patient's medication record and chart

For a bolus injection

- Extension set
- 10-ml syringe filled with normal saline solution
- Clamp
- Syringe containing prescribed drug
- Optional: a sterile needle filled with heparin flush solution

For a continuous infusion

- Prescribed I.V. solution or drug
- I.V. administration set
- Filter, if ordered
- Extension set
- Clamp

Understanding vascular access ports

Typically, a vascular access port (VAP) is used to deliver intermittent infusion of medication, chemotherapy, or blood products. Because the device is completely covered by the patient's skin, it reduces the risk of extrinsic contamination. Patients sometimes prefer this type of central line because it doesn't alter body image and it requires less routine catheter care.

The VAP consists of a catheter connected to a small reservoir. A septum designed to withstand multiple punctures seals the reservoir.

VAPs come in two basic designs: top-entry and side-entry. In a top-entry port, the needle is inserted perpendicular to the reservoir. In a side-entry port, the needle is inserted into the septum nearly parallel to the reservoir. (A needle stop prevents the needle from coming out the other side.)

Top-entry VAP

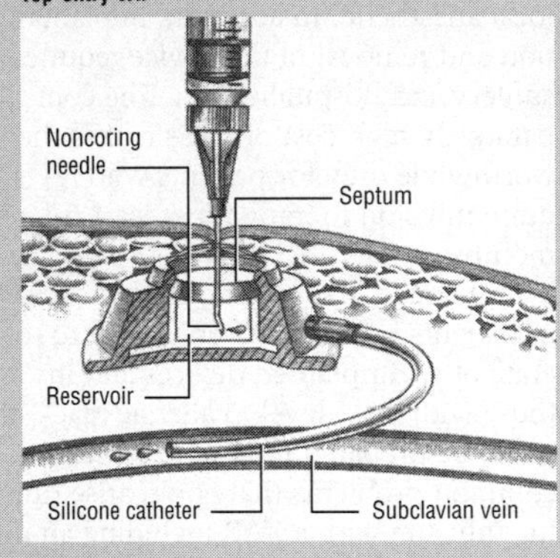

Side-entry VAP

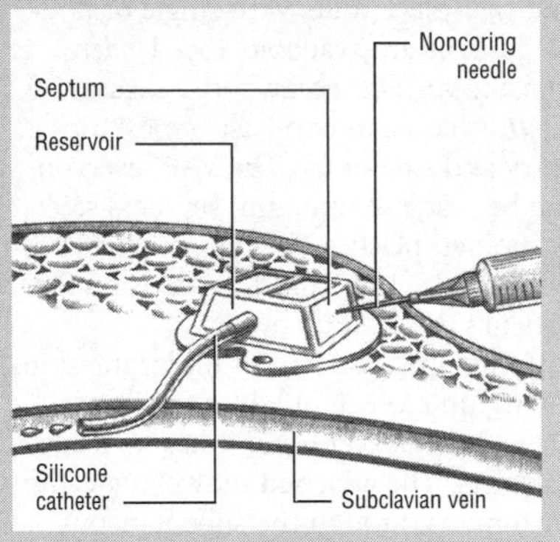

- 10-ml syringe filled with normal saline solution
- Antimicrobial ointment
- Adhesive tape
- Sterile 2″ × 2″ gauze pad
- Sterile tape
- Transparent semipermeable dressing

Some facilities use an implantable-port access kit.

Implementation

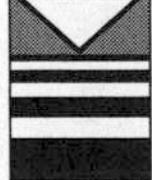

Key point The VAP can be used immediately after placement, although some edema and tenderness might persist for about 72 hours. This makes the device initially difficult to palpate and slightly uncomfortable for the patient.

- Using aseptic technique, inspect the area around the port for signs of infection or skin breakdown.
- Place an ice pack over the area for several minutes to alleviate possible discomfort from the needle puncture. Or you can administer a local anesthetic after cleaning the area (see below).
- Wash your hands thoroughly and put on sterile gloves. Keep the gloves on throughout the procedure.
- Clean the area with an alcohol pad, starting at the center of the port and working outward with a firm, circular motion over a 4″ to 5″ (10- to 13-cm) diameter. Repeat this procedure twice.
- If your facility's policy calls for a local anesthetic, check the patient's record for possible allergies. As indicated, anes-

thetize the insertion site by injecting 0.1 ml of lidocaine (without epinephrine).

Accessing a top-entry port

- Palpate the area over the port to locate the port septum.
- Anchor the port with your nondominant hand. Then, using your dominant hand, aim the needle at the center of the device.
- Insert the needle perpendicular to the port septum. Push the needle through the skin and septum until you reach the bottom of the reservoir.
- Check needle placement by aspirating for blood return.
- If you're unable to obtain blood, remove the needle and repeat the procedure. Inability to obtain blood may indicate that the catheter is lodged against the vessel's wall. Ask the patient to raise his arms, perform Valsalva's maneuver (if not contraindicated), or change position to free the catheter. If you still don't get a blood return, notify the physician; a coating of fibrin (fibrin sleeve) on the distal end of the catheter may be occluding the opening.
- Flush the device with normal saline solution. If you detect swelling or the patient reports pain at the site, remove the needle and notify the physician.

Accessing a side-entry port

- To gain access to a side-entry port, follow the same procedure as with a top-entry port; however, insert the needle parallel to the reservoir instead of perpendicular to it.

Giving a bolus injection

- Attach the 10-ml syringe filled with saline solution to the end of the extension set and remove all the air. Next, attach the extension set to the noncoring needle. Check for blood return. Then flush the port with normal saline solution, according to your facility's policy. (Some require flushing the port with a sterile needle containing heparin solution first.)
- Clamp the extension set and remove the saline syringe.
- Connect the drug syringe to the extension set. Open the clamp and inject the drug, as ordered.
- Examine the skin surrounding the needle for signs of infiltration, such as swelling or tenderness. If you note these signs, stop the injection and intervene appropriately.
- Assess the implant site for signs of infection, device rotation, or skin erosion. You don't need to apply a dressing to the wound site except during infusions or to maintain an intermittent infusion device.
- While the patient is hospitalized, a luer-lock injection cap may be attached to the end of the extension set to provide ready access for intermittent infusions.
- If your patient is receiving an intermittent infusion, flush the port periodically with heparin solution. When the VAP isn't being used, flush it every 4 weeks. During the course of therapy, you might have to clear a clotted VAP, as ordered.
- When the injection is complete, clamp the extension set and remove the syringe.
- Open the clamp and flush with 5 ml of normal saline solution after each drug injection to minimize drug incompatibility reactions.
- Flush with heparin solution, as your facility's policy directs.

Giving a continuous infusion

- Remove all air from the extension set by priming it with an attached syringe of normal saline solution. Next, attach the extension set to the noncoring needle.
- Flush the port system with normal saline solution. Clamp the extension set and remove the syringe.

- Connect the administration set, and secure the connections with sterile tape if necessary.
- Unclamp the extension set and begin the infusion.
- Apply a small amount of antimicrobial ointment to the insertion site.
- Affix the needle to the skin. Then apply a transparent semipermeable dressing.
- Examine the site carefully for infiltration. If the patient complains of stinging, burning, or pain at the site, discontinue the infusion and intervene appropriately.
- When the solution container is empty, obtain a new I.V. solution container as ordered.
- Flush with heparin solution as your facility's policy directs.
- Change the dressing and needle every 5 to 7 days. Also change the tubing and solution as you would for a long-term CV infusion.

Complications

Infection and bleeding are possible complications of a VAP.

Patient teaching

- Teach the patient and his family proper VAP care.
- Instruct the patient to report any signs of infection, such as redness or swelling.

Documentation

Document the date and time the VAP was accessed as well as the reason for using the port. Note the condition of the site.

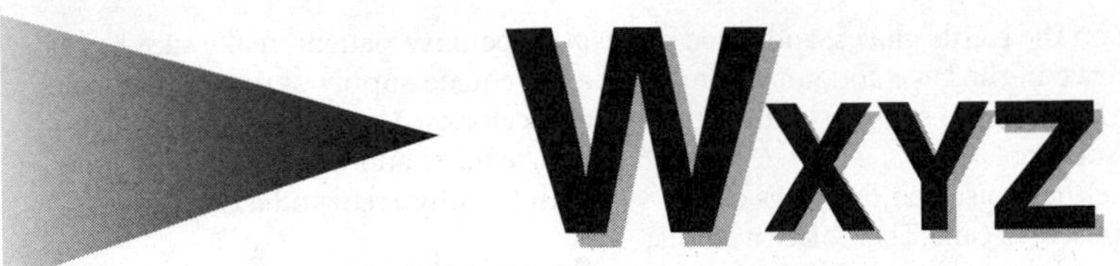

Wound dehiscence

Although the typical surgical wound heals without incident, occasionally the edges of a wound may fail to join, or they may separate even after they appear to be healing normally. This development, called wound dehiscence, may lead to evisceration, an even more serious complication, in which a portion of the viscera (usually a bowel loop) protrudes through the incision. Evisceration, in turn, can lead to peritonitis and septic shock. Dehiscence and evisceration are most likely to occur 6 or 7 days after surgery. By then, sutures may have been removed and the patient can cough easily and breathe deeply—both of which strain the incision.

Older people are at increased risk for this condition because of age-related changes that delay wound healing. Several other factors can contribute to these complications. Poor nutrition—whether from inadequate intake or a condition such as diabetes mellitus—may hinder wound healing, as may chronic pulmonary or cardiac disease, which deprives the injured tissue of sufficient nutrients and oxygen. Localized wound infection may limit closure, delay healing, and weaken the incision. Also, stress on the incision from coughing or vomiting may cause abdominal distention or severe stretching; for example, a patient with a midline abdominal incision has a high risk of developing wound dehiscence.

Supplies

- Two sterile towels
- 1 L normal sterile saline solution
- Sterile irrigation set (basin, a solution container, and a 50-ml catheter-tip syringe)
- Several large abdominal dressings
- Sterile, waterproof drape
- Linen-saver pads
- Sterile gloves

If returning to operating room

- I.V. administration set and I.V. fluids
- Equipment for nasogastric intubation
- Prescribed sedative
- Suction apparatus

Implementation

- Provide reassurance and support to ease the patient's anxiety. Tell him to stay in bed. If possible, stay with him while someone else notifies the doctor and collects the necessary equipment.
- Place a linen-saver pad under the patient to keep the sheets dry when you moisten the exposed viscera.
- Using aseptic technique, unfold a sterile towel to create a sterile field. Open the package containing the irrigation set, and place the basin, solution container, and 50-ml syringe on the sterile field.
- Open the bottle of normal saline solution and pour about 400 ml into the solution container. Also pour about 200 ml into the sterile basin.
- Open several packages containing large abdominal dressings, and place the dressings on the sterile field.

▶ Put on the sterile gloves, and place one or two of the large abdominal dressings in the basin to saturate them with saline solution.
▶ Place the moistened dressings over the exposed viscera. Then place a sterile, waterproof drape over the dressings to prevent the sheets from getting wet.
▶ Moisten the dressings every hour by withdrawing saline solution from the container through the syringe and then gently squirting the solution onto the dressings.
▶ When you moisten the dressings, inspect the color of the viscera. If it appears dusky or black, notify the physician immediately. A protruding organ may become ischemic and necrotic if its blood supply is interrupted.
▶ Keep the patient on absolute bed rest in low Fowler's position (no more than 20 degrees elevation) with his knees flexed. This prevents injury and reduces stress on an abdominal incision.
▶ Monitor the patient's vital signs every 15 minutes to detect shock.
▶ If necessary, prepare the patient to return to the operating room. Gather the necessary equipment and start an I.V. infusion as ordered.
▶ Insert a nasogastric tube and connect it to continuous or intermittent low suction, as ordered.
▶ Administer preoperative drugs to the patient as ordered.
▶ Depending on the circumstances, some routine procedures may not be done at the bedside. For instance, nasogastric intubation may make the patient gag or vomit, causing further evisceration. For this reason, the doctor may choose to have the tube inserted in the operating room with the patient under anesthesia.
▶ Continue to reassure the patient while you prepare him for surgery. Be sure he has signed a consent form and the operating room staff has been informed about the procedure.
▶ As always, the best treatment is prevention. If you're caring for an older postoperative patient, make sure he gets an adequate supply of protein, vitamins, and calories. Monitor him for dietary deficiencies, and discuss any problems with the physician and a dietitian.

Complications

Infection, which can lead to peritonitis and possibly septic shock, is a complication of wound dehiscence and evisceration. If the wound isn't immediately treated, the patient may also suffer impaired circulation and necrosis of the affected organ.

Patient teaching

▶ Explain to the patient why it's necessary to keep the wound clean and moist until surgical repair.
▶ Tell him the importance of maintaining bed rest with the head of the bed no higher than 20 degrees.

Documentation

Note when the problem occurred, the patient's activity preceding the problem, his condition, and the time the doctor was notified. Describe the appearance of the wound or eviscerated organ; the amount, color, consistency, and odor of any drainage; and any nursing actions taken. Record the patient's vital signs, his response to the incident, and the doctor's actions. Remember to change the patient's care plan to reflect nursing actions needed to promote proper wound healing. Document your patient teaching measures and their effect.

WOUND IRRIGATION

Irrigation cleans tissues and flushes cell debris and drainage from an open wound. Irrigation with an antiseptic or antibiotic solution helps the wound heal properly from the inside tissue layers outward to the skin surface; it also helps prevent premature surface healing over an abscess pocket or infected tract.

Wound irrigation requires strict aseptic technique. After irrigation, open wounds usually are packed to absorb additional drainage. Take care not to damage healthy tissue, and remember that older adults heal at a slower pace and fight infection less efficiently than younger people. Also, be sure to guard the patient's privacy and protect him from hypothermia by exposing only the involved body part.

Supplies

- Waterproof trash bag
- Linen-saver pad
- Emesis basin
- Clean gloves or sterile gloves
- Gown and goggles (if splashing is possible)
- Prescribed irrigant (such as sterile normal saline solution or commercial wound cleansing solution)
- Sterile water or normal saline solution
- Soft rubber or plastic catheter
- 50- to 60-ml piston syringe
- Sterile container
- Materials needed for wound care
- Sterile irrigation and dressing set

Implementation

- Try to coordinate wound irrigation with the physician's visit so he can inspect the wound.
- Assemble all equipment in the patient's room. Check the expiration date on each sterile package, and inspect each one for tears. Check the sterilization date and the date that each bottle of irrigating solution was opened; don't use any solution that has been open longer than 24 hours.
- Using aseptic technique, dilute the prescribed irrigant to the correct proportions with sterile water or normal saline solution, if necessary. Let the solution stand until it reaches room temperature, or warm it to between 90° and 95° F (32° and 35° C).
- Open the waterproof trash bag and place it near the patient's bed to avoid reaching across the sterile field or the wound when disposing of soiled articles. Form a cuff by turning down the top of the trash bag to provide a wide opening and to prevent contamination by touching the bag's edge.
- Check the physician's order, and assess the patient's condition. Identify any allergies, especially to topical solutions or drugs.
- Explain the procedure to the patient, provide privacy, and position the patient correctly for the procedure. Place the linen-saver pad under the patient to catch any spills and avoid linen changes. Place the emesis basin below the wound so the irrigating solution flows from the wound into the basin.
- Wash your hands thoroughly. If necessary, put on a gown to protect your clothing from wound drainage and contamination. Put on clean gloves.
- Remove the soiled dressing; then discard the dressing and gloves in the trash bag.
- Establish a sterile field with all the equipment and supplies you'll need for irrigation and wound care. Pour the prescribed amount of irrigating solution into a sterile container so you won't contaminate your sterile gloves later by picking up unsterile containers. Put on sterile gloves, gown, and goggles if splashing is possible.
- Fill the syringe with the irrigating solution; then connect the catheter to the syringe. Gently instill a slow, steady stream of irrigating solution into the wound until the syringe empties. Another method of cleaning the wound is to use a commercial product in a spray bottle that delivers the product at 8 psi. Avoid exceeding this force to prevent damage to healing tissues. Make sure the solution flows from the clean to the dirty area of the wound to prevent contamination of clean tissue by exudate. Also make sure the solution reaches all areas of the wound.
- Refill the syringe, reconnect it to the catheter, and repeat the irrigation.

▶ Continue to irrigate the wound until you've administered the prescribed amount of solution or until the solution returns clear. Note the amount of solution administered. Then remove and discard the catheter and syringe in the waterproof trash bag.

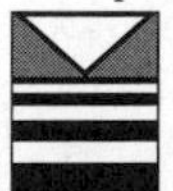

Key point Irrigate with a bulb syringe only if a piston syringe is unavailable; the piston syringe reduces the risk of aspirating drainage. If the wound is small or not particularly deep, you may want to use just the syringe for irrigation. A syringe with a 30G through-the-needle catheter delivers irrigating solutions at 8 psi.

▶ Keep the patient positioned to allow further wound drainage into the basin.

▶ Clean the area around the wound with a cleaning agent to help prevent skin breakdown and infection.

▶ Pack the wound, if ordered, and apply a sterile dressing. Discard your gloves, gown, and goggles.

▶ Make sure the patient is comfortable.

▶ Properly dispose of drainage, solutions, and trash bag, and clean or dispose of soiled equipment and supplies according to your facility's policy. To prevent contamination of other equipment, don't return unopened sterile supplies to the sterile supply cabinet.

▶ Use only the irrigant specified by the doctor because others may be erosive or otherwise harmful.

▶ Remember to follow your facility's policy concerning wound and skin precautions, as appropriate.

Complications

Wound irrigation increases the risk of infection. The patient may also suffer excoriation and increased pain.

Patient teaching

▶ Explain the procedure to the patient and the importance of keeping the wound clean.

▶ Tell him to immediately report any increasing pain during the procedure.

▶ If the wound must be irrigated at home, teach the patient or a family member how to irrigate using strict aseptic technique. Ask for a return demonstration of the proper technique.

▶ Provide written instructions.

▶ Arrange for visiting nurses and delivery of home health supplies, as appropriate.

▶ Urge the patient to call his physician if he detects signs of infection.

Documentation

Record the date and time of irrigation, the amount and type of irrigant, the appearance of the wound, any sloughing tissue or exudate, the amount of solution returned, any skin care performed around the wound, any dressings applied, and the patient's tolerance of the treatment. Document your patient teaching measures and their effect.

YOGA THERAPY

Among the oldest known health practices, *yoga* (meaning "union" in Sanskrit) is the integration of physical, mental, and spiritual energies to promote health and wellness. It's practiced by young and old alike, individually or in groups, and can be started at any age.

Based on the idea that a chronically restless or agitated mind causes poor health and decreased mental strength and clarity, yoga outlines specific regimens for lifestyle, hygiene, detoxification, physical activity, and psychological practices. By integrating these practices, yoga aims to raise the individual's physical vitality and spiritual awareness.

There are several styles of yoga, the most common in the West being Hatha yoga. It combines physical postures and exercises (called *asanas*), breathing techniques (called *pranayamas*), relaxation, diet, and "proper thinking."

Asanas fall into two categories, meditative and therapeutic. Meditative asanas promote proper blood flow through the body by bringing the spine and body into perfect alignment. The mind and body are brought into a state of relaxation and stillness, which facilitates concentration during meditation. These asanas also keep the heart, glands, and lungs properly energized. Therapeutic asanas are commonly prescribed for joint pain. The "cobra," "locust," "spinal twist," and "shoulder stand" are examples.

The goal of a properly executed asana is to create a balance between movement and stillness, which is the state of a healthy body. Very little movement is needed. Instead, the mind provides discipline, awareness, and a relaxed openness to maintain the posture and properly execute the asana. Using these asanas, the individual learns to regulate autonomic functions such as heartbeat and respirations, while relaxing physical tensions.

Pranayamas focus on disciplined breathing. Pranayama exercises regulate the flow of *prana* (breath and electromagnetic force), keeping the individual healthy. Pranayama has been shown to aid digestion, regulate cardiac function, and alleviate a variety of other physical ailments. It can be especially effective at reducing the frequency of asthma attacks.

The goal of breathing in yoga is to make the process as smooth and regular as possible. The assumption is that the rhythm of the mind is mirrored in the rhythm of breathing. By keeping respirations steady and rhythmic, the mind will remain calm and focused.

Samadhi, or spiritual realization, is an additional component of Eastern yoga. Yoga practitioners compare samadhi to a fourth state of consciousness, separate from the normal states of waking, dream, and sleep. The technique called *Hong-Sau* uses meditation to develop the powers of concentration. Thought and energy are withdrawn from outer distractions and focused on any goal or problem the individual chooses. The *Aum* technique expands the individual's awareness beyond the limitations of the body and mind, allowing the user to experience what is called the "Divine Consciousness," which is believed to underlie and uphold all life.

Among yoga's measured benefits are improvement in the individual's health,

A simple pranayama exercise

The following pranayama exercise is called purification of the channels (nadi shodhana). You can easily teach it to a patient.

- Have the patient sit upright on a cushion or in a firm chair with his head, neck, and body aligned.
- Tell him to breathe from his diaphragm, in a relaxed fashion, taking care to keep his inhalation and exhalation even and slow.
- Instruct him to begin by exhaling through his left nostril and inhaling through his right one. Have him use the thumb and forefinger of his right hand to alternately close one nostril. He should continue alternating for three cycles, inhaling through the same nostril each time.
- At the end of the third cycle, he should change the pattern to inhale through the nostril he was originally using for exhalation. Have him alternate, for three cycles, now inhaling and exhaling through the opposite nostrils he used in the beginning.
- Then have him place both hands on his knees, and inhale and exhale through both nostrils for three cycles.

As the patient practices this technique, have him try to lengthen the duration of his inhalation and exhalation, always keeping them even.

Encourage him to practice nadi shodhana twice each day, in the morning and evening.

vitality, and peace of mind. It is successfully used to alleviate stress and anxiety, lower blood pressure, relieve pain, improve motor skills, treat addictions, increase auditory and visual perception, and improve metabolic and respiratory function. Yoga has also been effective in the treatment of metabolic disorders and lung ailments. It can increase lung capacity and lower respiratory rates.

Yoga has been credited with decreasing serum cholesterol and increasing histamine levels to fight allergies. Its ability to help the user regulate blood flow is being studied in cancer therapy. Scientists are eager to see if restricted blood flow to the tumor region will slow growth.

Implementation

- Provide a private, quiet environment, which is free of distractions.
- Participants should have enough room to move without touching or distracting other members.
- Each participant will need a small blanket or large towel to use in some of the postures.
- Explain the purpose of the session and describe the planned exercises and their benefits. (See *A simple pranayama exercise,* page 619.)
- Answer any questions, and remind the participants that they don't have to engage in any posture that may be uncomfortable.
- When the group is ready, talk them through the positions or breathing techniques, demonstrating each one.
- After they've all assumed the position or begun the breathing pattern, circulate among the students to adjust their technique, as needed.
- Offer praise for all of their efforts.
- After you've led them through all of the planned exercises, close the session by having everyone take slow, deep breaths.
- Document the session, the techniques used, and the patients' responses.

Special considerations

- Some of the more physical aspects of yoga can cause muscle injury if they're not properly performed, or if the older adult tries to force his body into position. Caution patients to attempt the various techniques and postures cautiously, and remind them that very few people are able to perform all of the techniques in the beginning.
- There are yoga techniques to fit the needs of all people regardless of their physical condition. Individuals who can't perform some of the more physically demanding postures can still benefit from the breathing or meditation techniques.

Appendices
Selected references
Index

Appendix A
Physiologic changes in aging

Aging is characterized by the loss of some body cells and reduced metabolism in other cells. These processes cause a decline in body function and changes in body composition. This chart will help you recognize the gradual changes in body function that normally accompany aging so you can adjust your assessment techniques accordingly.

Body system	Age-related changes
Nutrition	▪ Protein, vitamin, and mineral requirements usually unchanged ▪ Energy requirements possibly decreased by about 200 calories per day because of diminished activity ▪ Loss of calcium and nitrogen (in patients who aren't ambulatory) ▪ Diminished absorption of calcium and vitamins B_1 and B_2 due to reduced pepsin and hydrochloric acid secretion ▪ Decreased salivary flow and decreased sense of taste (may reduce appetite) ▪ Diminished intestinal motility and peristalsis of the large intestine ▪ Brittle teeth due to thinning of tooth enamel ▪ Decreased biting force ▪ Diminished gag reflex ▪ Limited mobility (may affect ability to obtain or prepare food)
Skin	▪ Facial lines resulting from subcutaneous fat loss, dermal thinning, decreasing collagen and elastin, and 50% decline in cell replacement ▪ Delayed wound healing due to decreased rate of cell replacement ▪ Decreased skin elasticity (may seem almost transparent) ▪ Brown spots on skin due to localized melanocyte proliferation ▪ Dry mucous membranes and decreased sweat gland output (as the number of active sweat glands declines) ▪ Difficulty regulating body temperature because of decrease in size, number, and function of sweat glands and loss of subcutaneous fat
Hair	▪ Decreased pigment, causing gray or white hair ▪ Thinning as the number of melanocytes declines ▪ Pubic hair loss resulting from hormonal changes ▪ Facial hair increase in postmenopausal women and decrease in men
Eyes and vision	▪ Baggy and wrinkled eyelids due to decreased elasticity, with eyes sitting deeper in sockets ▪ Thinner and yellow conjunctivae; possible pingueculae (fat pads) ▪ Decreased tear production due to loss of fatty tissue in lacrimal apparatus ▪ Corneal flattening and loss of luster ▪ Fading or irregular pigmentation of iris ▪ Smaller pupil, requiring three times more light to see clearly; diminished night vision and depth perception ▪ Scleral thickening and rigidity; yellowing due to fat deposits ▪ Vitreous degeneration, revealing opacities and floating debris ▪ Lens enlargement; loss of transparency and elasticity, decreasing accommodation ▪ Impaired color vision due to deterioration of retinal cones ▪ Decreased reabsorption of intraocular fluid, predisposing to glaucoma

Body system	Age-related changes
Ears and hearing	■ Atrophy of the organ of Corti and the auditory nerve (sensory presbycusis) ■ Inability to distinguish high-pitched consonants ■ Degenerative structural changes in the entire auditory system
Respiratory system	■ Nose enlargement from continued cartilage growth ■ General atrophy of tonsils ■ Tracheal deviation due to changes in the aging spine ■ Increased anteroposterior chest diameter as a result of altered calcium metabolism and calcification of costal cartilage ■ Lung rigidity; decreased number and size of alveoli ■ Kyphosis ■ Respiratory muscle degeneration or atrophy ■ Declining diffusing capacity ■ Decreased inspiratory and expiratory muscle strength; diminished vital capacity ■ Lung tissue degeneration, causing decrease in lungs' elastic recoil capability and increase in residual capacity ■ Poor ventilation of the basal areas (from closing of some airways), resulting in decreased surface area for gas exchange and reduced partial pressure of oxygen ■ Oxygen saturation decreased by 5% ■ 30% reduction in respiratory fluids, heightening risk of pulmonary infection and mucus plugs ■ Lower tolerance for oxygen debt
Cardiovascular system	■ Slightly smaller heart size ■ Loss of cardiac contractile strength and efficiency ■ 30% to 35% diminished cardiac output by age 70 ■ Heart valve thickening, causing incomplete closure (systolic murmur) ■ 25% increase in left ventricular wall thickness between ages 30 and 80 ■ Fibrous tissue infiltration of the sinoatrial node and internodal atrial tracts, causing atrial fibrillation and flutter ■ Vein dilation and stretching ■ 35% decrease in coronary artery blood flow between ages 20 and 60 ■ Increased aortic rigidity, causing increased systolic blood pressure disproportionate to diastolic, resulting in widened pulse pressure ■ Electrocardiogram changes: increased PR, QRS complex, and QT interval; decreased amplitude of QRS complex; shift of QRS axis to the left ■ Heart rate takes longer to return to normal after exercise ■ Decreased strength and elasticity of blood vessels, contributing to arterial and venous insufficiency ■ Decreased ability to respond to physical and emotional stress
GI system	■ Diminished mucosal elasticity ■ Reduced GI secretions, affecting digestion and absorption ■ Decreased motility, bowel wall and anal sphincter tone, and abdominal wall strength ■ Liver changes: decreases in weight, regenerative capacity, and blood flow ■ Decline in hepatic enzymes involved in oxidation and reduction, causing less efficient metabolism of drugs and detoxification of substances

Body system	Age-related changes
Renal system	■ Decline in glomerular filtration rate ■ 53% decrease in renal blood flow secondary to reduced cardiac output and atherosclerotic changes ■ Decrease in size and number of functioning nephrons ■ Reduction in bladder size and capacity ■ Weakening of bladder muscles, causing incomplete emptying and chronic urine retention ■ Diminished kidney size ■ Impaired clearance of drugs ■ Decreased ability to respond to variations in sodium intake
Male reproductive system	■ Reduced testosterone production, resulting in decreased libido as well as atrophy and softening of testes ■ 48% to 69% decrease in sperm production between ages 60 and 80 ■ Prostate gland enlargement, with decreasing secretions ■ Decreased volume and viscosity of seminal fluid ■ Slower and weaker physiologic reaction during intercourse, with lengthened refractory period
Female reproductive system	■ Declining estrogen and progesterone levels (about age 50) cause: – cessation of ovulation; atrophy, thickening, and decreased size of ovaries – loss of pubic hair and flattening of labia majora – shrinking of vulval tissue, constricted introitus, and loss of tissue elasticity – vaginal atrophy; thin and dry mucus lining; more alkaline pH of vaginal environment – shrinking uterus – cervical atrophy, failure to produce mucus for lubrication, thinner endometrium and myometrium – pendulous breasts; atrophy of glandular, supporting, and fatty tissue – nipple flattening and decreased size – more pronounced inframammary ridges.
Neurologic system	■ Degenerative changes in neurons of central and peripheral nervous system ■ Slower nerve transmission ■ Decrease in number of brain cells by about 1% per year after age 50 ■ Hypothalamus less effective at regulating body temperature ■ 20% neuron loss in cerebral cortex ■ Slower corneal reflex ■ Increased pain threshold ■ Decrease in stage III and IV of sleep, causing frequent awakenings; rapid eye movement sleep also decreased
Immune system	■ Decline beginning at sexual maturity and continuing with age ■ Loss of ability to distinguish between self and nonself ■ Loss of ability to recognize and destroy mutant cells, increasing incidence of cancer ■ Decreased antibody response, resulting in greater susceptibility to infection ■ Tonsillar atrophy and lymphadenopathy ■ Lymph node and spleen size slightly decreased ■ Some active blood-forming marrow replaced by fatty bone marrow, resulting in inability to increase erythrocyte production as readily as before in response to such stimuli as hormones, anoxia, hemorrhage, and hemolysis ■ Diminished vitamin B_{12} absorption, resulting in reduced erythrocyte mass and decreased hemoglobin level and hematocrit

Body system	Age-related changes
Musculoskeletal system	■ Increased adipose tissue ■ Diminished lean body mass and bone mineral contents ■ Decreased height from exaggerated spinal curvature and narrowing intervertebral spaces ■ Decreased collagen formation and muscle mass ■ Increased viscosity of synovial fluid, more fibrotic synovial membranes
Endocrine system	■ Decreased ability to tolerate stress ■ Blood glucose concentration increases and remains elevated longer than in a younger adult ■ Diminished levels of estrogen and increasing levels of follicle-stimulating hormone during menopause, causing coronary thrombosis and osteoporosis ■ Reduced progesterone production ■ 50% decline in serum aldosterone levels ■ 25% decrease in cortisol secretion rate

Appendix B
Laboratory Value Changes in Elderly Patients

Standard normal laboratory values reflect the physiology of adults ages 20 to 40. However, normal values for older patients usually differ because of age-related physiologic changes.

Certain test results, however, remain unaffected by age. These include partial thromboplastin time, prothrombin time, serum acid phosphatase, serum carbon dioxide, serum chloride, aspartate aminotransferase, and total serum protein. You can use this chart to interpret other, changeable test values in your elderly patients.

Test values ages 20 to 40	Age-related changes	Considerations
Serum		
Albumin 3.5 to 5 g/dl	Under age 65: Higher in males Over age 65: Equal levels that then decrease at same rate	Increased dietary protein intake needed in older patients if liver function is normal; edema: a sign of low albumin level
Alkaline phosphatase 13 to 39 IU/L	Increases 8 to 10 IU/L	May reflect liver function decline or vitamin D malabsorption and bone demineralization
Beta globulin 2.3 to 3.5 g/dl	Increases slightly	Increases in response to decrease in albumin if liver function is normal; increased dietary protein intake needed
Blood urea nitrogen Men: 10 to 25 mg/dl Women: 8 to 20 mg/dl	Increases, possibly to 69 mg/dl	Slight increase acceptable in absence of stressors, such as infection or surgery
Cholesterol 120 to 220 mg/dl	Men: Increases to age 50, then decreases Women: Lower than men until age 50, increases to age 70, then decreases	Rise in cholesterol level (and increased cardiovascular risk) in women as a result of postmenopausal estrogen decline; dietary changes, weight loss, and exercise needed
Creatine kinase 17 to 148 U/L	Increases slightly	May reflect decreasing muscle mass and liver function
Creatinine 0.6 to 1.5 mg/dl	Increases, possibly to 1.9 mg/dl in men	Important factor to prevent toxicity when giving drugs excreted in urine
Creatinine clearance 104 to 125 ml/min	Men: Decreases; formula: (140 − age) × kg body weight/ 72 × serum creatinine Women: 85% of men's rate	Reflects reduced glomerular filtration rate; important factor to prevent toxicity when giving drugs excreted in urine

Test values ages 20 to 40	Age-related changes	Considerations
Serum *(continued)*		
Glucose tolerance (fasting plasma glucose) 1 hr: 160 to 170 mg/dl 2 hr: 115 to 125 mg/dl 3 hr: 70 to 110 mg/dl	Rises faster in first 2 hours, then drops to baseline more slowly	Reflects declining pancreatic insulin supply and release and diminishing body mass for glucose uptake (Rapid rise can quickly trigger hyperosmolar hyperglycemic nonketotic syndrome. Rapid decline can result from certain drugs, such as alcohol, beta-adrenergic blockers, and monoamine oxidase inhibitors.)
Hematocrit Men: 45% to 52% Women: 37% to 48%	May decrease slightly (unproven)	Reflects decreased bone marrow and hematopoiesis, increased risk of infection (because of fewer and weaker lymphocytes and immune system changes that diminish antigen-antibody response)
Hemoglobin Men: 13 to 18 g/dl Women: 12 to 16 g/dl	Men: Decreases by 1 to 2 g/dl Women: Unknown	Reflects decreased bone marrow, hematopoiesis, and (for men) androgen levels
High-density lipoprotein 80 to 310 mg/dl	Levels higher in women than in men but equalize with age	Compliance with dietary restrictions required for accurate interpretation of test results
Lactate dehydrogenase 45 to 90 U/L	Increases slightly	May reflect declining muscle mass and liver function
Leukocyte count 4,300 to 10,800/µl	Decreases to 3,100 to 9,000/µl	Decrease proportionate to lymphocyte count
Lymphocyte count T cells: 500 to 2,400/µl B cells: 50 to 200/µl	Decreases	Decrease proportionate to leukocyte count
Platelet count 150,000 to 350,000/ mm^3	Change in characteristics: decreased granular constituents, increased platelet-release factors	May reflect diminished bone marrow and increased fibrinogen levels
Potassium 3.5 to 5.5 mEq/L	Increases slightly	Requires avoidance of salt substitutes composed of potassium, vigilance in reading food labels, and knowledge of hyperkalemia's signs and symptoms
Thyroid-stimulating hormone 0.3 to 5 µIU/ml	Increases slightly	Suggests primary hypothyroidism or endemic goiter at much higher levels
Thyroxine 4.5 to 13.5 µg/dl	Decreases 25%	Reflects declining thyroid function
Triglycerides 40 to 150 mg/dl	Range widens: 20 to 200 mg/dl	Suggests abnormalities at any other levels, requiring additional tests such as serum cholesterol

Test values ages 20 to 40	Age-related changes	Considerations
Serum *(continued)*		
Triiodothyronine 90 to 220 ng/dl	Decreases 25%	Reflects declining thyroid function
Urine		
Glucose 0 to 15 mg/dl	Decreases slightly	May reflect renal disease or urinary tract infection (UTI); unreliable check for older diabetics because glucosuria may not occur until plasma glucose level exceeds 300 mg/dl
Protein 0 to 5 mg/dl	Increases slightly	May reflect renal disease or UTI
Specific gravity 1.032	Decreases to 1.024 by age 80	Reflects 30% to 50% decrease in number of nephrons available to concentrate urine

Appendix C
Levels of care

Many care and service options, including those described below, are available to elderly people to help them maintain their independence and to provide care when they can no longer care for themselves.

Multipurpose senior centers

▶ Provide a wide variety of services to active, independent adults in the community, including health screening and promotion programs, social and recreational programs, tax assistance, and educational programs

Homemaker services

▶ Help with such activities as light cleaning, cooking, shopping, and laundry

▶ Possible discount available through Area Agency on Aging

Home maintenance and repair

▶ Provide help with home repairs and chores for those unable to perform these tasks independently

▶ Costs sometimes underwritten by Area Agency on Aging

▶ May also be provided by service groups, such as church youth groups, Scouts, or adult volunteer groups

Check-in services

▶ Offer telephone check-in to ascertain patient status and provide social contact through volunteers from senior centers, churches, and other community agencies

▶ Provide periodic scheduled visits by friendly visitors to provide social contact, assistance with correspondence and, possibly, transportation to a community activity

Community-based adult day care

▶ Offers numerous services for frail or cognitively compromised older adults in a variety of settings

▶ Provides structured activities, personal care, recreation and socialization, nutritional support, and health care; social services and caregiver support frequently a part of these programs

▶ Allows family members and other caregivers to maintain their jobs and to postpone or avoid institutionalizing the older person

▶ Charges based on patient's ability to pay

Respite care

▶ Trained individuals provide relief (for a brief, limited period of a few hours, days, or weeks) for family members who care for an elderly patient at home

▶ Can be offered in the home, through a day-care program, or within a facility

Hospice care

▶ Offered in an institutional or home setting for the terminally ill patient and family

▶ May be covered by medical insurance

▶ May be provided by the pastoral care department of the affiliated hospital, a home health agency, the patient's church, or the parish nurse

▶ Bereavement services for grieving family offered by many agencies

Acute care

- Hospital setting that provides care for acute illness or acute exacerbations of chronic illness
- Geriatric units with specially trained interdisciplinary staff (nurses, pharmacists, social workers, rehabilitation therapists and mental health professionals) available in some hospitals

Subacute care

- Available in some hospitals and nursing homes
- Usually for people who require short-term care, such as those recuperating from surgery or illness and those with a chronic illness that requires short-term skilled nursing care
- Usually includes rehabilitation and social activities
- Goal of discharging the patient to home

Home health care

- Services provided by Medicare and Medicaid to those who meet eligibility criteria for skilled care
- Services that include registered nurse; physical, occupational, or speech therapist; home health aide; or social worker on short-term episodic basis
- Maintenance level programs that provide personal care services and periodic nursing assessments to support the frail elderly in the home setting

Assisted living

- Allows the elderly person to remain in his own home
- Provides meals, assistance with activities of daily living (ADLs), health care, 24-hour supervision, and other supportive systems
- Not regulated by federal government; licensing guidelines developed by each state
- Goal of maintaining the patient's independence, individuality, freedom of choice, privacy, and dignity

Long-term care

- Provides around-the-clock nursing care for chronically ill or cognitively impaired individuals, most of whom have four or five limitations in performing ADLs
- Regulated by the state and federal government
- Fees paid by Medicare, Medicaid, the patient, and insurance companies

Appendix D
Using antipsychotics in long-term care facilities

The Centers for Medicare and Medicaid Services has guidelines for using antipsychotics in long-term care facilities.

Guidelines for use

Before initiating antipsychotic therapy in any patient, take nonpharmacologic steps to modify his behavior and environment. If such measures are unsuccessful, you may use an antipsychotic provided that your patient has one of the following conditions:

1. schizophrenia
2. schizoaffective disorder
3. delusional disorder, which may include characteristics of other disorders
4. psychotic mood disorders, including mania or depression with psychotic features
5. acute psychotic episodes
6. brief reactive psychosis (related to an event and lasting less than 1 month)
7. schizophreniform disorder
8. atypical psychosis (covers psychotic disorders not otherwise specifically diagnosed)
9. Tourette syndrome
10. Huntington's disease
11. symptomatic 7-day treatment of hiccups, nausea, vomiting, or pruritus; residents with nausea and vomiting secondary to cancer or cancer chemotherapy possibly treated longer
12. organic mental syndromes — including dementia, delirium, and amnestic and other cognitive disorders — accompanied by psychotic or agitated behaviors.

However, behaviors must be quantitatively (number of episodes) and objectively (for example, hitting, kicking, scratching) documented and mustn't be caused by preventable reasons. Behaviors must present a danger to the resident or others or involve continuous crying, screaming, yelling, or pacing if these behaviors impair functional capacity. Also, psychotic symptoms (hallucinations, paranoia, delusions) must not otherwise be related to the above behaviors, which cause distress to the resident or impair functional capacity.

If a patient has a history of recurring psychotic symptoms and has 1 of the first 10 conditions — and if that condition has been stabilized with an antipsychotic with no significant adverse effects — dosage doesn't need to be reduced for a finding that dosage reduction is contraindicated. If the patient has an organic mental disease, such as Alzheimer's, attempt gradual dosage reductions twice per year. If attempts are unsuccessful, a finding that further attempts at dosage reduction are contraindicated must be established and documented.

Don't use an antipsychotic if one of the following is the only indication: agitated behaviors that don't pose a danger to resident or others, anxiety, depression (without psychotic features), fidgeting, indifference to surroundings, insomnia, memory impairment, nervousness, poor self care, restlessness, uncooperativeness, unsociability, or wandering.

Guidelines for dosing

The table of daily doses on the next page is only for patients with organic mental syndromes. Avoid exceeding the total daily dose, unless higher doses are necessary to maintain or improve the patient's functional status — and unless evidence of that need is documented. Reduce dosage for a patient taking an antipsychotic, unless doing so is contraindicated. Monitor any patient taking an antipsychotic for adverse effects, such as tardive dyskinesia, orthostatic hypotension, cognitive or behavioral impairment, akathisia, and parkinsonism.

Generic name (brand name)	Daily dose (mg/day)
chlorpromazine (Thorazine)	75
clozapine (Clozaril)	50
fluphenazine (Prolixin, Permitil)	4
haloperidol (Haldol)	4
loxapine (Loxitane)	10
mesoridazine (Serentil)	25
molindone (Moban)	10
olanzapine (Zyprexa)	10
perphenazine (Trilafon)	8
prochlorperazine* (Compazine)	10
quetiapine (Seroquel)	200
risperidone (Risperdal)	2
thioridazine (Mellaril)	75
thiothixene (Navane)	7
trifluoperazine (Stelazine)	8

*May exceed dose for up to 7 days when treating nausea and vomiting.

Adapted with permission from American Society of Consultant Pharmacists, *Nursing Home Survey Procedures and Interpretive Guidelines*, 2nd edition, 1999.

Appendix E
Using anxiolytics and sedatives in long-term care facilities

According to the Center For Medicare and Medicaid Services, a health care provider must consider, rule out, and document other reasons for distress before treating a patient in a long-term care facility with an anxiolytic or sedative. If used, the drug must maintain or improve the patient's functional status — and documentation must support its use.

Short-acting benzodiazepines and other anxiolytics and sedatives

These drugs may only be used for sleep disorders and the following indications:

- generalized anxiety disorder
- organic mental syndromes, including dementia, accompanied by a quantitatively and objectively documented agitated state that's a source of distress or dysfunction to the patient or that poses a danger to the patient or others
- panic disorder
- symptomatic anxiety that's accompanied by another diagnosed psychiatric disorder, such as depression or adjustment disorder.

Limit daily use of the drugs in the table below to less than 4 consecutive months, unless one or more dosage reductions are unsuccessful. If two attempts at dosage reduction in 1 year are unsuccessful, reduction is contraindicated. Don't exceed the total daily dose, unless doing so is necessary to maintain or improve functional status.

Generic name (brand name)	Daily dose (mg/day)
alprazolam (Xanax)	0.75
chloral hydrate (Noctec)	750
diphenhydramine (Benadryl)	50
hydroxyzine (Atarax, Vistaril)	50
lorazepam (Ativan)	2
oxazepam (Serax)	30

Long-acting benzodiazepines

Avoid using long-acting benzodiazepines, unless short-acting benzodiazepines have failed. Limit daily use of drugs listed in the table below to less than 4 consecutive months, unless gradual dosage reductions are unsuccessful. If two attempts at dosage reduction in 1 year are unsuccessful, dosage reduction is contraindicated. For patients receiving duplicate therapy — that is, more than one drug with the same effect — monitor for adverse reactions.

Don't exceed the total daily dose, unless doing so is necessary to maintain or improve functional status. Exceptions include diazepam (Valium) for neuromuscular syndromes (such as cerebral palsy, tardive dyskinesia, and seizure disorders); clonazepam (Klonopin) for bipolar disorders, tardive dyskinesia, nocturnal myoclonus, and seizure disorders; and any long-acting benzodiazepines if used to withdraw patients from short-acting benzodiazepines.

Generic name (brand name)	Daily dose (mg/day)
chlordiazepoxide (Librium)	20
clonazepam (Klonopin)	1.5
clorazepate (Tranxene)	15
diazepam (Valium)	5
flurazepam (Dalmane)	15

Drugs to induce sleep

Before considering drug therapy to treat insomnia, first eliminate the external causes of the condition — for example, noise, light, caffeine, pain, and depression. Then initiate hypnotic drug therapy as appropriate to induce sleep with lower doses, and increase doses only gradually when necessary. Avoid exceeding the total daily dose, unless it can be shown that higher doses are necessary to maintain or improve the patient's functional status. Limit daily use of the drugs listed in the table below to less than 10 continuous days, unless gradual dosage reduction is unsuccessful. If three attempts at dosage reduction in 6 months are unsuccessful, dosage reduction is contraindicated.

Generic name (brand name)	Daily dose (mg/day)
alprazolam (Xanax)	0.25
chloral hydrate* (Noctec)	500
diphenhydramine* (Benadryl)	25
estazolam (ProSom)	0.5
hydroxyzine* (Atarax, Vistaril)	50
lorazepam (Ativan)	1
oxazepam (Serax)	15
temazepam (Restoril)	7.5
triazolam (Halcion)	0.125
zolpidem (Ambien)	5

*Not a drug of choice for sleep disorders, but it may be used.

Anxiolytics and sedatives to avoid

Certain anxiolytics and sedatives shouldn't be used for patients in long-term care facilities, including amobarbital (Amytal), amobarbital-secobarbital (Tuinal), butabarbital (Butisol and others), ethchlorvynol (Placidyl), glutethimide (Doriden), meprobamate (Equanil, Miltown), paraldehyde (many brands), pentobarbital (Nembutal), phenobarbital (many brands), and secobarbital (Seconal).

To help eliminate or modify the symptoms for which such a drug is prescribed, reduce the patient's dosage; however, a newly admitted patient may have an adjustment period before his dosage is reduced. If two attempts at dosage reduction in 1 year are unsuccessful, reduction is contraindicated. Because rapid withdrawal of such drugs may result in severe physiological symptoms, reduce all dosages gradually.

Adapted with permission from American Society of Consultant Pharmacists, *Nursing Home Survey Procedures and Interpretive Guidelines,* 2nd edition, 1999.

APPENDIX F
UNNECESSARY DRUGS IN LONG-TERM CARE FACILITIES

The Centers for Medicare and Medicaid Services (CMS) has guidelines for using unnecessary drugs in long-term care facilities. Such drugs are characterized as either high severity or low severity, with severity being defined as "a combination of both the likelihood that an adverse outcome would occur and the clinical significance of that outcome should it occur."

High severity

The following drugs are inappropriate for geriatric patients and are characterized as high severity:

- anticholinergics for patients with bening prostatic hypertrophy (BPH), including anticholinergic antidepressants; anticholinergic antihistamines and GI antispasmodics that are used more frequently than every 3 months for 7 days (a surveyor must review drug use that's more frequent); and antiparkinsonians
- aspirin, dipyridamole (Persantine), nonsteroidal anti-inflammatory drugs (NSAIDs), or ticlopidine (Ticlid) for residents taking anticoagulants
- hypnotics or sedatives for residents with chronic obstructive pulmonary disease (COPD); short-acting benzodiazepines are acceptable for patients with mild COPD
- metoclopramide (Reglan) for patients with seizures or epilepsy
- NSAIDs for patients with active or recurrent gastritis, peptic ulcer disease, or gastroesophageal reflux disease (GERD); COX-2 inhibitors, such as celecoxib (Celebrex), not included on the CMS list of NSAIDs
- tricyclic antidepressants in patients with arrhythmias, if started within past month.

The following drugs may be inappropriate for geriatric patients because of the high potential for severe adverse reactions:

- amitriptyline (Elavil); may be used for neurogenic pain if another tricyclic antidepressant, such as desipramine (Norpramin), failed
- chlorpropamide (Diabinese)
- digoxin (Lanoxin); unless an atrial arrhythmia is being treated, dosages greater than 0.125mg/day increase the risk of adverse reaction without improving outcomes; high severity is considered if started within the past month
- disopyramide (Norpace)
- doxepin (Sinequan)
- GI antispasmodics (belladonna alkaloids, clidinium, dicyclomine, hyoscyamine, propantheline) that are used more frequently than every 3 months for 7 days (a surveyor must review drug use that's more frequent)
- meperidine (Demerol), oral; high severity considered if started within the past month
- meprobamate (Equanil, Miltown)
- methyldopa (Aldomet); high severity is considered if started within the past month.
- pentazocine (Talwin)
- ticlopidine; may be used for patients who are intolerant of aspirin or who have had a previous stroke or evidence of stroke precursors (for example, transient ischemic attacks).

Low severity

The following drugs are inappropriate for geriatric patients and are characterized as low severity:

- antipsychotics in patients with seizures or epilepsy; treatment of acute psychosis for 72 hours or less is permissible.
- corticosteroids in patients with diabetes, if started within past month
- narcotics and bladder relaxants, such as oxybutynin (Ditropan) and bethanechol (Urecholine), in patients with BPH; no need for a surveyor to review drug use if drug is used for 7 days or less once every 3 months for symptoms of an acute self limiting condition
- potassium supplements or aspirin (dosages exceeding 325 mg/day) in patients with active or recurrent gastritis, peptic ulcer disease, or GERD; use of potassium supplements to treat low potassium levels until they return to normal range permissible in these patients if the health care provider determines that using fresh fruits and vegetables or other dietary supplementation is inadequate or impossible.

The following drugs may worsen constipation:

- anticholinergic antidepressants
- anticholinergic antihistamines; no need for a surveyor to review drug use if drug is used for 7 days or less once every 3 months for symptoms of an acute self-limiting condition
- antiparkinsonians
- GI antispasmodics
- narcotics; no need for a surveyor to review drug use if drug is used for 7 days or less once every 3 months for symptoms of an acute self-limiting condition.

The following drugs may worsen insomnia:

- beta agonists
- decongestants
- monoaminase oxidase inhibitors
- selective serotonin reuptake inhibitors and desipramine (Norpramin)
- theophylline.

The following drugs may be inappropriate for geriatric patients because of the high potential for less severe adverse outcomes:

- antihistamines with anticholinergic properties
- digoxin (Lanoxin); unless an atrial arrhythmia is being treated, increased risk of adverse reaction without improving outcomes with dosages exceeding 0.125mg/day; low severity considered if therapy exceeds 1 month
- diphenhydramine (Benadryl); no need for a surveyor to review drug use if drug is used for 7 days or less once every 3 months for treatment of allergies
- dipyridamole (Persantine)
- indomethacin (Indocin); may be used for 1 week to treat acute gouty arthritis
- meperidine (Demerol), oral; low severity is considered if therapy exceeds 1 month
- methyldopa (Aldomet); low severity is considered if therapy exceeds 1 month
- muscle relaxants, such as carisoprodol (Soma), chlorzoxazone (Paraflex), cyclobenzaprine (Flexeril), dantrolene (Dantrium), methocarbamol (Robaxin); no need for a surveyor to review drug use if drug is used for 7 days or less once every 3 months for acute self-limiting condition
- trimethobenzamide (Tigan).

Adapted with permission from American Society of Consultant Pharmacists, *Nursing Home Survey Procedures and Interpretive Guidelines,* 2nd edition, 1999.

Appendix G
Preventing adverse drug reactions in older patients

A drug's action in the body and its interaction with body tissues (pharmacodynamics) change significantly in older people. In the chart below, you'll find the information you need to help prevent adverse drug reactions in your elderly patients.

Pharmacology	Indications	Special considerations
Adrenergics, direct- and indirect-acting		
Exert excitatory actions on the heart, glands, and vascular smooth muscle and peripheral inhibitory actions on smooth muscles of the bronchial tree	■ Hypotension ■ Cardiac stimulation ■ Bronchodilation ■ Shock	■ An elderly patient may be more sensitive to therapeutic and adverse effects of some adrenergics and may require lower doses.
Adrenocorticoids, systemic		
Stimulate enzyme synthesis needed to decrease the inflammatory response	■ Inflammation ■ Immunosuppression ■ Adrenal insufficiency ■ Rheumatic and collagen diseases ■ Acute spinal cord injury	■ These drugs may aggravate hyperglycemia, delay wound healing, or contribute to edema, insomnia, or osteoporosis in an elderly patient. ■ Decreased metabolic rate and elimination may cause increased plasma levels and increase the risk of adverse effects. Monitor the elderly patient carefully.
Alpha-adrenergic blockers		
Block the effects of peripheral neurohormonal transmitters (norepinephrine, epinephrine) on adrenergic receptors in various effector systems	■ Peripheral vascular disorders ■ Hypertension ■ Benign prostatic hyperplasia	■ Hypotensive effects may be more pronounced in an elderly patient. ■ These drugs should be administered at bedtime to reduce potential for dizziness or light-headedness.
Aminoglycosides		
Inhibit bacterial protein synthesis	■ Infection caused by susceptible organisms	■ The elderly patient may have decreased renal function and thus be at greater risk for nephrotoxicity, ototoxicity, and superinfection (common).
Angiotensin-converting enzyme (ACE) inhibitors		
Prevent the conversion of angiotensin I to angiotensin II Decrease vasoconstriction and adrenocortical secretion of aldosterone	■ Hypertension ■ Heart failure	■ Diuretic therapy should be discontinued before ACE inhibitors are started to reduce the risk of hypotension. ■ An elderly patient may need lower doses because of impaired drug clearance.

Pharmacology	Indications	Special considerations
Anticholinergics		
Exert antagonistic action on acetylcholine and other cholinergic agonists within the parasympathetic nervous system	■ Hypersecretory conditions ■ GI tract disorders ■ Sinus bradycardia ■ Dystonia and parkinsonism ■ Perioperative use ■ Motion sickness	■ These drugs should be used cautiously in an elderly adult, who may be more sensitive to the effects of these drugs; a lower dosage may be indicated.
Antihistamines		
Prevent access and subsequent activity of histamine	■ Allergy ■ Pruritus ■ Vertigo ■ Nausea and vomiting ■ Sedation ■ Cough suppression ■ Dyskinesia	■ An elderly patient is usually more sensitive to the adverse effects of antihistamines; he's especially likely to experience a greater degree of dizziness, sedation, hypotension, and urine retention.
Barbiturates		
Decrease presynaptic and postsynaptic excitability, producing central nervous system (CNS) depression	■ Seizure disorders ■ Sedation (including preanesthesia) ■ Hypnosis	■ An elderly patient and a patient receiving subhypnotic doses may experience hyperactivity, excitement, or hyperanalgesia. Use with caution.
Benzodiazepines		
Act selectively on polysynaptic neuronal pathways throughout the CNS; synthetically produced sedative-hypnotic	■ Seizure disorders ■ Anxiety, tension, insomnia ■ Surgical adjuncts for conscious sedation or amnesia ■ Skeletal muscle spasm, tremor	■ These drugs should be used cautiously in an elderly patient, who is sensitive to the drugs' CNS effects; parenteral administration is more likely to cause apnea, hypotension, bradycardia, and cardiac arrest.
Beta-adrenergic blockers		
Compete with beta agonists for available beta-receptor sites; individual agents differ in their ability to affect beta receptors	■ Hypertension ■ Angina ■ Arrhythmias ■ Glaucoma ■ Myocardial infarction ■ Migraine prophylaxis	■ Increased bioavailability or delayed metabolism in the elderly patient may require a lower dosage; an elderly patient may also experience enhanced adverse effects.
Calcium channel blockers		
Inhibit calcium influx across the slow channels of myocardial and vascular smooth muscle cells, causing dilation of coronary arteries, peripheral arteries, and arterioles and slowing cardiac conduction	■ Angina ■ Arrhythmias ■ Hypertension	■ These drugs should be used cautiously in an elderly patient because the half-life of calcium channel blockers may be increased as a result of decreased clearance.

Pharmacology	Indications	Special considerations
Cardiac glycosides		
Directly increase myocardial contractile force and velocity, atrioventricular node refractory period, and total peripheral resistance Indirectly depress sinoatrial node and prolong conduction to the atrioventricular node	■ Heart failure ■ Arrhythmias ■ Paroxysmal atrial tachycardia or atrioventricular junctional rhythm ■ Myocardial infarction (MI) ■ Cardiogenic shock ■ Angina	■ These drugs should be used cautiously in an elderly patient with renal or hepatic dysfunction or with electrolyte imbalance that may predispose him to toxicity.
Cephalosporins		
Inhibit bacterial cell wall synthesis, causing rapid cell lysis	■ Infection caused by susceptible organisms	■ Because the elderly patient commonly has impaired renal function, he may require a lower dosage. ■ An older adult is more susceptible to superinfection and coagulopathies.
Coumarin derivatives		
Interfere with the hepatic synthesis of vitamin K–dependent clotting factors II, VII, IX, and X, decreasing the blood's coagulation potential	■ Treatment for or prevention of thrombosis or embolism	■ An older adult has an increased risk of hemorrhage because of altered hemostatic mechanisms or age-related deterioration of hepatic and renal function.
Diuretics, loop		
Inhibit sodium and chloride reabsorption in the ascending loop of Henle and increase excretion of potassium, sodium, chloride, and water	■ Edema ■ Hypertension	■ An elderly or debilitated patient is more susceptible to drug-induced diuresis and can quickly develop dehydration, hypovolemia, hypokalemia, and hyponatremia, which may cause circulatory collapse.
Diuretics, potassium-sparing		
Act directly on the distal renal tubules, inhibiting sodium reabsorption and potassium excretion	■ Edema ■ Hypertension ■ Diagnosis of primary hyperaldosteronism	■ An older patient may need a smaller dosage because of his susceptibility to drug-induced diuresis and hyperkalemia.
Diuretics, thiazide and thiazide-like		
Interfere with sodium transport, thereby increasing renal excretion of sodium, chloride, water, potassium, and calcium	■ Edema ■ Hypertension ■ Diabetes insipidus	■ Age-related changes in cardiovascular and renal function make the elderly patient more susceptible to excessive diuresis, which may lead to dehydration, hypovolemia, hyponatremia, hypomagnesemia, and hypokalemia.

Pharmacology	Indications	Special considerations
Estrogens		
Promote development and maintenance of the female reproductive system and secondary sexual characteristics; inhibition of the release of pituitary gonadotropins	■ Moderate to severe vasomotor symptoms of menopause ■ Atrophic vaginitis ■ Carcinoma of the breast and prostate ■ Prophylaxis of postmenopausal osteoporosis	■ A postmenopausal woman on long-term estrogen therapy has an increased risk of developing endometrial cancer.
Histamine-2 receptor antagonists		
Inhibit histamine's action at histamine-2 receptors in gastric parietal cells, reducing gastric acid output and concentration, regardless of the stimulatory agent or basal conditions	■ Duodenal ulcer ■ Gastric ulcer ■ Hypersecretory states ■ Reflux esophagitis ■ Stress ulcer prophylaxis	■ These drugs should be used cautiously in an elderly patient because of his increased risk of developing adverse reactions, particularly those affecting the CNS.
Insulin		
Increases glucose transport across muscle and fat-cell membranes to reduce blood glucose levels Promotes conversion of glucose to glycogen Stimulates amino acid uptake and conversion to protein in muscle cells Inhibits protein degradation Stimulates triglyceride formation and lipoprotein lipase activity; inhibits free fatty acid release from adipose tissue	■ Diabetic ketoacidosis ■ Diabetes mellitus ■ Diabetes mellitus inadequately controlled by diet and oral antidiabetic agents ■ Hyperkalemia	■ Insulin is available in many forms that differ in onset, peak, and duration of action; the physician will specify the individual dosage and form. ■ Blood glucose measurement is an important guide to dosage and management. ■ The elderly patient's diet and his ability to recognize hypoglycemia are important. ■ A source of diabetic teaching should be provided, especially for the elderly patient, who may need follow-up home care.
Iron supplements, oral		
Are needed in adequate amounts for erythropoiesis and efficient oxygen transport; essential component of hemoglobin	■ Iron deficiency anemia	■ Iron-induced constipation is common among elderly patients; stress proper diet to minimize constipation. ■ An elderly patient may also need higher doses because of reduced gastric secretions and because achlorhydria may lower his capacity for iron absorption.

Pharmacology	Indications	Special considerations
Nitrates		
Relax smooth muscle; generally used for vascular effects (vasodilatation)	■ Angina pectoris ■ Acute MI	■ Severe hypotension and cardiovascular collapse may occur if nitrates are combined with alcohol. ■ Transient dizziness, syncope, or other signs of cerebral ischemia may occur; instruct the elderly patient to take nitrates while sitting.
Nonsteroidal anti-inflammatory drugs (NSAIDs)		
Interfere with prostaglandins involved with pain; anti-inflammatory action that contributes to analgesic effect	■ Pain ■ Inflammation ■ Fever	■ A patient over age 60 may be more susceptible to the toxic effects of NSAIDs because of decreased renal function; these drugs' effects on renal prostaglandins may cause fluid retention and edema, a drawback for a patient with heart failure.
Opioid agonists		
Act at specific opiate receptor–binding sites in the CNS and other tissues; alteration of pain perception without affecting other sensory functions	■ Analgesia ■ Pulmonary edema ■ Preoperative sedation ■ Anesthesia ■ Cough suppression ■ Diarrhea	■ Lower doses are usually indicated for elderly patients, who tend to be more sensitive to the therapeutic and adverse effects of these drugs.
Opioid agonist-antagonists		
Act, in theory, on different opiate receptors in the CNS to a greater or lesser degree, thus yielding slightly different effects	■ Pain	■ Lower doses may be indicated in patients with renal or hepatic dysfunction to prevent drug accumulation.
Opioid antagonists		
Act differently, depending on whether an opioid agonist has been administered previously, the actions of that opioid, and the extent of physical dependence on it	■ Opioid-induced respiratory depression ■ Adjunct in treating opiate addiction	■ These drugs are contraindicated for narcotic addicts, in whom they may produce an acute abstinence syndrome.
Penicillins		
Inhibit bacterial cell-wall synthesis, causing rapid cell lysis; most effective against fast-growing susceptible organisms	■ Infection caused by susceptible organisms	■ An elderly patient (and others with low resistance from immunosuppressants or radiation therapy) should be taught the signs and symptoms of bacterial and fungal superinfection.

Pharmacology	Indications	Special considerations
Phenothiazine		
Believed to function as dopamine antagonists, blocking postsynaptic dopamine receptors in various parts of the CNS; antiemetic effects resulting from blockage of the chemoreceptor trigger zones	■ Psychosis ■ Nausea and vomiting ■ Anxiety ■ Severe behavior problems ■ Tetanus ■ Porphyria ■ Intractable hiccups ■ Neurogenic pain ■ Allergies and pruritus	■ An older adult needs a lower dosage because he's more sensitive to these drugs' therapeutic and adverse effects, especially cardiac toxicity, tardive dyskinesia, and other extrapyramidal effects. ■ Dosage should be titrated to patient response.
Salicylates		
Decrease formation of prostaglandins involved in pain and inflammation	■ Pain ■ Inflammation ■ Fever	■ A patient over age 60 with impaired renal function may be more susceptible to these drugs' toxic effects. ■ The effect of salicylates on renal prostaglandins may cause fluid retention and edema, a significant disadvantage for a patient with heart failure.
Serotonin-reuptake inhibitors		
Inhibit reuptake of serotonin; have little or no effect on other neurotransmitters	■ Major depression ■ Obsessive compulsive disorder ■ Bulimia nervosa	■ These drugs should be used cautiously in a patient with hepatic impairment.
Sulfonamides		
Inhibit folic acid biosynthesis needed for cell growth	■ Bacterial and parasitic infections ■ Inflammation	■ These drugs should be used cautiously in an elderly patient, who is more susceptible to bacterial and fungal superinfection, folate deficiency anemia, and renal and hematologic effects because of diminished renal function.
Tetracyclines		
Inhibit bacterial protein synthesis	■ Bacterial, protozoal, rickettsial, and fungal infections ■ Sclerosing agent	■ Some elderly patients have decreased esophageal motility; administer tetracyclines with caution and monitor for local irritation from slowly passing oral forms.
Thrombolytic enzymes		
Convert plasminogen to plasmin for promotion of clot lysis	■ Thrombosis, thromboembolism	■ Patients age 75 and older are at greater risk for cerebral hemorrhage because they're more apt to have pre-existing cerebrovascular disease.

Pharmacology	Indications	Special considerations
Thyroid hormones		
Have catabolic and anabolic effects Influence normal metabolism, growth and development, and every organ system; vital to normal CNS function	■ Hypothyroidism ■ Nontoxic goiter ■ Thyrotoxicosis ■ Diagnostic use	■ In a patient over age 60, the initial hormone replacement dose should be 25% less than the recommended dose.
Thyroid hormone antagonists		
Inhibit iodine oxidation in the thyroid gland through a block of iodine's ability to combine with tyrosine to form thyroxine	■ Hyperthyroidism ■ Preparation for thyroidectomy ■ Thyrotoxic crisis ■ Thyroid carcinoma	■ Serum thyroid-stimulating hormone should be monitored as a sensitive indicator of thyroid hormone levels. Dosage adjustment may be required.
Tricyclic antidepressants		
Inhibit neurotransmitter reuptake, resulting in increased concentration and enhanced activity of neurotransmitters in the synaptic cleft	■ Depression ■ Obsessive compulsive disorder ■ Enuresis ■ Severe, chronic pain	■ Lower doses are indicated in an elderly patient because he's more sensitive to both the therapeutic and adverse effects of tricyclic antidepressants.

Appendix H
Adverse reactions misinterpreted as age-related changes

Some conditions result from aging, others from drug therapy. However, some can result from aging and drug therapy. The chart below indicates drug classes and their associated adverse reactions.

Body system

Drug classifications	Agitation	Anxiety	Arrhythmias	Ataxia	Changes in appetite	Confusion	Constipation	Depression	Difficulty breathing	Disorientation	Dizziness	Drowsiness	Edema	Fatigue	Hypotension	Insomnia	Memory loss	Muscle weakness	Restlessness	Sexual dysfunction	Tremors	Urinary dysfunction	Visual changes
$Alpha_1$-adrenergic blockers		■					■	■			■	■	■	■	■	■				■		■	■
Angiotensin-converting enzyme inhibitors						■	■	■			■			■	■	■				■			■
Antianginals	■	■	■			■					■		■	■	■	■			■	■		■	■
Antiarrhythmics			■				■		■		■		■	■									
Anticholinergics	■	■	■			■	■	■		■	■	■		■	■		■	■	■			■	■
Anticonvulsants	■		■	■	■	■	■	■	■		■	■	■	■	■	■					■	■	■
Antidepressants, tricyclic	■	■	■	■	■	■	■		■	■	■	■		■	■	■			■	■	■	■	■
Antidiabetics, oral											■			■									
Antihistamines					■	■	■			■	■	■		■							■	■	■
Antilipemics							■				■			■		■		■		■		■	■
Antiparkinsonians	■	■		■	■	■	■	■		■	■	■		■	■	■		■			■	■	■
Antipsychotics	■	■	■	■	■	■	■	■			■	■		■	■	■			■	■	■	■	■
Barbiturates	■	■	■			■			■	■		■		■	■				■				
Benzodiazepines	■			■		■	■	■	■	■	■	■		■		■	■	■			■	■	■
Beta-adrenergic blockers		■	■					■	■		■			■	■		■			■	■	■	■
Calcium channel blockers		■	■				■		■		■		■	■	■	■				■		■	■
Corticosteroids	■					■		■					■	■		■		■					■
Diuretics						■					■			■	■			■				■	
Nonsteroidal anti-inflammatory drugs		■				■	■	■			■	■		■		■		■					■
Opioids	■	■				■	■	■	■	■	■	■		■	■	■	■		■	■		■	■
Skeletal muscle relaxants	■	■		■		■		■			■	■		■	■	■					■		
Thyroid hormones			■		■											■					■		

Appendix I
Resources for geriatric care

Government agencies

Administration on Aging
Department of Health and Human Services
330 Independence Ave., S.W.
Washington, DC 20201
www.aoa.dhhs.gov

National Association of Area Agencies on Aging
927 15th St., N.W., 6th Floor
Washington, DC 20005
www.n4a.org

National Council on the Aging
409 Third St., S.W., Suite 200
Washington, DC 20024
www.ncoa.org

National Institute on Aging
Building 31, Room 5C27
31 Center Dr., MSC 2292
Bethesda, MD 20892
www.nia.nih.gov

Health organizations

American Association for Geriatric Psychiatry
7910 Woodmont Ave., Suite 1050
Bethesda, MD 20814-3004
www.aagpgpa.org

American Geriatrics Society
Empire State Building
350 Fifth Ave., Suite 801
New York, NY 10018
www.americangeriatrics.org

American Health Care Association
1201 L St., N.W.
Washington, DC 20005-4014
www.ahca.org

American Society for Geriatric Dentistry
211 E. Chicago Ave., 5th Floor
Chicago, IL 60611
www.aoa.dhhs.gov

Gerontological Society of America
1030 15th St., N.W., Suite 250
Washington, DC 20005-1503
www.geron.org

National Association for Home Care
228 Seventh St., S.E.
Washington, DC 20003
www.nahc.org

National Gerontological Nursing Association
7794 Grow Dr.
Pensacola, FL 32514-7072
www.ngna.org

National Hospice Organization
1901 N. Moore St., Suite 901
Arlington, VA 22209
www.nho.org

Social welfare organizations

American Association of Retired Persons
601 E. St., N.W.
Washington, DC 20049
www.aarp.org

American Bar Association
Commission on Legal Problems of the Elderly
740 15th St., N.W.
Washington, DC 20005-1019
www.abanet.org/elderly/home.html

Children of Aging Parents
1609 Woodbourne Rd., Suite 302-A
Levittown, PA 19057
www.careguide.net

Gray Panthers
733 15th St., N.W., Suite 437
Washington, DC 20005
www.graypanthers.org

Institute for Retired Professionals
New School for Social Research
66 W. 12th St.
New York, NY 10011
www.newschool.edu

National Caucus and Center on Black Aged
1424 K St., N.W., Suite 500
Washington, DC 20005
www.ncba-blackaged.org

National Council on the Aging
409 Third St., S.W., Suite 200
Washington, DC 20024
www.ncoa.org

National Institute on Adult Daycare
(c/o National Council on the Aging)
409 Third St., S.W., Suite 200
Washington, DC 20024
www.ncoa.org/nadsa/ads_factsheet.htm

National Senior Citizens Law Center
1101 14th St., N.W., Suite 400
Washington, DC 20005
www.nsclc.org

Older Women's League
666 11th St., N.W.
Washington, DC 20001
www.members.aol.com/owlil

Selected references

Administration on Aging, U.S. Department of Health and Human Services. A Profile of Older Americans: 2001. *www.aoa.dhhs.gov/aoa/stats/profile/default.htm.*

Administration on Aging, U.S. Department of Health and Human Services. Elder Abuse Prevention. *www.aoa.gov/factsheets/abuse.html.*

Albers, G.W., et al. "Addendum to the Supplement to the Guidelines for the Management of Transient Ischemic Attacks," *Stroke* 31(4):1001, April 2000.

Allison, M., and Keller, C. "Physical Activity in the Elderly: Benefits and Intervention Strategies," *Nurse Practitioner* 22(8):53-54, 56, 58, August 1997.

American Dietetic Association. "Nutrition, Aging, and the Continuum of Care: Position of ADA." *Journal of the American Dietetic Association,* 100(5):580-95, May 2000.

Assessment Made Incredibly Easy, 2nd ed. Springhouse, Pa.: Springhouse Corp., 2001.

Borton, D. "Fighting the Flu," *Nursing2000* 30(10):14, October 2000.

Bubien, R.S. "A New Beat on an Old Rhythm," *AJN* 100(1):42-50, January 2000.

Connolly, K. "New Directions in Heart Failure," *Nurse Practitioner* 25(7):23, 27-28, 31-34, July 2000.

Deblinger, L. "Alcohol Problems in the Elderly," *Patient Care* 34(19):70-72, 75-76, 79-80, October 2000.

Fuller, G. "Falls in the Elderly," *American Family Physician* 61(7):2159-168, 2173-174, April 2000.

Grossan, M. "Safe Effective Techniques for Cerumen Removal," *Geriatrics* 55(1):80, 83-86, January 2000.

Handbook of Diseases, 2nd ed. Springhouse, Pa.: Springhouse Corp., 2000.

Handbook of Geriatric Drug Therapy. Springhouse, Pa.: Springhouse Corp., 2000.

Hazzard, W.R., et al., eds. *Principles of Geriatric Medicine and Gerontology,* 4th ed. New York: McGraw–Hill Health Professional Division, 1999.

Hoban, S., and Kearney, K. "Emergency: Elder Abuse and Neglect," *American Journal of Nursing* 100(11):49-50, November 2000.

Hwang, M.Y. "Growing Older in Good Health," *JAMA Patient Page: Aging* 283(4):560, January 2000.

Joint Commission on Accreditation of Healthcare Organizations. "JCAHO Revises Restraints Standards," *Contemporary Long Term Care* 23(8):9, August 2000.

Lewis, L. "Optimal Treatment for COPD," *Patient Care* 34(10) 60-64, 66, 69-70, May 2000.

Lowe, F.C., and Fageman, E. "Using Complementary Medications to Treat BPH…Benign Prostatic Hyperplasia," *Patient Care* 34(7):191-92, 195, 199-203, April 2000.

Martin, J.H., and Haynes, L.C.H. "Depression, Delirium, and Dementia in the Elderly Patient," *AORN Journal* 72(2):209-13, 216-21, 223, August 2000.

Morris, M.R. "As America Ages. Elder Abuse: What the Law Requires," *RN* 61(8):52-54, August 1998.

National Center on Elder Abuse. "The Basics: What is Elder Abuse?" *www.elderabusecenter.org/basic/index.html.*

National Comprehensive Cancer Network. Breast Cancer Treatment Guidelines for Patients. *www.nccn.org.*

National Osteoporosis Foundation. Medications and Osteoporosis. *www.nof.org/patientinfo/medications.htm.*

The Johns Hopkins Medical Letter. "A New Sight Saving Option," *Health After 50*, 11(12):1-2, February 2000.

Wallis, M.A. "Looking at Depression through Bifocal Lenses," *Nursing2000* 30(9):58-61, September 2000.

Young, M.G. "Chronic Pain Management in the Elderly," *Patient Care* 34(18):31-32, 35-36, 37-38, September 2000.

Index

i refers to an illustration; t refers to a table.

B

i refers to an illustration; t refers to a table.

i refers to an illustration; t refers to a table.

D

i refers to an illustration; t refers to a table.

i refers to an illustration; t refers to a table.

i refers to an illustration; t refers to a table.

i refers to an illustration; t refers to a table.

i refers to an illustration; t refers to a table.

i refers to an illustration; t refers to a table.

Q

R

i refers to an illustration; t refers to a table.

i refers to an illustration; t refers to a table.

i refers to an illustration; t refers to a table.

i refers to an illustration; t refers to a table.